INTRODUCTION TO AUDIOLOGY

FOURTH EDITION

INTRODUCTION
TO AUDIOLOGY

Frederick N. Martin

The University of Texas at Austin

PRENTICE HALL Englewood Cliffs, New Jersey 07632

Library of Congress Cataloging-in-Publication Data

Martin, Frederick N.
    Introduction to audiology / Frederick N. Martin. -- 4th ed.
        p.   cm.
    Includes bibliographical references.
    Includes indexes.
    ISBN 0-13-477605-4
    1. Hearing disorders. 2. Audiometry.   I. Title.
    [DNLM: 1. Audiometry. 2. Hearing Disorders. 3. Hearing Tests.
WV 270 M3791]
RF290.M34 1991
617.8--dc20
DNLM/DLC
for Library of Congress   90-7690
                                                              CIP

Editorial/production supervision and
   interior design: Sabrina Fuchs and Mary McKinley
Cover design: Richard Puder
Prepress buyer: Herb Klein
Manufacturing buyer: Dave Dickey

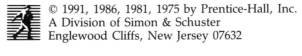 © 1991, 1986, 1981, 1975 by Prentice-Hall, Inc.
A Division of Simon & Schuster
Englewood Cliffs, New Jersey 07632

Printed in the United States of America

10 9 8 7 6

ISBN 0-13-477605-4

Prentice-Hall International (UK) Limited, *London*
Prentice-Hall of Australia Pty. Limited, *Sydney*
Prentice-Hall Canada Inc., *Toronto*
Prentice-Hall Hispanoamericana, S.A., *Mexico*
Prentice-Hall of India Private Limited, *New Delhi*
Prentice-Hall of Japan, Inc., *Tokyo*
Simon & Schuster Asia Pte. Ltd., *Singapore*
Editora Prentice-Hall do Brasil Ltda., *Rio de Janeiro*

To Cathy, Leslie Anne, David and April

CONTENTS

PREFACE   xiii

HOW TO USE THIS BOOK   xv

Part 1   *Elements of Hearing and Sound*

1 THE HUMAN EAR AND SIMPLE TESTS OF HEARING   1

Chapter Objectives   *1*
Anatomy and Physiology of the Ear   *2*
Pathways of Sound   *3*
Conductive Hearing Loss   *3*
Sensorineural Hearing Loss   *3*
Mixed Hearing Loss   *4*   Hearing Tests   *5*
Tuning-Fork Tests   *5*   Summary   *10*
Glossary   *10*   Study Questions   *11*
Suggested Reading   *14*

2 SOUND AND ITS MEASUREMENT

Chapter Objectives   *15*   Sound   *16*
Waves   *16*   Vibrations   *19*   Frequency   *21*
Resonance   *22*   Sound Velocity   *23*
Wavelength   *24*   Phase   *24*   Intensity   *26*
The Decibel   *29*   Complex Sounds   *35*
Impedance   *36*   Sound Measurement   *39*
Environmental Sounds   *51*
Psychoacoustics   *51*   Summary   *54*
Glossary   *55*   Study Questions   *59*
References   *62*   Suggested Reading   *62*

Part 2   *Audiometry*

3 PURE TONE AUDIOMETRY   63

Chapter Objectives   *63*
The Pure-Tone Audiometer   *64*
Test Environment   *66*
The Patient's Role in Manual Pure-Tone
    Audiometry   *70*
The Clinician's Role in Manual Audiometry Pure-Tone
    Audiometry   *71*
Air-Conduction Audiometry   *73*
Bone-Conduction Audiometry   *79*
Audiogram Interpretation   *85*   Masking   *91*
The Audiometric Weber Test   *102*
Automatic Audiometry   *105*
Computerized Audiometry   *105*
Audiometric Response Simulators   *107*
Summary   *108*   Glossary   *109*
Study Questions   *111*   References   *112*
Suggested Readings   *113*

4 SPEECH AUDIOMETRY   114

Chapter Objectives   *114*
The Speech Audiometer   *115*

Test Environment   115
The Patient's Role in Speech Audiometry   116
The Clinician's Role in Speech Audiometry   117
Speech-Threshold Testing   117
Masking for SRT   126
Bone-Conduction SRT   128
Most Comfortable Loudness Level   129
Uncomfortable Loudness Level   130
Speech-Discrimination Testing   131
Computerized Speech Audiometry   143
Summary   147   Glossary   147
Study Questions   149   References   151
Suggested Readings   155

5 AUDITORY TESTS FOR SITE OF LESION   **157**

Chapter Objectives   157
Loudness Recruitment   158
Implications of Loudness Recruitment   160
Differential Intensity Discrimination   164
Tone Decay   168   Békésy Audiometry   172
Acoustic Immittance   177
Auditory Evoked Potentials   195
Summary   205   Glossary   207
Study Questions   210   References   212
Suggested Readings   214

Part 3   *Anatomy and Physiology*
of the Auditory System:
Pathology, Etiology, and Therapy

6 THE OUTER EAR   **215**

Chapter Objectives   215
Anatomy of the Outer Ear   216
Development of the Outer Ear   220
Hearing Loss and the Outer Ear   220
Disorders of the External Ear and Their
    Treatment   221   Summary   229

Glossary   *230*   Study Questions   *231*
References   *232*   Suggested Readings   *232*

7 THE MIDDLE EAR   **233**

Chapter Objectives   *233*
Anatomy of the Middle Ear   *234*
Development of the Middle Ear   *241*
Hearing Loss and the Middle Ear   *241*
Disorders of the Middle Ear and Their Treatment   *241*
Other Causes of Middle-Ear Hearing Loss   *273*
Summary   *275*   Glossary   *275*
Study Questions   *278*   References   *280*
Suggested Readings   *280*

8 THE INNER EAR   **281**

Chapter Objectives   *281*   The Inner Ear   *282*
Hearing Loss and the Inner Ear   *295*
Disorders of the Cochlea   *295*
Causes of Inner-Ear Disorders   *295*
Summary   *314*   Glossary   *316*
Study Questions   *320*   References   *320*
Suggested Readings   *322*

9 THE AUDITORY NERVE AND CENTRAL AUDITORY PATHWAYS   **324**

Chapter Objectives   *324*
The Auditory Nerve and Ascending Auditory Pathways   *324*
The Descending Auditory Pathways   *328*
Development of the Auditory Nerve and Central Auditory
   Nervous System   *329*
Summary of the Auditory Pathways   *329*
Hearing Loss and the Auditory Nerve and Central Auditory
   Pathways   *330*
Disorders of the Auditory Nerve   *330*
Disorders of the Cochlear Nuclei   *341*
Disorders of the Higher Auditory Pathways   *343*
Tests for Central Auditory Disorders   *344*

Summary   *355*   Glossary   *356*
Study Questions   *358*   References   *359*
Suggested Readings   *361*

Part 4   *Special Problems in Audiology*

10 PSEUDOHYPACUSIS   363

Chapter Objectives   *363*   Terminology   *364*
Patients with Pseudohypacusis   *364*
Tests for Pseudohypacusis   *369*
Management of the Patient with
    Pseudohypacusis   *379*   Summary   *380*
Glossary   *381*   Study Questions   *382*
References   *384*
Suggested Readings   *382*

11 THE PEDIATRIC PATIENT   385

Chapter Objectives   *385*
Auditory Responses   *386*
Testing Infants under Three Months   *387*
Testing Children from Birth to One Year of Age   *391*
Testing Children One to Five Years of Age   *395*
Language Disorders   *403*
Psychological Disorders   *405*
Identifying Hearing Loss in the Schools   *406*
Pseudohypacusis in Children   *410*
Management of Hearing-Impaired Children   *441*
Summary   *418*   Glossary   *418*
Study Questions   *420*   References   *421*
Suggested Readings   *423*

12 MANAGEMENT OF
   THE HEARING-IMPAIRED PATIENT   425

Chapter Objectives   *425*
Patient Histories   *425*
Referral to Other Specialists   *428*

Hearing Aids   *432*
Selecting Hearing Aids   *442*
Assistive Listening Devices and Systems (ALDS)   *448*
Management of Tinnitus   *450*
Counseling   *451*
Management of the Hearing-Impaired Adult   *453*
Auditory Training   *455*   Speechreading   *457*
Summary   *458*   Glossary   *458*
Study Questions   *459*   References   *460*
Suggested Readings   *461*

Appendixes

**I INSTRUCTIONS FOR TAKING
THE HEARING EXAMINATION**   **463**

**II WORD LISTS FOR USE
IN SPEECH AUDIOMETRY**   **465**

Spondaic Words   *465*   PB Word Lists   *466*
Kindergarten PB Word Lists   *467*
CNC Word Lists   *468*
California Consonant Test Items   *470*
High Frequency Consonant Discrimination Word List   *471*
Children's Picture-Identification Test   *471*
Synthetic Sentences   *472*
Competing-Sentence Test   *472*

**III COMMON AUDIOLOGICAL PREFIXES,
SUFFIXES, AND ABBREVIATIONS**   **475**

Prefixes   *475*   Suffixes   *476*
Abbreviations   *476*

INDEXES   **479**

Author Index   *479*
Subject Index   *485*

PREFACE

Since its initial development more than four and a half decades ago, the science of audiology has grown and changed in ways that could not have been predicted. A constant stream of scientific breakthroughs keeps audiology exciting and challenging. Nevertheless, its initial mission, to assist the hearing impaired, has remained unchanged.

Before rehabilitation of the hearing-impaired individual can begin, the audiologist must have a firm understanding of hearing disorders. For this reason, diagnostics are essential to proper management. Diagnosis is useless without treatment, but treatment is impossible without diagnosis. This book is designed to help prepare persons entering the field of communication sciences to understand and assess hearing disorders, and to comprehend the implications of aural rehabilitation. The emphasis on diagnostic procedures in portions of this book should not be perceived as a one-sided approach to audiology. The rehabilitative aspects described, however briefly, should serve as a springboard for further education on patient management.

A great deal of information is required before any person can enter the field of clinical audiology. Largely through the efforts of the American Speech-Language-Hearing Association (ASHA), which has historically served as the parent organization for audiologists, most states now require licensing for audiological practice. Requirements for both a state license and ASHA's Certificate of Clinical Competence include at least a master's degree, with specific course work in audiology and related areas. Today, a new emphasis on increased training is emerging. A proposal for a professional doctorate in audiology has been fostered by the newly formed American Academy of Audiology. Just how these new events will develop is, at the time of this writing, unclear, but there is little doubt that audiologists will increasingly take their rightful places as important members of the hearing health team.

Whether readers of this book are primarily interested in audiology, otology, speech-language pathology or education of hearing-impaired children, a fundamental knowledge of audiology is essential to successful clinical practice. The attributes of clinicians working in any of these areas must transcend academic and scientific acumen. Those who choose the professions that work with the communicatively handicapped must care, nurture, and empathize. Humanism and science must combine as never before.

I wish to extend thanks to the following individuals who read the manuscript in its early stages and offered suggestions: Ron D. Chambers, University of Illinois; Faith Loven, University of Minnesota, Duluth; Ross J. Roeser, The University of Texas, Dallas; and David M. Lipscomb.

As in the previous three editions of this book, much help has been gratefully received from friends, colleagues and former students. They are very special people. To my family, my wife Cathy, my son David, and my daughter, Leslie Anne, I owe my thanks for their patience and their love.

Frederick N. Martin

HOW TO USE THIS BOOK

The chapter arrangement in this book differs somewhat from traditional texts in audiology in several ways. The usual approach is to present the anatomy and physiology of the ear and then to present auditory tests. This book, however, first presents a superficial look at how the ear works. With this conceptual beginning, details of auditory tests can be understood as they relate to the basic mechanisms of the ear. Thus, with a grasp of the test principles, the reader is better prepared to benefit from the many examples of theoretical test results that illustrate different disorders in the auditory system. Presentations of anatomy and physiology, designed for greater detail and application, accompany the descriptions of auditory disorders.

The organization of this book has proved useful because it facilitates early comprehension of what is often perceived as new and difficult material. Readers who wish a more traditional approach may simply rearrange the sequence in which they read the chapters. Chapters 6 through 9, on the anatomy, physiology, disorders, and treatments of different parts of the auditory apparatus, can simply be read before Chapters 3 through 5 on auditory tests. At the completion of the book the same information will have been covered.

The teacher of an introductory audiology course may feel that the depth of coverage of some subjects in this book is greater than desired. If this is the case, the major and secondary headings allow for easy identification of sections which may be deleted. The book may be read in modules so that only specified materials are covered.

Each chapter in this book begins with an introduction to the subject matter and a statement of the instructional objectives. Liberal use is made of headings and subheadings. A summary at the end of each chapter iterates the important portions. Terms that may be new or unusual appear in **boldface** print and are defined in a glossary at the end of each chapter, thus eliminating the reader's need to underscore important words or concepts. In addition, review tables summarize the highlights of each chapter. Readers wishing to test their understanding of different materials may find the questions at the end of each chapter useful to check their grasp of new information. Some subjects may be explored in greater detail by pursuing the references and suggested readings.

The figures and other visuals used in this book are the result of student feedback indicating the desire for examples of specific materials. In no case do figures provide information or explanations not given in the text, unless this is specified.

The indexes at the back of the book are intended to help readers find desired materials rapidly. In the Author Index, page numbers in *italics* direct the reader to complete book or journal references by a particular author. Numbers in *italics* in the Subject Index identify the page on which a term is briefly defined in a glossary. The Appendixes contain helpful instructions for taking the hearing examination, as well as lists of test materials and commonly used prefixes, suffixes, and abbreviations.

1

THE HUMAN EAR AND SIMPLE TESTS OF HEARING

Anatomy is concerned with how the body is structured, and physiology is concerned with how it functions. To facilitate understanding, the anatomist neatly divides the mechanism of hearing into separate compartments, at the same time realizing that these units actually function as one. Sound impulses pass through the **auditory** tract, where they are converted from acoustical to mechanical to hydraulic to chemical and electrical energy, until finally they are received by the brain, which makes the signal discernible.

We test human hearing by two sound pathways, **air conduction** and **bone conduction**. Tests of hearing utilizing **tuning forks** are by no means modern, but they illustrate hearing via these two pathways. Tuning-fork tests may compare the hearing of the patient to that of an examiner, relative sensitivity by air conduction and bone conduction, the effects on bone conduction of closing off the opening into the ear, and the ability to hear a sound in one ear or the other by bone conduction.

CHAPTER OBJECTIVES

The purpose of this chapter is to present a simplified explanation of the mechanism of human hearing and to describe tuning-fork tests that provide information about hearing. The reader will learn a basic vocabulary relative to the ear, acquire a background for study of more sophisticated hearing tests, and gain exposure to details of the anatomy of hearing. Because of the structure of this chapter, some of the statements have been oversimplified. These basic concepts are expanded on in later chapters in this book.

ANATOMY AND PHYSIOLOGY OF THE EAR

A simplified look at a coronal section through the ear (Figure 1.1) illustrates the division of the hearing mechanism into three parts. The **outer ear** comprises a shell-like protrusion from each side of the head; a canal through which sounds travel; and, at the end of the canal, the eardrum membrane. The **middle ear** consists of an air-filled space with a chain of tiny bones, the third of which, the stapes, is the smallest in the human body. The portion of the **inner ear** that is responsible for hearing is called the **cochlea**; it is filled with fluids and many microscopic components, all of which serve to convert waves into a message that travels to the stem (base) of the brain via the **auditory nerve**. The brain stem is not coupled to the highest auditory center in the cortex by a simple neural connection. Rather, there is a series of waystations that receive, analyze, and transmit impulses along the auditory pathway.

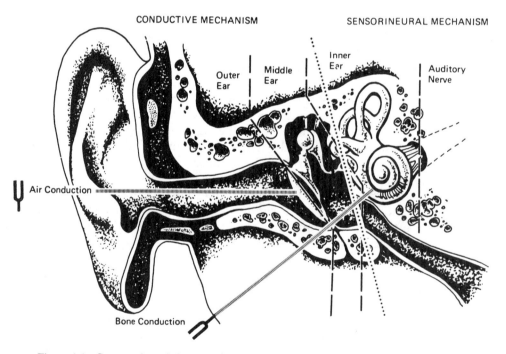

Figure 1.1 Cross-section of the ear showing the air-conduction pathway and the bone-conduction pathway.

Conductive   sensorineural
outer   inner &
middle   auditory nerve

PATHWAYS OF SOUND

Those persons whose primary interests are in the measurement of hearing sometimes divide the hearing mechanism differently than the anatomists do. Audiologists and physicians separate the ear into the conductive portion, consisting of the outer and middle ears, and the sensorineural portion, consisting of the inner ear and the auditory nerve. This type of breakdown is illustrated in the block diagram in Figure 1.2A.

Any sound that courses through the outer ear, middle ear, inner ear, and beyond is heard by air conduction. It is possible to bypass the outer and middle ears by vibrating the skull mechanically and stimulating the inner ear directly. In this way the sound is heard by bone conduction. Therefore, hearing by air conduction depends on the function of the outer, middle, and inner ear, and of the neural pathways beyond; hearing by bone conduction depends on the function of the inner ear and beyond.

CONDUCTIVE HEARING LOSS

A decrease in the strength of a sound is called **attenuation**. Sound attenuation is precisely the result of a conductive hearing loss. Whenever a barrier to sound is present in the outer ear or middle ear, some loss of hearing will result. Individuals will find that their sensitivity to sounds that are introduced by air conduction is impaired by such a blockage. If the sound is introduced by bone conduction, it bypasses the obstacle and goes directly to the sensorineural mechanism. Because the inner ear and the other sensorineural structures are unimpaired, the hearing by bone conduction will be normal. This impaired air conduction with normal bone conduction is called a **conductive hearing loss** and is diagrammed in Figure 1.2B. In this illustration the **hearing loss** is due to damage to the middle ear. Outer-ear abnormalities produce the same relationship between air and bone conduction.

SENSORINEURAL HEARING LOSS

If the disturbance producing the hearing loss is situated in some portion of the sensorineural mechanism, such as the inner ear, a hearing loss by air conduction will result. However, because the attenuation of the sound occurs along the bone-conduction pathway, the hearing loss by bone conduction will be as great as the hearing loss by air conduction. When a hearing loss exists in which there is the same amount of attenuation for both air conduction and bone conduction, the conductive mechanism is eliminated as a possible cause of the difficulty. A diagnosis of **sensorineural hearing loss** can then be made (see Figure 1.2C). In Figure 1.2C the inner ear was selected to illustrate a sensorineural disorder, although the same principle would hold if the auditory nerve were damaged.

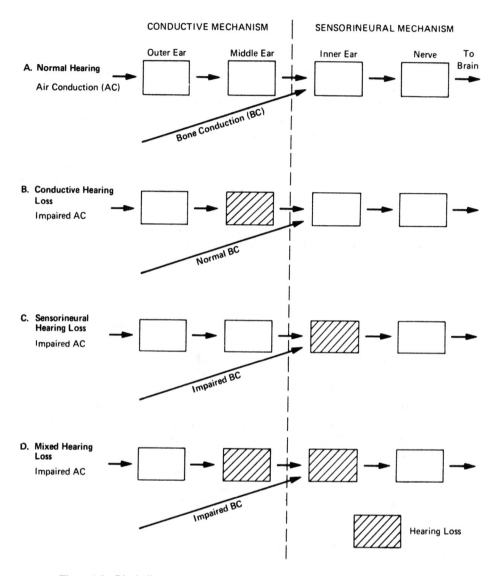

Figure 1.2 Block diagram of the ear. A conductive hearing loss is illustrated by damage to the middle ear. Damage to the outer ear would produce the same effect. Similarly, a sensorineural hearing loss could be illustrated by damage to the nerve as well as to the inner ear.

MIXED HEARING LOSS

Problems can occur simultaneously in both the conductive and sensorineural mechanisms, as illustrated in Figure 1.2D. This results in a loss of hearing sensitivity by bone conduction due to the sensorineural abnormality, but an even greater loss of sensitivity by air conduction. This is true because the loss of hearing by air conduction must include the loss by bone conduction in the sensorineural portion plus the attenuation in the conductive portion. In other words, sound traveling the bone-conduction pathway will be attenuated only by the defect in the inner ear, but sound traveling the air-conduction pathway will be attenuated by both middle-ear and inner-ear problems. This type of impairment is called a **mixed hearing loss**.

HEARING TESTS

Some of the earliest tests of hearing probably consisted merely of producing sounds of some kind, such as clapping the hands or making vocal sounds, to see if an individual could be made aware of the sounds. Asking people if they could hear the ticking of a watch or the clicking of two coins together may have suggested to the examiner that primarily the upper pitch range was being sampled. Obviously these tests provided little information of either a quantitative or a qualitative nature.

TUNING-FORK TESTS

The tuning fork (Figure 1.3) is a device, usually made of steel, magnesium, or aluminum, that is used to tune musical instruments or, by singers, to obtain certain pitches. A tuning fork emits a tone at a particular pitch and has a clear

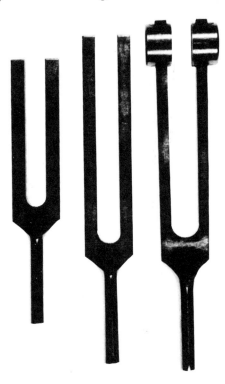

Figure 1.3 Several tuning forks. The larger forks vibrate at lower frequencies than the smaller forks.

musical quality. When the tuning fork is vibrating properly, the tines move alternately away from and toward each other (Figure 1.4), and the stem moves with a piston action. The air-conduction tone emitted is relatively pure, meaning that it is free of overtones (more on this in Chapter 2).

Tuning forks have been used by otologists (ear specialists) for some time in the diagnosis of hearing disorders. They are rarely used by audiologists, who prefer more sophisticated electronic devices. Tuning-fork tests serve, however, to illustrate the principles involved in certain modern tests. The tuning fork is set into vibration by holding the stem in the hand and striking one of the tines against a firm but resilient surface. The rubber heel of a shoe does nicely for this purpose, although many physicians prefer the knuckle, knee, or elbow. If the fork is struck against too solid an object, dropped, or otherwise abused, its vibrations may be considerably altered.

The tuning fork was adopted as an instrument for testing hearing over a hundred years ago. It held promise then because it could be quantified, at least in terms of the pitch emitted. Several forks are available that correspond to notes on the scientific C scale. By using tuning forks with various known properties, hearing sensitivity through several pitch ranges may be sampled. However, any diagnostic statement made on the basis of a tuning-fork test is absolutely limited to the pitch of the fork used, because hearing sensitivity is often different for different pitches.

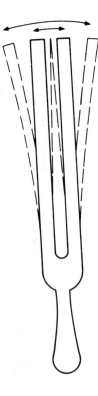

Figure 1.4 Vibration pattern of tuning forks.

The Schwabach Test

The **Schwabach test**, introduced in 1890, is a test for bone conduction. It compares the hearing sensitivity of a patient with the sensitivity of the examiner. The tuning fork is set into vibration, and the stem is placed alternately against the **mastoid process** (the bony protrusion behind the ear) of the patient and of the examiner (Figure 1.5A). Each time the fork is pressed against the patient's head, the patient makes a signal if the tone is heard. The vibratory energy of the tines of the fork decreases over time, making the tone softer. When the patient no longer hears the tone, the examiner immediately places the stem of the tuning fork behind his or her own ear and, using a watch, notes the number of seconds that the tone is audible after the patient stops hearing it.

This test assumes that the examiner has normal hearing, and it is less than worthless unless this is true. If both examiner and patient have normal hearing, then both will stop hearing the tone emitted by the fork at approximately the same time. This is called a *normal Schwabach*. If patients have sensorineural hearing loss; hearing by bone conduction is impaired, and they will stop hearing the sound much sooner than will the examiner. This is called a *diminished Schwabach*. The test can be quantified to some degree by recording the number of seconds the examiner continues to hear the tone after the patient has stopped hearing it. If the examiner hears the tone for 10 seconds longer than does the patient, the patient's hearing is "diminished 10 seconds." If patients have a conductive hearing loss, bone conduction is normal and they will hear the tone for at least as long as the examiner, and sometimes longer. In some conductive hearing losses, the patient's hearing in the low-pitch range may appear to be better than normal. When this occurs, the result is called a *prolonged Schwabach*.

Difficulties arise in the administration and interpretation of the Schwabach test. Interpretation of test results in cases of mixed hearing losses is especially difficult. Because both inner ears are very close together and are embedded in the bones of the skull, it is virtually impossible to stimulate one without simultaneously stimulating the other. Therefore, if there is a difference in sensitivity between the two inner ears, the patient will probably respond to sound heard through the better ear. Thus, the examiner may have difficulty determining which ear is actually being tested.

The Rinne Test

Performance of the **Rinne test** compares patients' hearing sensitivity by bone conduction to their sensitivity by air conduction. This is done by asking them to state whether the tone is louder when the tuning-fork stem is held against the bone behind the ear, as in the Schwabach test (Figure 1.5A), or when the tines of the fork that are generating an air-conducted sound are held next to the opening of the ear (Figure 1.5B).

Because air conduction is a more efficient means of sound transmission to the inner ear than is bone conduction, people with normal hearing will hear the tone as louder when the fork is at the ear than when it is behind the ear. This is called a *positive Rinne*. A positive Rinne also occurs in patients with sensorineural hearing loss. The attenuation produced by a problem in the sensorineural mechanism produces the same degree of loss by air conduction as by bone conduction (see Figure 1.2C).

If patients have more than a mild conductive hearing loss, their bone-conduction hearing is normal (Figure 1.2B), and they will hear the tone louder with the stem of the fork behind the ear (bone conduction) than with the tines at the ear (air conduction). This is called a *negative Rinne*. Sometimes patients manifest what has been called the *false negative Rinne*, which occurs when the inner ear not deliberately being tested responds to the tone. As mentioned in the discussion of the Schwabach test, this may happen readily during bone-conduction tests. For example, if the right ear is the one being tested, the loudness of the air-conducted tone in the right ear may inadvertently be com-

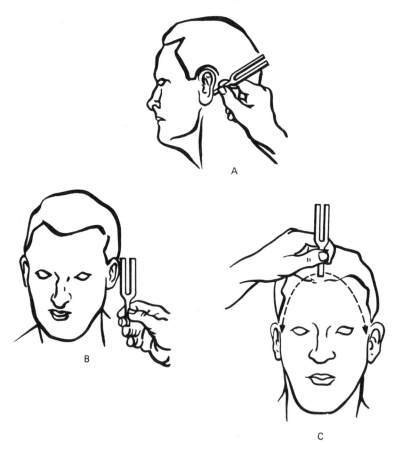

Figure 1.5 Positions of the tuning fork during tuning-fork tests (Courtesy of The Ear and Nose-Throat Clinic, P.A. Little Rock, Arkansas.)

pared to the loudness of the bone-conducted tone in the left ear. If the left-ear bone conduction is more sensitive than the right-ear bone conduction, a false negative Rinne may result, giving rise to improper diagnosis of conductive hearing loss.

The Bing Test

For some time it has been known that when persons with normal hearing close off the opening into the ear canal, the loudness of a tone presented by bone conduction increases. This phenomenon has been called the **occlusion effect**, and it is observed primarily for low-pitched sounds. This effect is also evident in patients with sensorineural hearing loss, but it is absent in patients with conductive hearing loss. This is the premise of the **Bing test**.

In performance of the Bing test, the tuning-fork handle is held to the mastoid process behind the ear (Figure 1-5A) while the examiner alternately closes and opens the ear canal with a finger. For normal hearers and those with sensorineural hearing loss, the result is a pulsating sound, or a sound that seems to get louder and softer. For the patient with a conductive hearing loss, no change in the loudness of the sound is noticed.

The Bing test must be performed carefully, and precautions must be taken against suggesting to patients what their responses should be. As in the Schwabach and Rinne tests, the dangers of the nontest ear's responding to the tone are ever present.

The Weber Test

Since its introduction in 1834 the **Weber test** has retained such popularity that it has been modified by many audiologists for use with modern electronic testing equipment. It is a test of **lateralization**; that is, patients must state where they hear the tone (left ear, right ear, both ears, or in the midline).

In performance of the Weber test, the tuning fork is set into vibration and the stem is placed on the midline of the patient's skull. The illustration in Figure 1.5C shows placement on the forehead, which is probably the most popular location. Other sites are also used, such as the top or the back of the head, the chin, or the upper teeth. (In most cases, surprisingly, using the upper teeth produces the loudest bone-conducted sound.) Patients are simply asked in which ear they hear the sound as louder. Often the reply is that they hear it in only one ear.

People with normal hearing or with equal amounts of the same type of hearing loss in both ears (conductive, sensorineural, or mixed) will report a midline sensation. They may say that the tone is equally loud in both ears, that they cannot tell any difference, or that they hear the tone as if it originated somewhere in the middle of the head. Patients with sensorineural hearing loss in one ear will hear the tone in their better ear. Patients with conductive hearing loss in one ear will hear the tone in their poorer ear.

The midline sensation is easy to understand. If the ears are equally sensitive and equally stimulated, then equal loudness should logically result.

One explanation of the Weber effect in sensorineural cases is based on the Stenger effect. The **Stenger principle** states that if two tones that are identical in all ways except loudness are introduced simultaneously into both ears, only the louder tone will be perceived. When the bone-conduction sensitivity is poorer in one ear than in the other, the tone being introduced to both ears with equal energy will be perceived as softer or will not be perceived at all in the poorer ear.

The Weber results are most poorly understood in conductive hearing losses. The explanation for the tone being heard as louder in the ear with a conductive loss than in the normal ear is probably based on the same phenomenon as prolonged bone conduction, described briefly in the discussion of the Schwabach test.

The Weber test is quick, easy, and often helpful, although, like most auditory tests, it has some drawbacks. Clinical experience has shown that many patients with a conductive hearing loss in one ear report hearing the tone in their better ear because what they are actually experiencing seems incorrect or even foolish to them. Again, care must be taken not to lead patients into giving the kind of response they think they should. Interpretation of the Weber test is also difficult in mixed hearing losses.

SUMMARY

The mechanisms of hearing may roughly be broken down into conductive and sensorineural portions. Tests by air conduction measure sensitivity through the entire hearing pathway. Tests by bone conduction sample the sensitivity of the structures from the inner ear and beyond, up to the brain. The Schwabach test compares the bone-conduction sensitivity of the patient to that of a presumed normal (the examiner); the Rinne tuning-fork test compares patients' own hearing by bone conduction to their hearing by air conduction in order to sample for conductive versus sensorineural loss; the Bing test samples for conductive hearing loss by testing the effect of occluding the ear; and the Weber test checks for lateralization of a bone-conducted tone presented to the midline of the skull to determine if a loss in only one ear is conductive or sensorineural.

GLOSSARY

Air conduction The course of sounds that are conducted to the inner ear by way of the outer ear and middle ear.

Attenuation The reduction of energy (e.g., sound).

Auditory Reference to the sense of hearing.

Auditory nerve The VIIIth cranial nerve that connects the inner ear to the brain stem.

Bing test   A tuning-fork test that utilizes the occlusion effect to test for the presence or absence of conductive hearing loss.

Bone conduction   The course of sounds that are conducted to the inner ear by way of the bones of the skull.

Cochlea   That portion of the inner ear responsible for converting sound waves into an electrochemical signal that can be sent to the brain for interpretation.

Conductive hearing loss   The loss of sound sensitivity produced by abnormalities of the outer ear and/or middle ear.

Hearing loss   Any loss of sound sensitivity, partial or complete, produced by abnormality anywhere in the auditory system.

Inner ear   That portion of the hearing mechanism, buried in the bones of the skull, that converts mechanical energy into electrochemical energy for transmission to the brain.

Lateralization   The impression that a sound introduced directly to the ears is heard in the right ear or the left ear.

Mastoid process   The bony prominence behind the outer ear.

Middle ear   An air-filled cavity containing three small bones, the function of which is to carry sound energy from the outer ear to the inner ear.

Mixed hearing loss   The sum of the hearing losses produced by abnormalities in both the conductive and sensorineural mechanisms of hearing.

Occlusion effect   The impression of increased loudness of a bone-conducted tone when the outer ear is tightly covered or occluded.

Outer ear   The outermost portion of the hearing mechanism, filled with air. Its primary function is to carry sounds to the middle ear.

Rinne test   A tuning-fork test that compares hearing by air conduction with hearing by bone conduction.

Schwabach test   A tuning-fork test that compares an individual's hearing by bone conduction with the hearing of an examiner (who is presumed to have normal hearing).

Sensorineural hearing loss   The loss of sound sensitivity produced by abnormalities of the inner ear or nerve pathways beyond the inner ear to the brain.

Stenger principle   When two tones are presented to both ears simultaneously, only the louder one is perceived.

Tuning fork   A metal instrument with a stem and two tines. When struck, it vibrates, producing an audible, near-perfect tone.

Weber test   A tuning-fork test performed in cases of hearing loss in one ear to determine if the impairment in the poorer ear is conductive or sensorineural.

STUDY QUESTIONS

1. Sketch a diagram of the ear.   Mark the conductive and sensorineural areas.
2. What information is derived from bone conduction that cannot be inferred from air conduction?

3. Why is it a good idea to use more than one tuning fork when doing tuning-fork tests?
4. Why are statements regarding the results of different tuning-fork tests limited to the pitch of the fork used?
5. What are the probable results on the four tuning-fork tests described in this chapter on a person with a conductive hearing loss in the right ear? State results for both ears when indicated.
6. What is implied if a person's hearing sensitivity is reduced by air conduction but is normal by bone conduction?
7. What is implied if a person's hearing sensitivity is reduced by air conduction and is reduced the same amount by bone conduction?
8. What are some of the problems with tuning-fork tests?

REVIEW TABLE 1.1   TYPES OF HEARING LOSS

ANATOMICAL AREA	PURPOSE	TYPE OF LOSS
Outer ear	Conduct sound energy	Conductive
Middle ear	Conduct sound energy and intensify sound	Conductive
Inner ear	Convert mechanical to hydraulic to electrochemical energy	Sensorineural
Auditory nerve	Transmit electrochemical (nerve) impulses to brain	Sensorineural

REVIEW TABLE 1.2 TUNING-FORK TESTS

TEST	PURPOSE	PLACEMENT OF FORK	NORMAL HEARING	CONDUCTIVE LOSS	SENSORINEURAL LOSS
Schwabach	Compare patient's BC to normal	Mastoid process	*Normal Schwabach:* Patient hears tone for as long as examiner	*Normal or Prolonged Schwabach:* Patient hears tone as long as, or longer, than examiner	*Diminished Schwabach:* Patient hears tone for shorter time than examiner
Rinne	Compare patient's AC to BC	Alternately mastoid process and at ear opening	*Positive Rinne—* Louder at ear	*Negative Rinne—* Louder behind ear	*Positive Rinne:* Louder at ear
Bing	Determine presence or absence of occlusion effect	Mastoid process	*Positive Bing:* Tone sounds louder with ear opening occluded	*Negative Bing:* Tone does not sound louder with ear opening occluded	*Positive Bing:* Tone sounds louder with ear opening occluded
Weber	Determine conductive vs. sensorineural loss (in unilateral losses)	Midline of head	Tone heard equally in both ears	Tone louder in poorer ear	Tone louder in better ear

AC = air conduction; BC = bone conduction.

REVIEW TABLE 1.3 RELATIONSHIPS BETWEEN AIR CONDUCTION AND BONE CONDUCTION FOR DIFFERENT HEARING CONDITIONS

Normal air conduction	Normal
Normal bone conduction	Normal or conductive
Air–bone gap	Conductive or mixed
No air–bone gap	Normal or sensorineural

SUGGESTED READING

JOHNSON, E. W. (1970). Tuning forks to audiometers and back again. *Laryngoscope, 80,* 49–68.

SOUND AND ITS MEASUREMENT

It is impossible to study abnormalities of human hearing without a basic understanding of the physics of sound and some of the properties of its perception and measurement. Sound is generated by vibration and is carried through the air around us in the form of pressure waves. It is only when a sound wave strikes the ear that hearing may take place.

Many factors may affect sound waves during their creation and propagation through the air. Many of these factors may be specified physically in terms of the frequency, intensity, and spectrum of vibrations. Human reactions to sound are psychological and reflect such subjective experiences as pitch, loudness, sound quality, and the ability to tell the direction of a sound source.

CHAPTER OBJECTIVES

Understanding this chapter requires no special knowledge of mathematics or physics, although a background in either or both of these disciplines would surely be helpful. From this chapter readers should be able to learn about sound waves, their common attributes, expression, and measurement. They should also come to understand the basic interrelationships among the measurements and be able to do simple calculations—for example, determining a given number of decibels developed in a sound system. At this point, however, it is more important to grasp the concepts than to gain skill in working equations.

SOUND

Sound may be defined in terms of either psychological or physical phenomena. In the psychological sense a sound is an auditory experience—the act of hearing something. In the physical sense, sound is a series of disturbances of molecules within an elastic medium.

If an elastic object is distorted, it will return to its original shape. The rate at which this occurs is determined by the **elasticity** of the object. Sound may travel through any elastic medium, although the immediate concern is the propagation of sound in air. Every cubic inch of the air that surrounds us is filled with billions and billions of tiny molecules. These particles move about randomly, constantly bouncing off each other. The elasticity, or springiness, of any medium is increased as the distance between the molecules is decreased. Molecules are packed more closely together in a solid than in a liquid and more closely in a liquid than in a gas. Therefore, a solid is more elastic than a liquid, and a liquid is more elastic than a gas.

The rapid and random movement of air particles is called **Brownian motion** and is affected by the heat in the environment. As the heat is increased, the particle velocity is increased. When water is heated in a kettle, the molecules are caused to bounce around, which in turn causes them to move further apart from each other. The energy increases until steam is created, resulting in the familiar teakettle whistle as the molecules are forced through a small opening. As long as there is any heat in the air, there is particle vibration.

A word might be said here regarding units of measurement. The metric centimeter gram second (cgs) has been most popular among scientists in the United States for many years, but it is gradually being replaced by the meter kilogram second (MKS) system. What may eventually be used exclusively is the International System of Units, abbreviated SI, taken from the French *Le Système International d'Unites.*

WAVES

Whenever air molecules are disturbed by a body set into **vibration**, they move from the point of disturbance, striking and bouncing off adjacent molecules. Because of their elasticity, the original molecules bounce back to their points of rest after having forced their neighbors from their original points. When the molecules are pushed close together, they are said to be condensed or compressed. When a space exists between areas of compression, this area is said to be rarefied. The succession of molecules being shoved together and then strung out sets up a motion called **waves**. Waves through the air, therefore, are made up of successive **compressions** and **rarefactions**. Figure 2.1A illustrates such wave motion and shows the different degrees of particle density. Figure 2.1B illustrates the same wave motion as a function of time.

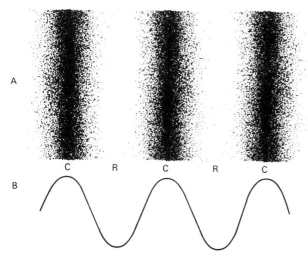

Figure 2.1 Simple wave motion in air showing (A) particle displacement (movement of pressure waves through space) and (B) and sinusoidal waveform (the pressure wave displayed as a function of time). Note the compressions (C) and rarefactions (R).

Transverse Waves

In **transverse waves** the molecular motion is perpendicular to the direction of wave motion. The example of water is often useful in understanding transverse wave motion. If a pebble is dropped into a water tank, the effect is that a hole is made in the area of water through which the pebble falls (Figure 2.2A). Water from the surrounding area flows into the hole to fill it, leaving a circular trough around the original hole (Figure 2.2B). Water from an area surrounding the trough then flows in to fill the first trough (Figure 2.2C). As the circles widen, each trough becomes shallower, until the troughs are barely perceptible. As the water flows in, the waves move out. A float anywhere on the surface of the water moves only up and down. In water, then, a float would illustrate a fixed point of the surface, which could be seen to bob only up and down. In fact the movement of the float would describe a circle or ellipse on a vertical axis.

Longitudinal Waves

Another kind of wave, more important in the understanding of sound, is the **longitudinal wave**. This wave is illustrated by the motion of wheat blowing in a field, with the tips of the stalks representing the air particles. The air molecules, like the grains of wheat, move along the same axis as the wave itself.

Sine Waves

Sound waves pass through the air without being seen. Indeed, they are real even if there is no one there to hear them. It is useful to depict sound waves in a graphic way to help explain them. Figure 2.3 assists in such a

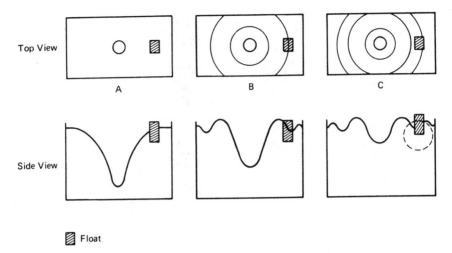

Top View

A   B   C

Side View

▨ Float

Figure 2.2 Wave motion in water as an example of transverse waves. A hole in the water is produced by a pebble (A); the first trough is produced when water flows in to fill the hole (B); the second trough is produced when water flows in to fill the first trough (C). A cork on the surface bobs up and down in a circular fashion.

pictorial representation if the reader will concede a bird's-eye view of a bucket of paint suspended by a string above a sheet of paper. If the bucket is pushed forward and backward, a small hole in its bottom allows a thin stream of paint to trace a line on the paper. We assume that forward motions of the bucket stand for compressions of molecules and backward motions for rarefactions. If the bucket continues to swing at the same rate, and if the paper is moved

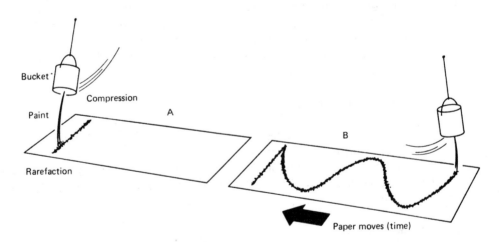

Bucket

Compression

Paint   A

Rarefaction

B

Paper moves (time)

Figure 2.3 Sine-wave motion. Bird's-eye view of a stream of paint from a bucket tracing a line forward (compression) and backward (rarefaction) on a sheet of paper (A). When the paper is moved to the left to represent the passage of time (B), the paint traces a sinusoidal wave.

in a leftward direction to represent the passage of time, a smooth wave is painted on the paper; this represents each **cycle**, consisting of its compression and rarefaction as a function of time. If the movement of the paper takes one second during which two complete cycles take place, the **frequency** is two cycles per second (cps), and so forth.

A body moving back and forth is said to **oscillate**. One cycle of vibration, or oscillation, begins at any point on the wave and ends at the identical point on the next wave, lending itself to a number of mathematical analyses which are important in the study of acoustics. Such waves are called **sine waves** or **sinusoidal** (sine-like) waves. When a body oscillates sinusoidally, showing only one frequency of vibration with no tones superimposed, it is said to be a **pure tone**. The number of complete sine waves that occur within one second constitutes the frequency of that wave.

The compression of a sine wave is usually shown by the curve extending upward and the rarefaction by the curve extending downward.

One cycle may be broken down into 360 degrees (Figure 2.4). Looking at a sine wave in terms of degrees is useful, as is seen later in this chapter. When a wave begins at 90 degrees rather than at zero degrees, it is called a **cosine wave**, but it is still circular in nature.

VIBRATIONS

Given the proper amount of energy, a mass can be set into vibration. The properties of its vibration may be influenced by a number of factors.

Effects of Energy on Vibration

Figure 2.5 illustrates the effects of energy on a sine wave. When the oscillating body has swung from point A to point B, it must come to a stop before the onset of the return swing, as the paint bucket in Figure 2.3 must cease its forward swing before it can swing back. At this point there is no **kinetic** (moving) energy, but rather all the energy is **potential**. As the vibrating

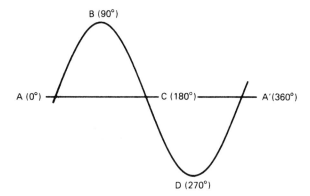

Figure 2.4 Denotation of a sine wave into 360 degrees.

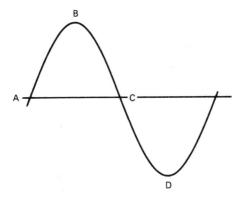

Figure 2.5 The effects of energy on a sine wave. At point B maximum excursion has taken place and all motion stops prior to the return swing. At point B all energy is potential with zero kinetic energy. At point C maximum velocity is reached, so all energy is kinetic and none is potential. Swinging slows down as point C is approached (the same as at point B, and when point D is reached all energy is potential again).

body picks up speed going from B to D, it passes through point C, where there is maximum kinetic energy and no potential energy. As point D is approached, kinetic energy decreases and potential energy increases, as at point B.

Free Vibrations

An object that is allowed to vibrate—for example, a weight suspended at the end of a string (Figure 2.6A)—will encounter a certain amount of opposition to its movement offered by the molecules in the air. This small amount of friction converts some of the energy involved in the initial movement of the object into heat. The friction has the effect of slowing down the distance of the swing until eventually all swinging will stop. If no outside force is added to perpetuate the swinging, the movement is called a **free vibration**. When

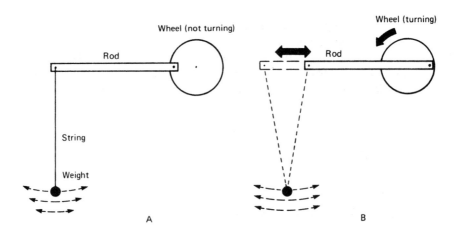

Figure 2.6 Free and forced vibrations. If the weight at the end of the string in A is pushed, the swinging back and forth will decrease until it stops. If the rod is caused to move back and forth because of the motion of the wheel (B) the distance of the swing of the weight will remain uniform until the wheel ceases to turn. A illustrates free vibration; B, forced vibration.

the vibrations of a mass decay gradually over time, the system is said to be *lightly damped*. *Heavy* **damping** causes the oscillations to cease rapidly. When the oscillations cease before a single cycle, the system is said to be *critically damped*.

Forced Vibrations

If an outside force is added to a swinging motion that controls the vibration (Figure 2.6B), swinging will continue unaltered until the outside force is removed. Such movement is called **forced vibration**. When the external force is removed, the object simply reverts to a condition of free vibration, decreasing the length of its swing until it becomes motionless. In both free and forced vibrations, the number of times the weight moves to and fro (the frequency) is unaltered by the distance of the swing (the amplitude). As the amplitude of movement decreases, the velocity of movement also decreases.

FREQUENCY

Nothing may transpire without the passage of time. It may be questioned how often or how frequently an event may occur during some unit of time. Occurrences may be rated using units such as the day or minute; in acoustics, however, when referring to events per unit of time, the duration usually used is the second. Consider the familiar metronome, whose pendulum swings back and forth. It can be considered that any time the pendulum has moved from any still position to the far right, past the original position to the far left, and then back to the point of origin, one cycle has occurred. Other motions, such as from far left to far right and back again, would also constitute one cycle. If the time required to complete a cycle is one second, it could be said that the frequency is one cycle per second (cps). The metronome may be adjusted so that the swings of the pendulum occur twice as often. In this way each journey of the pendulum can be made in half the time. This would mean that the time required for each cycle (the **period**) is cut to one-half second. Consequently, the frequency is doubled to 2 cps. This reciprocal relationship between frequency and period always exists and may be expressed as

$$\text{Period} = \frac{1}{\text{Frequency}}$$

In recent years the term **hertz (Hz)**, instead of cps, has been adopted in honor of the nineteenth-century German physicist Heinrich Hertz.

Effects of Length on Frequency

Through the use of a little imagination, the swinging of an object suspended at the end of a string can be seen to move slowly back and forth (Figure 2.7A). If the length of the string were suddenly shortened by holding it closer

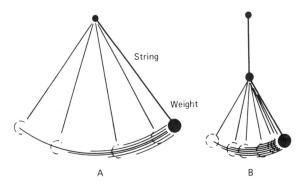

Figure 2.7 Effects of length of a pendulum on frequency of vibration. Given a length of string, the weight at the end will swing back and forth a specific number of times per second. If the string is shortened (B), the weight will swing faster (increase in frequency).

to the weight (Figure 2.7B), the number of swings per second would increase, causing the weight to swing back and forth more frequently. Thus, as length decreases, frequency increases. Conversely, as length increases, the number of hertz decreases. The musical harp exemplifies the effects of length on frequency: As the strings get shorter, they are easily seen (and heard) to vibrate at a higher frequency.

Effects of Mass on Frequency

A greater mass of an oscillating system results in a decrease in velocity so as to keep the kinetic energy constant. Simply stated, as the mass is increased, the frequency of vibration is decreased, unlike the pendulum example in Figure 2.7 in which mass does not affect frequency. For example, consider that the increased thickness of the larger strings of a harp produces lower notes.

Effects of Stiffness on Frequency

As a body vibrates, it exhibits a certain amount of compliance (the reciprocal of stiffness). As the compliance increases, the frequency at which the body is most easily made to vibrate (the resonant frequency) decreases. Systems that are stiffer (have more elasticity) vibrate better at higher frequencies than at lower frequencies.

RESONANCE

Any mass, regardless of size, may be set into vibration. Because of its inherent properties, each mass has a frequency at which it vibrates most naturally—that is, the frequency at which it is most easily set into vibration and at which the magnitude of vibration decays most slowly. The natural rate of vibration of a mass is called its **resonant frequency**. Although a mass may be set into vibration by a frequency other than its resonant frequency, when the external force is removed, the oscillation will revert to the resonant frequency until it is damped.

Musical notes have been known to shatter a drinking glass. This is accomplished if the resonant frequency of the glass is reached and the **amplitude** of the sound (the pressure wave) is increased until the glass is set into vibration that is sympathetic to (the same as) the sound source: If the glass is made to vibrate with sufficient amplitude, its shape becomes distorted and it may shatter.

SOUND VELOCITY

The **velocity** of a sound wave is the speed with which it travels from the source to another point. Sound velocity is determined by a number of factors, one of the most important of which is the density of the medium. As stated earlier, molecules are packed closer together in a solid than in a liquid or gas, and more closely in some solids (or liquids or gases) than in others. The closer together the molecules, the shorter the journey of each one before it strikes its neighbor, and the more quickly the adjacent molecules can be set into motion. Therefore, sounds travel faster through a solid than through a liquid and faster through a liquid than through a gas. In audiology our concern is with the movement of sound through air. The velocity of sound in air is approximately 344 meters (1130 feet) per second at standard temperature-pressure conditions (20 degrees Celsius at sea level). When temperature and humidity are increased, the speed of sound is increased. At higher altitudes the speed of sound is reduced because the distance between molecules is greater.

The velocity of sound may be determined at a specific moment in time; this is called the *instantaneous velocity*. In many cases sound velocity fluctuates as the wave moves through a medium. In such cases the *average velocity* of the wave may be determined by dividing the distance traveled by the time interval required for passage. Although we often think of velocity in miles per hour (mph), we can shift our thinking to meters per second (m/s) or centimeters per second (cm/s). When velocity is increased, *acceleration* takes place. When velocity is decreased, *deceleration* is experienced.

As a solid object moves through air, it pushes the air molecules it strikes out of the way, setting up a wave motion. As soon as the object itself exceeds the speed of sound, it causes a great compression ahead of itself, leaving a partial vacuum behind. The compressed molecules rushing in to fill the vacuum result in the sudden overpressure called the *sonic boom*. An aircraft flying faster than the speed of sound is first seen to pass by, followed by the boom, followed by the sound of the aircraft approaching, flying overhead, and departing. The loud sound of a gun discharging is made not so much by the explosion of gunpowder as by the bullet's breaking the sound barrier (exceeding the speed of sound) as it leaves the barrel.

WAVELENGTH

A characteristic of sound proportionately related to frequency is **wavelength**. The length of a wave is measured from any point on a sinusoid (any degree from zero to 360) to the exact same point on the next cycle of the wave (Figure 2.8). The formula for determining wavelength is $\lambda = c/f$, where λ = wavelength, c = the velocity of sound, and f = frequency. To solve for velocity, the formula $c = f\lambda$ may be used; to solve for frequency $f = c/\lambda$ may be used. As frequency goes up, wavelength decreases. For example, the wavelength of a 250 Hz tone is 4.5 feet ($\lambda = 1130/250$), whereas the wavelength of an 8000 Hz tone is 0.14 feet ($\lambda = 1130/8000$). Expressed in the metric system, the wavelength for a 250 Hz tone is 1.4 meters ($\lambda = 344/250$) and for an 8000 Hz tone is 0.04 meters ($\lambda = 344/8000$).

PHASE

It is convenient to discuss the relationships among corresponding points on different waves in terms of the angular measurements used to describe circular motion. Any point on a sine wave (expressed in degrees) may be compared to a standard. This standard is considered to be zero degrees. If an oscillation has a beginning at zero (or 360) degrees, it is said to be in phase with the

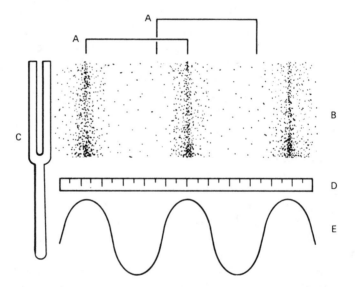

Figure 2.8 A wavelength (A) is measured from any point on the sine wave to the exact same point (in degrees) on the next wave. Pressure waves (B) are set up in the air by the vibrating tines of the tuning fork (C). These waves move a given distance as measured by the meter stick (D) and also may be displayed as a function of time (E).

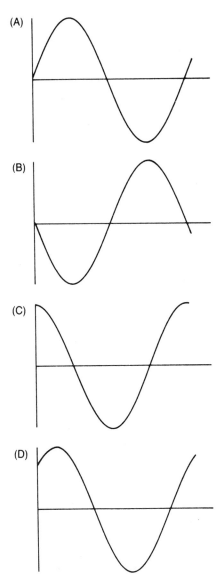

Figure 2.9 Relationship of phase on four waves of identical frequency.

standard (Figure 2.9A). Tones presented out of phase (Figure 2.9B, C, and D) are discussed in terms of differences in degrees from the standard.

Interference

Whenever more than one tone is introduced, there are interactions among sound waves. Such interactions are determined by the frequency, intensity, and phase relationships of the different waves. At any given moment in time the instantaneous amplitudes of concurrent sound waves must be summed. Two tones of the same frequency and phase relationship will reinforce each other, increasing the amplitude. Two tones of identical frequency but 180 degrees out of phase will cancel each other out, resulting in zero amplitude at any given moment. Away from laboratory conditions, there are usually more than two concomitant signals, so complete **cancellation** rarely occurs.

Beats

When two tones of almost identical frequency are presented (e.g., 1000 and 1003 Hz), there will be a noticeable increase and decrease in the resulting sound intensity, which is determined by the difference in frequency (in this illustration, three times per second). These changes are perceived as **beats**. When two tones of different frequency are presented and the difference between the two frequencies is increased, the number of beats per second increases, changing to a pulsing, then to a roughness, and finally to a series of complex sounds. Depending on the starting frequency, when the difference in Hz between two tones becomes large enough, the ear recognizes a number of tones, including the higher one, the lower one, **different tones,** and summation tones, all expressed in Hz.

INTENSITY

Up to this point we have concerned ourselves with the frequency of vibration of an oscillating body and its related functions. It is important that we know not only how fast but also how hard a body vibrates—its **intensity**. Figure 2.10A shows two tones of identical frequency; however, a difference exists in the maximum excursions of the two waves. Obviously a greater force has been applied to the wave on top than to the wave on the bottom to cause this difference to occur. The distance the mass moves from the point of rest is called its amplitude. Because our concern is with particle motion in air, it is assumed that if a greater force is applied to air molecules, they will move further from their points of rest, causing greater compressions and greater rarefactions, increasing the particle displacement and therefore the amplitude. Figure 2.10B shows two tones of identical amplitude and starting phase but of different frequency, and Figure 2.10C shows two tones with the same amplitude and frequency but different phase.

Force

When a vibrating body, such as the tines of a tuning fork, moves to and fro, it exerts a certain amount of **force** on adjacent air molecules. The greater the force, the greater the displacement by the tines, and therefore the greater

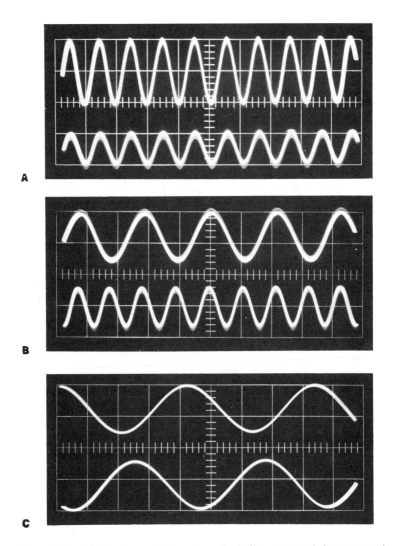

Figure 2.10 (A) Two tones of different amplitude (frequency and phase constant); (B) two tones of different frequency (amplitude and phase constant); and (C) two tones differing in phase (amplitude and frequency constant).

the amplitude of the sound wave. Because of the extreme sensitivity of the human ear to sound, only very small amounts of force are required to stimulate hearing. The **dyne (d)** is a convenient unit of measurement. One dyne is a force sufficient to accelerate a mass of 1 gram at 1 centimeter per second squared. If a mass of 1 gram (one-thirtieth of an ounce) is held at sea level, the force of gravity on this mass is about 1000 dynes. The **Newton (N)** has been used more recently as a force measurement in the United States. One Newton is a force that will accelerate a 1 kg mass at 1 m/s^2.

Pressure

Pressure is generated whenever force is distributed over a surface area. An example of this is the number of pounds per square inch used in tire-pressure measurements. Normal atmospheric pressure is 14.7 lb/in.², 1 million dynes/cm², or 10^5 **pascals (Pa)**. If a given area remains constant, the pressure increases as the force is increased. In the cgs system, pressure is expressed in dynes/cm² and in the SI system as pascals. Due to the sensitivity of human hearing, micropascals (millionths of a pascal [μPa]) are used. The smallest pressure variation required to produce a just-audible sound to healthy young ears is approximately 0.0002 dyne/cm², or 20 μPa. Sound waves that may be damaging to the ear have a pressure of about 2×10^8 μPa.

Work

When any mass, such as a group of air particles, is moved, a certain amount of **work** is done as energy is expended. The amount of work done may be expressed as the force exerted times the distance the mass is moved. One unit of work, the **erg (e),** is the amount of work done when 1 dyne force displaces an object by 1 cm; one **joule (J)** is 10 million ergs.

Power

Power is the capacity to exert physical force or energy and is expressed as the rate at which energy is expended. Familiar units of power are horsepower and watts. Because human hearing is extremely sensitive, small units of power, such as the erg/second, are used in acoustics. One watt is equal to 1 million ergs/second or 10^{-1} joule/second and 1 horsepower is equal to 746 watts. Power is a common measure of the magnitude of a sound. As the distance from the source is increased, the sound energy that reaches a given point decreases because it is spread out over a larger area.

Intensity of a Sound Wave

In any vibration, more air particles are displaced as the distance from the vibrating source increases. When the intensity of sound is measured, interest is centered on a small area at the point of measurement. The intensity of a sound wave is the amount of force per unit area. Although in any vibration the intensity of the sound decreases proportionately to the square of the distance of the sound source (the **inverse square law**), an intensity of 10^{-12} watt/m² at 1000 Hz will produce a just-audible sound if that intensity reaches the ear.

Assuming that sound radiates in a spherical pattern from a source, this relationship can be expressed by the following formula:

$$\text{Intensity (watts/cm}^2 \text{ or watts/m}^2) = \frac{\text{Power (watts)}}{4\pi \times \text{Radius}^2 \text{ (cm or m)}}$$

Common units of measurement, such as the pound or the mile, are additive in nature. As an example, ten one-pound weights equal exactly ten pounds. However, because the range of human hearing is so great, using such units results in very large numbers and becomes cumbersome. It is convenient to discuss one intensity in terms of the number of times it is *multiplied* by another intensity—that is, in terms of a ratio between the two. The **decibel (dB)** is useful for this purpose.

THE DECIBEL

A convenient way of expressing a ratio between two numbers is to use the logarithm to eliminate very lengthy figures. One unit easily adapted for such purposes is the **Bel**, named for Alexander Graham Bell, renowned educator of hearing-impaired children and inventor of the telephone. Because a Bel may have a rather large value, the decibel (dB), which is one-tenth of a Bel, is the unit of measurement of intensity used in acoustics and in audiometrics.

Five important aspects of the decibel must be remembered: (1) it involves a ratio; (2) it involves a logarithm; (3) it is therefore nonlinear; (4) it is expressed in terms of various reference levels, which *must* be specified; (5) it is a relative unit of measure.

Logarithms

A **logarithm** (log) is simply a number expressed as an **exponent**, which tells how often another number (the base) will be multiplied by itself. In the expression 10^2 (ten squared), the log (^{2}) tells that the base (10) will be multiplied by itself one time ($10 \times 10 = 100$). The exponent is the power, which tells how many times the base will be used in multiplication (e.g., $10^3 = 10 \times 10 \times 10 = 1000$).

Although any base may be used, in acoustics the base 10 is most common. This is convenient because the log simply tells how many zeros appear after the 1. Table 2.1 (*A* and *B*) shows a natural progression of logarithms with the base 10. It is important to note that *the log of 1 is zero.*

Ratios. The logarithm is useful in expressing a **ratio** between two numbers. Remember that a ratio is shown when any number is divided by another number. If a number is divided by itself (e.g., 25/25), the ratio is always one to one (1:1), a fact that obtains regardless of the magnitude of the numbers. When numbers with identical bases are used in division, the log of the denominator is subtracted from the log of the numerator (e.g., $10^3/10^2 = 10^1$). These mathematics do not change, regardless of whether the numerator or the denominator is the larger (e.g., $10^2/10^3 = 10^{-1}$). When a ratio is expressed as a fraction, the denominator becomes the reference to which the numerator is compared. Ratios expressed without a specific reference are totally meaningless, as in those commercial ads that claim a product is twice as good, three

TABLE 2.1 RATIOS, LOGARITHMS, AND OUTPUTS FOR DETERMINING NUMBER OF DECIBELS WITH INTENSITY AND PRESSURE REFERENCES

A RATIO	B LOG	C INTENSITY OUTPUTS (I_O) CGS (watt/cm²)	C SI (watt/m²)	D dB IL*	E EQUAL AMPLITUDES	F dB SPL†	G PRESSURE OUTPUTS (P_O) CGS (dyne/cm²)	G SI (µ Pa)
1:1	0	10^{-16}	10^{-12}	0	Threshold of Audibility	0	.0002	20.0(2 × 10^1)
10:1	1	10^{-15}	10^{-11}	10				
100:1	2	10^{-14}	10^{-10}	20		20	.002	200.0(2 × 10^2)
1,000:1	3	10^{-13}	10^{-9}	30				
10,000:1	4	10^{-12}	10^{-8}	40		40	.02	2,000.0(2 × 10^3)
100,000:1	5	10^{-11}	10^{-7}	50				
1,000,000:1	6	10^{-10}	10^{-6}	60		60	.2	20,000.0(2 × 10^4)
10,000,000:1	7	10^{-9}	10^{-5}	70				
100,000,000:1	8	10^{-8}	10^{-4}	80		80	2.0	200,000.0(2 × 10^5)
1,000,000,000:1	9	10^{-7}	10^{-3}	90				
10,000,000,000:1	10	10^{-6}	10^{-2}	100		100	20.0	2,000,000.0(2 × 10^6)
100,000,000,000:1	11	10^{-5}	10^{-1}	110				
1,000,000,000,000:1	12	10^{-4}	10^{0}	120		120	200.0	20,000,000.0(2 × 10^7)
10,000,000,000,000:1	13	10^{-3}	10^{1}	130	Threshold of Pain			
100,000,000,000,000:1	14	10^{-2}	10^{2}	140		140	2000.0	200,000,000.0(2 × 10^8)

*The number of dB with an intensity reference ($I_R = 10^{-12}$ watt/m²) uses the formula: dB (IL) $= 10 \times \log (I_O/I_R)$.

†The number of dB with a pressure reference ($P_R = 20$ µPa) uses the formula: dB (SPL) $= 20 \times \log (P_O/P_R)$.

times as bright, or 100% faster without saying what it is better, brighter, or faster than.

Intensity Level

Under some circumstances it is useful to express the decibel with an intensity reference. A practical unit in such cases is the watt per meter squared (watt/m^2). The intensity reference in a given system may be expressed as I_R (the number of **watts** of the reference intensity). The output, as of a loud-speaker, of the system may be expressed as I_O so that a ratio may be set up between the intensity reference and the intensity output. In solving for the number of decibels using an intensity reference, the formula used is:

$$dB = 10 \times \log (I_O/I_R)$$

The usual intensity reference (I_R) is 10^{-12} watt/m^2, although this may be changed if desired. In an expression like 10^{-12}, the exponent tells the number of places the decimal points must be moved to the right or left of the number 1. If the exponent is positive (or unsigned), the number of zeros is added following the 1. If the exponent is negative, the number of zeros placed before the 1 is equal to the exponent minus 1, with a decimal point before the zeros. If the exponent is positive, it suggests a large number; if it is negative, it suggests a small number, less than 1. Therefore, 10^{-12} watt/m^2 is an extremely small quantity (0.000000000001 watt/m^2).

If the intensity reference of a sound system (I_R) is known, the preceding equation may be used to determine the number of decibels of the output above (or below) the reference. As mentioned earlier, it is essential that the reference always be stated. When the reference is 10^{-12} watt/m^2, the term **intensity level** (IL) may be used as shorthand to imply this reference.

If the intensity output and the intensity reference are exactly the same ($I_O = I_R$), the ratio is 1:1. Because the log of 1 is 0, use of the formula shows the number of decibels to be 0. Therefore, 0 dB does not mean the absence of sound but rather that the intensity output is the same as the intensity reference. If I_O were changed to 10^1 watt/m^2, the number of decibels (IL) would be 130. Table 2.1 shows that as the intensity output (C) increases, the ratio (A) increases, raising the power of the log (B) and increasing the number of decibels (D).

The decibel, remember, is a logarithmic expression. When the intensity of a wave is doubled—for example, by adding a second loudspeaker with a sound of identical intensity to the first—the number of decibels is not doubled but is increased by three. This is because the intensity outputs of the two signals, and not the number of decibels, are added algebraically according to the principles of wave interference. For example, if loudspeaker A creates a sound of 60 dB IL (10^{-6} watt/m^2) and loudspeaker B also creates a sound of 60 dB IL (10^{-6} watt/m^2) to the same point in space, the result is 63 dB IL (2×10^{-6} watt/m^2).

Sound-Pressure Level

Audiologists and acousticians are more accustomed to making measurements of sound in pressure than in intensity. Such measurements are usually expressed as **sound-pressure level (SPL).** Because pressure ratios are known to be proportional to the square root of intensity ratios (intensity $\sim$ pressure^2), the conversion from intensity to pressure may be made as follows:

$$\text{Intensity reference dB (IL)} = 10 \times \log(I_O/I_R)$$

$$\text{Pressure reference dB (SPL)} = 10 \times \log(P_O^2/P_R^2)$$

Because intensity is proportional to pressure squared, when determining the number of decibels from a pressure reference, I_R may be written as $P_R{}^2$ (pressure reference) and I_O may be written as $P_O{}^2$ (pressure output). It is a mathematical rule that when a number is squared, its log is multiplied by 2; therefore the formula for dB SPL may be written:

$$\text{dB (SPL)} = 10 \times \log(P_O{}^2/P_R{}^2)$$

or

$$\text{dB (SPL)} = 10 \times 2 \times \log(P_O/P_R)$$

or

$$\text{dB (SPL)} = 20 \times \log(P_O/P_R)$$

As in the case of decibels with an intensity reference, when P_O is the same as P_R, the ratio between the two is 1:1 and the number of decibels (SPL) is zero. Just as in the case of intensity, zero dB SPL does not mean silence; it means only that the output pressure is zero dB above the reference pressure.

One dyne/cm^2 is equal to 1 **microbar** (one millionth of normal barometric pressure at sea level), so the two terms are frequently expressed interchangeably. The pressure of 0.0002 dyne/cm^2 has been the sound-pressure reference for use in physics and acoustics for some time. It is, however, being replaced by its SI equivalent, 20 micro pascals (μPa). This is the reference used for most **sound-level meters.** These devices are used to measure the sound-pressure levels in various acoustical environments (Figure 2.11). Therefore, 20 μPa is zero dB SPL. The threshold of pain at the ear is reached at 140 dB SPL. The term *dB SPL* implies a pressure reference of 20 μPa. Table 2.1 shows that increases in the number of μPa (or dyne/cm^2) (G) is reflected in the ratio (A), the log (B), and the number of dB SPL (F).

Because the decibel expresses a ratio between two sound intensities or two sound pressures, decibel values cannot be simply added and subtracted. Therefore, 60 dB plus 60 dB does not equal 120 dB. When sound-pressure values are doubled, the number of decibels is increased by six. Therefore, 60 dB (20,000 μPa) plus 60 dB (20,000 μPa) equals 66 dB (40,000 μPa). This point has been confusing to students because an increase in the number of decibels with an intensity reference results in an identical increase in decibels with a

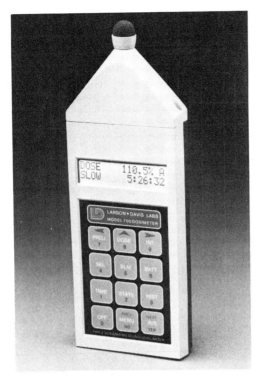

Figure 2.11 A commercial sound-level meter. (Courtesy of Larson-Davis Laboratory.)

pressure reference. The SPL will increase by a factor of 3 dB unless the two waves are in perfect correspondence. Also, because of the special relationship that exists between intensity and sound pressure, a 6 dB increase will be shown if the number of loudspeakers is quadrupled.

Note that the amplitude of a wave, whether expressed in decibels with an intensity reference or a pressure reference (Table 2.1, columns C and G), is the same as long as the number of decibels is the same. Intensity and pressure are simply different ways of looking at the same wave. Column E of Table 2.1 is designed to illustrate this point.

Hearing Level

The modern pure-tone audiometer was designed as an instrument to test human hearing sensitivity at a number of different frequencies. Originally each audiometer manufacturer determined the SPL required to barely stimulate the hearing of an average normal-hearing individual. Needless to say, there were some differences from make to make. Several studies have been conducted (Beasley, 1938) in which the hearing of many young adults was carefully measured, eventually culminating in the standard adopted in 1951 by the American Standards Association (ASA), summarized in Table 2.2.

The lowest sound intensity that stimulates normal hearing has been variously called zero hearing loss and zero **hearing level (HL)**. Because the ear

TABLE 2.2 STANDARD REFERENCE SOUND-PRESSURE LEVELS FOR 0 dB HEARING LEVEL*

FREQUENCY (Hz)	ASA-1951 W.E. 705A EARPHONE	ANSI-1969 (ISO-1964) W.E. 705A EARPHONE	ANSI-1969 (ISO-1964)** TDH-39 EARPHONE	TDH-49*** EARPHONE
125	54.5	45.5	45.0	47.5
250	39.5	24.5	25.5	26.5
500	25.0	11.0	11.5	13.5
1000	16.5	6.5	7.0	7.5
1500	16.5+	6.5	6.5	7.5
2000	17.0	8.5	9.0	11.0
3000	16.0+	7.5	10.0	9.5
4000	15.0	9.0	9.5	10.5
6000	17.5+	8.0	15.5	13.5
8000	21.0	9.5	13.0	13.0

*According to ASA-1951, ISO-1964, ANSI-1969, and a new proposed standard. Levels shown are those measured in a standard 6 cm³ coupler (NBS 9A).

**ISO-1964 values for TDH-39 earphone were obtained from the loudness balance data of Cox and Bilger (1960).

***+ Interpolations. Values for TDH-49 earphones are proposed SPLs.

shows different amounts of sensitivity to different frequencies (being most sensitive in the 1000 to 4000 Hz range), different amounts of pressure are required for zero HL at different frequencies. Even early audiometers were calibrated so that hearing could be tested over a wide range of intensities up to 100 or 110 dB HL (above normal hearing thresholds) at some frequencies. The pressure reference for decibels on an audiometer calibrated to ASA-1951 specifications was therefore different at each frequency, but the hearing-level dial was calibrated with reference to normal hearing (audiometric zero).

Audiometers manufactured in different countries had slightly different SPL values for audiometric zero until a standard close to what had been used in England was adopted by the International Organization for Standardization. This new standard, which was called ISO-1964, showed normal hearing to be more sensitive than the 1951 ASA values, resulting in a lowering of the SPL values averaging approximately 10 dB across frequencies. The ISO-1964 values are shown in Table 2.2. Differences between the two standards probably occurred because of differences in the studies during which normative data were compiled, in terms of test environment, equipment, and procedure.

Audiologists who had experience testing normal-hearing persons on the ASA standard had noted that many such subjects had hearing better than the zero reference, often in the −10 dB HL range, and welcomed the conversion to the new standard. More recently a new American standard has been published by the American National Standards Institute (ANSI, formerly ASA) showing SPL values for normal hearing the same as the ISO levels using the usual audiometer earphones.

Sensation Level

Another reference for the decibel may be to the auditory **threshold** of a given individual. The threshold of a pure tone is usually defined as the level at which the tone is so soft that it can only be perceived 50% of the time it is introduced, although the 50% response criterion is purely arbitrary. The number of decibels of a sound above the threshold of a given individual is that number of decibels **sensation level (SL)**.

If a person can barely hear a tone at 0 dB HL at a given frequency, a tone presented at 50 dB HL will be 50 dB above his or her threshold, or, stated another way, 50 dB SL. The same 50 dB HL tone presented to a person with a 20 dB threshold will have an SL of 30 dB. It is important to recognize that a tone presented at threshold has an SL of 0 dB. In order to state the number of dB SL, the threshold of the individual (the reference) must be known.

COMPLEX SOUNDS

Pure tones, as described in this chapter, seldom appear in nature. When they are created, it is usually by devices like tuning forks or electronic sine-wave generators. Most sounds, therefore, are composed of a number of different tones having different frequencies, amplitudes, and phase relationships. A mathematician by the name of Fourier first showed that any complex wave can be analyzed into its sinusoidal **components**.

Fundamental Frequency

Some complex sounds repeat over time, as do many of the sounds of speech and music. Such sounds are called **periodic**. When a number of pure tones are presented, one of them will naturally have a frequency lower than the others. The lowest frequency of vibration in the spectrum of a complex periodic sound is called the **fundamental frequency** and is determined by the physical properties of the vibrating body. **Aperiodic** sounds are random, do not have fundamental frequencies, and are usually perceived as noise.

Harmonics

In a periodic complex sound, all frequencies present are whole-number multiples of the fundamental. These tones, which occur over the fundamental, are called **harmonics** or **overtones**. The spectrum of a sound with a 100 Hz fundamental would therefore contain only higher frequencies of 200, 300, 400 Hz, and so on. With respect to periodic signals, the only difference between overtones and harmonics is the way in which they are numbered: The first harmonic is the fundamental frequency, the second harmonic is twice the fundamental, and so on. The first overtone is equal to the second harmonic, and further overtones are numbered consecutively.

Spectrum of a Complex Sound

When two or more pure tones of different frequencies are generated simultaneously, their combined amplitudes must be summed at each instant in time. This is illustrated in Figure 2.12, which shows that a new and slightly different wave shape appears. Adding a fourth and fifth tone would further alter the wave shape. **Complex waves** of this nature can be synthesized in the laboratory and constitute, in essence, the opposite of a **Fourier analysis**.

Although the fundamental frequency determines all the harmonic frequencies, the harmonics do not all have equal amplitude (Figure 2.13A). In any wind instrument the fundamental frequency is determined by a vibrating body: in a clarinet, the reed; in a trombone, the lips within the mouthpiece; and in that peculiar wind instrument called the human vocal tract, the vocal folds in the larynx. The length and cross-sectional areas of any of these wind instruments may be varied: in the trombone, by moving the slide; in the clarinet, by depressing keys; and in the vocal tract, by raising or lowering the tongue and moving it forward or back. In this way, even though the fundamental and harmonic frequencies may be the same, the amplitudes of different harmonics vary from instrument to instrument, resulting in the different harmonic spectrum (Figure 2.13B and C) and characteristic **qualities** of each.

Without changing the fundamental frequency during speech, changing the size and shape of the vocal tract, mostly by moving the tongue, results in some harmonics being emphasized and others being suppressed. The resulting wave form has a series of peaks and valleys. Each of the peaks is called a **formant**, and it is precisely this phenomenon that aids in the recognition of different vowel sounds. The peaks are numbered consecutively and are expressed as the lowest or first formant (F_1), the second formant (F_2), and so on. The spectrum of a musical wind instrument may be similar to that of a vowel and is similarly determined by the resonances of the acoustic systems.

Once the harmonic structure of a wave has been determined by the fundamental, the fundamental is no longer critical for the clear perception of a sound. This is exemplified by the telephone, which does not allow frequencies below about 300 Hz to pass through. Although a man's fundamental vocal frequency averages about 85 to 150 Hz and a woman's about 175 to 250 Hz (both the consequences of laryngeal size, shape, and subglottal pressure), the sex of the speakers as well as their identity is evident over a telephone even though the fundamental frequency is filtered out.

IMPEDANCE

Any moving object must overcome a certain amount of **resistance** to its movement. A sound wave moving through air will strike surfaces that impede or retard its progress. The **impedance** of a medium is the opposition it offers to the transmission of acoustic energy.

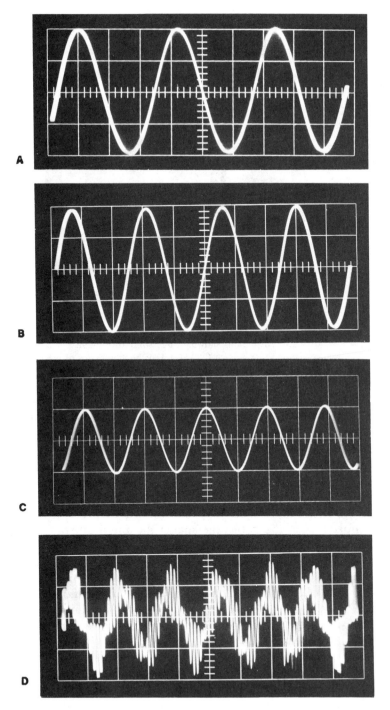

Figure 2.12 Synthesis of a complex, waveform (D) from three sine waves (A, B, C) of different frequency and amplitude. Note that the amplitudes are summed at each moment in time, resulting in a new waveform.

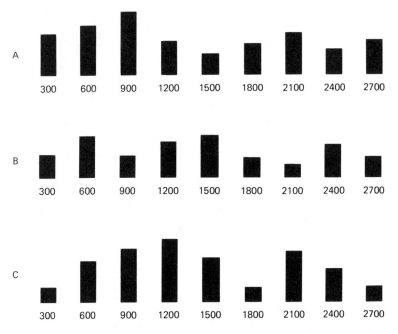

Figure 2.13 Histograms showing three wind instruments. The fundamental frequency is the same in each (300 Hz), but the amplitudes of the harmonics differ.

As a general rule, the denser a surface that is placed in the path of a sound wave, the greater the impedance offered to the wave. For example, when a sound strikes a closed door, some of the energy will be reflected because the door is so much denser than the air on either side of it. If the sound is to be carried to the adjacent room, the door itself must be set into vibration, whereupon the opposite side of the door, moving against the air molecules in the next room, generates new sound waves. The amount of impedance of the door will determine the amplitude of the waves in the next room. The greater the impedance of the door, the smaller the amplitude of the waves transmitted to the adjacent room.

Given sufficient energy to overcome its inertia, a mass may be set into vibration. The resonant characteristics of a body or medium determine the frequencies of most efficient and least efficient vibration. **Resonance** is determined by the mass, elasticity, and frictional characteristics of an object (or medium). Therefore, resonance characteristics are defined by impedance.

Total impedance (Z) is determined by two factors. The first is simple resistance (R)—that is, resistance that is not influenced by frequency of vibration. This simple resistance is analogous to electrical resistance in a direct-current electrical system, such as a battery, in which electrons move in a single direction from a negative to a positive pole. The second factor is complex resistance or **reactance**. Reactance is influenced by frequency so that the opposition to energy transfer varies with frequency. Reactance is seen in alternating-current electrical systems, such as household current, in which the flow of electrons is periodically reversed.

Total reactance is determined by two subsidiary factors called *mass reactance* and *stifffness reactance*. As either the physical mass (*M*) of an object or the frequency (*f*) at which the object vibrates is increased, so does the mass reactance. In other words, mass reactance is directly related to both mass and frequency. Stiffness reactance behaves in an opposite manner. As the physical **stiffness** (*S*) of an object increases, so does stiffness reactance. However, as frequency increases, stiffness reactance decreases (an inverse relationship).

Together, simple resistance, mass reactance, and stiffness reactance all contribute to the determination of total impedance. All four terms are given the same unit of measurement, the **ohm (Ω)**. The formula for computing total impedance is:

$$Z = \sqrt{R^2 + \left(2\pi fM - \frac{S}{2\pi f}\right)^2}$$

in which *Z* is the total impedance, *R* is the simple resistance, $2\pi fM$ is the mass reactance, and $S/2\pi f$ is the stiffness reactance. This equation shows that mass reactance and stiffness reactance combine algebraically.

SOUND MEASUREMENT

Audiologists are generally interested in making two kinds of measurements: those of the hearing ability of patients with possible disorders of the auditory system and those of sound-pressure levels in the environment.

The first modern step toward quantifying the amount of a patient's hearing loss came with the development of the pure-tone audiometer. Use of this device allows for comparison of any person's hearing threshold to that of an established norm. Hearing threshold is frequently defined as the intensity at which a tone is barely audible. Hearing sensitivity is expressed as the number of decibels above (or below) the average normal-hearing person's thresholds for different pure tones. Speech audiometers have been designed to measure thresholds for the spoken word, in addition to other things.

The Pure-Tone Audiometer

A pure-tone audiometer is diagrammed in Figure 2.14. It consists of an audio oscillator, which generates pure tones of different frequencies, usually at discrete steps of 125, 250, 500, 750, 1000, 1500, 2000, 3000, 4000, 6000, and 8000 Hz. Each tone is amplified to a maximum of about 110 dB HL in the frequency range of 500 to 4000 Hz, with less output above and below that range.

The tones are attenuated with the use of a dial, which is numbered (contrary to attenuation) in decibels above the normal threshold for each fre-

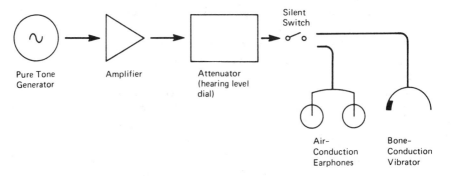

Figure 2.14 Block diagram of a pure-tone audiometer.

quency. As the number of decibels is increased, the attenuation is decreased. The audiometer is provided with a silent switch that can introduce or interrupt a tone. The signal is routed via an output selection control to a right or left earphone or to a bone-conduction vibrator. A photograph of a pure-tone audiometer is shown in Figure 2.15.

Air Conduction. Earphones are held in place by a steel headband that fits across the top of the head. The phones themselves are connected to the headband via two small metal yokes. The earphone consists of a magnetic device that transduces the electrical translations supplied by the audiometer to a small diaphragm that vibrates according to the acoustic equivalents in terms of frequency and intensity. Around the earphone is a rubber cushion that may fit around the ear (circumaural) or, more usually, over the ear (supraaural). The movement of the earphone diaphragm generates the sound, which enters

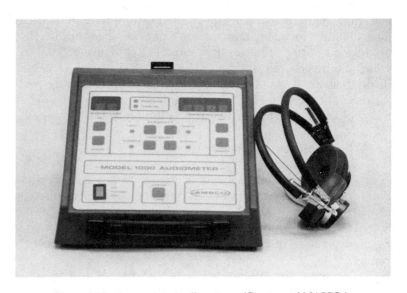

Figure 2.15 A pure-tone audiometer. (Courtesy of MAICO.)

the ear directly, resulting in an air-conduction signal. Standard audiometric earphones are shown in Figure 2.16.

For some time it has been recognized that there are distinct advantages to using earphones for air-conduction testing that are inserted into the external ear canal. These advantages will be discussed in some detail later in this book, but one of them includes a significant increase in comfort to the patient. Insert earphones that are appropriate for audiometry have only recently been perfected and are shown in Figure 2.17.

Bone Conduction. Selection of the bone-conduction output of the audiometer causes the signal to terminate in a small plastic device with a slight concavity on one side for comfortable fit against the skull. The principle of the bone-conduction vibrator is the same as that of the air-conduction receiver except that instead of moving a waferlike diaphragm, the plastic shell of the vibrator must be set into motion. Because they must vibrate a greater mass (the skull), bone-conduction vibrators require greater energy than air-conduction receivers do to generate a level high enough to stimulate normal hearing. For this reason the maximum power outputs are considerably lower, usually not exceeding 65 dB HL. Frequencies of 250 through 4000 Hz are those usually found available for bone-conduction testing.

The bone-conduction vibrator is held against the skull at either the forehead or the mastoid process. When the forehead is the placement site, a plastic strap, which circles the head, is used. When the bone behind the ear is the desired place for testing, a spring-steel headband, which goes across the top of the skull, is employed. A bone-conduction vibrator is shown in Figure 2.18.

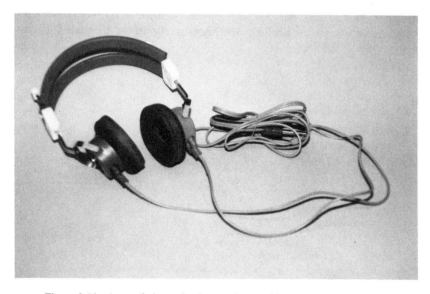

Figure 2.16 A set of air-conduction receivers. (Courtesy of Starkey Labs.)

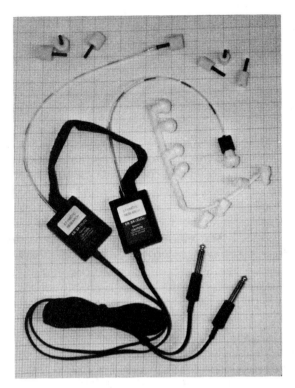

Figure 2.17 A pair of insert receivers. (Courtesy of Etymotic Research, Elk Grove Village, IL)

The Speech Audiometer

As is discussed later, measurements made with speech stimuli are very helpful in the diagnosis of auditory disorders. A speech audiometer is required for such measurements. The speech audiometer, along with a pure-tone audiometer, may be part of a clinical audiometer (Figure 2.19) or it may be a separate unit.

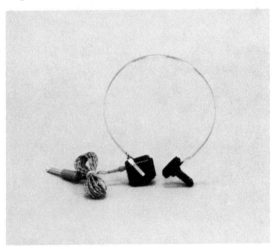

Figure 2.18 A bone conduction vibrator. (Courtesy of Starkey Labs.)

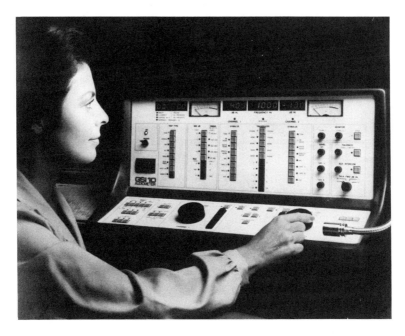

Figure 2.19 A diagnostic audiometer. (Courtesy of GSI and Eckle, Ind.)

The diagram in Figure 2.20 shows that a speech audiometer can have an input signal provided by a microphone, a phonograph, or a tape recorder. The loudness of the speech signal is monitored by an averaging voltmeter called a VU (volume units) meter. Such a meter reads in dB VU, implying an electrical reference in watts. The signal is amplified and attenuated as in a pure-tone audiometer, with the hearing-level dial calibrated in decibels with reference to

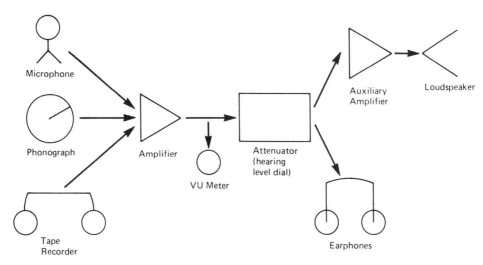

Figure 2.20 Block diagram of a speech audiometer.

SOUND AND ITS MEASUREMENT   43

audiometric zero for speech (20 dB SPL on the ANSI–1969 standard for a TDH–49 earphone).

Air Conduction. Most of the measurements made on speech audiometers are accomplished through air-conduction receivers. Testing may be carried out by selecting the right ear, the left ear, or both ears. The usual range is from −10 to 110 dB HL.

Sound Field. It is often desirable to make measurements of speech in the sound field—that is, to feed the speech signal into the room using a loudspeaker rather than earphones. The signal generated with the audiometer is designed for the air-conduction earphone and does not have sufficient power to drive a larger loudspeaker. When the speaker output of the audiometer is selected, the speech signal is usually fed to an auxiliary amplifier, which augments the intensity of the signal, developing the additional power necessary.

Sound-Level Meters

As mentioned earlier, airborne sounds are measured by devices called sound-level meters. These consist of a microphone, amplifier, attenuator, and meter to pick up and transduce the pressure waves in the air so that they can be measured electrically and read out in decibels. The usual reference for sound-level meters is 20 μPa.

Because the human ear responds differently to different frequencies, many sound-level meters contain systems called *weighting networks*, which are filters to alter the response of the instrument much as the ear does at different levels. The **phon** lines (Figure 2.21) show that the ear does not respond well to low frequencies at low SPLs, and that as the sound increases in intensity, the ear is capable of better and better low-frequency response. The three usual weighting networks of sound-level meters are shown in Figure 2.22 and illustrate how the meter responds at relatively low levels (A weighting), moderate levels (B weighting), and high levels (C scale with no weighting).

Sound-level meters are useful in the study of acoustics and are becoming common tools in industry as concern over noise pollution grows. Background noise levels can play a major role in the testing of hearing because, if they are sufficiently high, they may interfere with accurate measurement by causing **masking.** Whenever hearing testing is undertaken, especially of persons with normal or near-normal hearing, the background noise levels should be known.

Acceptable Noise Levels for Audiometry

Table 2.3 shows the maximum room noise allowable for air- and bone-conduction testing on the ANSI–1969 scale. To determine the allowable levels for bone-conduction testing, the attenuation provided by the usual audiometer earphone and cushion must be subtracted from the maximum allowable levels for air conduction because the ear remains uncovered during bone-conduction audiometry.

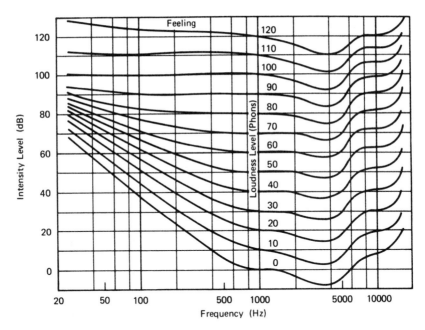

Figure 2.21 Equal loudness contours showing the relationship between loudness level (in phons) and intensity (in dB).

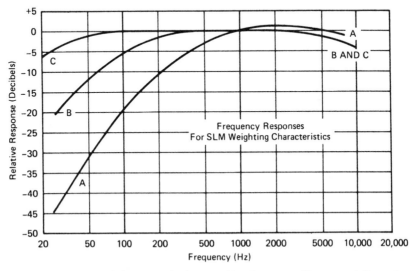

Figure 2.22 Weighting networks for sound-level meter. (Courtesy of General Radio Corporation.)

TABLE 2.3 MAXIMUM ALLOWABLE OCTAVE BAND AND ONE-THIRD OCTAVE BAND LEVELS FOR NO MASKING ABOVE ZERO HEARING LEVEL DIAL SETTINGS FOR AUDIOMETERS CALIBRATED TO THE ANSI—1969 STANDARD*

TEST FREQUENCY (Hz)	125	250	500	750	1000	1500	2000	3000	4000	6000	8000
Air conduction (ears covered**)											
Octave band levels	34.5	23.0	21.5	22.5	29.5	29.0	34.5	39.0	42.0	41.0	45.0
One-third octave band levels	29.5	18.0	16.5	17.5	24.5	24.0	29.5	34.0	37.0	36.0	40.0
Bone conduction (ears not covered)											
Octave band levels		18.5	14.5	12.5	14.0	10.5	8.5	8.5	9.0		
One-third octave band levels		13.5	9.5	7.5	9.0	5.5	3.5	3.5	4.0		

*Levels are in decibels with reference to 20 μPa (ANSI—1977).

**Ears covered with an earphone mounted in an MX—41/AR cushion.

Calibration of Audiometers

Although periodic factory checks on audiometer calibration are desirable, many audiologists also perform frequent checks on the operation of their equipment on site in the clinic. In the early days of audiometers, checks on the reliability of the hearing level were conducted by testing a group of subjects with known normal hearing. Known as the psychoacoustic method, this is done by taking the median of the results and posting a correction chart on the audiometer to remind the audiologist to correct any readings obtained on a patient by the number of decibels the audiometer had drifted out of calibration. This procedure is still quite common.

Many audiology clinics today are equipped with meters and couplers so that the task of level checking may be accomplished electroacoustically. The earphone is placed over a carefully machined coupler, usually containing a cavity of precisely 6 cm^3. A weight of 500 grams or a spring with equivalent tension holds the receiver in place. Sounds emanating from the diaphragm of the receiver are picked up by a sensitive microphone at the bottom of the coupler (the coupler is often called the **artificial ear**), amplified, and read in dB SPL on a sound-level meter. In order to be certain that the meter is reading the level of the tone (or other signal) from the receiver and not from the ambient room noise, the level of the signal is usually high enough to avoid this possibility. Hearing levels of 70 dB are convenient for this purpose, and the readout should correspond to the number of decibels required for threshold of the particular signal plus 70 dB. A form designed for level checking with an artificial ear is shown in Figure 2.23, and a commercial testing unit is shown in Figure 2.24.

When one is calibrating a speech audiometer, a signal must be fed through one of the inputs. A pure tone, a noise containing approximately equal intensity at all frequencies or a sustained vowel sound, may be used. The signal is adjusted so that the VU meter reads zero. With the hearing-level dial set at 70 dB and with the earphone on the coupler, the signal should read 90 dB SPL on the meter (70 dB HL plus 20 dB SPL required for audiometric zero for speech on the ANSI–1969 standard) for the most commonly used earphone.

In addition to level checking, it is important on pure-tone audiometers to check for changes in frequency to be sure that the ANSI frequency limitations (the nominal frequency ± 3%) have not been exceeded. This may be done with a frequency counter.

The linearity of the attenuator dial is most easily tested electronically with a volt meter. Checks should be made through the entire intensity range to be certain that when the hearing-level dial is moved a given number of decibels, the level changes by this precise amount ± 1.5 dB per 5 dB step, the tolerance allowed by the ANSI–1969 standard. In addition, the total error in the hearing-level dial linearity cannot exceed ± 3 to 5 dB, depending on frequency.

Even though the audiometer generates a pure tone, it is likely that distortion in the system (often the earphone) will result in the second harmonic of the tone's being emitted; that is, if a 1000 Hz tone is generated, some energy

For TDH-49 Earphone

University of Texas Speech and Hearing Center
AUDIOMETER CALIBRATION

Calibrated By ______________ Audiometer ______________ Serial No. ______________ Date ______________

	Frequency					Right Air Output*			Left Air Output*				Mastoid Output #			Forehead Output #		
Obs.	Attn. HL	Err.	Dial	Count	HL	Obs.	Cor.	Err.	Obs.	Cor.	Err.	HL	Obs.	Cor.	Err.	Obs.	Cor.	Err.
	110																	
	105		125		70		117.5			117.5		—		—			—	
	100																	
	95		250		70		96.5			96.5		25		66.4			79.9	
	90																	
	85		500		70		83.5			83.5		40		70.7			85.7	
	80																	
	75		750		70		78.5			78.5		40		59.3			71.8	
	70																	
	65		1000		70		77.5			77.5		40		56.9			66.9	
	60																	
	55		1500		70		77.5			77.5		40		55.4			66.4	
	50																	
	45		2000		70		81.0			81.0		40		48.1			56.6	
	40																	
	35		3000		70		79.5			79.5		40		46.6			54.1	
	30																	
	25		4000		70		80.5			80.5		40		51.2			57.7	
	20																	
	15		6000		70		83.5			83.5		—		—			—	
	10																	
	5		8000		70		83.0			83.0		—		—			—	
	0																	
	Ttl Err.		Speech		70		90.0			90.0		40		( )			( )	

FUNCTIONAL CHECKS WITH TOLERANCES:

Rise Time (20 — 100 milliseconds) ______________ .

Fall Time (5 — 100 milliseconds) ______________ .

Overshoot and ringing (± 1dB) ______________ .

Total Harmonic Distortion (max. —30dB) ______________ .

Comments:

*Figures in this column are dB re 20 μPa for proposed ANSI standards for use with TDH-49 receivers mounted in MX-41/AR cushions.

#These figures include corrections for the B&K Model 4930 artificial mastoid for a B—70A bone-conduction vibrator.

FNM/80

Figure 2.23 Sample of form for field check of audiometer air- and bone-conduction level and frequency.

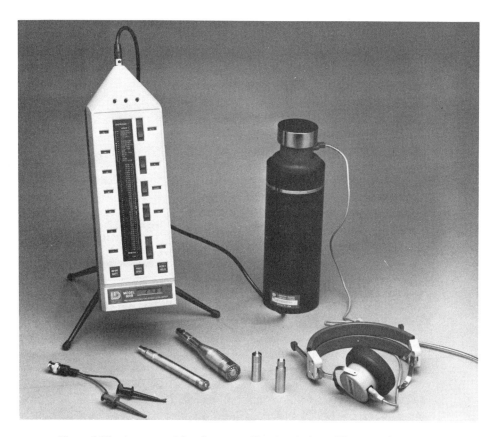

Figure 2.24 A commercial audiometer calibration device. (Courtesy of Larson-Davis Laboratory.)

at 2000 Hz will be present. ANSI standards specify that the second harmonic be at least 30 dB below the fundamental (the nominal frequency). This can be checked with special equipment.

Calibration of the bone-conduction systems of audiometers may be accomplished in several ways. The most popular method of field calibration involves the use of several patients with known sensorineural losses. Their air- and bone-conduction thresholds are compared and median values for the differences taken at each frequency. The amounts by which the bone-conduction thresholds differ from the (calibrated) air-conduction thresholds are averaged and corrections are posted on the audiometer.

Recent years have seen the development of the **artificial mastoid** (Figure 2.25), a device that allows for electronic calibration of the bone-conduction system of an audiometer. The procedure is similar to that for testing air conduction for calibration. The bone-conduction vibrator is placed on the artificial mastoid and vibrations are transduced into electrical currents, which are then converted to decibels for direct readout. The form shown in Figure

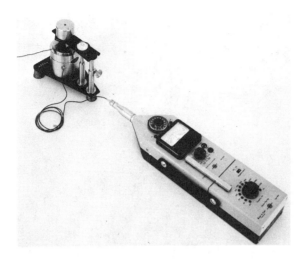

Figure 2.25 An artificial mastoid assembly. (Courtesy of B & K instruments.)

2.23 allows for calibration to the ANSI (1972; 1981) standard for bone-conduction testing on either the forehead or the mastoid.

Calibration of a loudspeaker system with an audiometer requires either the testing of a number of normal-hearing subjects or the use of a sound-level meter. A heavy chair that is difficult to move should be placed before the speaker at a distance of about three times the diameter of the loudspeaker, plus one foot. This allows the subject to be placed in the "far field." The sound-level meter should be placed in the same position as the head of a patient seated in that same chair. If the hearing-level dial is set to 70 dB, the sound-level meter should read 70 dB plus 20 dB for audiometric zero for speech minus 6 dB. Six dB are subtracted, because data from several older studies showed that thresholds for pure tones determined under earphones, called the Minimum Audible Pressure (MAP) (Sivian & White, 1933), were slightly poorer than thresholds determined in a free sound field, the Minimum Audible Field (MAF) (Fletcher & Munson, 1933). Wilber (1985, p. 138) recommends that the loudspeaker output for 0 dB HL in the sound field should be 13 dB SPL or produce equivalent spondee thresholds to earphone measurements. Because an auxiliary amplifier is usually required to power the loudspeaker, its volume control may be adjusted to acquire the proper level.

Whenever the audiometer differs from the required level at any frequency by more than 2.5 dB, a correction may be added to the hearing-level dial setting during audiometric testing. Corrections are rounded out to the nearest multiple of 5 dB. If the calibration procedure reveals that the system is putting out too low a level, the number of decibels of deviation is *subtracted* from the hearing-level dial setting during any given test. If the intensity is too high, the correction is *added* during testing. Whenever level calibration reveals marked differences from specification, the audiometer should be seen for recalibration. Audiologists should never assume that their audiometers are in proper calibration, even new units, unless they have verified this for themselves. One study (Thomas et al., 1969) revealed that of 100 audiometers placed in public schools and physicians' offices, not one was in proper calibration.

ENVIRONMENTAL SOUNDS

Earlier we saw that the range of sound intensities from threshold of audibility to pain is extremely wide. All of the sounds that normal-hearing persons may hear without discomfort must be found within this range. Table 2.4 gives examples of some ordinary environmental sounds and their approximate intensities. This table may help the reader to develop a framework from which to approximate the intensities of other sounds.

PSYCHOACOUSTICS

Thus far in the present chapter, attention has been focused on physical acoustics. These factors are the same with or without human perception. It is important that some brief space be allocated here to psychoacoustics, the study of the relationship between physical stimuli and the psychological responses to which they give rise.

Pitch

Pitch is a term used to describe the subjective impressions of the "highness" or "lowness" of a sound. Pitch relates to frequency in that, as the frequency of vibration increases, so does pitch, at least within the range of

TABLE 2.4 SCALE OF INTENSITIES FOR ORDINARY ENVIRONMENTAL SOUNDS*

0 dB	Just audible sound
10 dB	Soft rustle of leaves
20 dB	A whisper at 4 feet
30 dB	A quiet street in the evening with no traffic
40 dB	Night noises in a city
50 dB	A quiet automobile 10 feet away
60 dB	Department store
70 dB	Busy traffic
60–70 dB	Normal conversation at 3 feet
80 dB	Heavy traffic
80–90 dB	Niagara Falls
90 dB	A pneumatic drill 10 feet away
100 dB	A riveter 35 feet away
110 dB	Hi-fidelity phonograph with a 10 watt amplifier, 10 feet away
115 dB	Hammering on a steel plate 2 feet away

*The reference is 10^{-16} watt/cm² (Van Bergeijk, Pierce, & David, 1960).

human hearing, from about 20 to 20,000 Hz. The Western world uses the **octave** scale in its music. When frequency is doubled, it is raised one octave, but raising (or lowering) a sound one octave does not double (or halve) its pitch. Intensity also contributes to the perception of pitch, although to a lesser extent than frequency.

The subjective aspect of pitch can be measured using a unit called the **mel**. One thousand mels is the pitch of a 1000 Hz tone at 40 dB SL. Frequencies can be adjusted so that they sound twice as high (2000 mels), half as high (500 mels), and so on. Except for the fact that the number of mels increases and decreases with frequency, apart from 1000 Hz, the numbers do not correspond. Although the task sounds formidable, pitch scaling can be accomplished on cooperative normal-hearing subjects with great accuracy after a period of training. The mel scale is illustrated in Figure 2.26.

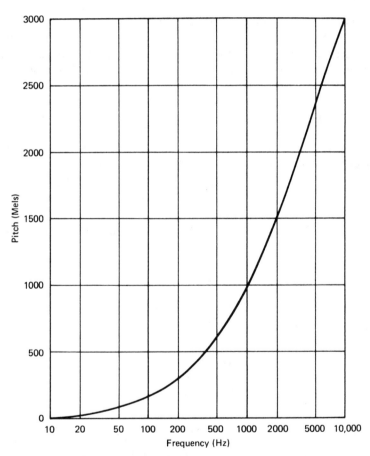

Figure 2.26 The mel scale, showing the relationship between pitch (in mels) and frequency (in hertz).

Loudness

Loudness is a subjective experience, as contrasted with the purely physical force of <u>intensity.</u> The thinking reader has realized, to be sure, that a relationship exists between increased intensity and increased loudness. The decibel, however, is *not* a unit of loudness measurement, and so such statements as "The noise in this room is 60 decibels loud" are erroneous. The duration and frequency of sounds contribute to the sensation of loudness.

As stated earlier, the ear is not equally sensitive at all frequencies. It is also true that the subjective experience of loudness changes differently at different frequencies. Comparing the loudness of different frequencies to the loudness of a 1000 Hz tone at a number of intensity levels determines the **loudness level** of the different frequencies. Figure 2.21 shows that loudness grows faster for low-frequency tones (and certain high-frequency tones) than for midfrequencies. The unit of loudness level is the phon.

The term **sone** refers to the comparison of the loudness of a 1000 Hz tone at different intensities. One sone is the loudness of 1000 Hz at 40 dB SL. The intensity required for subjects to perceive half the loudness of 1 sone is 0.5 sones, the intensity for twice the loudness is 2 sones, and so forth. Loudness level (in phons) can therefore be related to loudness (in sones); but, as Figure 2.27 shows, the measurements do not correspond precisely.

Localization

Hearing is a distance sense, unaffected by many barriers that interfere with sight, touch, and smell. Sound can bend around corners with little distortion, although as frequencies get higher, they become more unidirectional. Under many conditions it is possible, even without seeing the source of a sound, to tell the direction from which it comes. This ability, called **localization**, is a complex phenomenon resulting from the interaction of both ears. The localization of sound, which warned our ancestors of possible danger, was probably a major contributor to the early survival of our species.

Localization is possible because of the relative intensities of sounds and their times of arrival at the two ears (i.e., phase). The greatest single contributors to our ability to localize are interaural phase differences in the low frequencies (below 1500 Hz) and intensity differences in the higher frequencies. Naturally, in an acoustical environment with hard surfaces the sound may **reverberate** and be heard to come from a direction other than its source. An area in which there are no hard surfaces to cause reverberation is called a **free field**. Free fields actually exist only in such exotic areas as mountaintops and specially built **anechoic chambers** (Figure 2.28).

Masking

When two sounds are heard simultaneously, the intensity of one sound may be sufficient to cause the other to be inaudible. This change in the

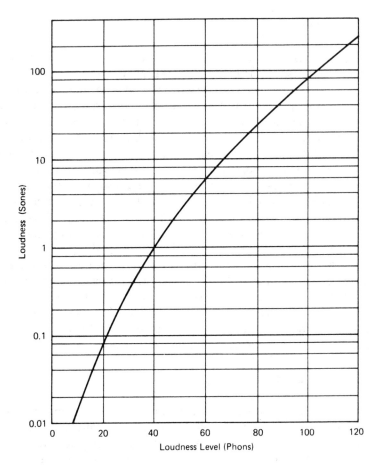

Figure 2.27 Loudness function showing the relationship between loudness (in sones) and loudness level (in phons).

threshold of a sound caused by a second sound with which it coexists is called masking. There is surely no one who has not experienced masking in noisy situations in the form of speech interference. The noise that causes the interference is called the masker and the affected signal the maskee. Because masking plays an important role in some aspects of clinical audiology, it is discussed in detail in subsequent chapters of this book.

SUMMARY

Sound may be regarded objectively if we consider its waves in terms of their frequency, intensity, phase, and spectrum. Sounds may also be studied subjectively in terms of pitch, loudness, or the interactions of signals producing masking or localization. In discussing sounds it is always important to specify

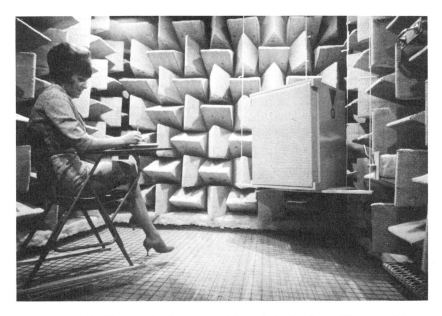

Figure 2.28 Photograph of a commercial anechoic chamber. (Courtesy of Industrial Acoustics Company, Inc.)

precisely their various aspects and appropriate measurement references, such as Hertz, decibels (IL, SPL, HL, or SL), mels, sones, or phons.

GLOSSARY

Amplitude The extent of the vibratory movement of a mass from its position of rest to that point furthest from the position of rest.

Anechoic chamber A specially built room with large wedges of sound-absorbing material on all walls, floor, and ceiling. The purpose of the room is to provide maximum sound absorption and to keep reverberation to an absolute minimum.

Aperiodic wave A waveform that does not repeat itself over time.

Artificial ear A device for calibrating air-conduction earphones. It consists of a 6 cm^3 coupler to connect an earphone to a condenser microphone with cathode follower and a meter that reads in dB SPL.

Artificial mastoid A device for calibrating bone-conduction vibrators. It consists of a resilient surface that simulates the vibrating properties of the mastoid process of the skull and an accelerometer. It is connected to a meter that reads in either decibels or units of force.

Beats Periodic variations of the amplitude of a tone when a second tone of slightly different frequency is superimposed.

Bel A unit for expressing ratios in base 10 logarithms.

Brownian motion The constant colliding movement of molecules in a medium.

Cancellation The reduction of the amplitude of a sound wave to zero. This results when two tones of the same frequency and amplitude are introduced 180 degrees out of phase.

Complex wave A sound wave made up of a number of different waves, each having unique frequencies.

Component A pure-tone constituent of a complex wave.

Compression That portion of a sound wave where the molecules of the medium become compressed together.

Cosine wave A sound wave representing simple harmonic motion that begins at 90 (or 270) degrees.

Cycle The complete sequence of events of a single sine wave through 360 degrees.

Damping Progressive diminution in the amplitude of a vibrating body. Systems are said to be heavily damped when the amplitude decays rapidly, lightly damped when the amplitude decays slowly over time, and critically damped if all vibration ceases before the completion of one cycle.

Decibel (dB) A unit for expressing the ratio between two sound pressures or two sound powers. One-tenth of a Bel.

Difference tone The perceived pitch of a tone resulting from the simultaneous presentation of two tones of different frequencies. The tone perceived has a frequency equal to the difference in Hz between the other two tones.

Dyne (d) A unit of force just sufficient to

accelerate a mass of 1 gram at 1 cm/sec^2.

Elasticity The ability of a mass to return to its natural shape.

Erg (e) A unit of work. One erg results when 1 dyne force displaces an object by 1 centimeter.

Exponent A logarithm.

Force The impetus required to institute or alter the velocity of a body.

Forced vibration The vibration of a mass controlled and maintained by an external force.

Formant A concentration of energy in the spectrum of a vowel sound.

Fourier analysis The mathematical breakdown of any complex wave into its component parts, consisting of simple sinusoids of different frequencies.

Free field An acoustic environment with no reverberating surfaces.

Free vibration The vibration of a mass independent of any external force.

Frequency The number of complete oscillations of a vibrating body per unit of time. In acoustics the unit of measurement is cps or Hz.

Fundamental frequency The lowest frequency of vibration in a complex wave.

Harmonic Any whole-number multiple of the fundamental frequency of a complex wave. The fundamental frequency equals the first harmonic.

Hearing level (HL) The number of decibels above an average normal threshold for a given signal. The hearing-level dial of an audiometer is calibrated in dB HL.

Hertz (Hz)   Cycles per second (cps).

Impedance   The opposition to sound-wave transmission. It comprises frictional resistance, mass, and stiffness, and is influenced by frequency.

Intensity   The amount of sound energy per unit area.

Intensity level (IL)   An expression of the power of a sound per unit area. The reference level in decibels is 10^{-12} watt/m^2.

Inverse square law   The intensity of a sound decreases as a function of the square of the distance from the source.

Joule (J)   The work obtained when a force of 1 Newton displaces an object 1 meter. (One J is equal to 10 million ergs.)

Kinetic energy   The energy of a mass that results from its motion.

Localization   The ability of an animal to determine the specific location of a sound source.

Logarithm   The exponent that tells the power to which a number is raised. The number of times that a number (the base) is multiplied by itself.

Longitudinal wave   A wave in which the particles of the medium move along the same axis as the wave.

Loudness   The subjective impression of the power of a sound. The unit of measurement is the sone.

Loudness level   The intensity above the reference level for a 1000 Hz tone that is subjectively equal in loudness. The unit of measurement is the phon.

Masking   The process by which the threshold of a sound (maskee) is elevated by the simultaneous introduction of another sound (masker).

Mel   A unit of pitch measurement. One thousand mels is the pitch of a 1000 Hz tone at 40 dB SL. Two thousand mels is the subjective pitch exactly double 1000 mels, and so on.

Microbar   A pressure equal to one-millionth of standard atmospheric pressure. (One μ bar equals 1 dyne/cm^2.)

Newton (N)   The force required to give a 1 kg mass an acceleration of 1 m/sec^2. (One N equals 100,000 dynes.)

Octave   The difference between two tones separated by a frequency ratio of 2:1.

Ohm   One acoustic ohm of impedance is the opposition to a sound when a pressure of 1 microbar produces a volume velocity of 1 cubic cm/sec.

Oscillation   The back-and-forth movement of a vibrating body.

Overtone   Any whole-number multiple of the fundamental frequency of a complex wave. It differs from the harmonic only in the numbering used (e.g., the first overtone is equal to the second harmonic, etc.).

Pascal (Pa)   A unit of pressure equal to 1 N/m^2.

Period   The duration (in seconds) of one cycle of vibration. The period is the reciprocal of frequency (e.g., the period of a 1000 Hz tone is 1/1000 second).

Periodic wave   A waveform that repeats itself over time.

Phase   The relationship in time between two or more waves.

Phon   The unit of loudness level. It corresponds to the loudness of a signal at other frequencies equal to the intensity at numbers of points along the scale of a 1000 Hz tone.

Pitch The subjective impression of the highness or lowness of a sound.

Potential energy Energy resulting from a fixed and relative position, as a coiled spring.

Power The rate at which work is done. Units of measurement are watts or ergs per second.

Pressure Force over an area of surface.

Pure tone A tone of only one frequency (i.e., no harmonics).

Quality The sharpness of resonance of a sound system. The vividness or identifying characteristics of a sound. The subjective counterpart of spectrum. (Synonyn: *timbre*.)

Rarefaction That portion of a sound wave where the molecules become less dense.

Ratio The mathematical result of a quantity divided by another quantity of the same kind, often expressed as a fraction.

Reactance The contributions of mass, stiffness, and frequency to impedance.

Resistance The opposition to a force.

Resonance The ability of a mass to vibrate at a particular frequency with a minimum application of external force.

Resonant frequency The frequency at which a mass vibrates with the least amount of external force. The natural frequency of vibration of a mass.

Reverberation A short-term echo or the continuation of a sound in a closed area after the source has stopped vibrating. This results from reflection and refraction of sound waves.

Sensation level (SL) The number of decibels above the hearing threshold of a given subject for a given signal.

Sinusoid or sine waves The waveform of a pure tone showing simple harmonic motion.

Sone The unit of loudness measurement. One sone equals the loudness of a 1000 Hz tone at 40 dB SL.

Sound-level meter A device designed for measurement of the intensity of sound waves in air. It consists of a microphone, an amplifier, a frequency weighting circuit, and a meter calibrated in decibels with a reference of 20 μPa.

Sound-pressure level (SPL) An expression of the pressure of a sound. The reference level in decibels is 20 μPa.

Spectrum The sum of the components of a complex wave.

Stiffness (acoustic) The quantity that, when divided by $2\pi f$ (frequency), yields compliant reactance.

Threshold In audiology, the least audible sound-pressure level. Often defined operationally as the level of a sound at which it can be heard by an individual 50% of the time.

Transverse wave A wave in which the motion of the molecules of the medium is perpendicular to the direction of the wave.

Velocity The speed of a sound wave in a given direction.

Vibration The to-and-fro movements of a mass. In a free vibration the mass is displaced from its position of rest and allowed to oscillate without outside influence. In a forced vibration the mass is moved back and forth by applying an external force.

Watt   A unit of power.

Wave   A series of moving impulses set up by a vibration.

Wavelength   The distance between the exact same point (in degrees) on two successive cycles of a tone.

Work   Energy expended by displacement of a mass.   The unit of measurement is the erg or joule.

STUDY QUESTIONS

1. What is wrong with the statement, "The signal has a loudness of 40 dB"?   *amplitude*

2. Why may two complex waves with components of identical frequency have different waveforms?

3. What determines the frequency of vibration of a mass?

4. List ten units of measurement. Describe what they measure and their references when applicable.

5. Give examples of periodic and aperiodic sounds.

6. Explain why two sounds with SPLs of 60 dB each do not total 120 dB when presented simultaneously. What is the total SPL and why?

7. How is an audiometer-level calibration accomplished for air conduction, bone conduction, speech, sound field?

8. Define the threshold of a sound.

9. What is the number of dB IL with a power output of 10^{-1} watt/m^2? What is the number of dB SPL with a pressure output of 2×10^4 μPa? Check your answers in Table 2.1, and generate more problems if you did not answer these correctly.

10. List the factors that contribute to acoustic impedance.

REVIEW TABLE 2.1 COMMON UNITS OF MEASUREMENT IN ACOUSTICS

MEASUREMENT	UNIT		ABBREVIATION		EQUIVALENTS
	CGS	SI	CGS	SI	
Length	centimeter	meter	cm	m	1 cm = 0.01 m 1 m = 100 cm
Mass	gram	kilogram	g	kg	1 g = 0.001 kg 1 kg = 1000 g
Area	square centimeter	square meter	cm²	m²	1 cm² = 0.0001 m² 1 m = 10,000 cm²
Work	erg	joule	e	J	1 e = 0.0000001 1 J = 10,000,000 e
Power	ergs per second watts	joules per second watts	e/sec w	J/sec w	1 e/sec = 0.0000001 J/sec 1 J/sec = 10,000,000 e/sec 1 w = 1 J/sec 1 w = 10,000,000 e/sec
Force	dyne	Newton	dyn	N	1 dyn = 0.00001 N 1 N = 100,000 dyn
Intensity	watts per square centimeter	watts per square meter	w/cm²	w/m²	1 w/cm² = 10,000 w/m² 1 w/m² = 0.0001 w/cm²
Pressure	dynes per square centimeter	*Newtons per square meter Pascal	dyn/cm²	N/m² Pa	1 dyn/cm² = 0.1 Pa 1 Pa = 10 dyn/cm² 1 Pa = 1 N/m²
Speed (Velocity)	centimeters per second	meters per second	cm/sec	m/sec	1 cm/sec = 0.01 m/sec 1 m/sec = 100 cm/sec
Acceleration	centimeters per square second	meters per second squared	cm/sec²	m/sec²	1 cm/sec² = 0.01 m/sec² 1 m/sec² = 100 cm/sec²

*Related to but not strictly on the SI scale.

REVIEW TABLE 2.2 FACTORS CONTRIBUTING TO PSYCHOLOGICAL PERCEPTIONS OF SOUND

PHYSICAL FACTORS		
Percept	*Prime Determinant*	*Other Determinants*
Pitch	Frequency	Intensity
Loudness	Intensity	Frequency, duration
Quality	Spectrum	
Protensity	Duration	Intensity

REVIEW TABLE 2.3 Psychological Measurements of Sound

MEASUREMENT	UNIT	REFERENCE	PHYSICAL CORRELATE
Pitch	Mel	1000 mels (1000 Hz at 40 dB SL)	Frequency
Loudness	Sone	1 sone (1000 Hz at 40 dB SL)	Intensity
Loudness level	Phon	0 phons (corresponding to threshold at 1000 Hz)	Intensity
Quality			Spectrum

REVIEW TABLE 2.4 Physical Measurements of Sound

MEASUREMENT	UNIT	REFERENCE	FORMULA	PSYCHOLOGICAL CORRELATE
Frequency	cps (Hz)			Pitch
Intensity level	dB IL	10^{-16} watt/cm² (CGS) 10^{-12} watt/m² (SI)	$NdB = 10 \log I_O I_R$	Loudness
Sound-pressure level	dB SPL	0.0002 dyne/cm² (CGS) 20 μPa (SI)	$NdB = 20 \log P_O P_R$	Loudness
Hearing level	dB HL	ANSI–1969	$NdB = 20 \log P_O/P_R$	Loudness
Sensation level	dB SL	Hearing threshold of subject	$NdB = 20 \log P_O/P_R$	Loudness
Impedance	Ohm (Z)		$Z = \sqrt{R^2 + \left(2\pi fM - \dfrac{S}{2\pi f}\right)^2}$	

REFERENCES

AMERICAN NATIONAL STANDARDS INSTITUTE. (1972). *Specifications for audiometers.* ANSI S3.6–1969. New York: Author.

———. (1972). *Artifical head-bone for the calibration of audiometer bone vibrators.* ANSI S3.13–1972. New York: Author.

———. (1977). *Criteria for permissible ambient noise during audiometric testing.* ANSI S3.1–1977. New York: Author.

———. (1981). *Reference equivalent threshold force levels for audiometric bone vibrators.* ANSI S3.26–1981. New York: Author.

———. (1951). *American standard specification for audiometers for general diagnostic purposes,* A24.5–1951. New York: Author.

BEASLEY, W. C. (1938). National Health Survey (1935–1936), preliminary reports. *Hearing Study Series Bulletin,* 1–7. Washington, DC: U.S. Public Health Service.

COX, J. R., JR., & BILGER, R. D. (1960). Suggestion relative to the standardization of loudness-balance data for the telephonics TDH–39 earphones. *Journal of the Acoustical Society of America, 32,* 1081–1082.

FLETCHER, H., & MUNSON, W. A. (1933). Loudness, its definition, measurement, and calculation. *Journal of the Acoustical Society of America, 5,* 82–107.

INTERNATIONAL ORGANIZATION FOR STANDARDIZATION. (1964). *Standard Reference Zero for the Calibration of Pure-Tone Audiometers.* ISO Recommendation R389. New York: American National Standards Institute.

SIVIAN, L. J., & WHITE, S. D. (1933). On minimum audible sound fields. *Journal of the Acoustical Society of America, 4,* 288–321.

THOMAS, W. G., PRESLAR, M. J., SUMMERS, R., & STEWART, J. L. (1969). Calibration and working condition of 100 audiometers. *Public Health Report, 84,* 311–327.

VAN BERGEIJK, W. A., PIERCE, J. R. & DAVID, E. E. (1960). *Waves and the ear.* New York: Doubleday.

WILBER, L. A. (1985). Calibration, puretone, speech and noise signals. In J. Katz (Ed.), *Handbook of clinical audiology* (pp. 116–150). Baltimore: Williams & Wilkins.

SUGGESTED READING

YOST, W. A., & NIELSEN, D. W. (1977). *Fundamentals of hearing: An introduction.* New York: Holt, Rinehart & Winston.

Part 2: Audiometry

[handwritten note: Schwabach — tuning fork test. Compares clients hearing by bone conduction w/ that of examiner. (for sensorineural)]

3

PURE-TONE AUDIOMETRY

[handwritten note: Rinne — tuning fork test. Compares hearing by air c. by bone conduction (for conductive)]

[handwritten margin note: look up from Ch1]

Pure-tone tests of hearing performed with an audiometer are electronic extensions of the same concepts developed in such tuning-fork tests as the Schwabach and Rinne. When such tests are carried out, the procedure is called *audiometry*. The main disadvantage of the tuning-fork tests is that they are difficult to quantify. That is, although the Schwabach might suggest sensorineural sensitivity that is poorer than normal, it does not tell how much poorer; although the Rinne might suggest the presence of a conductive component, it does not tell how large that component is.

The purpose of examining hearing is to aid in the process of making decisions regarding the type and extent of a patient's hearing loss. Because some of these decisions may have profound effects on the patient's medical, social, educational, and psychological status, accurate performance and careful interpretation of hearing tests are mandatory. The reliability of any test is based on interrelationships among such factors as calibration of equipment, test environment, patient performance, and examiner sophistication. In the final analysis, it is not *hearing* that we measure but, rather, *responses* to a set of acoustic signals that we interpret as representing hearing.

CHAPTER OBJECTIVES

Upon completion of this chapter, the reader should have a fundamental understanding of pure-tone audiometry and should understand the basic ingredients of a reliable audiogram and how different pure-tone tests are performed. The vocabularies obtained through reading chapters 1 and 2 are relied on extensively here, and the reader is exposed to new concepts and problems. Some of these problems can be solved; others can only be compensated for and understood. A basic understanding of this chapter should enable the reader to perform and interpret several pure-tone tests, assuming access to an audiometer in good working condition and the opportunity for supervised experience are provided.

def
pure tone - a tone of only 1 frequency - no harmonics.

THE PURE-TONE AUDIOMETER

Pure-tone **audiometers** have been in use for nearly a hundred years as devices for determining hearing thresholds, which are then compared to established norms at various frequencies. The original audiometers were electrically driven tuning forks that generated a number of pure tones of different frequencies. In later designs the tones were generated electrically. With the advent of the electronic era, audiometers incorporated vacuum tubes, then transistors, and then the integrated circuits of today. Like other commercial items, audiometers vary considerably in cost. ANSI specifications are imposed on all audiometers so that price differences should not reflect differences in quality of manufacture, although some manufacturers adhere more closely to minimum standards accepted by ANSI than do others. *American Nat'l Standards Institute*
(Pg34)

Kinds of Audiometers

→ Pure-Tone Audiometers ⟩

A common type of audiometer, which is sometimes portable, tests hearing sensitivity by **air conduction** and **bone conduction**. A switch allows for easy selection of pure tones. The testable frequencies for these audiometers usually include 125, 250, 500, 750, 1000, (1500,) 2000, 3000, 4000, 6000, and 8000 Hz. The range of intensities begins at −10 dB and goes to 110 dB HL at frequencies between 500 and 6000 Hz, with slightly lower maxima at 125, 250, and 8000 Hz. *know these*

record patient's threshold at each frequency

A matched pair of earphones is provided with threshold audiometers. An output switch directs the tone to either earphone. Usually only the range from 250 through 4000 Hz may be tested by bone conduction. The maximum testable hearing level for bone conduction is considerably lower than for air conduction, not exceeding 50 dB at 250 Hz and 70 or 80 dB at 500 Hz and above. Maximum outputs for bone conduction are lower than for air conduction, for several reasons. The power required to drive a bone-conduction vibrator is greater than for an air-conduction earphone. In addition, when the bone-conduction vibrator is driven at high intensities, harmonic distortion takes place, especially in the low frequencies.

In addition to air- and bone-conduction capability, a *masking* control is often provided that allows for introduction of a noise to the nontest ear as needed during audiometry. Often the masking noise is not of a specific spectrum and is not well calibrated for practical clinical purposes. Persons who rely solely on portable air- and bone-conduction audiometers are often unso-

Swschabach — SN
Rennie — Cond.
← know

Pure tone tests

type of loss

how much loss

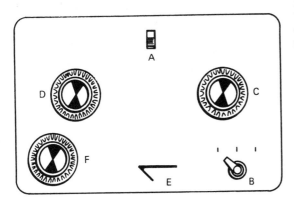

Figure 3.1 Typical face of a pure-tone audiometer (A) *On-off power switch.* (B) *Output selector switch.* Selects *Right Ear, Left Ear,* or *Bone Conduction.* Masking delivered to nontest earphone for air conduction and to left earphone for bone conduction. (C) *Frequency selector dial* Air conduction selects 125, 250, 500, 750, 1000, 1500, 2000, 3000, 4000, 6000, and 8000 Hz. Bone conduction selects 250, 500, 750, 1000, 1500, 2000, 3000, and 4000 Hz. (D) *Hearing-level dial.* Air conduction range: −10 to 110 dB (500 to 6000 Hz), −10 to 90 dB (250 to 8000 Hz). −10 to 80 dB (125 Hz). Bone-conduction range: −10 to 50 dB (250 Hz). −10 to 70 dB (500 Hz). −10 to 80 dB (750 to 4000 Hz). (E) *Tone-presentation bar.* Introduces tone with prescribed rise and fall time with no audible sound from the switch. (F) *Masking-level dial.* Controls intensity of masking noise in the nontest ear: Spectrum and intensity range vary with manufacturer.

phisticated about the need for and proper use of masking. Some pure-tone audiometers, however, contain excellent masking-noise generators and can be used for a variety of pure-tone audiometric procedures (Figure 3.1).

Automatic Audiometers > (Békésy)

Audiometers have been devised that allow a patient to track his or her own auditory threshold while it is automatically recorded in the form of a graph on a special form. The first such device was perfected by Reger (1952), based on the work of Békésy (1947). During automatic audiometry, patients hold a switch in their hands that they press whenever they hear a tone. The tone is automatically increased in intensity until the switch is pressed, whereupon it automatically decreases in intensity until the switch is released. In this way patients bracket their own hearing thresholds (Figure 3.2).

Some automatic audiometers are used extensively in screening programs. They provide pure tones at discrete frequencies for approximately 2 minutes each. The test is performed first in one ear and then in the other. The tones are automatically pulsed on and off to make them more recognizable. Such audiometers rarely test by bone conduction.

Other models of automatic audiometers provide a tone that is continuously variable in frequency, and they are capable of sweeping either up or down in frequency from 100 to 10,000 Hz, using either a continuous or automatically pulsed tone. The information provided with regard to the amount of hearing loss at each frequency is obviously much more detailed in continuously variable

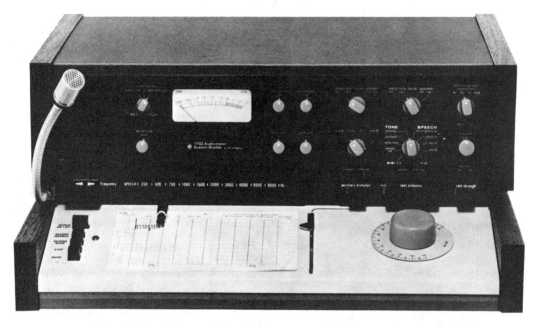

Figure 3.2 A commercial automatic audiometer. (Courtesy of Grason-Stadler Co.)

frequency audiometers than in discrete frequency audiometers. In addition, other valuable diagnostic audiometric information is available from automatic audiometry, which is discussed in Chapter 5.

TEST ENVIRONMENT

Table 2.3 shows the maximum ambient sound-pressure levels allowable for air-conduction and bone-conduction testing. Rooms in which such standards can be met are not readily available. This is true in the case of hearing test sites provided in industry or in the public schools. Regardless of the practical limitations imposed by a given situation, the person responsible for audiometric results must realize that background room noise may affect audiometric results by elevating auditory thresholds. There are three major ways in which ambient room noise may be attenuated: by using specially designed earphone enclosures, by testing through receivers that insert into the ear, and by constructing sound-treated chambers.

Earphone Attenuation Devices

A photograph of a commercial earphone enclosure device is shown in Figure 3.3. The standard audiometer earphone and cushion are mounted within the large cup, which fits over the ear. A fluid-filled cushion helps to achieve a tight seal against the head. Such enclosures are often quite effective.

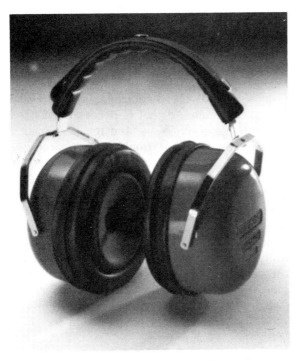

Figure 3.3 Commercial earphone enclosure device used to attenuate room noise during threshold audiometry. (Audiocups courtesy of American Overseas Trading Corporation.)

Problems with regard to **calibration** are encountered in the use of some earphone enclosures. The phones cannot be placed on the usual 6 cm³ coupler of an artificial ear. If the earphone is checked and found to be in proper calibration before it is mounted, mounting may alter the calibration slightly, especially in the low frequencies. Because bone-conduction testing is done with the ears uncovered, the masking effects of room noise may affect these test results without affecting the air-conduction results, possibly causing a misdiagnosis. Children often find these earphone devices heavy and uncomfortable.

Insert Earphones

Testing hearing with receivers that insert directly into the ear (Figure 2.17) has a number of advantages audiometrically. In addition, Clark and Roeser (1988) have shown that when the foam tips are placed into the ears, attenuation of background noise is increased over use of the standard earphone-cushion arrangement. If the foam is inserted deep into the ear, just short of causing discomfort, even more attenuation is obtained. It is desirable to have patients open and close their mouths three or four times to ensure proper seating of the cushion. Insert earphones can be used for testing children as well as adults. Problems with room noise masking remain unsolved for bone-conduction testing even if insert earphones are used for air conduction.

Sound-isolated Chambers

The term *soundproof room* is often used erroneously. Totally soundproofing a room is a formidable task indeed. All that is necessary in clinical audiometry is to keep the noise in the room below the level of masking that would cause a threshold shift in persons with normal hearing. Sound-isolated rooms may be specially constructed or purchased commercially.

The primary objective in sound treating a room is to isolate it acoustically from the rest of the building in which it is housed. This usually involves the use of mass (such as cinderblock), insulating materials (such as Fiberglas), and dead-air spaces. The door must be solid and must close with a tight acoustic seal. Sometimes two doors are used, one opening into the room and the other opening out. The inside walls are covered with soft materials, such as acoustic tile, to help absorb sound and limit reverberation. Some such chambers contain large wedge-shaped pieces of soft material, such as Fiberglas, on all walls, the ceiling, and the floor, with a catwalk provided for the subject. Rooms in which reverberation is markedly diminished are called anechoic chambers; an example of one such room is shown in Figure 2.28.

Audiometric suites may be designed for either one-room or two-room use. In the one-room arrangement, examiners, their equipment, and the patient are all seated in the same room. In the two-room arrangement, the examiner and audiometer are in the test room and the patient is in the examining room. Windows provide visual communication between the rooms. As a rule there are several panes of glass to attenuate the sounds that emanate from the test room. Moisture-absorbing materials must be placed between the panes of glass to keep the windows from fogging. Electrical connections between the rooms are necessary so that signals can be directed from the audiometer to the earphones. In addition, a talkback device consisting of a microphone, amplifier, and speaker and/or earphone enables the examiner to hear patients when they speak.

In customizing sound-isolated rooms, a great deal of attention is often paid to attenuating sound from adjoining spaces outside the walls of the room, but insufficient care is given to building-borne vibrations that may enter the room from floor or ceiling. It does little good to have 3 foot walls of solid concrete when footsteps can be heard from the floor above.

When sufficient space, money, and architectural know-how are available, custom sound rooms may be the proper choice. Contemporary audiology centers, however, seem to be leaning more toward the commercially prefabricated sound room, which is made of steel panels and can be more easily installed, with wiring included for two-room operation (Figure 3.4). Remember that the manufacturer does not guarantee the noise level within the sound room after installation, but guarantees only the amount of attenuation the room will provide. It is therefore necessary to prepare the room that will enclose

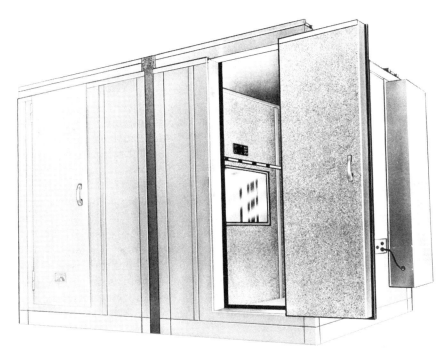

Figure 3.4 A commercial double-room sound-treated audiometric test chamber. (Courtesy of Tracoustics, Austin, Texas)

the prefabricated booth by making this area as quiet and nonreverberant as possible.

Prefabricated sound booths are available in one- and two-room suites. Windows with several panes of glass are installed to enable the examiner to observe the patient. The inside walls of the booth are constructed of perforated steel and filled with sound-absorbing materials. Some booths are double-walled; that is, there is one booth inside another larger one. Prefabricated booths are free-standing, touching none of the walls of the room in which they stand, and are isolated from the ceiling by air and from the floor by specially constructed sound rails.

One of the great weaknesses of audiometric rooms, whether custom or commercial, is their ventilation systems. Rooms that are to be tightly closed must have adequate air circulation, requiring the use of fans and motors. Sometimes the air-intake system is coupled directly with the heating and air-conditioning ducts of the building. In such cases care must be taken to minimize the introduction of noise via the ventilation system.

Lighting for both kinds of rooms should be incandescent, but if the use of fluorescent lighting cannot be avoided, the starters must be remotely mounted. Starters for fluorescent tubes often put out an annoying hum, which can be heard by the patient or picked up by the audiometer.

Patients seeking hearing tests vary a great deal in age, intelligence, education, motivation, and willingness to cooperate. The approach to testing will be very different for an adult than for a child, for a bright individual than for a retarded person, and for an interested person than for one who is frightened, shy, or even hostile. Procedures must also vary depending on the degree of the patient's spoken language. Test results are most easily obtained when a set of instructions can be given orally to a patient who then complies. As any experienced audiologist will testify, things do not go equally well with all patients.

In pure-tone audiometry, regardless of how the message is conveyed, patients must learn to accept their responsibility in the test if results are to be valid. Spoken instructions, written instructions, gestures, and/or demonstrations may be required. In any case, patients must become aware that they are to indicate when they hear a tone, even when that tone is very soft. The level at which tones are perceived as barely audible is the **threshold** of auditory sensitivity. The thresholds at different frequencies form the basis for pure-tone audiometry.

Patient Response

After patients understand the instructions and know what they are listening for they must be told some way of indicating that they have heard.

Some audiologists request that patients raise one hand when a tone is heard. They then lower the hand when they no longer hear the tone. Sometimes patients are asked to raise their right hands when they hear the tone in the right ear and their left hands when they hear the tone in the left ear. The hand signal is probably the most popular response system used in pure-tone audiometry. Many audiologists like this method because they can observe both how the patient responds and the hearing level that produces the response. Often, when the tone is close to threshold, patients will raise their hands more hesitatingly than when it is clearly audible. Problems occur with this response system when patients either forget to lower their hands or keep them partially elevated.

As with the hand signal, the patient may simply raise one index finger when the tone is heard and lower it when it is not heard. This system has the same advantages and disadvanatages as the hand-signal system. Also, it is sometimes difficult to see from an adjacent control room when the patient raises only a finger.

The patient may be given a signal button with instructions to press it when the tone is heard and release it when the tone goes off. Pressing the button illuminates a light on the control panel of the audiometer and/or sounds a buzzer. The use of signal buttons limits the kind of subjective information the audiologist may glean from observing hand or finger signals because the push-button is an all-or-none type of response. Use of the push-button technique does have the advantage of training the patient in this response method, which is mandatory in some of the special tests described in Chapter 5. Patient reaction time is sometimes another important drawback to push-button signaling, as some people may be slow in pushing and releasing the button. Often, if the button is tapped very lightly, the panel light may only flicker, and the response may be missed. Push-buttons are usually not a good idea for children or the physically handicapped, although they are standard equipment on many audiometers.

Some audiologists prefer a vocal response like "now" or "yes" or "I hear it" whenever the tone is heard. This procedure is often useful with children, although some patients have complained that their own voices "ring" in the earphones after each utterance, making tones close to threshold difficult to hear.

Play and other motivational techniques are often necessary when testing children or other difficult-to-test persons. Some of these methods are discussed in the chapter on pediatric audiology (Chapter 11).

False Responses

False responses are common during behavioral audiometry, and the alert clinician is always on guard for them because they can be misleading and can cause serious errors in the interpretation of test results.

A common kind of false response occurs when patients fail to indicate that they have heard a tone. Some patients may have misunderstood or forgotten their roles in the test. Such **false negative responses**, which tend to suggest that hearing is worse than it actually is, are also seen in patients who deliberately feign or exaggerate a hearing loss.

False positive responses, wherein the patient responds when no tone has been presented, are often more irritating to the clinician than are false negatives. Most patients will respond with some false positives if long silent periods occur in the test, especially if they are highly motivated to respond. When false positive responses obscure accurate test results, the clinician must slow down the test to watch for them, which encourages even more false positives. Sometimes even reinstruction to the patient fails to alleviate this vexing situation.

THE CLINICIAN'S ROLE IN MANUAL PURE-TONE AUDIOMETRY

As implied earlier, the first step in manual pure-tone testing is to make patients aware of their task in the procedure. If verbal instructions are given, they may be something like this:

You are going to hear a series of tones, first in one ear and then in the other. When you hear a tone, no matter how high or low in pitch and no matter how loud or soft, please signal that you have heard it. Raise your hand when you first hear the tone, and keep it up as long as you hear it. Put your hand down quickly when the tone goes away. Remember to signal every time you hear a tone. Are there any questions?

If a different response system is preferred, it may be substituted. There is an advantage to asking the patient to signal quickly to both the onset and the offset of the tone. This permits two responses to each presentation of the tone to be observed. If the patient responds to both the introduction and the discontinuation of the tone, the acceptance of false responses may be avoided.

There are some distinct advantages to providing written instructions to patients before they undergo a hearing evaluation. These instructions can be mailed to patients so that they can be read at home before patients arrive at the audiology clinic, or they can be provided when the patients check in with the receptionist, to be read while waiting to be seen by the audiologist. In addition to augmenting verbal instructions, printed instructions have the advantage that they can be retained for reference after the patient leaves the clinic, to help clarify what the different tests were intended to measure. Printed instructions should never be used to replace verbal instructions. A sample of patient instructions for the basic test battery may be found in Appendix I.

Patient Position During Testing

It is of paramount importance that the patient never be in a position to observe the clinician during pure-tone testing. Even small eye, hand, or arm movements on the clinician's part may cue patients into signaling that they have heard a tone when they have not. In one-room situations, patients should be seated so that they are at right angles to the audiometer (Figure 3.5). Some audiologists prefer to have the patient's back to the audiometer to eliminate any possibility of visual cues; however, this is disconcerting to some patients

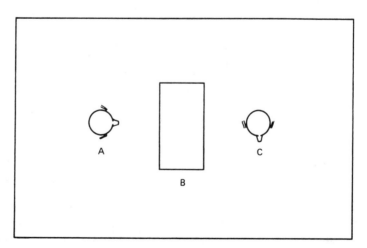

Figure 3.5 Proper positioning during pure-tone audiometry for (A) examiner, (B) audiometer, (C) patient.

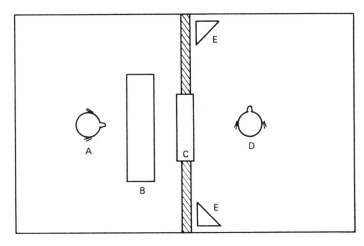

Figure 3.6 Proper positioning during pure-tone audiometry conducted in a two-room suite for (A) examiner, (B) audiometer, (C) window separating rooms, (D) patient, and (E) loudspeakers.

and eliminates observation of the patient's facial expression, which is often helpful to the audiologist in interpreting responses.

Even if the audiologist and patient are in different rooms, care must be taken to ensure that the patient cannot observe the clinician's movements. Figure 3.6 illustrates one satisfactory arrangement. Of course, the patient must always be clearly observable by the audiologist.

AIR-CONDUCTION AUDIOMETRY

The purpose of air-conduction audiometry is to specify the amount of a patient's hearing sensitivity at various frequencies. If a loss of hearing is present, air-conduction test results can specify the degree of loss but cannot indicate whether the deficit is produced by abnormality in the conductive mechanism, the sensorineural mechanism, or both.

Proper placement of earphones is shown in Figure 3.7. The headband should be placed directly over the top of the head. Eyeglasses should be removed when possible, as they sometimes lift the cushion of the earphone away from the ear and cause pressure on the temple bar of the eyeglass, which may be uncomfortable. Earrings should also be removed when possible.

Most earphone cushions are the hard rubber, supra-aural type, fitting tightly against the external ear. The phones should be positioned so that their diaphragms are aimed directly at the opening into the ear canal. The yokes that hold the phones may be pulled down so that the headset is in its most extended position. While the clinician is holding the phones against the ears, the size of the headset can be readjusted for a tight fit. All interfering hair should be pushed out of the way.

not what type of loss —

just if a loss exists (extent c. (extent) at what frequencies)

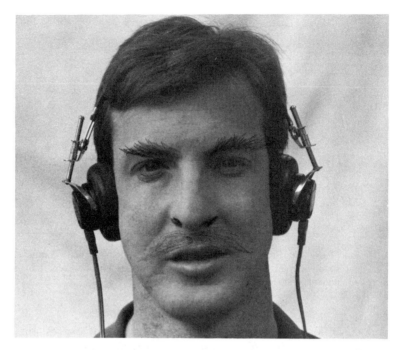

Figure 3.7 Properly placed air-conduction earphones.

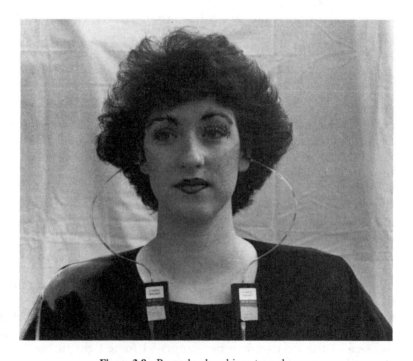

Figure 3.8 Properly placed insert earphones.

Some patients' outer ears collapse because of the pressure of the earphones. This creates an artificial conductive hearing loss, which usually shows poorer sensitivity in the higher frequencies and which can be misleading in diagnosis. When this occurs, or when the clinician suspects that it may occur because the ear seems particularly supple, certain steps can be taken to overcome the difficulty. One easy solution is to place a short length of plastic tubing in the ear; the canal may collapse around the tube, but the sound can still travel through it. A short length of strong thread should be placed through the tube and extended out of the ear for easy removal. Such placement must be made with the utmost care, of course, to avoid injury to the patient.

Insert receivers (Figure 2.17) may be used for air-conduction testing when collapsing ear canals are a potential problem. The foam insert must be compressed with the fingers and can be slipped into a small plastic sleeve to maintain this compression until insertion is made into the ear canal. After the insert is in place, the foam quickly expands and holds the device in place. The transducer itself is mounted at the end of a 250 mm plastic tube and may be clipped to the patient's clothing. As with standard phones, insert receivers are colored red and blue for testing the right and left ears, respectively. Properly placed insert earphones are shown in Figure 3.8.

Procedure for Air-Conduction Audiometry

The selection of which ear to test first is purely arbitrary. Although the American Speech-Language-Hearing Association, formerly the American Speech and Hearing Association, or ASHA recommends testing the better ear first, it cannot be proved that this has any real effect on test results. Likewise, frequency order probably does not affect results, although most audiologists prefer to test at 1000 Hz initially, test higher frequencies in ascending order, retest 1000 Hz, and then test lower frequencies in descending order (1000, 2000, 4000, 8000, 1000, 500, 250 Hz, etc.). Some audiologists feel that useful information is gained from the 125 Hz threshold; others believe that thresholds at this frequency can be predicted from the 250 Hz results. Some clinicians also prefer to test 6000 rather than 8000 Hz because of the calibration difficulties sometimes encountered at the higher frequency. Many audiologists only sample hearing at octave points, whereas still others prefer the detail resulting from testing the mid-octave frequencies (750, 1500, 3000, and 6000 H). In its guidelines for manual pure-tone audiometry, ASHA (1978) sensibly recommends that mid-octave points be tested when a difference of 20 dB or more is seen in the thresholds at adjacent octaves.

Over the years, a number of different procedures have been devised for determining pure-tone thresholds. Some audiologists have used automatically pulsing tones, and some have used manually pulsed tones. Some have used a descending technique whereby the tone is presented above threshold and lowered in intensity until patients signal that they can no longer hear the tone. Others have used an ascending approach, increasing the level of the tone from below threshold until a response is given. Still others have used a bracketing procedure to zero in on the threshold of a tone.

Carhart and Jerger (1959) investigated several pure-tone test procedures and found that there were no real differences in test results obtained with different methods. Nevertheless, they recommended that a particular procedure be followed, and this procedure appears to have been widely accepted.

The procedure recommended here, based on Carhart and Jerger's suggestion, is to begin testing at 1000 Hz because this frequency is easily heard by most people and has been said to have high test–retest reliability. In practice, it may be advisable in some cases to begin testing at other frequencies, perhaps lower ones, in cases of severe hearing loss in which no measurable hearing may be found at 1000 Hz and above.

Following the ASHA (1978) procedure, a pure tone is presented initially at 30 dB HL. If a response is obtained, this suggests that the 30 dB tone is above the patient's threshold. If no response is seen, the level is raised to 50 dB, and then raised in 10 dB steps until a response is obtained or the limit of the audiometer is reached for the test frequency.

After a response is obtained, the level is lowered in 10 dB steps. Each time a tone is introduced, it is maintained for one or two seconds. The hearing-level dial is never moved while the tone is in the *on* position, as a scratching sound may occur in the earphone, causing the patient to respond as if to a tone. All ascending movements of the hearing-level dial from this point are made in steps of 5 dB. When the tone is lowered below the patient's threshold, it is then raised in 5 dB steps until it is audible again, then lowered in 10 dB steps and raised in 5 dB steps until the 50% threshold response criterion has been met. The threshold is the lowest level at which the patient can correctly identify three out of a theoretical six tones. This usually, but not always, implies that a point 5 dB above this level will evoke more than 50% response. Levels accepted as threshold are often in the 75% to 100% response range.

As the thresholds are obtained at each frequency, they must be recorded on a data sheet. Some audiologists prefer to record the results directly onto a graph called an **audiogram**, using symbols to depict the threshold of each ear as a function of frequency and intensity (with reference to normal threshold). Others prefer to record their results numerically on a specially prepared score sheet. The form shown in Figure 3.9 has proved to be very useful, especially in the training of new clinicians. This form allows for recording the audiometric data numerically before plotting the graph. The form in Figure 3.9 allows for retest of 1000 Hz and, if necessary, retest of all frequencies. Accuracy criteria must be satisfied before the graph is drawn.

Any audiometric worksheet should have some minimal identifying information—the patient's name, age, and sex, as well as the date of examination, equipment used, and examiner's name. Some estimate of the test reliability should also be noted. After the air-conduction thresholds have been recorded, the average threshold levels for each ear at 500, 1000, and 2000 Hz should be recorded. This is called the **pure-tone average (PTA)**, and it is useful for predicting the threshold for speech as well as for establishing the degree of

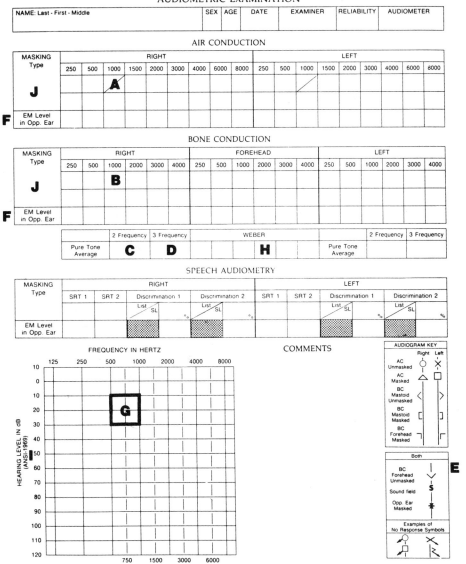

SPEECH AND HEARING CENTER
The University of Texas at Austin 78712
AUDIOMETRIC EXAMINATION

Figure 3.9 Example of an audiometric worksheet. Note the identifying information regarding the patient's name, sex, and age; examiner's name; date of examination; and description of the audiometer used. The following information is included on the worksheet: (A) air-conduction thresholds (recorded numerically); (B) bone-conduction thresholds (recorded numerically) for either the forehead or the mastoid; a second set of boxes is provided for repeated measurements of air-conduction or bone-conduction tests with opposite-ear masking, if that is necessary; (C) two-frequency pure-tone average (lowest two thresholds at 500, 1000, and 2000 Hz); (D) three frequency pure-tone average (500, 1000, and 2000 Hz); (E) symbols used for plotting the audiogram; (F) effective masking levels in the nontest ear used, when necessary, during air-conduction or bone-conduction tests; (G) a square to illustrate that the distance of one octave (across) is the same as 20 dB (down); (H) audiometric Weber results; (I) indication that the hearing levels are with reference to ANSI–1969 values; (J) type of noise used in asking for pure-tone tests.

TABLE 3.1 SCALE OF HEARING IMPAIRMENT BASED ON THE PURE-TONE AVERAGE AT 500, 1000, AND 2000 HZ*

PTA (dB)	DEGREE OF HANDICAP	CONSIDER HEARING AID	CONSIDER SPEECHREADING
~~-10-15~~ 10-25	None	No	No
~~16-25~~	Slight (Normal)	Possibly	Possibly
26-40	Mild	Probably	Probably
41-65	Moderate	Definitely	Definitely
66-95	Severe	Definitely	Definitely
>96	Profound	Definitely	Definitely

*Hearing levels are with reference to the ANSI (1969) scale.

[handwritten margin notes:]

0-25 in normal range says prof.

Know frequency threshold frequencies tested by — air & bone masking Bekesy (log) audiometry (automatic) reliability of test earphones background noise sound rooms (preparation) instructions for tests (how) (pure tone) E. finding threshold false neg. " pos. test rt ear 1st or better ear

handicap imposed by a hearing loss, although this can be misleading. Table 3.1 shows the degree of hearing impairment created by various degrees of sensitivity loss. Even though this table is based in part on the recommendations made by Stewart and Downs (1984) for children, it has applications for adults as well. The two-frequency pure-tone average (lowest two thresholds at 500, 1000, and 2000 Hz) may be recorded as well.

Many laypersons are accustomed to expressing degree of hearing impairment in percentage form because they are unfamiliar with the concepts of frequency, intensity, and the like. Many physicians also use the percentage concept, probably because it is easier for their patients to understand. Although percentage of hearing impairment is an outmoded concept, its continued use mandates mention here for the edification of the reader, but for practical application in the counseling of patients it is considered inappropriate and even misleading in many cases.

The weakness in the concept of percentage of hearing impairment is that it ignores audiometric configuration and looks only at the *average* hearing loss. The addition of 3000 Hz to the formula by the American Academy of Ophthalmology and Otolaryngology (AAOO) (1979) improves the situation somewhat. The formula, modified slightly from the description by Sataloff, Sataloff, and Vassallo (1980) works as follows:

1. Compute the average hearing loss (in decibels) from the threshold responses at 500, 1000, 2000, and 3000 Hz for each ear.
2. Subtract 25 dB—considered to be the lower limit of normal hearing by the AAOO.
3. Multiply the remaining number by 1.5% for each ear. This gives the percentage of hearing impairment for each ear.
4. Multiply the percentage of hearing impairment in the better ear by 5, add this figure to the percentage of hearing impairment in the poorer ear, and divide this total by 6. This gives the binaural (both ears) hearing impairment in percentage form.

Obviously, in addition to being somewhat misleading, the computation of percentage of hearing impairment is time-consuming. It is likely that patients are frequently confused by what they have been told about their hearing losses. For example, Table 3.1 indicates that a 25 dB pure-tone average constitutes a slight hearing impairment, but such a loss would prove to be 0% using the AAOO method, which would suggest to patients that their hearing is normal. Likewise, it can be seen that a 92 dB pure-tone average would be shown as 100% impairment, which would suggest total deafness to many laypersons. A 92 dB hearing level often proves to be considerable residual hearing in auditory rehabilitation.

When an audiogram is used, the graph should conform to specific dimensions. As Figure 3.9 illustrates, frequency (in Hz) is shown on the abscissa, and intensity (in dB HL) on the ordinate. The space horizontally for one octave should be the same as the space vertically for 20 dB, forming a perfect square (20 dB by one octave). Unlike most graphs, the audiogram is drawn with 0 at the top rather than the bottom. This is done so that as hearing thresholds get poorer, they are shown as being lower on the audiogram.

When a hearing threshold is obtained, a symbol is placed under the test frequency at a number corresponding to the hearing-level dial setting that represents threshold. The usual symbols for air conduction are a red circle representing the right ear and a blue X representing the left ear. After all the results are plotted on the audiogram, the symbols are usually connected using a solid red line for the right ear and a solid blue line for the left ear. When masking is used in the nontest ear, the symbol Δ (in red) is substituted for the right ear and the symbol □ (in blue) is used for the left ear. When no response is obtained at the highest output for the frequency being tested, the appropriate symbol is placed at the point on the intersection on the audiogram at the maximum testable level and the test frequency; an arrow pointing down indicates no response. ASHA (1974) has recommended a set of symbols that have been widely adopted. More recently, ASHA (1988) has proposed new symbols which are identical to the 1974 recommendations for air conduction and bone conduction, but slightly modify or add some other symbols. The currently used symbols are shown in Figure 3.10. The obvious reason for using standardized symbols is to improve communication and minimize confusion when audiograms are exchanged among different clinics.

Figure 3.11 shows an audiogram that illustrates normal hearing for both ears. Note that the normal audiometric contour is flat, because the normal threshold curve has been compensated for in calibration of the audiometer.

BONE-CONDUCTION AUDIOMETRY

The purpose of measuring hearing by bone conduction is to determine the patient's sensorineural sensitivity. The descriptions offered in Chapter 1 were very much oversimplified, as bone conduction is an extremely complex phe-

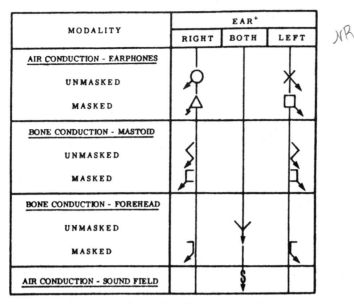

NR

+ The fine vertical lines represent the vertical axis of an audiogram.

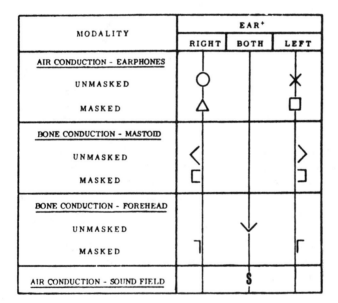

on test!

Figure 3.10 Symbols recommended by the American Speech, Language, and Hearing Association (1974) for use in pure-tone audiometry.

nomenon. Actually, hearing by bone conduction arises from an interaction of at least three different phenomena.

When the skull is set into vibration, as by a bone-conduction vibrator or a tuning fork, the bones of the skull become distorted, resulting in distortion of the structures of hearing in the inner ear. This distortion activates portions of the inner ear and gives rise to electrochemical activity that is identical to the

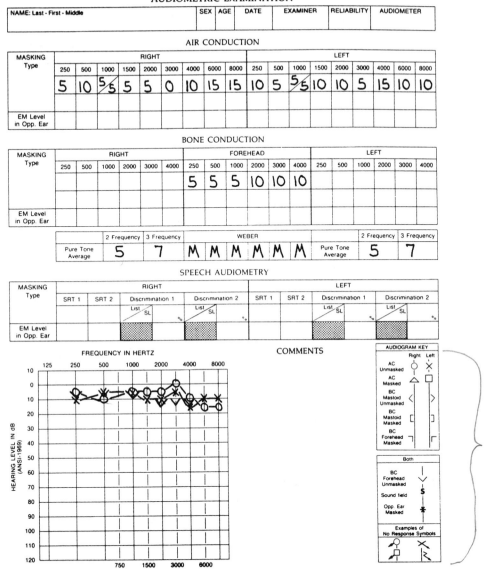

Figure 3.11 Audiogram illustrating normal hearing for both ears. Note that no hearing level by either air conduction or bone conduction exceeds 15 dBHL.

activity created by an air-conduction signal. This is called **distortional bone conduction**. While the skull is moving, the chain of tiny bones in the middle ear, owing to its inertia, lags behind so that the third bone, the stapes, moves in and out of an oval-shaped window into the inner ear. Activity is generated within the inner ear as in air-conduction stimulation. This mode of inner-ear stimulation is appropriately called **inertial bone conduction**. Simultaneously, oscillation of the skull causes vibration of the column of air in the outer-ear canal. Some of these vibrations pass out of the ear, while others go further down the canal, vibrating the eardrum membrane and following the same sound route as air conduction. This third mode is called **osseotympanic bone conduction**. Hearing by bone conduction results from an interaction of these three ways of stimulating the inner ear.

For many years the prominent bone behind the ear (the mastoid process) has been the place on the head from which bone-conduction measurements have been made. This place was probably chosen for two reasons: (1) because bone-conducted tones are loudest from the mastoid in normal-hearing persons and (2) because this site is close to the ear being tested. That the bone-conducted tone is loudest from behind the ear is probably because the chain of middle-ear bones is driven on a direct axis, taking maximum advantage of its hinged action. The notion that placing a vibrator behind the right ear results in stimulation of only the right inner ear is false, because vibration of the skull from any location results in approximately equal acoustic stimulation of both inner ears (Figure 3.12).

It has been demonstrated (Studebaker, 1962) that the forehead is in many ways superior to the mastoid process for measurement of clinical bone-conduction thresholds. Variations produced by vibrator-to-skull pressure, ar-

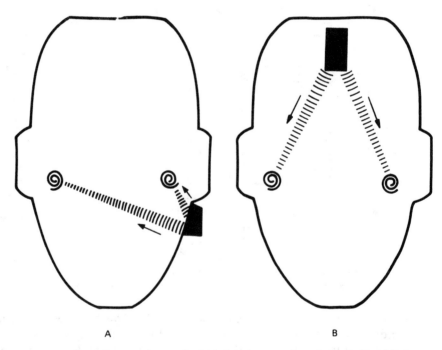

A   B

Figure 3.12 Vibrations of the skull result in bone-conducted stimulation of both inner ears, whether the vibrator is placed on (A) the mastoid or (B) the forehead.

tifacts produced by abnormalities of the sound-conducting mechanism of the middle ear, test–retest differences, and so on are all of smaller consequence when testing from the forehead than from the mastoid. The main disadvantage of testing from the forehead is that about 10 dB greater intensity is required to stimulate normal threshold, resulting in a decrease of the maximum level at which testing can be carried out. Although bone-conduction testing should sometimes be done from both the forehead and the mastoid, the forehead is recommended here for routine audiometry. Despite negative reports on mastoid test accuracy and other problems that go back many years (Barany, 1938), a national survey (Martin & Sides, 1985) shows that the mastoid process continues to be the preferred bone-conduction vibrator site among audiologists.

When the mastoid is the place of measurement, a steel headband crosses the top of the head (Figure 3.13A). If testing is to be done from the forehead, the bone-conduction vibrator should be affixed to the center line of the skull, just above the eyebrow line. A plastic strap encircles the head, holding the vibrator in place (Figure 3.13B). All interfering hair must be pushed out of the way, and the concave side of the vibrator must be placed against the skull.

Both ears must be uncovered during routine bone-conduction audiometry. When normal ears and those with sensorineural impairments are covered by earphones or occluded by other devices, there is an increase in the intensity of sound delivered by a bone-conduction vibrator to the inner ear, which occurs partly because of changes in osseotympanic bone conduction. This phenomenon, called the **occlusion effect (OE)**, occurs at frequencies of 1000 Hz and below. The occlusion effect is rare in patients with conductive hearing losses (e.g., problems in the middle ear) because the increase in sound pressure created by the occlusion is attenuated by the hearing loss. The occlusion effect (Table 3.2) explains the results on the Bing tuning-fork test described in Chapter

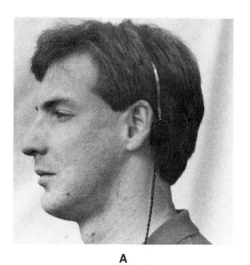
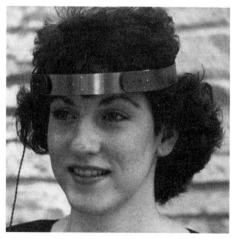

A   B

Figure 3.13 Bone-conduction vibrator placement on (A) the mastoid process and (B) the forehead.

TABLE 3.2 OCCLUSION EFFECT IN BONE CONDUCTION PRODUCED
WHEN A STANDARD EARPHONE-CUSHION ARRANGEMENT
(TDH−39 EARPHONE IN MX/41−AR CUSHION) IS PLACED
OVER THE EAR DURING BONE-CONDUCTION TESTS*

Frequency (Hz)	250	500	1000	2000	4000
Occlusion effect (dB)	30	20	10	0	0

*The amounts shown indicate central tendencies, and the range of occlusion
effects may be considerable. (Elpern & Naunton, 1963.)

1. Because there is a considerable amount of intrasubject variability in occluded
bone conduction, calibration difficulties have encouraged most audiologists to
prefer testing in the unoccluded state.

Procedure for Bone-Conduction Audiometry

The decision of which ear to test first in bone-conduction audiometry is
unimportant. As a matter of fact, as is illustrated in Figure 3.12, clinicians
really cannot be certain which inner ear they are testing. This is true regardless
of whether the mastoid or the forehead is the vibrator placement site. The
procedure for actual testing is identical to that for air conduction, although the
range of frequencies to be tested and the maximum intensities are more limited
for bone conduction than for air conduction.

Bone-conduction thresholds may be recorded in identical fashion to those
for air conduction, using the appropriate spaces on the audiometric worksheet.
Interpreting bone-conduction results from an audiogram is sometimes confusing, even though all audiograms should contain a key that tells the reader the
symbols used and what they represent. An arrowhead in red pointing to the
reader's left < is used for the right ear and in blue pointing to the reader's
right > for the left ear. If the printed page is viewed as the patient's face
looking at the reader, the symbols for right and left appear logical. When
masking is used in the opposite ear, the symbols are changed to square brackets,
[in red for the right ear and] in blue for the left ear. The symbol for forehead
bone conductions is ∨ when no masking is used and ⌐ (red) for the right ear
and ⌐ (blue) for the left ear when masking is applied to the nontest ear. Note
from Figure 3.14 that the bone-conduction symbols, except for unmasked forehead, are placed to the side of the ordinate.

Some audiologists prefer to connect the bone-conduction symbols on the
audiogram using a dashed red line for the right ear and a dashed blue line for
the left ear. Others prefer not to connect the symbols at all. The latter is the
preference in this book. At times, a patient may give no response at the
maximum bone-conduction limits of the audiometer. When this occurs, the
appropriate symbol should be placed under the test frequency where that line
intersects the maximum testable level. An arrow pointing down indicates no

response at the level. Figure 3.11 shows the recording of results and plotting of an audiogram for a hypothetical normal-hearing individual.

AUDIOGRAM INTERPRETATION

Whether the audiometric results have been recorded as numbers or plotted on the graph, they are interpreted in the same way. Results must be looked at in terms of (1) the amount of hearing loss by air conduction (the hearing level) at each frequency; (2) the amount of hearing loss by bone conduction; and (3) the relationship between air-conduction and bone-conduction thresholds.

The audiometric results depicted in Figure 3.14 illustrate a conductive loss of hearing in both ears. There is approximately equal loss of sensitivity at each frequency by air conduction. Measurements obtained by bone conduction show normal hearing at all frequencies. Therefore, the air-conduction results show the loss of sensitivity (about 35 dB); the bone-conduction results show the amount of sensorineural impairment (none); and the difference between the air- and bone-conduction thresholds, which is called the **air–bone gap (ABG)**, shows the amount of conductive involvement (35 dB).

Figure 3.15 shows an audiogram similar to that in Figure 3.14; however, Figure 3.15 illustrates a bilateral sensorineural hearing loss. Again, the air-conduction results show the total amount of loss (35 dB), the bone-conduction results show the amount of sensorineural impairment (35 dB), and the air–bone gap (0 dB) shows no conductive involvement at all.

The results shown in Figure 3.16 suggest a typical mixed loss of hearing in both ears. In this case the total loss of sensitivity is much greater than in the previous two illustrations, as shown by the air-conduction thresholds (60 dB). Bone-conduction results show that there is some sensorineural involvement (35 dB). The air–bone gap shows a 25 dB conductive component.

Sometimes high-frequency tones radiate from the bone vibrator when near-maximum levels are presented by bone conduction. If the patient hears these signals by air conduction, the false impression of an air–bone gap may be made. Sensorineural hearing losses have been misdiagnosed as mixed losses in such cases.

Interpretation of the air–bone relationships can be stated as a formula that reads: The air-conduction (AC) threshold is equal to the bone-conduction (BC) threshold plus the air–bone gap (ABG). Using this formula, the four audiometric examples just cited would read:

Formula: AC = BC + ABG

Figure 3.11   5   =   5   +   0 (normal)

Figure 3.14 35   =   0   + 35 (conductive loss)

Figure 3.15 35   = 35   +   0 (sensorineural loss)

Figure 3.16 60   = 35   + 25 (mixed loss)

SPEECH AND HEARING CENTER
The University of Texas at Austin 78712
AUDIOMETRIC EXAMINATION

NAME: Last - First - Middle	SEX	AGE	DATE	EXAMINER	RELIABILITY	AUDIOMETER

AIR CONDUCTION

MASKING Type	RIGHT									LEFT								
	250	500	1000	1500	2000	3000	4000	6000	8000	250	500	1000	1500	2000	3000	4000	6000	8000
	40	30	40	40	35	35	40	45	45	35	30	40	35	35	45	40	45	50
EM Level in Opp. Ear																		

BONE CONDUCTION

MASKING Type	RIGHT						FOREHEAD						LEFT					
	250	500	1000	2000	3000	4000	250	500	1000	2000	3000	4000	250	500	1000	2000	3000	4000
NB	0	-5	5	0	5	10									0	-5	5	0	5	10
	0*	-5*	5*	0*	5*	10*									0*	-5*	5*	0*	5*	10*
EM Level in Opp. Ear	35	30	40	35	45	40							40	30	40	35	35	40

	2 Frequency	3 Frequency	WEBER							2 Frequency	3 Frequency
Pure Tone Average	33	35	M	M	M	M	M		Pure Tone Average	33	35

SPEECH AUDIOMETRY

MASKING Type	RIGHT				LEFT			
	SRT 1	SRT 2	Discrimination 1	Discrimination 2	SRT 1	SRT 2	Discrimination 1	Discrimination 2
			List / SL %	List / SL %			List / SL %	List / SL %
EM Level in Opp. Ear								

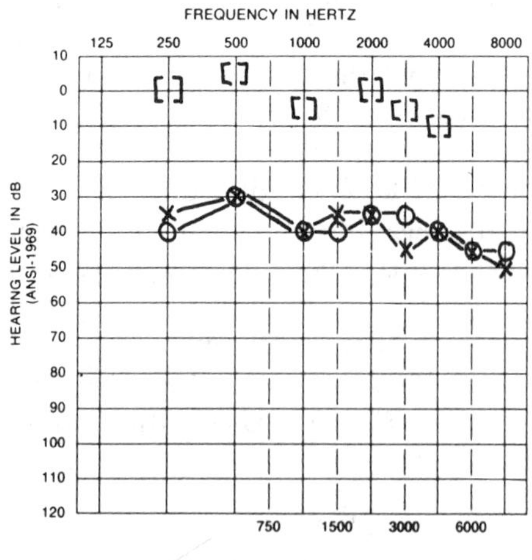

FREQUENCY IN HERTZ

COMMENTS

bone cond okay

air - hearing loss

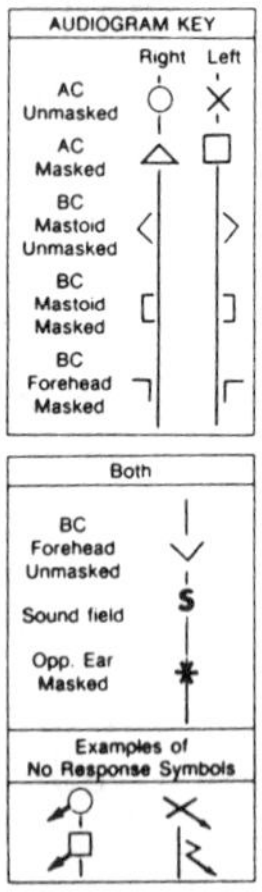

AUDIOGRAM KEY

Figure 3.14 Audiogram illustrating a conductive hearing loss in both ears. The air-conduction thresholds average 35 dB in each ear. Bone-conduction thresholds average 0 dB. There is an air–bone gap of 35 dB (conductive component) in both ears. Masking for bone conduction did not alter the original (unmasked) results. An asterisk is placed in a box denoting that opposite-ear masking was used when testing that frequency. No lateralization is seen on the Weber test at any frequency.

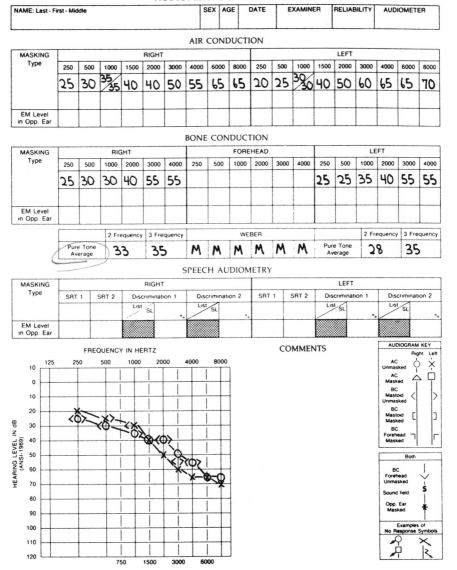

SPEECH AND HEARING CENTER
The University of Texas at Austin 78712
AUDIOMETRIC EXAMINATION

NAME: Last - First - Middle	SEX	AGE	DATE	EXAMINER	RELIABILITY	AUDIOMETER

AIR CONDUCTION

MASKING Type	RIGHT									LEFT								
	250	500	1000	1500	2000	3000	4000	6000	8000	250	500	1000	1500	2000	3000	4000	6000	8000
	25	30	35/35	40	40	50	55	65	65	20	25	30/30	40	50	60	65	65	70
EM Level in Opp. Ear																		

BONE CONDUCTION

MASKING Type	RIGHT						FOREHEAD						LEFT					
	250	500	1000	2000	3000	4000	250	500	1000	2000	3000	4000	250	500	1000	2000	3000	4000
	25	30	30	40	55	55							25	25	35	40	55	55
EM Level in Opp. Ear																		

		2 Frequency	3 Frequency	WEBER								2 Frequency	3 Frequency
Pure Tone Average		33	35	M	M	M	M	M	M	Pure Tone Average		28	35

SPEECH AUDIOMETRY

MASKING Type	RIGHT				LEFT			
	SRT 1	SRT 2	Discrimination 1	Discrimination 2	SRT 1	SRT 2	Discrimination 1	Discrimination 2
			List SL	List SL			List SL	List SL
EM Level in Opp. Ear								

FREQUENCY IN HERTZ

COMMENTS

AUDIOGRAM KEY

Figure 3.15 Audiogram illustrating sensorineural hearing loss in both ears. The air-conduction thresholds average 35 dB and the bone-conduction thresholds about the same (33 dB). Tones are heard in the midline at all frequencies on the Weber test.

NAME: Last - First - Middle	SEX	AGE	DATE	EXAMINER	RELIABILITY	AUDIOMETER

AIR CONDUCTION

MASKING Type	RIGHT									LEFT								
	250	500	1000	1500	2000	3000	4000	6000	8000	250	500	1000	1500	2000	3000	4000	6000	8000
	55	65	60/60	60	55	65	70	75	80	60	60	60/60	65	60	70	80	80	75
EM Level in Opp. Ear																		

BONE CONDUCTION

MASKING Type	RIGHT						FOREHEAD						LEFT					
	250	500	1000	2000	3000	4000	250	500	1000	2000	3000	4000	250	500	1000	2000	3000	4000
NB	25	35	35	35	40	45							25	35	35	35	40	45
	25*	35*	35*	35*	40*	45*							25*	35*	35*	35*	40*	45*
EM Level in Opp. Ear	60	60	60	60	70	80							55	65	60	55	65	70

	2 Frequency	3 Frequency	WEBER							2 Frequency	3 Frequency
Pure Tone Average	58	60	M	M	M	M	M	M	Pure Tone Average	60	60

SPEECH AUDIOMETRY

MASKING Type	RIGHT				LEFT			
	SRT 1	SRT 2	Discrimination 1	Discrimination 2	SRT 1	SRT 2	Discrimination 1	Discrimination 2
			List / SL	List / SL			List / SL	List / SL
EM Level in Opp. Ear								

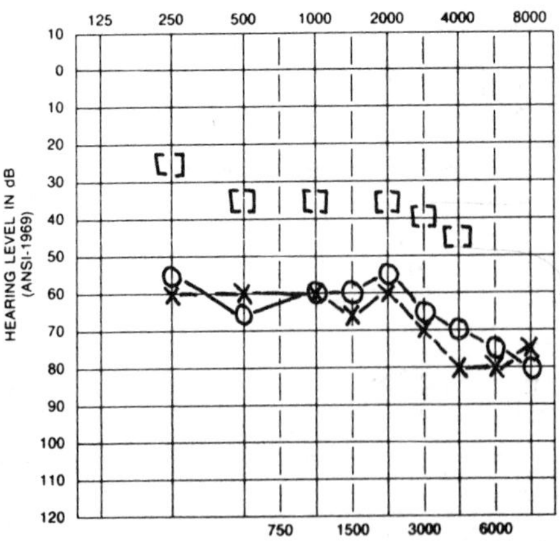

FREQUENCY IN HERTZ   COMMENTS

hearing loss · bone

hearing loss · air (worse)

Mixed below 25

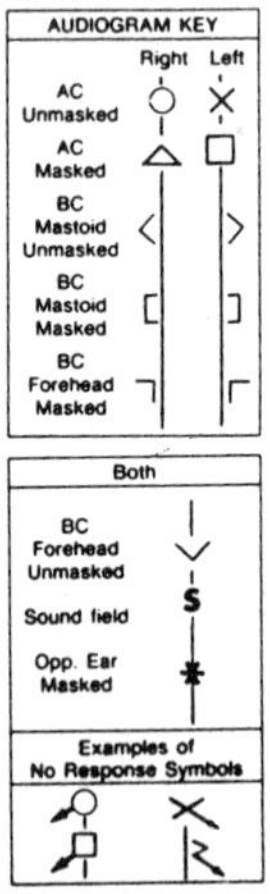

Figure 3.16 Audiogram illustrating a mixed-type hearing loss in both ears. The air-conduction thresholds average about 60 dB (total hearing loss), whereas the bone-conduction thresholds average 35 dB (sensorineural component). There is an air–bone gap of 25 dB (conductive component). Tones on the Weber Test do not lateralize.

Air–Bone Relationships

Figure 1.2 suggests that (1) hearing by bone conduction is the same as by air conduction in normal hearers and in those with sensorineural impairment (no air–bone gap); (2) hearing by air conduction is poorer than by bone conduction in patients with conductive or mixed hearing losses (some air–bone gap); but (3) hearing by bone conduction poorer than by air conduction should not occur, because both routes ultimately measure the integrity of the sensorineural structures. It has been shown that although assumptions 1 and 2 are correct, 3 may be false. There are several reasons why bone-conduction thresholds may be slightly poorer than air-conduction thresholds, even when properly calibrated audiometers are used. Some of these arise out of changes in the inertial and osseotympanic bone-conduction modes produced by abnormal conditions of the ears. In addition, Studebaker (1967b) has illustrated that slight variations are bound to occur based purely on normal statistical variability. Because no diagnostic significance is usually attached to air-conduction results' being better than those obtained by bone conduction, the insecure clinician may be tempted to alter the bone-conduction results to conform to the usual expectations. Such temptations are to be resisted because (in addition to any ethical reasons) they simply propagate the myth that air-conduction can never be better than bone-conduction.

Tactile Responses to Pure-Tone Stimuli

At times, when severe losses of hearing occur, it is not possible to know for certain whether responses obtained at the upper limits of the audiometer are auditory or **tactile**. Nober (1970) has shown that some patients feel the vibrations of the bone-conduction vibrator and respond when tones are introduced, causing the examiner to believe the patient has heard the tones. In such cases a severe sensorineural hearing loss may appear on the audiogram to be a mixed hearing loss, possibly resulting in unjustified surgery in an attempt to alleviate the conductive component. Martin and Wittich (1966) found that some children with severe hearing impairments often could not differentiate tactile from auditory sensations. Nober (1970) found that it is possible for patients to respond to tactile stimuli to both air- and bone-conducted tones, primarily in the low frequencies, when the levels are near the maximum outputs of the audiometer. When audiograms show severe mixed hearing losses, the validity of the test should be questioned and further tests, such as some of those described in Chapter 5, should be undertaken.

Cross-Hearing in Air- and Bone-Conduction Audiometry

It is logical to assume that if hearing sensitivity is considerably better in one ear than the other (say 50 dB) it is possible that before the threshold of the poorer ear is reached, the intensity of the signal may be great enough for the sound to escape from beneath the air-conduction earphone into the room and be heard by the better ear. Audiograms thus obtained have been called "shadow-grams." Sounds introduced by air conduction actually cross from one side of the head to the other primarily by means of bone conduction (Chaiklin, 1967; Martin & Blosser, 1970). It is probable that, whenever the intensity is raised to a high enough level, the air-conduction receiver vibrates sufficiently to cause deformations of the skull, giving rise to bone-conducted stimulation. If the level of a tone thus generated is above the bone-conduction threshold of the nontest ear during air-conduction audiometry, the patient will respond, signaling that the tone has been heard before the auditory threshold of the test ear has been reached.

As sounds travel from one side of the head to the other, a certain amount of energy is lost in transmission. This loss of intensity of a sound introduced to one ear and heard by the other is called **interaural attenuation (IA)**. Interaural attenuation for air conduction varies with frequency and from one individual to another. Results of two studies of interaural attenuation are shown in Table 3.3

The danger of **cross-hearing** for air-conducted tones presents itself whenever the level of the tone in the test ear (TE) by air conduction minus the interaural attenuation is equal to or higher than the bone-conduction threshold of the nontest ear (NTE). Stated as a formula:

$$AC_{TE} - IA \geq BC_{NTE}$$

Since it is not possible to know in advance the interaural attenuation of a given patient, it is advisable to adopt a conservative approach and consider 40 dB the minimum possible value.

Because there is rarely a way of knowing for certain which inner ear has been stimulated by a bone-conducted tone, regardless of where the vibrator is placed, cross-hearing during bone-conduction tests is always a possibility. Therefore, the minimum IA for bone conduction should be considered to be 0 dB. There are many approaches to this problem, only one of which is discussed in this book.

From a practical, clinical viewpoint, it seems important to ask, "Does it matter which ear has responded during pure-tone audiometry?" In the case of air conduction, the answer is an emphatic yes, for one must know for certain the hearing sensitivity of each ear. In the case of bone conduction, as illustrated in Figures 3.14 and 3.16, the answer is also yes, because the bone-conducted thresholds of each ear tell the amount of conductive involvement (by comparing

TABLE 3.3 INTERAURAL ATTENUATION FOR PURE TONES ACCORDING TO (A) COLES AND PRIEDE (1968) AND (B) ZWISLOCKI (1953)*

Frequency	250	500	1000	2000	4000
Interaural attenuation in dB (A)	61	63	63	63	68
Interaural attenuation in dB (B)	45	50	55	60	65

*The interaural attenuations shown are averages for the different frequencies. Interaural attenuations for individuals have been observed to be as low as 40 dB.

them to air conduction) and the amount of sensorineural involvement (by comparing them to 0 dB HL). If a bone-conduction response is obtained from the nontest ear, a completely incorrect diagnosis of the test ear may result. In the case of Figure 3.15, however, it really does not matter which ear has responded to the bone-conduction signal, because both ears show an absent air–bone gap, resulting in a diagnosis of bilateral sensorineural hearing loss. Therefore, cross-hearing in bone-conduction testing is of concern only when there is an air–bone gap in the test ear. Because there is a certain amount of normal variability between air- and bone-conduction thresholds, even among patients without conductive hearing losses, bone conduction often appears to be slightly better (or poorer) than air conduction. It seems practical, therefore, to consider an air–bone gap of 5 or 10 dB as insignificant. Thus, cross-hearing for bone conduction should be suspected whenever an air–bone gap greater than 10 dB is seen in the *test ear*:

$$ABG_{TE} > 10 \text{ dB}$$

MASKING

Whenever cross-hearing is suspected, it is necessary to remove the nontest ear from the test procedure to determine (1) if the original responses were obtained through the nontest ear and (2) when the original responses were obtained through the nontest ear, what is the true threshold of the test ear. The only way to do this is to deliver a noise to the nontest ear in order to remove it from the test procedure by **masking**.

The alert audiologist will probably suspect the possibility of cross-hearing more times than it actually occurs. This is good, for it is better to mask unnecessarily than to fail to mask when a signal has been heard in the nontest ear. In clinical audiology the rule should be, "When in doubt, mask."

As might be imagined, the relative effectiveness of a masking noise on a pure tone is determined by several variables, including the spectrum of the noise, how the masking-level dial is calibrated (that is, its decibel reference and the linearity of the dial), and the kind of earphone used to deliver the noise to the masked ear. When these variables are understood and controlled, the task of masking becomes considerably easier.

Noises Used in Pure-Tone Masking

Several different kinds of masking noises are available on commercial pure-tone audiometers. Each noise has a characteristic spectrum and therefore provides a different degree of masking efficiency at different frequencies.

Complex noise is often found in portable audiometers. It is relatively inexpensive to include and therefore keeps the price of the audiometer down. The noise is generated by a low-frequency pure tone with the harmonics present. There is usually less and less intensity as the harmonic frequencies increase, so that most of the masking is provided in the low frequencies. For a number of reasons, complex noise is not well accepted by audiologists as a good masker for pure tones.

It is possible to generate a noise that has approximately equal energy per cycle and covers a relatively broad range of frequencies. Because of its analogy to white light, which contains all the frequencies in the light spectrum, this noise has been called **white noise**. White noise sounds very much like a hissing sound and has also been called thermal and Gaussian noise. Since the earphones accompanying most audiometers are inexpensive, they do not provide much response in the higher frequencies and therefore limit the intensity of white noise above about 6000 Hz. Hence, that which is generated in the audiometer as white noise is more accurately termed *broad-band* or *wide-band* noise as it emanates from the earphone.

Pink noise has not been used much in masking for pure tones and is not available on commercial clinical audiometers. It provides a relatively broad spectrum with equal energy per octave below about 2000 Hz.

Because it has been proved that the masking of a pure tone is most efficiently accomplished by frequencies immediately surrounding that tone, the additional frequencies used in a broad-band noise are redundant. They supply additional sound pressure and loudness to the patient with no increase in masking effectiveness. Through the use of band-pass filters it is possible to shape the spectrum of a broad-band noise into **narrow-band noise**.

Surrounding every pure tone is a **critical band** of frequencies that provides maximum masking with minimum sound pressure. Narrowing the noise band to less than the critical band width requires greater intensity for masking a given level of tone. Conversely, adding frequencies outside the critical band increases intensity without increasing masking. Probably because of the expense of manufacture, the narrow noise bands found in most audiometers are usually considerably wider than the critical band.

The earphones usually employed to deliver a masking noise during clinical pure-tone testing are the ones provided with the audiometer, the TDH–39 or TDH–49 earphones with MX–41/AR (supra-aural) cushions. Some audiologists prefer to use earphones with circumaural (doughnut) cushions, which provide larger cavities, or smaller insert earphones. Because both these latter types of phones decrease the occlusion effect evident in bone conduction when an ear is covered, they have an advantage in masking during bone-conduction testing. In addition, because they are coupled to a smaller area of the skull, insert receivers provide 70 to 100 dB of interaural attenuation (Killion, Wilbur, & Dugmundsen, 1985), considerably more than the other two types.

Calibration of Pure-Tone Masking Noises

Calibration of the masking noise of an audiometer requires that the linearity of the masking-level dial be accurate and that the intensity reference be known.

Linearity calibration is best accomplished through the use of a device called an **electronic voltmeter**, which measures differences in decibels. By making measurements at the terminals of the earphones, the hearing-level dial can be moved in steps of 5 dB, and the accuracy of this 5 dB change can be checked throughout the entire range of the attenuator (-10 to 110 dB). At times, especially in the case of portable audiometers, the masking dial is so nonlinear that the appropriate corrections must be inscribed on the dial.

Some audiologists prefer that the decibel reference for masking be in SPL or HL. In recent years the concept of **effective masking (EM)** has become increasingly popular. Effective masking may be defined as the amount of threshold shift provided by a given level of noise. Thus, 20 dB EM at 1000 Hz is just enough noise to make a 20 dB HL 1000 Hz tone inaudible, 50 dB EM would just mask out a 50 dB tone, and so on. In the presence of 50 dB EM, a tone will not become audible until 55 dB HL, regardless of an individual's hearing loss (if it is less than 55 dB). This is true because any hearing loss attenuates both the tone and the masking noise equally.

The calibration of a noise in units of effective masking may be carried out electroacoustically on an artificial ear if the concept of the critical band is thoroughly understood. In many clinics this calibration is carried out psychoacoustically. Using about a dozen normal-hearing subjects, calibration for effective masking may be accomplished as follows:

1. Present a tone to one ear by air conduction at 1000 Hz at 30 dB HL. Interrupt to prevent auditory fatigue.
2. Present a noise (preferably narrow-band) to the same ear.
3. Raise the level of the noise in 5 dB steps until the 30 dB tone is no longer audible but the tone can be heard at 35 dB. Recheck several times for accuracy.
4. Take a median value of the masking-level dial setting at which the 30 dB tone was masked. This is 30 dB EM. Five to 10 dB may be added as a safety factor.
5. Post a correction chart showing the number of decibels that must be added to 0 dB HL to reach 0 dB EM.
6. Repeat this procedure for all audiometric frequencies.

Once calibration has been completed, any level at any frequency can be masked out (in the same ear) up to the maximum masking limits of the audiometer simply by introducing a level of effective masking equal to the level of the tone to be masked. If, for example, a $+25$ dB correction is needed for 0 dB EM, and a 40 dB tone is to be masked, the masking-level dial would be set to 65 dB HL (40 dB for the tone to be masked plus 25 dB correction).

Central Masking

It has been shown (Wegel & Lane, 1924) that a small shift is seen in the threshold of a pure tone when a masking noise is introduced to the opposite ear. This threshold shift increases with increased noise but averages about 5 dB. It is believed that the elevation of threshold is produced by inhibition that is sent down from the auditory centers in the brain and has, therefore, been called **central masking**. Central masking must be differentiated from **overmasking (OM)**, in which the noise is actually so intense in the masked ear that it crosses the skull and produces masking in the test ear.

Masking Methods for Air Conduction

Masking must be undertaken whenever the possibility of cross-hearing exists. A survey of clinical audiologists on contemporary clinical practices (Martin & Sides, 1985) showed more disagreement on masking methods and apparently greater insecurity than on any other clinical procedure.

The "Hit-or-Myth" Method. It is possible, in a large number of cases, for clinicians to mask using some fixed or arbitrary level of noise in the masked ear without really understanding what they are doing. In uncomplicated cases the procedure often appears to be satisfactory. Because of insufficient feedback about their errors, individuals performing hearing tests fail to profit by their mistakes and continue with such erroneous philosophies as, "Just use 70 dB of noise," with no recognition of the properties of the noise or of its effectiveness. Clinicians may be unaware of when they have used too little or too much masking noise. This ignorance is abetted by those audiometer manufacturers whose masking-level dials are nonlinear and whose noise spectra are irregular, inadvertently relegating the masking procedure to a relatively unimportant one.

The Minimum-Noise Method. Through calibration it is possible to determine the minimum amount of noise necessary to mask a pure tone. There is no need to burden the patient with any more noise than is necessary to get the job done. The best way to do this is to regard the masking in terms of decibels of effective masking.

Several methods have been developed using formulas for the determination of the minimum and maximum amounts of effective masking to be used (Liden, Nilsson, & Anderson, 1959; Studebaker, 1964). Although these formulas are accurate, they are time-consuming and not always practical for clinical use (Studebaker, 1967a). Martin (1974) has shown that the different formula approaches yield the same noise sound-pressure levels as does a simple, direct approach requiring almost no calculation. This book describes one method that does not require much computation and that can be applied rapidly.

When test results suggest the possibility of cross-hearing, they should be examined closely. Consider the example in Figure 3.17. The criteria for masking are met for the left ear by air conduction, since the threshold (60 dB) minus IA (40 dB) is greater than the bone-conduction threshold of the right ear (10 dB). It is known, since the test was presumably performed carefully, that the 60 dB response was a threshold. However, the question that arises is, "The threshold of which ear?" If the right (nontest) ear can be removed from the

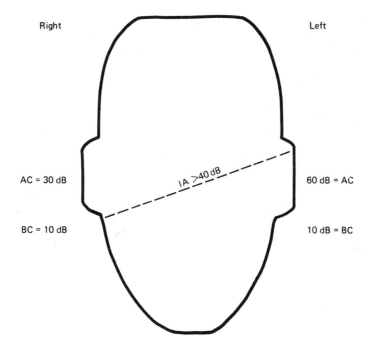

Right   **Left**

AC = 30 dB   IA ≥40 dB   60 dB = AC

BC = 10 dB   10 dB = BC

Figure 3.17 Illustration of the need to mask during air-conduction tests. Because the difference between the left-ear air conduction (10 dB) exceeds the minimum possible interaural attenuation (40 dB), cross-hearing is a possibility. Note that the minimum interaural attenuation for this patient must be 50 dB (AC left minus BC right). Masking needed for the right ear is 30 dB EM.

test by masking, and the threshold of the left (test) ear remains unchanged, this means that the original response was obtained through the test ear. If, on the other hand, eliminating the right ear from the test results in a failure of response at the left ear at the previous level, plus 5 dB for central masking, then the nontest ear provided the hearing for the original response, and further masking is required to determine the true threshold of the test ear.

The minimum amount of noise required for the screening described is an effective masking level equal to the threshold of the nontest ear and may be referred to as **initial masking (IM)**. This is just enough noise to shift the threshold of that ear 5 dB by both air conduction and bone conduction. If the threshold of the tone presented to the test ear was originally heard by bone conduction in the nontest ear, raising the bone-conduction threshold of the nontest ear with masking will eliminate the possibility of this response.

Maximum Masking. Just as the test tone can lateralize from test ear to nontest ear, given sufficient intensity, so can the masking noise lateralize from masked ear to test ear, both by bone conduction. A given individual's inter-aural attenuation cannot be less than the difference between the air-conduction level in the test ear and the bone-conduction level in the nontest ear at which threshold responses are obtained. For example, even though Figure 3.17 does not illustrate cross-hearing per se, but rather the danger of cross-hearing, the interaural attenuation for the individual illustrated cannot be less than 50 dB for the test frequency (air conduction of the test ear minus bone conduction of the opposite ear).

Whenever the level of effective masking presented to the masked ear, minus the patient's interaural attenuation, is above the bone-conduction threshold of the test ear, a sufficient amount of noise is delivered to the inner ear of the test ear to elevate its threshold. This is overmasking (OM) (Figure 3.18). The equation for overmasking for pure tones is:

$$EM_{NTE} \geq BC_{TE} + IA$$

Maximum masking is equal to the threshold of the test ear by bone conduction plus the interaural attenuation, minus 5 dB. When ears with large air–bone gaps are tested, minimum masking quickly becomes overmasking, sometimes making determination of masked pure-tone thresholds difficult. In such cases audiologists must recognize the problem and rely on other tests and observations to make their diagnoses.

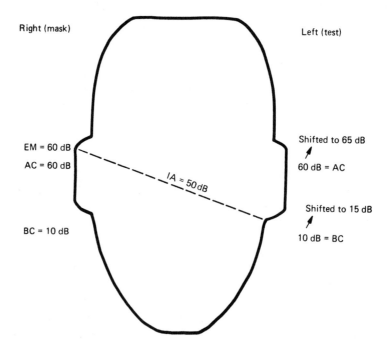

Figure 3.18 Example of overmasking. The effective masking level in the right ear (60 dB) is decreased by the interaural attenuation (50 dB) so that 10 dB EM is received by bone conduction in the left ear. This shifts the bone-conduction threshold to 15 dB, plus any additional shift for central masking. Adding more noise to the right ear results in increased masking at the left ear, with further threshold shifts. In this case the minimum amount of noise required to mask out the right ear produces overmasking.

The Plateau Method. Hood (1960) reported on a masking method that enjoys a great deal of popularity. When a tone seems to be heard through the nontest ear, a noise is delivered to that ear and the level of noise is increased in 5 dB steps until the tone is no longer audible. Then the threshold for the tone is measured again in the presence of the contralateral noise. The noise level is increased 5 dB and the threshold is measured again. This often results in necessary increases in the tone level of 5 dB for every 5 dB increase in noise in order to keep the tone audible. The assumption is that the threshold of the tone in the test ear has not been reached and that both tone and noise are heard by the nontest ear (Figure 3.19A). When the threshold of the tone for the test ear has been reached (Figure 3.19B), the level of noise can be increased several times without affecting the level of tone that evokes a response. This is the **plateau**. If the noise level is raised beyond a certain point (the bone-conduction threshold of the test ear plus the interaural attenuation), over-masking takes place and the tone and noise are mixed in the test ear. Further

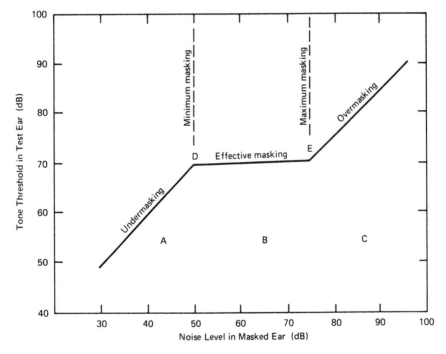

Figure 3.19 The plateau method for masking. (A) *Undermasking.* The tone (by cross-hearing) continues to be heard in the masked ear despite the noise, since the tone level is below the threshold of the test ear. (B) *The plateau.* The tone has reached the threshold of the test ear. Therefore, raising the masking level in the masked ear does not shift the threshold of the tone. (C) *Overmasking:* The masking level is so intense that it crosses to the test ear, resulting in continuous shifts in the threshold of the tone with increases in the masking noise. Minimum (D) and maximum (E) masking are found at either side of the plateau.

increases in noise will result in further shifts in the threshold of the tone (Figure 3.19C).

The plateau method is often used by introducing the noise at some low level or some arbitrary beginning point. It can be combined with the minimum masking method, beginning with the initial masking level (the air-conduction threshold of the masked ear). Problems of overmasking plague all the masking methods, including the plateau system, whenever large air–bone gaps exist in both ears. The larger the air–bone gap, the narrower the plateau, and the smaller the air–bone gap, the broader the plateau.

The width of the masking plateau is determined by three variables: (1) the air-conduction threshold of the nontest (masked) ear, (2) the bone-conduction threshold of the test ear, and (3) the interaural attenuation. The higher the air-conduction threshold of the masked ear, the greater must be the initial masking level; the higher that level is, the greater are the chances that the noise will cross to the test ear. The lower the bone-conduction threshold of the test ear, the greater is the likelihood that a noise, reaching that inner ear from a masking receiver on the opposite ear, will exceed its threshold, producing a threshold shift in the test ear. The smaller the interaural attenuation, the less is the attenuation of the noise and the greater are the chances that it will reach the nontest ear. By increasing interaural attenuation, insert receivers decrease the chances of overmasking and widen the masking plateau.

Martin (1980) has reduced the masking plateau for both air conduction and bone conduction to a series of models and formulas involving effective masking. Figure 3.20 shows (A) undermasking for air conduction, (B) undermasking for bone conduction, (C) minimum masking for air conduction, (D) minimum masking for bone conduction, (E) the plateau, (F) maximum masking (for air conduction and bone conduction), and (G) overmasking (for air conduction and bone conduction).

Masking Methods for Bone Conduction

Masking methods for bone conduction are very much the same as for air conduction, and their success depends on the training, interests, and motivation of the clinician. One problem in masking for bone conduction that does not arise for air conduction is the method for delivery of the masking noise. The matter is simple during air-conduction audiometry, as both ears have earphones already positioned, and one phone can deliver the tone while the other phone delivers the masking noise. Because both ears are uncovered during bone-conduction testing, an earphone must be placed over the nontest ear without covering the test ear. The test ear must not be covered because this may cause an occlusion effect and alter the zero reference for bone conduction. Figure 3.21 shows the proper positioning of standard receivers and insert for masking during bone conduction with the vibrator on the mastoid and also on the forehead.

When an earphone is placed over the nontest ear, an occlusion effect is usually created in that ear. This means that the intensity of the tone in the

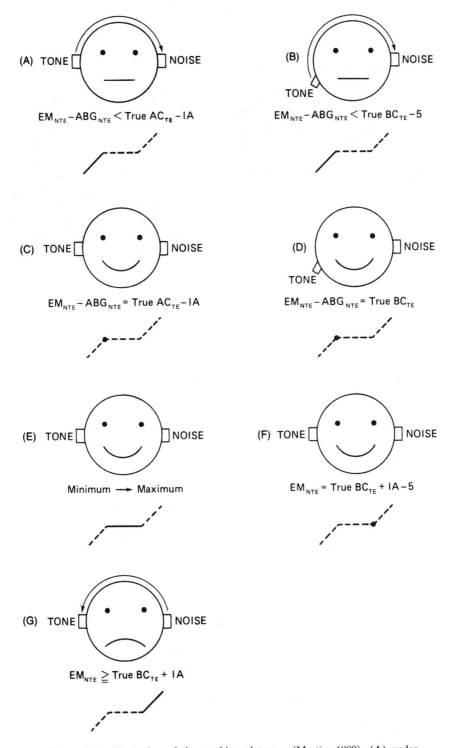

Figure 3.20 Illustration of the masking plateau. (Martin, 1980); (A) undermasking for air conduction; (B) undermasking for bone conduction; (C) minimum masking for air conduction; (D) minimum masking for bone conduction; (E) the plateau; (F) maximum masking (air and bone conduction); (G) overmasking (air and bone conduction).

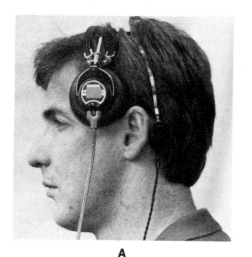 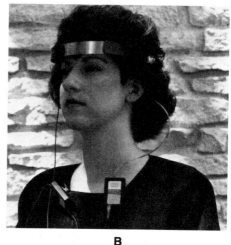

A **B**

Figure 3.21 Masking noise delivered to the nontest ear during bone-conduction audiometry performed from (A) the mastoid, using a standard earphone, and (B) the forehead, using an insert earphone.

low frequencies is actually increased in the nontest ear, increasing the likelihood that the nontest ear will respond to the tone. Of course, if the masked ear has a conductive hearing loss, no additional occlusion effect is evidenced, but it is not always possible to know whether or not a conductive loss exists in the masked ear. After all, if we knew the conditions of the auditory pathway before testing, the tests themselves would be unnecessary.

Because the masking earphone may make the bone-conducted tone appear louder in the masked ear, the initial effective masking level must be increased by the amount of the occlusion effect. Failure to do this will result in **under-masking** in a significant number of cases. The initial effective level for bone-conduction masking is the air-conduction threshold of the tone in the masked ear, plus the occlusion effect (OE) for the tested frequency. Initial masking for bone conduction can be expressed as:

$$EM = AC_{NTE} + OE$$

This increased amount of noise raises the chance of overmasking. In many cases it is advantageous to use insert receivers to deliver the masking noise because less noise needs to be delivered to offset the smaller occlusion effect. The increased interaural attenuation provided by these small phones decreases the probability of overmasking.

Martin, Butler, and Burns (1974) suggest a method by which the occlusion effect of the patient's masked ear may be determined and added to the initial masking level for air conduction. The procedure takes only moments and requires that, after the need to mask for bone conduction has been determined, an audiometric version of the Bing test be carried out. After the patient's unoccluded bone-conduction thresholds have been measured, the masking receiver is placed over the ear to be masked (no noise is presented). With the nontest ear occluded, the thresholds at 250, 500 and 1000 Hz are redetermined. The occluded thresholds for each frequency are substracted from the unoccluded thresholds. The difference is the patient's *own* occlusion effect. These differences may be added to the initial masking levels determined for air conduction. The bone-conduction vibrator may be placed either on the forehead or on the mastoid.

Use of the audiometric Bing test results in little or no additional masking for conductive losses where higher noise levels present the danger of overmasking. Where increased masking is required to offset the effect of having occluded the masked ear, the precise amount of noise may be added rather than some average figure that may be more or less masking than required for the individual patient.

The form shown in Figure 3.22 is useful for performing the audiometric Bing test. The results provide quantitative information about the amount of occlusion effect for each ear to be added to the initial effective masking level. In addition, the audiometric version can be interpreted in the same way as the original tuning-fork test to assist in the diagnosis of conductive versus sensorineural hearing loss.

SPEECH AND HEARING CENTER
THE UNIVERSITY OF TEXAS AT AUSTIN 78712

Name: Last-First-Middle	Sex	Age	Examiner	Reliability	Date

	AUDIOMETRIC BING TEST					
	RIGHT			LEFT		
Frequency (Hertz)	250	500	1000	250	500	1000
1) Unoccluded						
2) Occluded						
3) Occlusion Effect (1-2)						

Figure 3.22 Form for recording data obtained on the audiometric Bing test.

Plotting Masked Results on the Audiogram

Before any threshold data are entered on the audiometric worksheet for either air conduction or bone conduction, 5 dB may be subtracted from the values obtained with the nontest ear masked in order to compensate for central masking if a threshold shift of only 5 or 10 dB is seen. The appropriate symbols to indicate air conduction or bone conduction with and without masking are shown in the legend at the bottom of the audiogram. The graph should contain only symbols that represent accurate thresholds; otherwise the audiogram will be cluttered. The plotting of contralateral responses seems unnecessary, since they can readily be seen by examining the numerical insertions at the top of the audiometric worksheet.

Figure 3.23 illustrates a case of normal hearing in the right ear with a sensorineural hearing loss in the left ear. Note that the original test results suggested that the hearing loss in the left ear was conductive. The air–bone gap in the left ear was closed when proper masking was applied to the right ear.

The unmasked results shown in Figure 3.24 suggest a conductive loss in both ears, with poorer air conduction in the right ear. Using the criteria described earlier, masking was indicated for the right ear for air conduction and for both ears for bone conduction. Notice that the hearing loss in the left ear remains unchanged with masking, but the right ear actually has a severe mixed loss.

THE AUDIOMETRIC WEBER TEST

The Weber test, described in Chapter 1, can be accomplished using the bone-conduction vibrator of an audiometer. The vibrator is placed on the midline of the skull just as for forehead bone conduction, and the level of the tone is raised until it is above the patient's hearing threshold. Tones of different frequencies are then presented, and patients are asked to state whether they hear them in the left ear, in the right ear, or in the midline. Midline sensations are sometimes described as being heard in both ears or as unlateralized.

On the Weber test it is expected that tones will be referred to the poorer hearing ear in a conductive loss, to the better ear in a sensorineural loss, and to the midline in symmetrical losses. It has been suggested that the **audiometic Weber test** be used to determine which ear to mask during bone-conduction testing. This notion is not encouraged here, as there are several reasons that the Weber may be misleading. Weber results do help in the confirmation or denial of results obtained from standard pure-tone audiometry, and the probable results on this test are illustrated on all of the audiograms in this book.

AUDIOMETRIC EXAMINATION

NAME: Last - First - Middle	SEX	AGE	DATE	EXAMINER	RELIABILITY	AUDIOMETER

AIR CONDUCTION

MASKING Type	RIGHT									LEFT								
	250	500	1000	1500	2000	3000	4000	6000	8000	250	500	1000	1500	2000	3000	4000	6000	8000
NB	5	0	0/0	5	5	15	15	10	10	30	35	35/35	40	40	45	55	50	45
																55*		
EM Level in Opp. Ear																10		

BONE CONDUCTION

MASKING Type	RIGHT						FOREHEAD						LEFT					
	250	500	1000	2000	3000	4000	250	500	1000	2000	3000	4000	250	500	1000	2000	3000	4000
NB	5	0	5	5	15	10							5	5	5	10	15	10
													30*	35*	35*	40*	35*	55*
EM Level in Opp. Ear													60	50	35	35	40	55

	2 Frequency	3 Frequency	WEBER							2 Frequency	3 Frequency
Pure Tone Average	0	2	R	R	R	R	R	R	Pure Tone Average	35	37

SPEECH AUDIOMETRY

MASKING Type	RIGHT				LEFT			
	SRT 1	SRT 2	Discrimination 1	Discrimination 2	SRT 1	SRT 2	Discrimination 1	Discrimination 2
EM Level in Opp. Ear								

COMMENTS

Right air & bone test normal

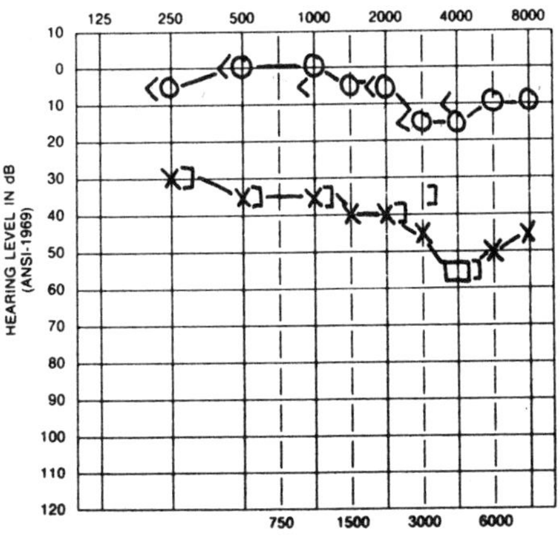

Left air & bone test same Moderate loss SN

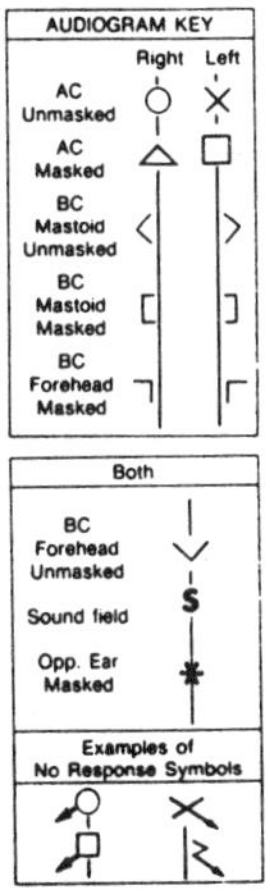

Figure 3.23 Audiogram showing normal hearing in the right ear and a sensorineural hearing loss in the left ear. The original (unmasked) results by air conduction and bone conduction suggested a conductive hearing loss in the left ear. When proper masking was administered to the right ear, the bone-conduction thresholds shifted, proving an absence of an air–bone gap in the left ear. Tones on the Weber test lateralize to the better-hearing right ear.

SPEECH AND HEARING CENTER
The University of Texas at Austin 78712
AUDIOMETRIC EXAMINATION

NAME: Last - First - Middle	SEX	AGE	DATE	EXAMINER	RELIABILITY	AUDIOMETER
-						

AIR CONDUCTION

MASKING Type	RIGHT									LEFT								
	250	500	1000	1500	2000	3000	4000	6000	8000	250	500	1000	1500	2000	3000	4000	6000	8000
NB	50	55	45/50	50	55	65	70	70	75	45	40	45/45	45	45	50	60	60	70
	55*	65*	70*	70*	75*	80*	85*	NR*	NR*									
EM Level in Opp. Ear	70	65	75	75	75	80	75	70	70									

BONE CONDUCTION

MASKING Type	RIGHT						FOREHEAD						LEFT					
	250	500	1000	2000	3000	4000	250	500	1000	2000	3000	4000	250	500	1000	2000	3000	4000
NB	10	5	10	15	20	25							5	0	10	15	10	20
	25*	35*	40*	45*	45*	50*							5*	0*	10*	15*	10*	20*
EM Level in Opp. Ear	65	75	70	75	75	70							55	65	70	75	80	85

	2 Frequency	3 Frequency	WEBER							2 Frequency	3 Frequency
Pure Tone Average	68	70	L	L	L	L	L	L	Pure Tone Average	42	43

SPEECH AUDIOMETRY

MASKING Type	RIGHT				LEFT			
	SRT 1	SRT 2	Discrimination 1	Discrimination 2	SRT 1	SRT 2	Discrimination 1	Discrimination 2
			List / SL %	List / SL %			List / SL %	List / SL %
EM Level in Opp. Ear								

left ear - cond loss

rt ear - Mixed

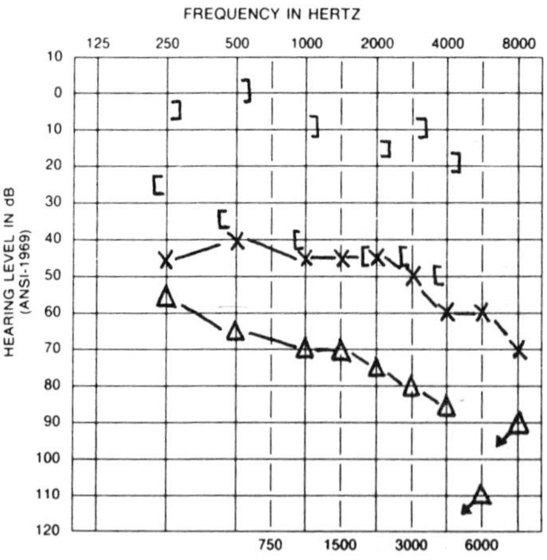

COMMENTS

bone masked left - Normal

left air - Mod loss

rt air severe loss
rt bone Mod loss

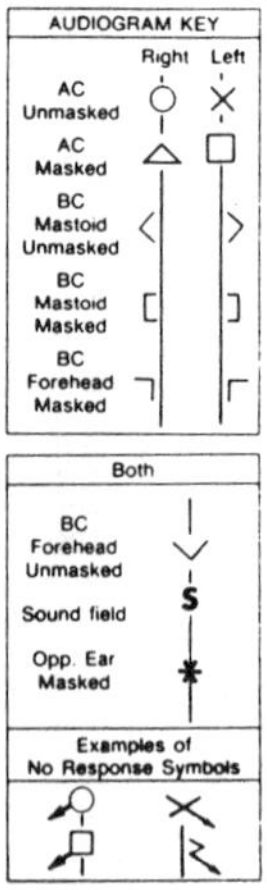

Figure 3.24 Audiogram showing a mixed hearing loss in the right ear and a conductive hearing loss in the left ear. Unmasked results showed conductive hearing losses in both ears. Masking for bone conduction was indicated for both ears, resulting in a threshold shift for the right ear. Masking was indicated for the right ear for air conduction, showing a slight threshold shift. The Weber refers consistently to the left ear, which has the better sensorineural sensitivity. Note that no response is obtained in the right ear by air conduction at 8000 Hz with masking in the left ear.

AUTOMATIC AUDIOMETRY

Automatic audiometers that utilize an oscillator with a range from 100 to 10,000 Hz may be used. The tones may be either automatically pulsed (200 msec on/200 msec off) or presented continuously. A special audiogram is placed on a movable stage on the audiometer or on a fixed stage beneath a moving stylus. When the motor is engaged, the tone gradually increases in frequency while the intensity increases. The pen traces the precise frequency and hearing level as the stage or pen moves. When patients hear the tone they press a hand switch, which reverses the motor on the attenuator, causing the signal to get weaker. When the tone becomes inaudible, the hand switch is released and the tone is allowed to increase in intensity again. Frequency continues to increase whether the intensity is increasing or decreasing. This procedure is called **Békésy audiometry**. Upon completion of the test, an audiogram has been drawn that represents the patient's thresholds over a continuous frequency range. The Békésy audiogram, illustrated in Figure 3.25, follows the same pattern as the manual audiogram for the left ear, seen in Figure 3.23.

Békésy audiometry can be carried out in either ear by reversing the test earphone or by using a switch to redirect the tone from one ear to the other. The chart speed and attenuation rate can be varied from slow to fast. If desired, frequency can be reversed, sweeping from 10,000 to 100 Hz, or an adjustment can be made to allow for continuous tracking of any single frequency within the range of the audiometer. A masking noise is available for the nontest ear. In one model, the entire sweep-frequency test for one ear takes from $3\frac{3}{4}$ to 15 minutes, depending on the chart speed.

Automatic discrete frequency audiometers are quite popular in hearing conservation programs, such as in industry. These units test for approximately 1 minute at each discrete frequency and automatically switch from the right ear to the left ear. Some of these units are now computerized.

In addition to providing detailed information regarding hearing sensitivity throughout the entire frequency range, Békésy audiometry has been found to be extremely valuable in the differential diagnosis of auditory disorders. This subject is discussed in detail in Chapter 5.

COMPUTERIZED AUDIOMETRY

A computer may be programmed to control all aspects of administering pure-tone air- and bone-conduction stimuli, recognize the need for masking, determine the appropriate level of masking, regulate the presentation of the masker to the nontest ear, analyze the subject's responses in terms of threshold-determination criteria, and present the obtained threshold values in an audi-

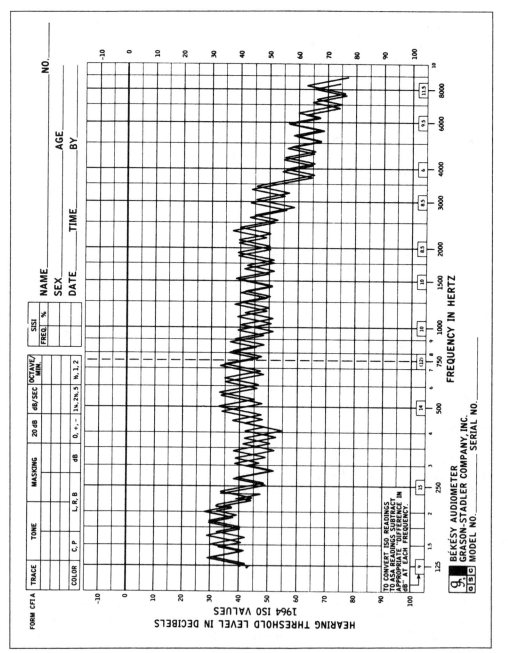

Figure 3.25 Békésy audiogram showing results for the left ear of the same hypothetical patient shown in Figure 3.24. The points at the bottom of each swing show where the patient presses the hand switch, signifying that the tone has been heard and causing it to decrease in intensity. The points at the top of the swing are where the patient releases the hand switch because the tone is no longer heard, allowing it to increase in intensity again.

ogram format at the conclusion of the test. **Computerized audiometry** may be performed on a device like the one shown in Figure 2.19. This instrument is microprocessor controlled, which allows it to be remotely operated by a computer; the audiometric data are "dumped" into a computer file for later retrieval.

Stach (1988) states that computerized audiometry is used successfully to a greater extent for military, industrial, and educational applications than for individual diagnostic purposes. In the former cases the advantages lie, in part, in the rapid storage and retrieval of data that computers allow.

In a pulse-count method the patient reports the number of tone pulses heard rather than the mere presence of the stimulus (Bragg & Collins, 1968; Gardner, 1947). This method has been successful in minimizing the number of false positive responses that many patients give. This pulse-count method has been computerized (Meyer, Sutherland, & Grogan, 1975) and found to compare favorably with traditional manual audiometry (Sutherland, Danford, & Gasaway, 1976).

It is highly unlikely that the computer will replace the clinical audiologist in the performance of pure-tone tests, although computerization of the audiometric process offers bright promise. The fact that computers can make step-by-step decisions in testing helps to prove that the majority of pure-tone tests can be carried out logically and scientifically.

AUDIOMETRIC RESPONSE SIMULATORS

One of the problems involved in training new clinicians is the clinical experience that is necessary to qualify them to do hearing tests on patients. In most university audiology centers, practice is usually obtained by having students test each other's hearing. After a number of hours of such practice, students may, under careful supervision, test actual patients. The problem with this training is that students soon become bored by testing subjects with predictably normal audiograms and must test a great number of clinical patients before a variety of different kinds of experience can be garnered.

Several companies now manufacture **audiometric response simulators** (Figure 3.26), which can be programmed like small computers to respond as patients do to pure-tone tests. False negative and false positive responses, as well as problems with cross-hearing and masking, can be programmed, thus simulating a wide variety of audiometric experiences. In this way students have instant feedback regarding their ability to perform tests and overcome difficulties. The use of such devices certainly seems desirable in training clinical audiologists.

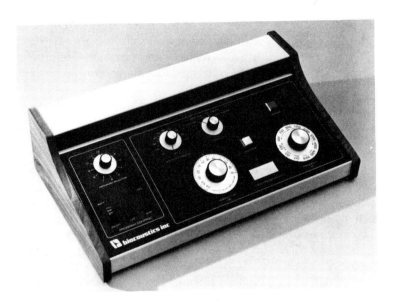

Figure 3.26 An audiometric response simulator. The device emits no sound but can be programmed to simulate any variety of pure-tone audiograms, including the need for masking and the plateau method. (Courtesy of Biocoustics, Inc.)

SUMMARY

Pure-tone hearing tests may be performed manually, with the clinician presenting the stimuli and the subject responding, thus providing data that are recorded by the clinician. Responses may also be recorded on an automatic audiometer. In order for hearing tests to be performed satisfactorily, control is needed over such factors as background noise levels, equipment calibration, patient understanding, and clinician expertise. The audiologist must be able to judge when responses are accurate and to predict when a sound may have contralateralized to the ear not being tested. When cross-hearing occurs, proper masking procedures must be instituted to overcome this problem. Although at times the performance of pure-tone hearing tests is carried out as an art, it should in most cases be approached with a scientific attitude, using rigid controls.

GLOSSARY

Air–bone gap (ABG) The amount by which the air-conduction threshold of a patient exceeds the bone-conduction threshold at any test frequency in the same ear. *fills conductive loss*

Air conduction The measurement made with the air-conduction earphones of an audiometer that checks the hearing sensitivity of the entire auditory system.

Audiogram A graphic representation of audiometric findings showing hearing levels as a function of frequency.

Audiometer (pure-tone) A device for determining the thresholds of hearing. Pure tones at various frequencies are generated, and their levels are increased and decreased until thresholds are found. Outputs may include earphones for air-conduction testing, a bone-conduction vibrator for bone-conduction testing, and one or more loudspeakers for sound-field testing.

Audiometric response simulator A device designed for the training of audiometrists. It has the outward appearance of an audiometer and can be programmed to simulate a variety of pure-tone configurations and hearing problems.

Audiometric Weber test An extension of the tuning-fork Weber test. The bone-conduction vibrator of the audiometer is applied to the forehead of a patient, and tones are presented above threshold. The patient is directed to respond by stating whether the tone was heard in the right ear, the left ear, or the midline.

Békésy audiometry Automatic audiometry wherein patients track their own auditory thresholds for pure tones by depressing a switch when the tone becomes audible and releasing it when the tone is inaudible. Results are traced in ink on a special audiogram blank.

Bone conduction The measurement made with the bone-conduction vibrator of an audiometer that theoretically checks the hearing sensitivity of the inner ear and auditory structures medial to the inner ear.

Calibration The electroacoustic or psychoacoustic determination that an audiometer is performing properly in terms of its acoustic output, attenuator linearity, frequency accuracy, harmonic distortion, and so on.

Central masking The shift in the auditory threshold of a tone produced by a noise in the opposite ear when the level of the noise is not sufficient to cause masking by cross-conduction.

Complex noise A broad band of frequencies created by generating a low-frequency tone with its harmonics. Each succeeding harmonic has less intensity.

Computerized audiometry The process of testing human hearing sensitivity by having computers programmed to present the stimuli and interpret the threshold results.

Contralateralization See *Cross-hearing.*

Critical band A portion of a continuous band of noise surrounding a pure tone. When the sound-pressure level of this narrow band is the same as the sound-pressure level of the tone, the tone is barely perceptible.

Cross-hearing   The reception of a sound signal during a hearing test (either by air conduction or bone conduction) at the ear opposite the ear under test.

Distortional bone conduction   The response to a sound stimulus evoked when the skull is deformed by a bone conduction vibrator, distorting the inner ear and giving rise to electrochemical activity within the inner ear.

Effective masking (EM)   The minimum amount of noise required just to mask out a signal (under the same earphone) at a given HL. (For example, 40 dB EM will just mask out a 40 dB HL signal.)

Electronic voltmeter   A device for measuring differences in decibels and voltages.

False negative responses   The failure of a patient to respond during a hearing test when he or she has in fact heard the stimulus.

False positive responses   Response from a subject when no stimulus has been presented or the stimulus is below threshold.

Inertial bone conduction   Stimulation of the inner ear caused by lag of the chain of middle ear bones or inner ear fluids when the skull is deformed, resulting in movement of the stapes in and out of the oval window.

Initial masking (IM)   The lowest level of effective masking presented to the nontest ear. For air-conduction tests this level is equal to the threshold of the masked ear; for bone-conduction tests

the IM is equal to the air-conduction threshold of the masked ear plus the occlusion effect at that frequency.

Interaural attenuation (IA)   The loss of energy of a sound presented by either air conduction or bone conduction as it travels from the test ear to the nontest ear. The number of decibels lost in cross-hearing.

Masking (clinical)   The introduction of a noise into the nontest ear in an attempt to eliminate cross-hearing.

Maximum masking   The highest level of noise that can be presented to one ear via an earphone before the noise crosses the skull and shifts the threshold of the opposite ear.

Narrow-band noise   A restricted band of frequencies surrounding a particular frequency to be masked. Obtained by band-pass filtering a broad-band noise.

Occlusion effect (OE)   The increase in the loudness of tones of 1000 Hz and below when the ears are occluded during bone-conduction testing. This effect is seen in normal hearers and patients with sensorineural hearing losses but is absent in patients with conductive hearing losses.

Osseotympanic bone conduction   The contribution to hearing by bone conduction created when the vibrating skull sets the air in the external ear canal into vibration, causing sound waves to pass down the canal, impinging upon the eardrum membrane, and being conducted through the middle ear to the inner ear.

Overmasking   Occurs when a masking noise presented to the nontest ear is of sufficient intensity to shift the threshold in the test ear beyond its true value. In overmasking, the masking noise crosses from the masked ear to the test ear by bone conduction.

Pink noise   A broad-spectrum noise with approximately equal energy per octave below 2000 Hz.

Plateau   The theoretical point in clinical masking at which the level of noise in the nontest ear may be raised or lowered about 15 dB without affecting the threshold of the signal in the test ear. The levels between undermasking and overmasking at which the true threshold of the test ear may be seen.

Pure-tone average (PTA)   The average of the hearing levels at frequencies 500, 1000, and 2000 Hz for each ear as obtained on a pure-tone hearing test.
to predict speech threshold

Tactile responses   The response obtained during bone-conduction (and occasionally air-conduction) audiometry to signals that have been felt rather than heard by the patient.

Threshold   In audiometry, the level at which a stimulus, such as a pure tone, is barely perceptible. Usual clinical criteria demand that the level be just high enough for the subject to be aware of the sound 50% of the times it is presented.

Undermasking   Occurs when a masking noise presented to the nontest ear is of insufficient intensity to prevent the test signal from being heard in that ear.

White noise   A broad-band noise with approximately equal energy per cycle.
hissing

STUDY QUESTIONS

1. Sketch an audiogram from memory. What is the proportional relationship between hearing level and the octave scale? Why?
2. Draw audiograms from memory illustrating normal hearing, a conductive hearing loss, sensorineural hearing loss, and mixed hearing loss. What would the results for these hypothetical patients be on the tuning-fork tests described in Chapter 1?
3. Name the parts of a pure-tone audiometer.
4. How would you calibrate for air conduction and bone conduction both with and without electroacoustic equipment?
5. How would you calibrate for effective masking for pure tones?
6. Why does the occlusion effect change the initial masking levels you might use for bone conduction?

REVIEW TABLE 3.1 SUMMARY OF PURE-TONE HEARING TESTS

TEST	AIR CONDUCTION (AC)	BONE CONDUCTION (BC)
Purpose	Hearing sensitivity for pure tones	Sensorineural sensitivity
When to mask	When difference between AC (test ear) and BC (nontest ear) exceeds minimal IA*	When there is an air–bone gap (more than 10 dB) in the test ear
How to mask	Initial maskng. IM = AC threshold in nontest ear. If tone not heard, plateau	Same as AC plus occlusion effect
Overmasking occurs	When EM level in masked ear minus IA is greater than BC of test ear at same frequency	Same as AC
Interpretation	Audiogram shows amount of hearing loss at each frequency	Air–bone gap shows amount of conductive impairment

*Minimal IA is considered to be 40 dB.

REFERENCES

AMERICAN ACADEMY OF OPHTHALMOLOGY AND OTOLARYNGOLOGY COMMITTEE ON HEARING AND EQUILIBRIUM AND THE AMERICAN COUNCIL OF OTOLARYNGOLOGY COMMITTEE ON THE MEDICAL ASPECTS OF NOISE. (1979). Guide for the evaluation of hearing handicap. *Journal of the American Medical Association, 241,* 2055–2059.

AMERICAN NATIONAL STANDARDS INSTITUTE. (1978). *Methods for manual pure-tone threshold audiometry.* S3.21–1978. New York: Author.

AMERICAN SPEECH AND HEARING ASSOCIATION. (1974). *Guidelines for audiometric symbols. Asha, 16,* 260–264.

———. (1978). Guidelines for manual pure-tone audiometry. *Asha, 20,* 297–301.

AMERICAN SPEECH-LANGUAGE-HEARING ASSOCIATION. (1988). *Guidelines for audiometric symbols. Asha, 30,* 39–42.

BARANY, E. A. (1938). A contribution to the physiology of bone conduction. *Acta Otolaryngologica* (Stockholm), Supplement 26.

BÉKÉSY, G. V. (1947). A new audiometer. *Acta Otolaryngologica* (Stockholm), *35,* 411–422.

BRAGG, V., & COLLINS, F. (1968, September). Audiometer modification and pulse-tone technic for pure-tone threshold determination. *SAM–TR–68–91.*

CARHART, R., & JERGER, J. F. (1959). Preferred method for clinical determination of pure-tone thresholds. *Journal of Speech and Hearing Disorders, 24,* 330–345.

CHAIKLIN, J. B. (1967). Interaural attenuation and cross-hearing in air-conduction audiometry. *Journal of Auditory Research, 7,* 413–424.

CLARK, J. L., & ROESER, R. J. (1988). Three studies comparing performance of the ER-3A tubephone with the TDH–50P earphone. *Ear and Hearing, 9,* 268–274.

Coles, R. R. A., & Priede, V. M. (1968). Clinical and subjective acoustics. *Institution of Sound and Vibration Research, 26,* Chap. 3A.

Elpern, B. S., & Naunton, R. F. (1963). The stability of the occlusion effect. *Archives of Otolaryngology, 77,* 376–382.

Gardner, M. B. (1947). A pulse-tone clinical audiometer. *Journal of the Acoustical Society of America, 19,* 592–599.

Hood, J. D. (1960). The principles and practice of bone-conduction audiometry: A review of the present position. *Laryngoscope, 70,* 1211–1228.

Killion, M. C., Wilber, L. A., & Dugmundsen, G. I. (1985). Insert earphones for more interaural attenuation. *Hearing Instruments, 36,* 34–36.

Liden, G., Nilsson, G., & Anderson, H. (1959). Narrow band masking with white noise. *Acta Otolaryngologica (Stockholm), 50,* 116–124.

———. (1974). Minimum effective masking levels in threshold audiometry. *Journal of Speech and Hearing Disorders, 39,* 280–285.

———. (1980). The masking plateau revisited. *Ear and Hearing, 1,* 112–116.

Martin, F. N., & Blosser, D. (1970). Crosshearing: Air-conduction or bone conduction. *Psychonomic Science, 29,* 231.

Martin, F. N., Butler, E. C., & Burns, P. (1974). Audiometric Bing test for determination of minimum masking levels for boneconduction tests. *Journal of Speech and Hearing Disorders, 39,* 148–152.

Martin, F. N., & Sides, D. G. (1985). Survey of current audiometric practices. *Asha, 27,* 29–36.

Martin, F. N., & Wittich, W. W. (1966). A comparison of forehead and mastoid tactile bone conduction thresholds. *The Eye, Ear, Nose and Throat Monthly, 45,* 72–74.

Meyer, C. R., Sutherland, H. C., Jr., & Grogan, F. (1975, December). The tone-count audiometric computer. *SAM–TR–75–50.*

Nober, E. H. (1970). Cutile air and bone conduction thresholds of the deaf. *Exceptional Children, 36,* 571–579.

Reger, S. N. (1952). A clinical and research version of the Békésy audiometer. *Laryngoscope, 62,* 1333–1351.

Sataloff, J., Sataloff, R. T., & Vassallo, L. A. (1980). *Hearing loss* (2nd ed.). Philadelphia: Lippincott.

Stach, B. A. (1988). Computers and audiologic instrumentation. *Hearing Instruments, 39,* 13–16.

Stewart, J. M., & Downs, M. P. (1984). Medical management of the hearing-handicapped child. In J. L. Northern (Ed.), *Hearing Disorders* (2nd ed.) (pp. 267–278). Boston: Little, Brown.

Studebaker, G. A. (1962). Placement of vibrator in bone conduction testing. *Journal of Speech and Hearing Research, 5,* 321–331.

———. (1964). Clinical masking in air- and bone-conducted stimuli. *Journal of Speech and Hearing Disorders, 29,* 23–35.

———. (1967a). Clinical masking of the nontest ear. *Journal of Speech and Hearing Disorders, 32,* 360–371.

———. (1967b). Intertest variability and the air–bone gap. *Journal of Speech and Hearing Disorders, 32,* 82–86.

Sutherland, H. C., Jr., Danford, R., Jr., & Gasaway, D. C. (1976, December). Comparison of TCAS and manual audiometry. *SAM–TR–77–8.*

Wegel, R. L., & Lane, G. I. (1924). The auditory masking of one pure tone by another and its probable relation to the dynamics of the inner ear. *Physiological Review, 23,* 266–285.

Zwislocki, J. (1953). Acoustic attenuation between ears. *Journal of the Acoustical Society of America, 25,* 752–759.

SUGGESTED READINGS

Dirks, D. D. (1985). Bone-conduction testing. In J. Katz (Ed.), *Handbook of Clinical Audiology* (pp. 202–223). Baltimore: Williams & Wilkins.

Yantis, P. A. (1985). Pure tone air-conduction testing. In J. Katz (Ed.), *Handbook of Clinical Audiology* (pp. 153–169). Baltimore: Williams & Wilkins.

_____ 4 ___ .

SPEECH AUDIOMETRY

It was not until the close of World War II that audiology got its start as an independent clinical discipline. This was brought about by the large numbers of military veterans who were discharged with service-connected disabilities. Not the least among these disabilities was hearing loss. The development of speech audiometry was accelerated because of a need for more diagnostic and corroborative information than was provided by pure-tone hearing tests.

Because difficulties in hearing and understanding speech evoke the greatest complaints from hearing-impaired patients, it is logical that tests of hearing function should be performed with speech stimuli. The hearing impairment inferred from a pure-tone audiogram cannot depict, beyond the grossest generalizations, the degree of handicap in speech communication caused by a hearing loss. Modern **speech audiometers**, which are devices for measuring various aspects of receptive speech communication, are shown in Figures 2.19 and 2.20. Using speech audiometers, audiologists set out to answer questions regarding patients' degree of hearing loss for speech, the levels required for their most comfortable and loudness levels, the range of comfortable loudness, and perhaps most important their ability to discriminate among the sounds of speech.

Sp. discrim
Comf. loudness level

CHAPTER OBJECTIVES   _Comf speech_
uncomfortable loudness level

Chapter 3 introduced the concept of pure-tone audiometry and described its administration and interpretation. Chapter 4 acquaints the reader with speech audiometry and some of its ramifications. Upon completion of this chapter, the new reader in audiology should have a fundamental knowledge of the measures obtained with speech audiometry, such as threshold for speech, most comfortable and most uncomfortable loudness levels, and speech discrimination ability. The reader should be able to interpret speech audiometric results; relate them to pure-tone threshold results; and, after some supervised practice with a speech audiometer, actually perform the tests described in this chapter. The vocabulary supplied in the text and reviewed in the glossary is indispensable for understanding the concepts that follow in this book.

THE SPEECH AUDIOMETER

Speech audiometers have been in use for about fifty years. Unlike some of the pure-tone audiometers, most speech audiometers are not portable, although the development of integrated circuitry has miniaturized them considerably. Most modern speech audiometers contain additional circuitry for pure-tone tests. These combination units save space in the audiometric control room and eliminate the need for changing earphones when switching from one type of test to the other.

Speech audiometers are either accompanied by or have auxiliary inputs for testing with microphones, phonographs, or tape recorders. A volume units (VU) meter is used to visually monitor the intensity of the input source. All speech audiometers contain a circuit for masking the nontest ear or for mixing a noise with the speech signal in the same ear. Tests can usually be carried out in either ear (**monaurally**) or in both ears simultaneously (**binaurally**). Hearing-level dials that usually have a range of 120 dB (from −10 to 110 dB according to ANSI–1969 values) are provided. The attenuators may be continuously variable or may be calibrated in steps of 2 or 5 dB, so that the dial clicks into position at each step. Outputs to auxiliary amplifiers are available so that speech can be channeled to one or more loudspeakers for testing in the sound field. A talkback system is available for use when the clinician and the patient are in separate rooms.

VU = volume units

TEST ENVIRONMENT

Most speech audiometry is carried out in two-room, sound-treated suites. This is mandatory when **monitored live-voice (MLV)** testing is used, because if examiners and patients are in the same room, there is no way to ensure that the patients are responding to sounds channeled to them through the audiometer rather than directly through the air in the room. If a tape recorder or phonograph is used, one-room operation is permissible. Problems of ambient noise levels are very much the same for speech audiometry as for pure-tone audiometry, as discussed in Chapter 3.

THE PATIENT'S ROLE IN SPEECH AUDIOMETRY

To use speech audiometry, patients must know and understand reasonably well the words with which they are to be tested. Depending on the type of test, a response must be obtainable in the form of an oral reply, a written reply, or the identification of a picture or object.

Although spoken responses are more necessary in some speech tests than in others, they have certain advantages and disadvantages. One advantage is in the speed with which answers can be scored. Also, a certain amount of rapport is maintained through the verbal interplay between the patient and the audiologist. One serious drawback is the possible misinterpretation of the patient's response. Many people seen for hearing evaluations have speech or language difficulties that make their responses difficult to understand. In addition, for reasons that have never become completely clear, the talkback systems on many speech audiometers are of poor quality, sounding very little better than inexpensive intercom systems. This creates an additional problem in interpreting responses.

Written responses lend themselves only to tests that can be scored upon completion. When responses require an instantaneous value judgment on the audiologist's part, written responses are undesirable. When used, however, written responses do eliminate errors caused by difficulties in discriminating the patient's speech; they also provide a permanent record of the kinds of errors made. Having patients write down or otherwise mark responses may slow down some test procedures and necessitate time at the end of the test for scoring. Difficulties with handwriting and spelling provide additional, though not insurmountable problems. In addition, Merrill and Atkinson (1965) have found that discrepancies occur in the scoring of some speech tests when verbal responses are obtained and the same tests using written responses, because audiologists tend to score some incorrect spoken responses as correct.

The use of pictures or objects is generally reserved for small children who otherwise cannot or will not participate in a test. Adults with special handicaps also are sometimes tested by this method, in which the patient is instructed to point to a picture or object that matches a stimulus word.

False responses may occur in speech audiometry as well as in pure-tone audiometry. False positive responses are theoretically impossible because patients cannot correctly repeat words that have been presented to them below their thresholds, unless, through the carelessness of the examiner, they have been allowed some visual cues and have actually lip-read the stimulus words. False negative responses, however, do occur. The audiologist must try to make certain that the patient completely understands the task and will respond in the appropriate manner whenever possible.

No matter how thorough the attempt to instruct patients, it is impossible to gain total control over the internal response criteria each individual brings to the test situation. It has been suspected, for example, that aging might affect the relative strictness of these criteria. Jerger, Johnson, and Jerger (1988), however, demonstrated that aging alone does not appear to affect the criteria that listeners use in giving responses to speech stimuli. All the alert clinician can do is to instruct patients carefully and be aware of overt signs of deviation from expected behaviors.

THE CLINICIAN'S ROLE IN SPEECH AUDIOMETRY

First and foremost in speech audiometry, through whatever means necessary, the audiologist must convey to patients what is expected of them during the session. A combination of written and verbal instructions is successful with adults and older children, whereas gestures and pantomine may be required for small children and certain adults. At times, the instructions are given to patients using their hearing aids, or, if this is not feasible, through a portable desk amplifier or the microphone circuit of the speech audiometer.

It is just as important that the patient not observe the examiner's face during speech audiometry as it is during pure-tone audiometry, and even more so if monitored live-voice testing is used. The diagram in Figure 3.6 shows a desirable arrangement.

SPEECH THRESHOLD TESTING

The logic of pure-tone threshold testing carries over to speech audiometry. If a patient's thresholds for speech can be obtained, they can be compared to an average normal-hearing individual's thresholds to determine the patient's degree of hearing loss for speech. Speech thresholds may be of two kinds, the **speech detection threshold** and the **speech recognition threshold**.

The terminology used in speech audiometry has been inconsistent. Konkle and Rintelmann (1983, p. 6) feel that the word *speech* itself may be too general and that the specific speech stimuli in any test should always be stated. Likewise, they are concerned with the conventional term *speech reception threshold*, since the listener is asked to *recognize* rather than *receive* the words used in the test. In the most recent *"Guidelines for Determining Threshold Level for Speech,"* ASHA (1988) also recommends the term *speech recognition threshold* as preferable to the traditional term *speech reception threshold*.

Speech Detection Threshold (SDT)

The speech detection threshold (SDT) may be defined as the lowest level (in decibels) at which a subject can barely detect the presence of speech and identify it as speech. The SDT is sometimes called the *speech awareness threshold (SAT)*. This does not imply that the speech is in any way understood—rather, merely that its presence is detected. One way of measuring the SDT is to present to the patient, through the desired output transducer, some continuous-discourse stimulus. The level of the speech is raised and lowered on the hearing-level dial until the patient indicates that he or she can barely detect the speech.

Sentences are preferable to isolated words or phrases for finding the SDT. The sentences should be read rapidly and monotonously so that there are few peaks above and below zero on the VU meter. The materials should be relatively uninteresting. One popular recording is commercially available.[1]

Whether the right ear or the left ear is tested first is an arbitrary decision. Sometimes tests of SDT are run binaurally or through the sound-field speakers, either with or without the use of a hearing aid. Patients may respond verbally, with hand or finger signals, or with a push-button, indicating the lowest level, in dB HL, at which they can barely detect speech.

Speech Recognition Threshold (SRT)

The speech recognition threshold (SRT) may be defined as the lowest hearing level at which speech can be understood. Most audiologists agree that the speech should be so soft that about half of it can be recognized. For a number of reasons, the SRT has become more popular with audiologists than the SDT, and is thus the preferred speech threshold test. In this book very little attention is paid to the SDT, although it has some clinical usefulness. SRTs have been measured with a variety of speech materials using both continuous discourse, as in measurement of the SDT, and isolated words.

Cold running speech, a form of continuous discourse, may be used to determine the SRT by modifying instructions to the patient and altering response criteria. Today most SRTs are obtained with the use of **spondaic words**, often called **spondees**. A spondee is a word with two syllables, both pronounced with equal stress and effort. In setting up their list of spondees, Hirsh et al. (1952) reduced the list of 84 words originated by Hudgins et al. (1947) to 36 words in order to increase their homogeneity of audibility and familiarity. Although spondees do not occur in spoken English, it is possible, by altering stress slightly, to force such common words as *baseball, hotdog,* and *toothbrush* to conform to the spondaic configuration. Whether the spondees are spoken into the microphone or introduced via tape or disk, both syllables of the word should peak at zero VU. Although it takes practice for the student to accomplish this equal peaking on the VU meter, most people can acquire the knack relatively quickly.

When a prerecorded list of spondaic words is to be used, it is common to find a calibration tone or signal recorded either before the list begins or, in the case of phonograph recordings, on a special band. The calibration signal is played long enough so that the gain control for the VU meter can be adjusted with the needle at zero VU. On some prerecorded spondee lists, a **carrier phrase** precedes each word, for example, "Say the word _____," followed

[1]Available as "Fulton Lewis, Jr., Reading the News," Technisonic Studios, 1201 South Brentwood Boulevard, Richmond Heights, Missouri 63117.

by the stimulus word.[2] In such cases the phrase is audible when the words are at threshold. This 10 dB difference must be subtracted from the hearing-level dial setting before the SRT is recorded on the audiometric worksheet. Although some clinicians prefer the use of a carrier phrase, many do not. When monitored live-voice testing is used, the carrier phrase should be omitted because the phrase and stimulus word would have to be delivered at the same level, making the phrase partially inaudible at threshold. No real advantage of using a carrier phrase with spondaic words has been proved. An alphabetized list of spondees may be found in the Appendix.

SRT Testing with Cold Running Speech. When continuous discourse is used to measure the SRT, patients are instructed to indicate the level at which the speech is so soft that they can barely follow what is being said. Sometimes this involves using a verbal or hand signal, or allowing the patient to control the hearing-level dial by using a hand switch, as was previously described for pure-tone automatic audiometry. The level of the speech may be raised and lowered in steps of 2 or 5 dB, depending on the preferences of the audiologist. Several measurements should be taken to ensure accuracy.

SRT Testing with Spondaic Words. The SRT is usually defined as the lowest hearing level at which 50% of a list of spondaic words is correctly identified. This definition appears incomplete, however, for it does not tell how many words are presented at threshold before the 50% criterion is invoked. Also, many methods used for SRT measurement in the past were rather vague, suggesting that the level should be raised and lowered but not giving a precise methodology.

For some reason, most SRTs had been obtained in 1 or 2 dB steps until Chaiklin and Ventry (1964) proved that, for clinical purposes, 5 dB steps are just as accurate. Using 5 dB steps speeds the procedure and makes decisions regarding threshold easier without sacrificing the quality of test results.

Tillman and Jerger (1959) showed that familiarizing the patient with the list of spondaic test words has the effect of lowering the SRT by 4 to 5 dB. Conn, Dancer, and Ventry (1975) found that only 15 of the original words from the 36 spondees in CID Auditory Test W–1 could be used without the effect of prior familiarization altering test results. Other studies (for example, Frank & McPhillips, 1976) have shown that fewer than half of the original words are similar with respect to the intensity required for intelligibility.

Practice with the SRT procedure has the effect of lowering the response interpreted as threshold by a very small amount, although guessing may lower that level more than 4 dB, at least for people with normal hearing. Burke and Nerbonne (1978) suggest that the guess factor should be controlled during SRT tests by asking the patient not to guess and thereby improving the agreement between the SRT and the PTA. Because no data have surfaced that reveal the effects of guessing on patients with actual hearing losses, the practice will

[2]Two such tests are CID Auditory Test W–1 and W–2, available from Technisonic Studios. (See the Appendix.)

probably continue to encourage guessing, to increase attentiveness to the test stimuli. It is considered advisable, whenever possible, to give the patient a list of the words before the test begins, together with printed instructions for the entire test procedure (see the Appendix).

Although written instructions may serve as an adjunct, they should not routinely replace spoken directions for taking a test. Instructions are of great importance in test results. One usable set of instructions follows:

instructions

> The purpose of this test is to determine the faintest level at which you can hear and repeat some words. Each word you hear will have two syllables, like *hotdog* or *baseball*, and will be selected from the list of words that you have been given. Each time you hear a word, just repeat it. Repeat the words even if they sound very soft. You may have to guess, but repeat each word if you have any idea what it is. Are there any questions?

Until the work of Chaiklin and Ventry (1964), most descriptions of the measurement of speech recognition threshold were rather vague. Clinicians and students had been advised simply to use an up–down method in search of threshold. Chaiklin and Ventry, however, proposed a systematic approach. Tillman and Olsen (1973) refined the SRT test methodology into a series of steps that led to the use of a formula for deciding on SRT, thereby taking the arbitrary decision out of the clinician's hands. The practicality of the Tillman-Olsen method was tested by Wilson, Morgan, and Dirks (1973), who recommended it as a standardized approach. Martin and Stauffer (1975) modified the Tillman-Olsen method so that it could be used without prior knowledge of the pure-tone results, thereby increasing its objectivity as an independent measurement of hearing.

ASHA (1988) has recently revised its guidelines for determing the SRT. There has been evidence that audiologists were not using the guidelines advanced earlier (ASHA, 1979), probably because of the time-consuming nature of the recommended procedure (Martin & Morris, 1989). The new ASHA guidelines are based on the findings of several studies (Beattie, Forrester, & Ruby, 1987; Huff & Nerbonne, 1982; Martin & Stauffer, 1975; Robinson & Koenige, 1979; Tillman & Olsen, 1973; Wall, Davis, & Myers, 1984; Wilson, Morgan, & Dirks, 1973).

The ASHA (1988) method for determining SRT involves the following steps: (1) familiarizing the listener with the spondaic words in the word list to be used, (2) ensuring that the vocabulary is familiar, (3) establishing that each word can be recognized auditorily, and (4) ascertaining that the patient's responses can be understood by the clinician. These goals can be accomplished by allowing the patient to listen to the words as presented through the speech audiometer. Words that present any difficulty should be eliminated from the list.

The ASHA method involves a descending procedure, which can be summarized as follows:

1. Set the *start level* at 30 to 40 dB above the estimated SRT. The pure-tone average can be used for this purpose; or, if this is not known, the start level can be set at 50 dB HL (Martin & Stauffer, 1975). One spondee is presented.
2. If no response or an incorrect response is obtained, raise the level in 20 dB steps until a correct response is given or the intensity limit of the equipment is reached.
3. If the patient responds correctly, descend in 10 dB steps, presenting one spondee at each level until an incorrect response is obtained.
4. When an incorrect response is given, present a second spondee at the same level.
5. Continue to decrease the intensity in 10 dB decrements until a level is reached at which two spondees are incorrectly recognized at the same level.
6. Following step 5, increase the level by 10 dB. This is the *starting level.* Present two spondees at this level.
7. Each time both spondees are correctly identified, decrease the intensity in 2 dB steps.
8. The test is completed when the subject fails to respond correctly to five of the last six words presented.
9. "Threshold is calculated by subtracting the total number of correct responses from the starting level and adding a correction factor of 1. This calculation is based on a statistical precedent (Spearman, 1908) for estimating threshold at the 50% point of the psychometric function" (ASHA, 1988, p. 87). Stated as a formula:

$$\text{SRT} = \text{starting level} - \text{\# correct} + \text{correction factor}$$

The ASHA method allows for substitution of five spondees and 5 dB steps in step #7, based on the recommendations of Martin and Stauffer (1975). Nevertheless, given the apparent reluctance with which previous ASHA methods have been adopted by the audiology profession (Martin & Forbis, 1978; Martin & Morris, 1989), there is reason to believe that this method may not be readily accepted.

Martin and Stauffer (1975) recommended beginning the SRT procedure at a given hearing level (50 dB), especially for cases in which pure-tone thresholds cannot be obtained. Additionally, if the SRT is to serve as an independent measurement of hearing and a check of the reliability of pure-tone thresholds, it should be accomplished without knowledge of the pure-tone thresholds with which it is compared. For this reason, Martin and Dowdy (1986) recommend a different procedure.

Martin and Dowdy found that SRTs obtained using the ASHA (1979) method and one similar to the ASHA (1978) guidelines for pure-tone audiometry yielded very similar results. The latter method, however, could be completed in a fraction of the time, with many fewer word presentations and no loss of accuracy. An advantage of the Martin and Dowdy method is that SRT can be determined before the pure-tone thresholds or in the absence of pure-tone results, as when testing hearing aids. The Martin and Dowdy procedure is summarized as follows:

1. Set start level at 30 dB HL. Present one spondee. If a correct response is obtained, this suggests that the word is above the patient's SRT.
2. If no correct response is obtained, raise the presentation level to 50 dB HL. Present one spondee. If there is no correct response, raise the intensity in 10 dB steps, presenting one spondee at each increment. Stop at the level at which either a correct response is obtained or the power limit of the equipment is reached.
3. After a correct response is obtained, lower the intensity 10 dB and present one spondee.
4. When an incorrect response is given, raise the level 5 dB and present one spondee. If a correct response is given, lower the intensity 10 dB. If an incorrect response is given, continue raising the intensity in 5 dB steps until a correct response is obtained.
5. From this point on the intensity is increased in 5 dB steps and decreased in 10 dB steps, with one spondee presented at each level until three correct responses have been obtained at a given level.
6. Threshold is defined as the lowest level at which *at least* 50% of the responses are correct, with a minimum of at least three correct responses at that intensity.

One reason for the selection of spondaic words for measuring SRT is that they are relatively easy to discriminate and can often be guessed with a high degree of accuracy. Once the threshold of spondees has been reached (50% response criterion), it does not take much increase in intensity before all the words can be identified correctly. This is illustrated by the curve in Figure 4.1, which shows the enhanced intelligibility of spondees as a function of increased intensity.

Recording SRT results. After SRTs for each ear have been obtained, they should be recorded in the appropriate space on the audiometric worksheet (Figure 4.2K). Many audiologists prefer to make routine measurements of the SRT binaurally or in the sound field. The audiometric worksheet used in the book does not provide for such notation, but many forms are available that do.

Relationship of SRT to SDT and the Pure-Tone Audiogram. The SRT is always higher (requires greater intensity) than the SDT. Egan (1948) showed that the magnitude of the difference between SRT and SDT does not normally exceed 12 dB. However, this difference may change with factors such as the shape of the pure-tone audiogram.

For many years different methods have been used to predict the SRT from the pure-tone audiogram. Although some of these procedures have been quite elegant, most audiologists have agreed that the SRT can be predicted by finding

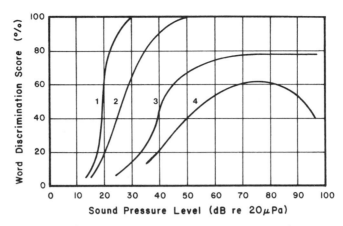

Figure 4.1 Theoretical performance-intensity (PI) functions for spondaic and PB words.

1. Spondaic words. Note that at about 5 dB above the 50% correct point, almost all of the words are intelligible. This shows an increase in discrimination of approximately 10% per decibel for scores between 20% and 80%.
2. PB words. Note the more gradual slope for PB words than for spondees. The increase in intelligibility for the W–22 word lists averages about 2.5% per decibel. The normal increase in word discrimination scores with increased intensity is to a maximum of approximately 100% (suggesting normal hearing or conductive hearing loss).
3. PB words. Note the increase in word discrimination scores with increased intensity to a maximum of less than 90% (suggesting sensorineural hearing loss).
4. PB words. Note the increase in word discrimination scores with increased intensity to a given level, beyond which scores decrease. This is the "rollover" effect and occurs in some ears when lesions in the higher auditory centers are present.

the average of the best two thresholds at 500, 1000, and 2000 Hz (Fletcher, 1950). Carhart and Porter (1971) found that the SRT can be predicted from the pure-tone audiogram by averaging the thresholds at 500 and 1000 Hz and subtracting 2 dB. Although 500, 1000, and 2000 Hz have been called the "speech frequencies," Wilson and Margolis (1983, p. 112) cautioned that such phrasing can be misleading if it is inferred that this narrow range of frequencies is all that is essential for the adequate discrimination of speech.

In some cases the SRT may be much lower (better) than the pure-tone average, such as when the audiogram fails precipitously in the high frequencies. In other cases the SRT may be higher (poorer) than even the three-frequency pure-tone average, for example with some elderly patients or those with disorders of the central auditory nervous system. The special significance of pure-tone–SRT disagreement regarding nonorganic hearing loss is discussed in Chapter 10.

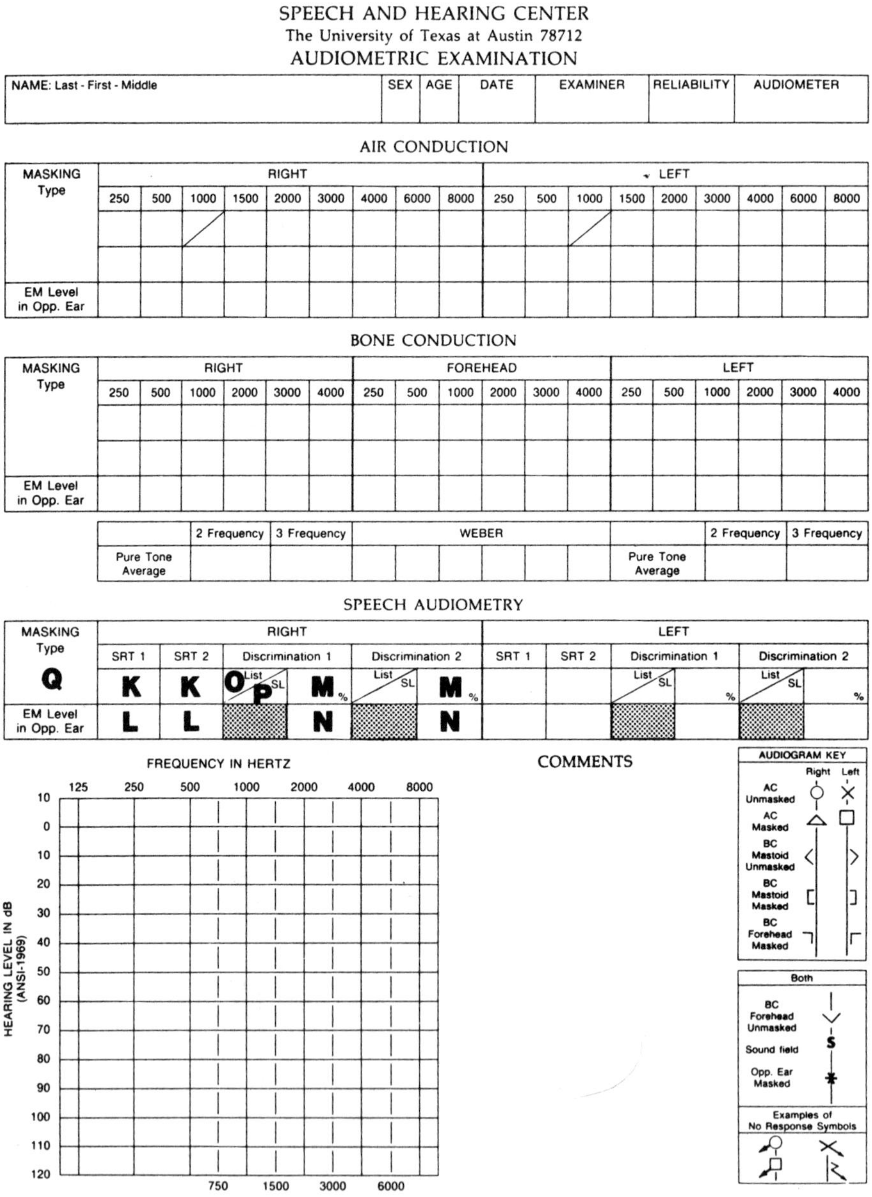

SPEECH AND HEARING CENTER
The University of Texas at Austin 78712
AUDIOMETRIC EXAMINATION

NAME: Last - First - Middle	SEX	AGE	DATE	EXAMINER	RELIABILITY	AUDIOMETER

AIR CONDUCTION

MASKING Type	RIGHT									← LEFT								
	250	500	1000	1500	2000	3000	4000	6000	8000	250	500	1000	1500	2000	3000	4000	6000	8000
EM Level in Opp. Ear																		

BONE CONDUCTION

MASKING Type	RIGHT						FOREHEAD						LEFT					
	250	500	1000	2000	3000	4000	250	500	1000	2000	3000	4000	250	500	1000	2000	3000	4000
EM Level in Opp. Ear																		

		2 Frequency	3 Frequency		WEBER				2 Frequency	3 Frequency
Pure Tone Average								Pure Tone Average		

SPEECH AUDIOMETRY

MASKING Type	RIGHT				LEFT			
Q	SRT 1	SRT 2	Discrimination 1	Discrimination 2	SRT 1	SRT 2	Discrimination 1	Discrimination 2
	K	**K**	**O** List **P** SL	**M** List SL %			List SL %	List SL %
EM Level in Opp. Ear	**L**	**L**	**N**	**N**				

FREQUENCY IN HERTZ

HEARING LEVEL IN dB (ANSI-1969)

COMMENTS

AUDIOGRAM KEY

	Right	Left
AC Unmasked	○	✕
AC Masked	△	☐
BC Mastoid Unmasked	‹	›
BC Mastoid Masked	⌐	⌐
BC Forehead Masked	⌐	⌐

Both

BC Forehead Unmasked

Sound field   **S**

Opp. Ear Masked

Examples of No Response Symbols

Figure 4.2 An example of an audiometric worksheet showing the following measurements, which can be made during speech audiometry: (K) SRT: (L) effective masking level in the nontest ear used, when necessary during SRT measurements; (M) word-discrimination scores (WDS); (N) effective masking level in the nontest ear used for WDS; (O) test list number used for WDS; (P) level above the SRT for WDS test (SL); (Q) type of noise used for masking during speech audiometry.

Cross-Hearing in SRT Tests. Problems involving cross-hearing exist for SRT measurements for the same reasons that they do for pure-tone air-conduction tests. In some cases the notion persists that a significant difference must exist between the SRTs of the two ears before suspicions of cross-hearing arise (Martin & Morris, 1989). This action ignores the current knowledge that sounds contralateralize by bone conduction rather than by air conduction. Cross-hearing is a danger whenever the SRT of the test ear, minus the interaural attenuation (conservatively set at 40 dB), is greater than or equal to the bone-conduction thresholds of the nontest ear. Because speech is a complex signal and bone-conduction thresholds are obtained with pure tones, it must be decided which frequency to use in computation. Martin and Blythe (1977) found that frequencies surrounding 250 Hz did not contribute to the recognition of spondees presented to the opposite ear, until levels were reached that considerably exceeded normal interaural attenuation values. Their research confirmed the recommendations made by ASHA (1988) that the SRT of the test ear should be compared to the lowest (best) bone-conduction threshold of the nontest ear at 500, 1000, 2000, or 4000 Hz.

$$SRT_{TE} - IA \geq Best\ BC_{NTE}$$

Figure 4.3 illustrates the possibility of cross-hearing for SRT.

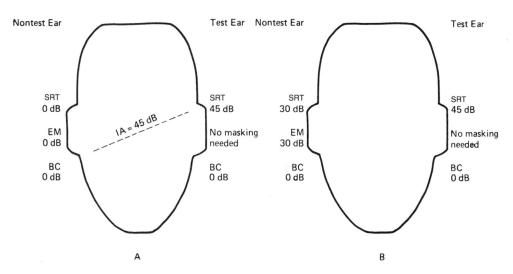

Figure 4.3 Possible cross-hearing during SRT testing. Both A and B show that the difference between the SRT of the test ear and the lowest bone-conduction threshold of the nontest ear exceed the minimum interaural attenuation found when speech sounds contralateralize (40 dB). Note that the SRT of the nontest ear in A is 0 dB and in B is 30 dB. The SRTs of the nontest ears are unrelated to the danger of cross-hearing for speech. The SRT of the test ear must be compared to the lowest bone-conduction threshold of the nontest ear. The initial effective masking level for the SRT is equal to the SRT of the nontest ear (i.e., 0 dB EH for A; 30 dB EM for B).

MASKING FOR SRT

Masking must be used in SRT testing to eliminate the influence of the nontest ear and to ascertain the true threshold of the test ear in precisely the same way as for pure-tone air-conduction audiometry. As in pure-tone testing, the audiologist should suspect the need to mask more often than cross-hearing actually occurs. Even in questionable cases of cross-hearing, masking is a prudent practice.

When in doubt Mask

Most speech audiometers provide only the standard earphone-cushion arrangements for testing and masking. The use of insert earphones can help to avoid some of the problems of overmasking, in large part because they increase interaural attenuation. The recent emphasis on their use holds promise for solving many masking dilemmas.

Noises Used in Masking for Speech

The types of masking noises used for speech audiometry are more limited than those used for pure tones. Because speech is a broad-spectrum signal, speech-masking noises must consist of a broad band of frequencies.

Complex noise is a usable noise for speech masking because most of the energy of speech is concentrated in the low frequencies. It is not considered ideal for masking speech, however, because of its relatively low energy in the high frequencies. *wide band*

Sawtooth noise has a fundamental frequency of 120 Hz, with equal intensity at all harmonics. This noise is adequate for masking speech and was the preferred masking noise on early speech audiometers. It is not as popular today as it was formerly and is rarely found on modern diagnostic audiometers.

White noise is available on many speech and combination speech and pure-tone audiometers. Because it is a broad-spectrum noise, it masks speech satisfactorily but is slightly less intense in the low frequencies.

Speech noise is obtained by filtering white noise above 1000 Hz at the rate of about 12 dB per octave and below 1000 Hz at 3 dB per octave. Speech noise provides more energy in the low-frequency spectrum than does white noise and is more like the overall spectrum of speech. Of the masking noises available on commercial audiometers, speech noise is usually preferred for masking speech.

Calibration of Speech-Masking Noises

All of the needs for adequate control of the masking system for pure tones are identical to those for speech. The linearity of the masking-level dial must be proved. If the masking circuit is calibrated in decibels of effective masking, procedures for masking speech can be carried out in the same way as those used for pure tones. Field calibration for effective masking may be carried out in the following fashion on a group of normal-hearing subjects:

1. Present a series of spondees at 30 dB HL.
2. Present a noise (preferably speech noise) to the same ear.
3. Raise the level of the noise in 5 dB steps until subjects miss more than 50% of the words. Recheck this several times on each subject.
4. Obtain a median for the dial reading on the noise attenuator that masked speech at 30 dB HL. This is 30 dB EM for speech.
5. Subtract 30 dB from what was determined (in step 4) to be 30 dB EM for speech. This is 0 dB EM.
6. Post a correction chart showing the amount of noise that must be added to 0 dB HL to reach 0 dB EM for speech. A safety factor of 5 or 10 dB should be added to ensure masking effectiveness for most cases.

Once calibration is completed, speech at any level can be masked out when an effective masking level equal to the SRT is introduced into the *test* ear. Any correction factors must be added.

Central Masking for Speech

It has been demonstrated that threshold shifts for continuous discourse (Martin, Bailey, & Pappas, 1965) and for spondaic words (Martin, 1966) occur when a noise is presented to the nontest ear under earphones. Because the levels of noise need not be high enough to cause peripheral masking by cross-conduction, it is assumed that the same central masking phenomenon exists for speech as for pure tones. Martin and DiGiovanni (1979) found smaller threshold shifts due to central masking than had been previously reported, but it should be expected that a threshold shift of about 5 dB will be seen for speech in the presence of a contralateral noise, even if that noise is of relatively low intensity (Konkle & Berry, 1983, p. 317).

Masking Methods for SRT

Figure 4.3 illustrates a case in which masking is needed for the nontest ear. The difference between the SRT of the test ear (45 dB) and the minimal interaural attenuation (40 dB) exceeds the bone-conduction threshold (0 dB) of the nontest ear. In this example, no specific frequency is referred to in terms of the bone-conduction threshold. In actual clinical practice, the SRT of the test ear is compared to the best (lowest) bone-conduction threshold of the nontest ear at 500, 1000, 2000, or 4000 Hz. If the nontest ear originally participated in the test, it should be removed by presenting an initial level of effective masking (IM) equal to the SRT of the masked ear. If the SRT of the test ear does not shift by more than 5 dB (for central masking), then the original threshold was correct as measured and masking is completed. This is true because the nontest ear was rendered incapable of test participation. If the threshold shifted by more than 5 dB, the implication is that the nontest ear did, in fact, play a role in unmasked results by cross-hearing. When original speech stimuli have been cross-heard, further testing, using the plateau method, is required.

Maximum masking for speech follows the same general rules noted previously for pure tones. If cross-hearing has taken place, the patient's interaural attenuation is no greater than the SRT of the test ear, minus the lowest bone-conduction threshold of the nontest ear. When a level of effective masking, minus the patient's interaural attenuation, is equal to or above the lowest bone-conduction threshold of the test ear, overmasking (OM) has occurred.

$$EM_{NTE} - IA \geq Best\ BC_{TE}$$

The Plateau Method

The plateau method described for pure tones in Chapter 3, and diagrammed in Figure 3.19 can be used when measuring the threshold for spondees. If the initial level of effective masking reveals that the SRT was obtained by cross-hearing, the SRT is determined with that level of noise in the nontest ear. Then the intensity of the noise is raised 5 dB in the nontest ear and spondaic words are presented to the test ear. If fewer than three out of six words can be repeated correctly, the level of the words is raised 5 dB, and so forth. The true SRT is reached when the intensity of the noise can be raised or lowered in at least three 5 dB steps without affecting the threshold for the words. As in the case of pure tones, the plateau for speech is influenced by the patient's interaural attenuation, the bone-conduction thresholds of the test ear, and the SRT of the masked ear.

Recording Masked SRT Results

Before SRTs are recorded on the audiometric worksheet, 5 dB may be subtracted from the SRT obtained with contralateral masking. The maximum level of effective masking required to obtain threshold should be recorded in the appropriate box below the SRT (Figure 4.2L).

BONE-CONDUCTION SRT

At times it is useful to determine the speech recognition threshold by bone conduction. Because the bone-conduction circuits on combination speech and pure-tone audiometers are not calibrated for speech, some degree of manipulation is required for bone-conduction speech audiometry (Barry & Gaddis, 1978). On some audiometers the speech input may be used with the bone-conduction output, but calibration corrections are required. The SRT by bone conduction may require up to 35 dB greater intensity than is needed for an air-conduction earphone.

Bone-conducted SRTs are especially useful in testing children who will "play a game" with words but not with tones. A comparison between their hearing thresholds for speech by bone conduction and by air conduction may provide useful information regarding a possible conductive hearing loss. Hahlbrock (1962) found this method helpful in separating auditory from tactile responses by bone conduction. Goetzinger and Proud (1955) found a high correlation between the pure-tone average by bone conduction at 500, 1000, and 2000 Hz and the bone-conducted SRT. Other researchers have found the bone-conducted SRT to be of clinical value (Edgerton, Danhauer, & Beattie, 1977; Merrill, Wolfe, & McLemore, 1973; Srinivasson, 1974). Of course, with bone-conducted speech audiometry there is no way to be certain which ear is being tested unless proper masking is invoked, which is impossible with some patients. However, even the limited information derived from this procedure and the inferences it allows often justify the use of bone-conducted speech audiometry.

MOST COMFORTABLE LOUDNESS LEVEL

Some audiologists gain useful information from determining the hearing level at which speech is most comfortably loud for their patients. Most people with normal hearing find speech comfortable at 40 to 55 dB above threshold. Kopra and Blosser (1968) found the level of **most comfortable loudness (MCL)** for speech to be a reliable measurement.

Measurement of MCL should be made with a continuous-discourse stimulus so that the patient has an opportunity to listen to speech as it fluctuates over time. The use of cold running speech, as described for SRT or SDT measurements, is practical for this purpose.

The patient is instructed to indicate when the speech is perceived to be at a comfortable level. The test may be begun at a hearing-level setting slightly above the SRT. From there the intensity is increased gradually. At each hearing level the patient should respond, indicating whether the speech is "too soft," "too loud," or "most comfortable." Several measurements should be made, approaching the MCL from both above and below the level first selected.

MCL may be determined monaurally or binaurally under earphones, or in the sound field. Martin and Morris (1989) found that most audiologists do not use the MCL measurement except in the evaluation of hearing aids.

Cross-Hearing and Masking in MCL Tests

Because in the MCL test the level of speech is raised above threshold, the probability increases that the threshold of the ear not being tested will be reached or exceeded. This often happens without the patient's awareness. In most cases the inclusion of the opposite ear in an MCL measurement does not affect either the results or their interpretation. If it is decided that the nontest ear must be absolutely excluded from the test, this can be done, in most cases, with masking. It must be remembered that a noise presented to one ear may have an effect on the subjective impression of the loudness of speech in the other ear. The following formula shows when masking may be needed for measuring MCL under earphones.

$$MCL_{TE} - IA \geq Best\ BC_{NTE}$$

As stated previously, masking is usually not used in determining the MCL. If it is desired, however, maximum masking should be used so the masking level can be set at the outset of the test and not varied thereafter. The maximum masking level for speech is equal to the best bone-conduction threshold of the test ear plus 40 dB for interaural attenuation. The equation for effective masking level for MCL is:

$$EM = Best\ BC_{TE} + 40\ dB$$

Recording the MCL Level Test Results

After the MCL results are obtained, they should be recorded in the space provided for this purpose on the audiometric worksheet, with the proper masking levels indicated when necessary.

UNCOMFORTABLE LOUDNESS LEVEL

Under some conditions, for example when a hearing aid is contemplated, it is of interest to find the level of speech that is uncomfortably loud for listeners. For normal-hearing subjects this intensity often extends to the upper limit of the speech audiometer (100 to 110 dB HL). In some patients with hearing disorders the **uncomfortable loudness level (UCL)** is much lower, especially when expressed in decibels above the SRT. Some patients find a given level of speech uncomfortable because of its loudness, others because of discomfort produced by the physical pressure of the sound. When possible, it is helpful to determine which effect is active in a given case. The UCL is also called the **threshold of discomfort (TD)**, the **tolerance level,** and the **loudness discomfort level (LDL)**.

Materials used for the UCL can be identical to those used for the MCL. Patients should be instructed to signal, either verbally or by whatever method is decided on, when the speech is uncomfortably loud. They should be reminded that the UCL may be considerably above the level at which they find the loudness of speech most enjoyable, but that they should signal only when exceeding a given level would be intolerable.

Cross-Hearing and Masking for UCL Level Tests

All the statements pertaining to cross-hearing and masking for MCL also pertain to UCL. Masking for UCL is not usually performed. However, if desired, the masking level may be determined in the same way as outlined for MCL.

Recording UCL Level Test Results

The audiometric form used in this book has no space devoted to the recording of the UCL. Appropriate space is provided on worksheets devised for sound-field speech audiometry used during hearing-aid evaluations. Audiologists who carry out UCL measurements under earphones design their audiometric data sheets accordingly.

Range of Comfortable Loudness

The **range of comfortable loudness (RCL)** is the arithmetic difference between the SRT and the UCL. This difference is also called the **dynamic range (DR)** for speech. A normal-hearing person has an RCL of 100 dB or more. The RCL determination is helpful in selecting hearing aids and in other rehabilitative measures. In situations where an SRT cannot be obtained, the difference between the SDT and the UCL provides a reasonable estimate of the RCL.

SPEECH DISCRIMINATION TESTING

A common primary complaint offered by patients is that they have difficulty in understanding what people are saying. This difficulty in discriminating among the sounds of speech plagues patients much more than does a reduction in loudness. Patients often state that their discrimination problems are solved when the speech is louder. Making speech louder can be accomplished by decreasing the distance from the listener to the speaker, by having the speaker increase his or her vocal loudness, or by using a system of sound amplification. Most patients with conductive hearing losses show improved discrimination when loudness is increased. Many patients with sensorineural problems, however, complain that even when sounds are made louder, they have difficulty with speech discrimination. These are the patients who claim, "I can hear, but I can't understand."

The development of materials for speech discrimination testing has been long and slow. For any test to be useful, it should be both reliable and valid. Reliability means that a test is able to reveal similar scores on subsequent administrations (test–retest reliability) and that different forms of the same test result in equivalent scores. The validity of any speech discrimination test relates to the following:

1. How well it measures what it is supposed to measure (a person's difficulties in understanding speech)
2. How favorably a test compares with other, similar measures
3. How the test stands up to alterations of the signal (such as by distortion or presentation with noise) that are known to affect other speech tests in specific ways.

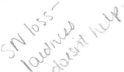
Conductive loss - louder helps

SN loss - loudness doesn't help

The quantitative determination of a patient's ability to discriminate speech helps the audiologist in several ways:

1. It determines the extent of the discrimination difficulty.
2. It aids in diagnosis of the site of the disorder in the auditory system.
3. It assists in the determination of the need for and proper selection of amplification systems.
4. It helps the clinician to make a prognosis for the outcome of rehabilitative efforts.

Through the years a number of different expressions have been used to describe the measurement of speech discrimination. The expression *speech recognition score* has appeared in the literature with greater frequency in recent years and may become the term of choice in the future. Konkle and Rintelmann (1983, p. 6) contend that the word *discrimination* in this context implies distinguishing between different stimuli, whereas *recognition* suggests the report of a patient on what has been heard after the presentation of a single item. For purposes of this book, the terms *speech discrimination score* (SDS) and *speech recognition score* (SRS) (not to be confused with SRT) will be used interchangeably to describe tests performed to determine an individual's understanding of speech stimuli.

Several methods have been advanced for measuring speech discrimination. These include testing with nonsense syllables, digits, monosyllabic words, and sentences. Procedures have included both open- and closed-response message sets. In the open-response set approach, the patient may respond by selecting an answer from an infinite number of possible utterances. On the other hand, in a closed-response system, the patient must choose the correct response from a group of words, sentences, or pictures from which the stimulus is selected.

Egan (1948) showed a relationship between the number of sounds in a word and the ability to discriminate that word. The more phonemes contained in a word, the more easily it is discriminated. Also, the more acoustic redundancy contained in a speech signal, the more easily it is recognized. Discrimination gets poorer as more and more high frequencies are eliminated from speech, which decreases intelligibility without affecting overall loudness very much. As frequencies below about 1900 Hz are removed from speech, the effect on discrimination is much less than that of removing higher frequencies (French & Steinberg, 1947).

Phonetically Balanced Word Lists

Original attempts at discrimination testing (Egan, 1948) involved compiling lists of words that are **phonetically balanced (PB)**—that is, words that contain all the phonetic elements of connected English discourse in their normal proportion to one another. Egan's work at the Psychoacoustic Laboratories at Harvard University resulted in 20 lists of 50 words each. When a weight of

2% per word was allowed, a discrimination score, in percentage terms, could be determined by counting the number of correct words out of 50 and multiplying this number by 2%. Formerly, some audiologists preferred the concept of speech discrimination loss, which was the number of incorrect words out of 50, multiplied by 2%. Most audiologists today prefer to record the **speech discrimination score (SDS)**, or the percentage of the speech material understood.

Hirsh and others (1952) eliminated most of Egan's original 1000 phonetically balanced words and were left with a total of 200 words, of which 180 were derived from Egan's list. These 200 words were divided into four lists of 50 words each, with each list scrambled into six sublists. The resultant PB word lists, known as CID Auditory Test W–22, are commercially available.[3] Ross and Huntington (1962) found some slight differences among the W–22 word lists in terms of discrimination scores, but showed that the magnitude of the differences among lists is small enough that they may be used interchangeably in clinical practice. Four PB word lists from CID Auditory Test W–22 are included in the Appendix.

Because many of the words contained in adult PB word lists are unfamiliar to children, Haskins (1949) developed four lists of 50 words, all within the vocabularies of small children. The test may be presented by tape or by monitored live voice, and is scored in the same way as PB words when adults or older children are tested.[4] Three PBK (for kindergarten) word lists are included in the Appendix; one of these (list 2) was found to be much easier than the other three and therefore is not included. The test increases sharply in difficulty for children younger than 3½ years (Sanderson-Leepa & Rintelmann, 1976).

Performance-Intensity Curves for PB Words. As was indicated earlier in this chapter, many of the word lists currently employed in speech recognition testing were developed during World War II to test the efficiency with which electronic communications systems could transmit speech. Thus, the primary objective was to design military communication systems that would, while transmitting a minimum of acoustic content, enable the listener to understand the message. Hence, the term *articulation* was used to express the "connection" achieved between the listener and the speaker—that is, the joining together of the two by means of a communication system. Use of the word *articulation* in this context is sometimes confusing to students of speech-language pathology, who learn to use this word to mean the manner in which speech sounds are produced with such organs as the tongue, lips, palate, and teeth.

Research has been conducted to determine the articulation-gain functions of PB word lists—that is, the percentage of correct identifications of the words at a variety of sensation levels. As Figure 4.1 illustrates, for normal-hearing

[3]Technisonic Studios, 1201 South Brentwood Boulevard, Richmond Heights, Missouri 63117.

[4]Auditec of St. Louis, 402 Pasadena Avenue, St. Louis, Missouri 63119.

individuals the maximum PB score (100%) is obtained about 35 to 40 dB above the SRT. For some people, especially those with sensorineural hearing losses, the maximum obtainable score is below 100%. The highest PB word score, in percentage terms, obtainable regardless of intensity, is called the **PB Max** (Eldert & Davis, 1951). The term **performance-intensity function** for PB wordlists **(PI-PB)** has replaced the old articulation-gain function terminology. PI-PB functions are discussed again in later chapters of this book, in terms of its diagnostic value.

Consonant-Nucleus-Consonant Word Lists

The phonetic construction of the English language is such that there is no way to truly balance a list of words phonetically, especially a relatively short list. This is because of the almost infinite number of variations that can be made on each phoneme (allophones) as it is juxtaposed with other phonemes. Lehiste and Peterson (1959) prepared ten 50-word lists that were phonemically balanced, a concept they judged to be more realistic than phonetic balancing. Each monosyllabic word contained a consonant, followed by a vowel or diphthong, followed by another consonant. The words were called **consonant-nucleus-consonant (CNC)** words and were scored the same way as the original PB word lists. Later, the CNC lists were revised (Lehiste & Peterson, 1962) by removing proper names, rare words, and the like. Duffy (1983) suggested scoring each of the three phonemes correctly identified, rather than using the correct-or-incorrect approach, in order to give patients credit for all the sounds that have been discriminated.

Tillman, Carhart, and Wilber (1963) took 95 words from the CNC lists (Lehiste & Peterson, 1959) and added 5 of their own, thereby generating two lists of 100 words each. Tillman and Carhart (1966) later developed four lists of 50 words each (Northwestern University Test No. 6), which they found to have high interest reliability. Each of the four lists is scrambled into four randomizations. The four main lists (alphabetized) are included in the Appendix. Auditory test NU–6 remains very popular and is commercially available.[5] It is important to remember, however, that patient responses to this test, as to other speech discrimination tests, may change on the basis of a number of variables, not the least of them being differences among the talkers who make the recordings. This problem is increased when the test is performed in the presence of background noise (Frank & Craig, 1984).

High-Frequency Emphasis Lists

Gardner (1971) developed two lists with 25 words on each (see the Appendix), with each word carrying a value of 4%. The test used with these lists is designed to measure the speech discrimination of patients with high-frequency hearing losses, who are known to have special difficulties in under-

---

[5]Available from Auditec of St. Louis.

standing speech. Each of the words contains the vowel /I/ (as in *kick*), and is preceded and followed by a voiceless consonant. Gardner suggested that the test is more useful if the words are spoken by a woman with a high-pitched voice. A similar approach to high-frequency word lists was taken by Pascoe (1975).

Nonsense-Syllable Lists

Edgerton and Danhauer (1979) developed two lists of 25 nonsense syllable items each. Each item contains a two-syllable utterance with each syllable produced by a consonant followed by a vowel (CVCV). Carhart (1965) originally suggested that nonsense words are too abstract and difficult for many patients to discriminate, and this is sometimes true of the CVCV test. It does have the advantage that each phenome can be scored individually, eliminating the obvious errors in the all-or-none scoring used in PB word tests. The advantages of such testing have also been supported by further research (Doyle, Danhauer, & Edgerton, 1980).

Testing Speech Discrimination with Half-Lists

A number of researchers (Elpern, 1961; Lynn, 1962; Resnick, 1962) have suggested that time can be saved in speech discrimination testing by limiting the test lists to 25 words, using one-half of each list with a weight of 4% per word. Opposition to this procedure (Grubb, 1963) is based on the following arguments: (1) that one half of a list may produce fewer audible sounds than the other half, (2) that there may be some real differences in difficulty of discrimination between the two halves of a list, but primarily that (3) splitting the lists causes them to lose their phonetic balance. Tobias (1964) pointed out that phonetic balancing is unnecessary in a "useful diagnostic test" and that half-lists do measure the same thing as full lists. The studies of Schwartz, Bess, and Larson (1977) and of Edgerton, Klodd, and Beattie (1978) have suggested that the use of half-lists is not advisable. On the other hand, Thornton and Raffin (1978) showed half-lists to be as reliable as the full 50 word lists. Martin and Morris (1989) found that most audiologists prefer to test with 25 word lists.

It has been demonstrated that very good or very poor speech recognition scores may be found using as few as 10 words (Hosford-Dunn, Runge, & Montgomery, 1983; Rose, Schreurs, & Miller, 1979) if the word list is rank-ordered. Because an entire list of 50 words, including the carrier phrases, takes less than 5 minutes to administer, the extensive arguments over time saving seem unfounded. Although this controversy is unresolved, it is probably advisable, when testing with monosyllables, to use all 50 words. When time is a factor, and a patient has achieved a high score on the first 25 words (that is, has missed no more than 2 words), the second half of the list may be eliminated if this high score is consistent with other audiometric data, such as the type and amount of hearing loss present.

Testing of Monosyllables Using a Closed Response Set

The closed-set paradigm for speech discrimination testing followed the development of a rhyme test developed by Fairbanks (1958). House and Colleagues (1965) developed the Modified Rhyme Test, in which the patients are supplied with six rhyming words from which they select the one they think they have heard. Fifty sets of items are presented to the patient, along with a noise in the test ear. Half of the word sets vary only on the initial phoneme, and the other half differ in the final phoneme. Variations on the rhyme test procedure have been proposed by Kreul and co-workers (1968).

A test designed to be sensitive to the discrimination problems of patients with high-frequency hearing losses is the **California Consonant Test** (Owens & Schubert, 1977). One hundred monosyllabic words are arranged in two scramblings to produce two test lists. The subject, selecting from four possibilities, marks a scoresheet next to the word that has been discriminated. Whereas normal-hearing individuals obtain high scores on this test, patients with high-frequency hearing losses show some difficulty. The increased difficulty found in the California Consonant Test was compared to that of the NU–6 lists for patients with high-frequency hearing losses by Schwartz and Surr (1979).

The **picture identification task (PIT)** was developed by Wilson and Antablin (1980) to test the speech discrimination of adults who could not produce verbal responses and had difficulty in selecting items from a printed worksheet. CNC words are represented by pictures that are arranged into sets of four rhyming words. The developers of the PIT found that it provides good estimates of speech discrimination for the nonverbal adult population.

Recognizing the need for testing the speech discrimination abilities of small children who are either unable or unwilling to respond in the fashion used with adults, Ross and Lerman (1970) developed the **Word Intelligibility by Picture Identification (WIPI)** test. The child is presented with a card that contains six pictures. Four of the six pictures are possibilities as the stimulus word on a given test, and the other two words on each card (which are never tested) act as foils to decrease the probability of a correct guess. Twenty-five such cards are assembled in a spiral binder. Children indicate which picture corresponds to the word they believe they have heard. This procedure is very useful in working with children whose discrimination for speech cannot otherwise be evaluated, provided that the stimulus words are within the children's vocabularies. Incorrect identification of words simply because they are not known is common with children under 3½ years of age (Sanderson-Leepa & Rintelmann, 1976). This test has been modified for use in sentence tests (Bench, Kovall, & Bamford, 1979; Weber & Reddell, 1976). The WIPI test just described is available commercially.[6] The test words are listed in the Appendix.

The *Northwestern University Children's Perception of Speech (NU-CHIPS)* test (Elliot & Katz, 1980) is similar to the WIPI. Each child is presented with a

[6]Stanwix House, Inc., Pittsburgh, Pennsylvania.

series of four picture sets, including 65 items with 50 words scored on the test. The use of this procedure appears to be gaining in popularity.

Testing Speech Discrimination with Sentences

Jerger, Speaks, and Trammell (1968) objected to the use of single words as a discrimination test on the basis that single words do not provide enough information regarding the time domain of speech. Normal connected speech is constantly changing in pattern over time, thus necessitating the use of a longer sample than single words can provide for a realistic test. Jerger, Speaks, and Trammell also iterated the problems inherent in testing using an open-message set. Other criticisms of sentence tests include the effects of memory and learning, familiarity with the items as a result of repetition, and the methods of scoring used. Much of the opposition to sentence tests is that their structure enables a listener who is a good guesser to make more meaning of a sentence than does another patient with similar speech recognition abilities.

A number of different sentence tests have been devised to measure speech recognition. One of the first was the Central Institute for the Deaf (CID) Everyday Sentence Test (Silverman & Hirsh, 1955), which was revised several times but never demonstrated the reliability necessary for a speech discrimination test.

Kalikow, Stevens, and Elliott (1977) developed a test made up of eight lists of 50 sentences each, with only the last word in each sentence as the test item, resulting in 200 test words (each of them a noun that appears twice). The test items are recorded on one channel of a two-channel tape, and a voice babble is recorded on the second channel. In this way the two hearing-level dials of a speech audiometer can control the ratio of the intensities of the two signals. This procedure, which has been called the **SPIN (Speech Perception in Noise)** test, continues to undergo attempts at standardization (Bilger, Nuetzel, Rabinowitz, & Rzeczkowski, 1984).

The test devised by Jerger, Speaks, and Trammell involves the development of a set of 10 synthetic sentences, each containing seven words. All items were selected from Thorndike's list of the 1000 most familiar words: The sentences, recorded on magnetic tape, are presented to patients, who indicate their responses by pushing a button corresponding to the sentences they have heard. Some sentences are more difficult than others. Because early experimentation showed that the test is not difficult enough when presented in quiet, a competing message of connected speech is presented in the test ear along with the synthetic sentences, and the intensity of the competing message is varied. Examples of 10 sentences used for **synthetic sentence identification (SSI)** are shown in the Appendix.

A test which appears to be increasing in popularity is the **Connected Speech Test (CST)** (Cox, Alexander, & Gilmore, 1987; Cox, Alexander, Gilmore, & Pusakulich, 1988). The most recent version of the test contains several practice passages and 48 test passages of continuous discourse, each approximately 30 seconds in length. On the second channel of a stereo recording tape is a babble of six simultaneous speakers, which is played to the same ear and thus serves as competition for the test sentences. Each passage contains 25 key words, which are used for scoring—5 words at each of five levels of difficulty. Listeners are instructed to repeat each sentence within a given passage in its entirety. Intelligibility scores are based on the number of key words repeated correctly. The CST appears to meet many of the criteria for reliability and validity not found in other sentence tests and thus holds promise as a diagnostic tool.

Cross-Hearing and Masking in Speech Discrimination Tests

When speech discrimination tests are delivered at suprathreshold levels, the danger of cross-hearing is even greater than during threshold tests. Because cross-hearing of an air-conducted signal occurs by bone conduction, the likelihood of opposite-ear participation in a discrimination test increases as the level of the test signal increases. In addition, the better the bone-conduction threshold in the nontest ear, the greater the probability that it will be stimulated by the speech. In other words, whenever the hearing level of the words minus the interaural attenuation equals or exceeds the bone-conduction threshold of the nontest ear, cross-hearing is a strong probability. Expressed as a formula:

$$\text{PBHL}_{\text{TE}} - \text{IA} \geq \text{Best BC}_{\text{NTE}}$$

As in the case of the SRT, the interaural attenuation is considered to be as little as 40 dB, and the bone-conduction threshold inserted in the formula is the lowest (that is, the best) one obtained in the nontest ear at any frequency. Whenever masking is needed during SRT testing, it will always be needed for discrimination testing for the same ear. Often, however, masking becomes necessary only when the level of speech is raised above the SRT for the discrimination test. Whatever masking noise is available for SRT should be used as well for finding the SDS. The noise should be calibrated as effective masking for speech. Although several masking methods have been suggested, I have found the one described here to be useful (Martin, 1972). The effective masking level for the masked ear is equal to the hearing level at which the discrimination test is performed (PBHL), minus 40 dB for interaural attenuation, plus the largest air–bone gap in the masked ear:

$$\text{EM} = \text{PBHL}_{\text{TE}} - \text{IA} + \text{ABG}_{\text{NTE}}$$

The effective masking level thus derived is just sufficient to mask speech at the nontest ear if the interaural attenuation is as low as 40 dB, and it is more than enough noise if the IA is greater than 40 dB (a probability). If the interaural attenuation can be computed on the basis of masking needs for SRT, the larger number should be used in the formula, which lowers the effective masking level and decreases the chance of overmasking.

The use of insert receivers for speech discrimination testing has several distinct advantages over the use of standard audiometer earphones. Presenting the words through the insert receiver increases the interaural attenuation from the test ear to the nontest ear. For example, substituting 70 dB for 40 dB as the minimum amount of interaural attenuation in the formula shown previously for determining the need to mask during speech recognition testing will eliminate masking entirely for a large number of subjects. When masking is required, if it is delivered through an insert receiver, the possibility of over-masking is reduced or eliminated because the interaural attenuation of the masking noise from nontest ear to test ear will likewise be increased. Seventy decibels can also replace 40 dB as interaural attenuation in the formulas used for determining the effective masking level needed for speech discrimination testing. Finally, the attenuation of background room noise that is provided by insert phones relative to standard phones may result in improved speech recognition when testing is done at low sensation levels.

Whenever the nontest ear is masked for speech discrimination, just as for other audiometric measures, the level of effective masking should be indicated on the audiometric worksheet (Figure 4.2N). In this way, if someone other than the examiner should review the test results, the precise masking level that was used in testing can be seen.

Compensation for Central Masking. If the SRT was obtained with contra-lateral masking, the central masking correction of 5 dB may have been subtracted before the result was recorded. This correction must be borne in mind when setting the hearing level for the speech discrimination test. If masking is required for finding the SDS but not for determining the SRT, the clinician should assume that a 5 dB shift would have occurred if masking had been used when finding the SRT. In such cases the hearing level should be increased for speech discrimination testing to compensate for the loss of loudness of the speech signal that results when noise is presented to the nontest ear. An example of proper masking for SDS will be shown in Figure 4.5.

Maximum Masking. Just as the need for masking increases as the hearing level is increased for the test stimuli, so does the necessary masking level increase. As the level of noise is raised in the masked ear, so is the possibility of overmasking. Rules for maximum masking and overmasking for speech have been expressed in the section on speech recognition threshold and should be scrutinized carefully when masking for speech discrimination tests.

Administration of Speech Discrimination Tests

In administering speech discrimination tests, audiologists must first help patients understand what is expected of them, what the test will consist of, and how they are to respond. Audiologists must decide on:

1. The method of delivery of the speech stimuli
2. The type of materials to be used
3. The method of response
4. The sensation level (in decibels in relation to the SRT) at which the test will be performed

5. Whether more than one level of testing is desired
6. Whether a noise is desired in the test ear (or loudspeaker) to increase the difficulty of the test and, if so, the intensity of the noise
7. Whether masking of the nontest ear is necessary and, if so, the amount and type of noise to use

Instructions to the patients should be delivered orally, even if printed instructions have been read prior to the test. Gestures and pantomimes or the use of sign language may be necessary, although it is likely that any patient who has insufficient language to comprehend oral instructions will be unable to participate in a speech discrimination test. If responses are to be given orally, the patients should be shown the microphone and the proper response should be demonstrated. If the responses are to be written, the proper forms and writing implements, as well as a firm writing surface, should be supplied. Determining that the patient understands the task at hand may save considerable time by avoiding test repetition.

Selection of Stimuli, Materials, and Response Method. Individual audiologists have their own preferences regarding whether to test speech discrimination using monitored live voice, tape, or phonograph recording. Regardless of the method used, the level should be properly controlled and monitored on the VU meter of the audiometer. If a recording is used, it must contain a calibration tone or noise of sufficient duration for the gain control of the VU meter to be adjusted so that the needle peaks at zero VU. If monitored live voice is used, proper microphone technique is very important. The audiologist should be seated in front of the microphone and should speak directly into the diaphragm from a distance of 6 to 12 inches. If monosyllables are being tested, a carrier phrase should be used to prepare the patient for the stimulus word. The last word of the carrier phrase should be at the proper loudness so that the needle of the VU meter will peak at zero, corresponding to the calibration signal. The test word should be uttered with the same monotonous stress and should be allowed to peak where it will, since words vary in power. Test words are not normally expected to peak at zero VU. Sufficient time (about 5 seconds) should be allowed between word presentations to permit the patient to respond.

Patients may respond by repeating the stimulus word, writing down their responses on a form (with 50 numbered spaces for PB words), pushing a button, circling or marking through the correct answer on a closed-message set test, or pointing to a picture or object. It is difficult to gauge the criteria that patients use in determining their responses—that is, whether they are relatively strict or lax in expressing their recognition of specific items. Jerger, Johnson, and Jerger (1988) studied these criteria in elderly hearing-impaired subjects and concluded that attempting to control for this variable is probably not essential. More research along these lines is obviously necessary.

Although no real satisfaction has been universally expressed for speech discrimination materials, audiologists have individual preferences. A recent survey (Martin & Morris, 1989) showed the W–22 PB word lists to be most popular, with the NU–6 lists a close second. The theoretical speech discrimination scores illustrated throughout this book are the probable results on auditory test NU–6. Some audiologists prefer one type of test material for routine hearing tests under earphones and another type for special diagnostic tests and hearing-aid evaluations.

Test Sensation Level. Some audiologists prefer to derive performance intensity functions for their discrimination tests. Others prefer to test at MCL or some fixed level above the SRT. Lezak (1963) recommended that discrimination tests be performed at the upper limits of comfortable loudness (ULCL) and found that discrimination scores obtained at that level were within 4% of the PB Max. Carhart (1965) has pointed out that, if testing is carried out at only one sensation level, there is no way to know that the SDS is the PB Max unless the score is 100%. Although there is no complete agreement on the ideal sensation level for SDS testing, I have found 30 dB to work out well for the initial test. At times other sensation levels (higher or lower) are tested following the first test in an attempt to obtain the maximum speech discrimination score.

Testing Speech Discrimination with Competition. Many audiologists feel that speech discrimination tests carried out in quiet do not tax patients' speech recognition abilities sufficiently to diagnose the kinds of communication problems that are experienced in daily life. For this reason, a noise is often added to the test ear to make discrimination more difficult. When this is done, the relative intensity of the signal (speech) and the noise is specified as the **signal-to-noise ratio (S/N)**. When the speech is 5 dB stronger than the noise, the S/N is +5 dB; when they are both presented at the same intensity, the S/N is zero decibels, and so on.

Signals used to help degrade the discrimination score include modulated white noise (Berry & Nerbonne, 1971), a mixture of noise in one or two speakers (Carhart, Tillman, & Greetis, 1969), one to three speakers (Carhart et al., 1975), two- and four-talker combinations (Young, Parker, & Carhart, 1975), a single speaker (Speaks & Jerger, 1965), or a multitalker babble (Cox, Alexander, & Gilmore, 1987; Cox et al., 1988; Kalikow et al., 1977). Speech has consistently been shown to be a better competing signal than electronically generated noise with a spectrum that resembles speech (Carhart et al., 1975).

Recording Speech Discrimination Test Results

After the speech discrimination tests are completed, the results are recorded on the audiometric worksheet in terms of the percentage of correctly identified words (Figure 4.2M), along with the test or list number (Figure 4.2O); the sensation level at which the test was performed (Figure 4.2P); and, if opposite ear masking was used, the effective masking level (Figure 4.2N) and the type of noise (Figure 4.2Q). If a second discrimination test is carried out with a masking noise in the same ear, the S/N ratio is indicated, along with results and other indentifying information.

Problems in Speech Discrimination Testing

Although the test–retest reliability of PB word tests is good for patients with normal hearing and conductive hearing losses, this reliability fails for patients with primarily sensorineural impairments (Engelberg, 1968). In the literature, estimates of expected test–retest agreement vary from 6% to 18%, but no justification has really been demonstrated for these estimates. Thornton and Raffin (1978) concluded that differences in speech discrimination scores for a given individual depend on the number of items in the test and the *true* score for that test. From a statistical viewpoint, the greatest variability in scores should be found in the middle range of scores (near 50%) and the smallest variability at the extremes (near 0% and 100%). In general, the variability may be assumed to decrease as the number of test items increases. Therefore, it is sometimes risky for audiologists to assume that an increase or decrease in a given patient's speech recognition scores represents a real change in speech discrimination ability.

Attempts have been made to relate the results obtained on speech discrimination tests to the kinds of difficulties experienced by patients. Statements such as "Our test shows you can understand 72% of what you hear" are oversimplified and naïve, for they ignore such important variables as contextual cues, lip-reading, ambient noise level, speaker intelligibility, and so on. Davis (1948) generated a table from which patients' **social adequacy index (SAI)** could be determined from their SRTs and speech discrimination scores. This procedure is not in common use today.

Bone-Conduction Speech Discrimination Testing

At times, in cases of severe mixed hearing loss, a patient's best possible discrimination score may not be attainable because of the severity of the air-conduction hearing loss. In many of these cases it is possible to test speech discrimination by bone conduction in the same way described earlier for testing SRTs. Goetzinger and Proud (1955) found PB word scores to be normal for bone-conducted speech at 25 dB SL in normal-hearing subjects. Discrimination

TABLE 4.1 GENERAL GUIDE FOR THE EVALUATION OF SPEECH DISCRIMINATION SCORES

DISCRIMINATION SCORES (IN PERCENTAGES)	GENERAL SPEECH DISCRIMINATION ABILITY
90%–100%	Normal limits
75%–90%	Slight difficulty, comparable to listening over a telephone
60%–75%	Moderate difficulty
50%–60%	Poor discrimination, marked difficulty in following conversation
<50%	Very poor discrimination; probably unable to follow running speech

Source: Goetzinger 1978.

testing by bone conduction has never become popular, but interest has been shown in this procedure from time to time.

Goetzinger (1978, p. 155) has generated a general guide for evaluating speech discrimination scores, which is presented in Table 4.1. This table, though helpful, should not be interpreted rigidly. Many patients perform considerably better on discrimination tests than they do in daily conversation, and others not nearly as well. Speech discrimination tests are helpful in diagnosis but are far from perfect in terms of predicting real-world communication.

COMPUTERIZED SPEECH AUDIOMETRY

Speech audiometry, like any behavioral measurement, must at times be practiced as more of an art than a science. In a majority of cases, however, it is possible to carry out these measurements in a methodical, scientific manner, using the process of logical decision making. To illustrate this, Wittich, Wood, and Mahaffey (1971) programmed a digital computer to administer SRT and SDS tests, including proper masking, to analyze the patient's responses and to present the results in an audiogram format at the conclusion of the test. Their results were compared to those of an experienced audiologist on a number of actual clinical patients, and very high correlations were observed.

Stach (1988) pointed out that the modern computer can improve the efficiency of speech audiometry in several ways. Speech materials may be pre-

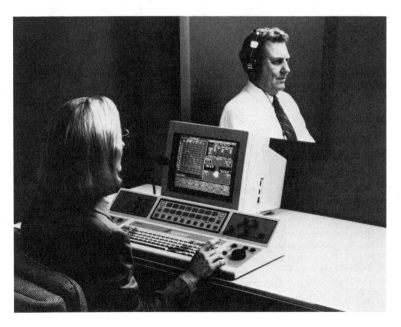

Figure 4.4 Photograph of a computerized audiometric work station. (Courtesy of Nicolet Instrument Corporation.)

AUDIOMETRIC EXAMINATION

NAME: Last - First - Middle			SEX	AGE	DATE	EXAMINER	RELIABILITY	AUDIOMETER

AIR CONDUCTION

MASKING Type	RIGHT									LEFT								
	250	500	1000	1500	2000	3000	4000	6000	8000	250	500	1000	1500	2000	3000	4000	6000	8000
	5	0	5/5	5	0	5	10	5	5	0	5	5/5	5	5	0	0	0	5
EM Level in Opp. Ear																		

BONE CONDUCTION

MASKING Type	RIGHT						FOREHEAD						LEFT					
	250	500	1000	2000	3000	4000	250	500	1000	2000	3000	4000	250	500	1000	2000	3000	4000
							0	5	5	5	5	0						
EM Level in Opp. Ear																		

	2 Frequency	3 Frequency	WEBER						2 Frequency	3 Frequency
Pure Tone Average	0	2	M	M	M	M	M		5	5
								Pure Tone Average		

SPEECH AUDIOMETRY

MASKING Type	RIGHT				LEFT			
	SRT 1	SRT 2	Discrimination 1	Discrimination 2	SRT 1	SRT 2	Discrimination 1	Discrimination 2
	0		1A List 30 SL 100 %	List SL %	5		2A List 30 SL 98 %	List SL %
EM Level in Opp. Ear								

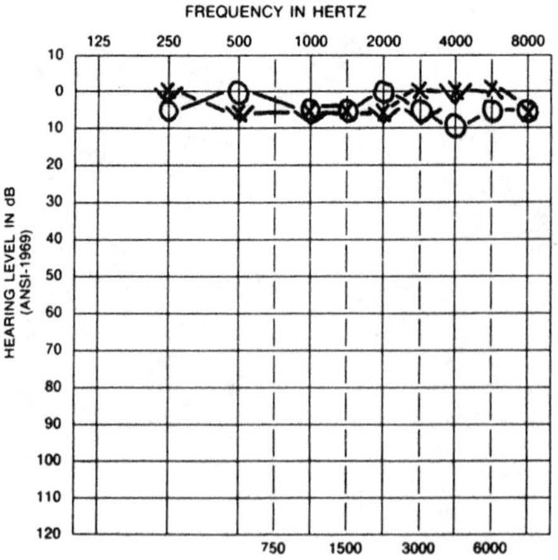

FREQUENCY IN HERTZ

COMMENTS

AUDIOGRAM KEY

	Right	Left
AC Unmasked	O	X
AC Masked	△	□
BC Mastoid Unmasked	<	>
BC Mastoid Masked	[	]
BC Forehead Masked	⌐	⌐

Both	
BC Forehead Unmasked	⋁
Sound field	S
Opp. Ear Masked	✳

Examples of No Response Symbols

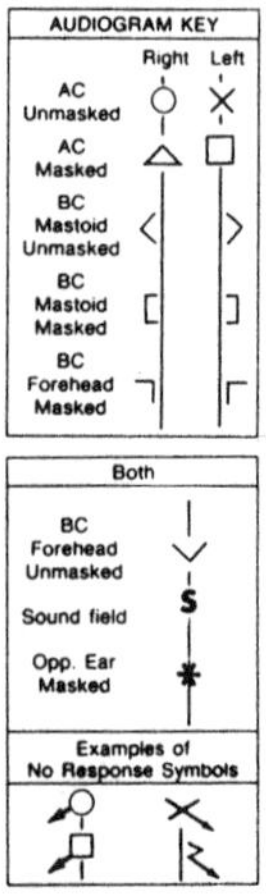

Figure 4.5 Audiogram illustrating normal hearing. Note that both the two- and three-frequency pure-tone averages compare favorably with the SRTs. The SDS in each ear is very high. No masking is indicated for any tests.

NAME: Last - First - Middle	SEX	AGE	DATE	EXAMINER	RELIABILITY	AUDIOMETER

AIR CONDUCTION

MASKING Type	RIGHT									LEFT								
	250	500	1000	1500	2000	3000	4000	6000	8000	250	500	1000	1500	2000	3000	4000	6000	8000
	35	40	45/45	40	40	50	45	50	55	40	40	45/45	45	50	55	55	60	60
EM Level in Opp. Ear																		

BONE CONDUCTION

MASKING Type	RIGHT						FOREHEAD						LEFT					
	250	500	1000	2000	3000	4000	250	500	1000	2000	3000	4000	250	500	1000	2000	3000	4000
NB	5*	5*	15*	20*	20*	15*	5	5	15	20	20	15	10*	5*	15*	20*	20*	20*
EM Level in Opp. Ear	40	40	45	50	55	55							50	40	45	40	50	60

	2 Frequency	3 Frequency	WEBER							2 Frequency	3 Frequency
Pure Tone Average	40	42	M	M	M	M	M	M	Pure Tone Average	43	45

SPEECH AUDIOMETRY

MASKING Type	RIGHT				LEFT			
	SRT 1	SRT 2	Discrimination 1	Discrimination 2	SRT 1	SRT 2	Discrimination 1	Discrimination 2
WB	45	45*	1A List/SL 30 100* %	List/SL %	45	45*	2A List/SL 30 98* %	List/SL %
EM Level in Opp. Ear		55	75			55	75	

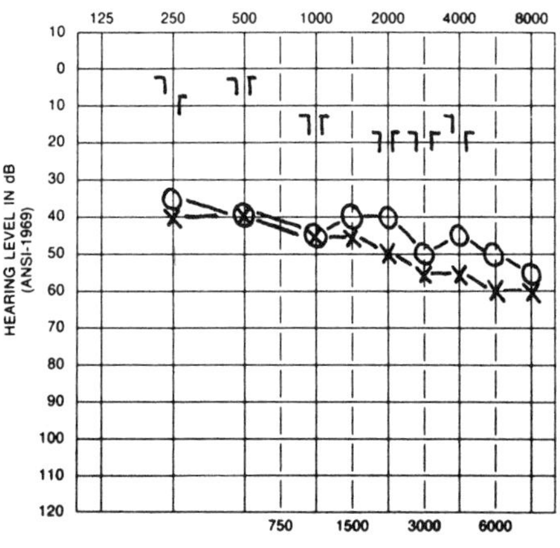

FREQUENCY IN HERTZ

COMMENTS

AUDIOGRAM KEY

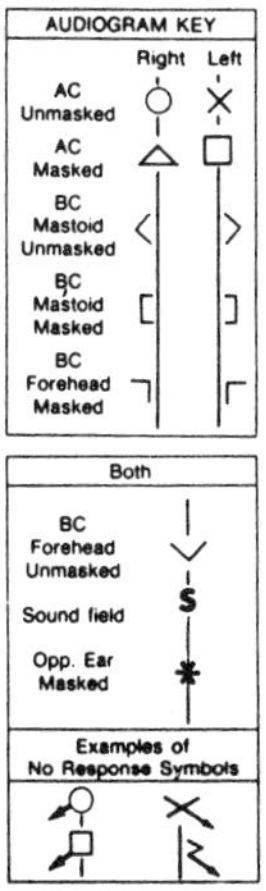

Figure 4.6 Audiogram illustrating conductive hearing loss in both ears. The pure-tone averages are in close agreement with the SRTs. The SDSs are high in both ears. Because of the difference between the SRTs and the opposite-ear bone-conduction thresholds, masking is required for testing SRTs and SDSs for both ears, although no evidence of cross-hearing was found. Wide-band noise was used for all speech masking.

SPEECH AND HEARING CENTER
The University of Texas at Austin 78712
AUDIOMETRIC EXAMINATION

NAME: Last - First - Middle	SEX	AGE	DATE	EXAMINER	RELIABILITY	AUDIOMETER

AIR CONDUCTION

MASKING Type	RIGHT									LEFT								
	250	500	1000	1500	2000	3000	4000	6000	8000	250	500	1000	1500	2000	3000	4000	6000	8000
	35	35	40/40	45	50	60	70	70	75	40	35	45/45	50	55	60	65	65	60
EM Level in Opp. Ear																		

BONE CONDUCTION

MASKING Type	RIGHT						FOREHEAD						LEFT					
	250	500	1000	2000	3000	4000	250	500	1000	2000	3000	4000	250	500	1000	2000	3000	4000
							40	35	40	50	55	65						
EM Level in Opp. Ear																		

	2 Frequency	3 Frequency	WEBER							2 Frequency	3 Frequency
Pure Tone Average	38	42	M	M	M	M	M	M	Pure Tone Average	40	45

SPEECH AUDIOMETRY

MASKING Type	RIGHT				LEFT			
	SRT 1	SRT 2	Discrimination 1	Discrimination 2	SRT 1	SRT 2	Discrimination 1	Discrimination 2
	35		1C List 30 SL 78 %	List SL %	40		2C List 30 SL 80 %	List SL %
EM Level in Opp. Ear								

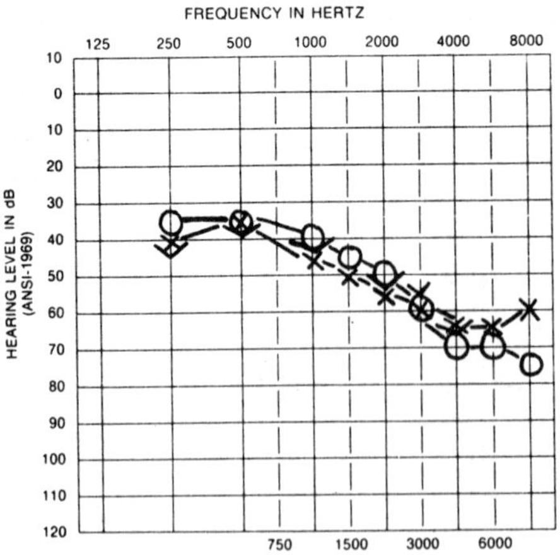

FREQUENCY IN HERTZ

COMMENTS

AUDIOGRAM KEY

bone & air same

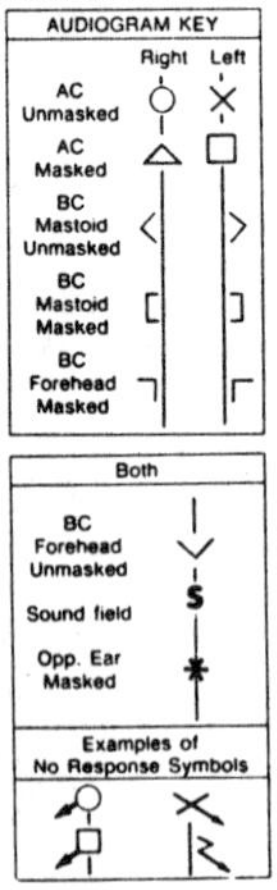

Figure 4.7 Audiogram illustrating a sensorineural hearing loss in both ears. The pure-tone averages of 500 and 1000 Hz agree closely with the SRTs. SDSs are impaired in both ears. No masking is required for any speech tests.

sented by means of a digital tape player (Kamm, Carteretta, Morgan, & Dirks, 1980), allowing for appropriate pacing of stimuli and thus providing the flexibility of live voice testing without its obvious limitations. Furthermore, the digital recordings do not deteriorate with time and use, and therefore the stimuli remain constant. Figure 4.4 shows a computer audiometer in use.

SUMMARY

Speech audiometry includes measurement of a patient's thresholds for speech—either speech recognition threshold (SRT), or speech detection threshold (SDT), most comfortable loudness level (MCL), uncomfortable loudness level (UCL or LDL), range of comfortable loudness (RCL or DR), and speech discrimination score (SDS). Measurements may be made either monaurally or binaurally under earphones, through a bone-conduction vibrator, or in the sound field through loudspeakers. Materials for speech audiometry may include connected speech, two-syllable (spondaic) words, monosyllabic words, or sentences. The materials may be presented by means of a microphone (using monitored live-voice), tape recorder, or phonograph. At times the sensitivity of the nontest ear by bone conduction is such that it may inadvertently participate in a test under earphones. When cross-hearing is a danger, a masking noise is presented to the nontest ear to eliminate its participation in the test.

Measurements using speech audiometry augment the findings of pure-tone tests and help to determine the extent of a patient's hearing loss, tolerance, and discrimination for speech. The knowledge gained from the use of speech audiometry is helpful in the diagnosis of site of lesion in the auditory system, as well as in the management of aural rehabilitation.

The audiograms depicted in Chapter 3 to illustrate normal hearing, conductive hearing loss, and sensorineural hearing loss are repeated in Figures 4.5, 4.6, and 4.7. These audiograms show the probable results obtained during speech audiometry, including the use of masking, where indicated.

GLOSSARY

Binaural Listening with both ears to either the same or different stimuli.

California Consonant Test A closed-message speech discrimination test with the emphasis on unvoiced consonants to tax the abilities of patients with high-frequency hearing losses.

Carrier phrase A phrase, such as "Say the word _____" or "You will say _____," which precedes the stim-

ulus word during speech audiometry. It is designed to prepare the patient for the test word and to assist the clinician (if monitored live voice is used) in controlling the input loudness of the test word.

Cold running speech Rapidly delivered speech, either prerecorded or by monitored live voice, such that the output is monotonous and the peaks of the words strike zero on the VU meter.

Connected speech   See *Cold running speech.*

Connected Speech Test (CST)   A procedure by which the intelligibility of speech passages is measured on a sentence-by-sentence basis in the presence of a related background babble.

Consonant-nucleus-consonant (CNC) words   Monosyllabic words used in testing word discrimination.   Each word comprises three phonemes; the initial and final phonemes are consonants, and the middle phoneme is a vowel or diphthong.

Dynamic range (DR) for speech   See *Range of comfortable loudness.*

Loudness discomfort level   See *Uncomfortable loudness level.*

Monaural   Listening with one ear.

Monitored live voice (MLV)   Introduction of a speech signal (as in speech audiometry) by use of a microphone. The loudness of the voice is monitored visually by means of a VU meter.

Most comfortable loudness (MCL)   The hearing level designated by a listener as the most comfortable listening level for speech.

PB Max   The highest speech discrimination score for PB words obtained on a performance intensity function regardless of level.

Performance-intensity function (PI-PB)   A graph showing the percentage correct of speech discrimination materials as a function of intensity.   The graph usually shows the discrimination score on the ordinate and the sensation level on the abscissa.

Phonetically balanced (PB) words   A list of monosyllabic words used for determination of word discrimination scores.   Theoretically, each list contains the same distribution of phonemes that occurs in connected American discourse.

Picture identification task (PIT)   A speech discrimination test using pictures of rhyming CNC words.

Range of comfortable loudness (RCL)   The difference, in decibels, between the threshold for speech and the point at which speech becomes uncomfortably loud.   It is determined by subtracting the SRT from the UCL.

Sawtooth noise   A noise made up of a fundamental frequency of 120 Hz, with equal amplitude at all the harmonic frequencies.

Signal-to-noise ratio (S/N) for speech   The difference in decibels between a signal (such as speech) and a noise presented to the same ear or both ears. When the speech has greater intensity than the noise, a positive sign is used; when the noise has greater intensity than the signal, a negative sign is used.

Social adequacy index (SAI)   A measurement of hearing handicap determined from the SRT and the SDS.

Speech audiometer   An audiometer calibrated in dB HL for speech.   It should be capable of presenting speech materials by monitored live voice, tape, or disk recording.   Signals may be fed into either or both earphones or into the sound field by means of one or more loudspeakers.

Speech detection threshold (SDT)   The hearing level at which a listener can just detect the presence of an ongoing speech signal and identify it as speech. Sometimes called the speech awareness threshold (SAT).

Speech discrimination score (SDS) The percentage of correctly identified items on a speech discrimination test.

Speech recognition threshold (SRT) The threshold of intelligibility of speech. The lowest HL at which 50% of a list of spondees are identified correctly.

Speech Perception in Noise (SPIN) test A sentence speech discrimination test recorded on magnetic tape with a voice babble recorded on the second channel of the same tape.

Spondaic word (spondee) A two-syllable word pronounced with equal stress on both syllables.

Synthetic sentence identification (SSI) test A method for determining speech discrimination by means of seven-word sentences that are grammatically correct but meaningless.

Threshold of discomfort (TD) See *Uncomfortable loudness level.*

Tolerance level See *Uncomfortable loudness level.*

Uncomfortable loudness level (UCL) That sound-pressure level (often referred to in dB HL) at which speech becomes uncomfortably loud.

Word Intelligibility by Picture Identification (WIPI) test A test that uses pictures to determine word discrimination ability in young children.

STUDY QUESTIONS

1. Sketch, from memory, performance-intensity functions for spondaic and PB words. How can you explain the differences in the curves on the basis of the words used?
2. Sketch audiograms illustrating conductive, sensorineural, and mixed hearing losses. Predict the probable SDSs and SRTs. Also predict the probable MCLs, UCLs, and RCLs.
3. What are the theoretical and practical values of the measures obtained in question 2?
4. Determine EM levels, if needed, for all speech tests in question 2.
5. List the different kinds of tests described in this chapter and the different materials used for each test.

REVIEW TABLE 4.1 SUMMARY OF TESTS USED IN SPEECH AUDIOMETRY*

TEST	PURPOSE	MATERIAL	UNIT	WHEN TO MASK	INITIAL MASKING	OVERMASKING	INTERPRETATION
SRT	HL for speech. Verify PTA.	Spondaic words. Cold running speech.	dB	$SRT_{TE} - 40 \geq BBC_{NTE}$	$EM = SRT_{NTE}$ If over 5 dB shift, plateau.	$EM_{NTE} - IA > BBC_{TE}$	± 10 dB of PTA
SDT	HL for speech awareness.	Cold running speech.	dB	$SDT_{TE} - 40 \geq BBC_{NTE}$	$EM = SDT_{NTE}$	$EM_{NTE} - IA > BBC_{TE}$	ST − 10 dB
MCL	Comfort level for speech. HL for WDS.	Cold running speech.	dB	$MCL_{TE} - 40 \geq BBC_{NTE}$	$EM = BBC_{TE} + 40$	$EM_{NTE} - IA > BBC_{TE}$	
UCL	Level at which speech becomes uncomfortably loud.	Cold running speech.	dB	$UCL_{TE} - 40 \geq BBC_{NTE}$	$EM = BBC_{TE} + 40$	$EM_{NTE} - IA > BBC_{TE}$	
RCL (DR)	Dynamic listening range for speech.	Cold running speech.	dB				
SDS	Discrimination for speech.	PB words. CNC words. Rhyming words. Sentences.	%	$HL_{TE} - 40 \geq BBC_{NTE}$	$HL_{TE} - IA + ABG_{NTE}$	$EM_{NTE} - IA > BBC_{TE}$	90%–100% normal or conductive. Below 90% sensorineural.

*TE = test ear; NTE = nontest ear; PTA = pure-tone average; EM = effective masking; IA = interaural attenuation; BBC = best bone-conduction threshold at 500, 1000, 2000, or 4000 Hz.

REFERENCES

AMERICAN SPEECH AND HEARING ASSOCIATION [ASHA]. (1979). Guidelines for determining the threshold level for speech. *Asha, 21,* 353–356.

AMERICAN SPEECH-LANGUAGE-HEARING ASSOCIATION. (1978). Guidelines for manual pure-tone audiometry. *Asha, 20,* 297–301.

———. (1988). Guidelines for determining threshold level for speech. *Asha, 30,* 85–88.

BARRY, S. J., & GADDIS, S. (1978). Physical and physiological constraints on the use of bone conduction speech audiometry. *Journal of Speech and Hearing Disorders, 43,* 220–226.

BEATTIE, R. C., FORRESTER, P. W., & RUBY, B. K. (1987). Reliability of the Tillman-Olsen procedure for determination of spondaic word threshold using recorded and live voice presentation. *Journal of the American Audiology Society, 2,* 159–162.

BENCH, J., KOVAL, A., & BAMFORD, J. (1979). The BKB (Bamford-Koval-Bench) sentence lists for partially-hearing children. *British Journal of Audiology, 13,* 108–112.

BERGER, K. W. (1969). Speech discrimination task using multiple choice key words in sentences. *Journal of Auditory Research, 9,* 247–262.

BERRY, R. C., & NERBONNE, C. P. (1971, October). *Comparison of the masking function of speech modulated and white noise.* Paper presented to the 82nd meeting of the Acoustical Society of America, Denver.

BILGER, R. C., NUETZEL, J. M., RABINOWITZ, W. M., & RZECZKOWSKI, C. (1984). Standardization of a test of speech perception in noise. *Journal of Speech and Hearing Research, 27,* 32–48.

BURKE, L. E., & NERBONNE, M. A. (1978). The influence of the guess factor on the speech reception threshold. *Journal of the American Auditory Society, 4,* 87–90.

CARHART, R. (1965). Problems in the measurement of speech discrimination. *Archives of Otolaryngology, 82,* 253–260.

CARHART, R., & JERGER, J. (1959). A preferred method for the clinical determination of pure tone thresholds. *Journal of Speech and Hearing Disorders, 24,* 330–345.

CARHART, R., JOHNSON, C., & GOODMAN, J. (1975, November). *Perceptual masking of spondees by combination of talkers.* Paper presented to the 90th meeting of the Acoustical Society of America, San Francisco.

CARHART, R., & PORTER, L. S. (1971). Audiometric configuration and prediction of threshold for spondees. *Journal of Speech and Hearing Research, 14,* 486–495.

CARHART, R., TILLMAN, T. W., & GREETIS, E. S. (1969). Perceptual masking in multiple sound backgrounds. *Journal of the Acoustical Society of America, 45,* 694–703.

CHAIKLIN, J. B., & VENTRY, I. M. (1964). Spondee threshold measurement: A comparison of 2- and 5-dB methods. *Journal of Speech and Hearing Disorders, 29,* 47–59.

CONN, M., DANCER, J., & VENTRY, I. M. (1975). A spondee list for determining speech reception threshold without prior familiarization. *Journal of Speech and Hearing Disorders, 40,* 376–388.

COX, R. M., ALEXANDER, G. C., & GILMORE, C. (1987). Development of the Connected Speech Test (CST). *Ear and Hearing, 8,* 1195–1265.

COX, R. M., ALEXANDER, G. C., GILMORE, C., & PUSAKULICH, K. M. (1980). Use of the Connected Speech Test with hearing-impaired listeners. *Ear and Hearing, 9,* 198–207.

DAVIS, H. (1948). The Articulation Area and the Social Adequacy Index for Hearing. *Laryngoscope, 58,* 761–768.

DOYLE, K. J., DANHAUER, J. L., & EDGERTON, B. J. (1980). Features from normal and sensorineural listeners' nonsense syllable test errors. *Ear and Hearing, 2,* 117–121.

DUFFY, J. K. (1983). The role of phoneme-recognition audiometry in hearing rehabilitation. *The Hearing Journal, 37,* 24–28.

EDGERTON, B. J., & DANHAUER, J. L. (1979). *Clinical implications of speech discrimination testing using nonsense stimuli.* Baltimore: University Park Press.

EDGERTON, B. J., DANHAUER, J. L., & BEATTIE, R. C. (1977). Bone conduction speech audiometry in normal subjects. *Journal of the American Audiology Society, 3*, 84–87.

EDGERTON, B. J., KLODD, D. A., & BEATTIE, R. C. (1978). Half-list speech discrimination measures in hearing aid evaluations. *Archives of Otolaryngology, 104*, 669–672.

EGAN, J. P. (1948). Articulation testing methods. *Laryngoscope, 58*, 955–991.

ELDERT, M. A., & DAVIS, H. (1951). The articulation function of patients with conductive deafness. *Laryngoscope, 61*, 891–909.

ELLIOT, L., & KATZ, D. (1980). Development of a new children's test of speech discrimination. St. Louis: Auditec.

ELPERN, B. S. (1961). The relative stability of half-list and full-list discrimination tests. *Laryngoscope, 71*, 30–35.

ENGELBERG, M. (1968). Test–retest variability in speech discrimination testing. *Laryngoscope, 78*, 1582–1589.

FAIRBANKS, G. (1958). Test of phonemic differentiation: The rhyme test. *Journal of the Acoustical Society of America, 30*, 596–601.

FLETCHER, H. (1950). Method of calculating hearing loss for speech from an audiogram. *Journal of the Acoustical Society of America, 22*, 1–5.

FRANK, T., & CRAIG, C. H. (1984). Comparison of the Auditec and Rintelmann recordings of the NU–6. *Journal of Speech and Hearing Disorders, 49*, 267–271.

FRANK, T., & MCPHILLIPS, M. A. (1976). *Relative intelligibility of the CID spondees for normal-hearing and hearing-impaired listeners.* Paper presented to the meeting of the American Speech and Hearing Association, 1976.

FRENCH, M. R., & STEINBERG, J. C. (1947). Factors governing the intelligibility of speech sounds. *Journal of the Acoustical Society of America, 19*, 90–119.

GARDNER, H. J. (1971). Application of a high frequency consonant discrimination word list in hearing-aid evaluation. *Journal of Speech and Hearing Disorders, 36*, 354–355.

GOETZINGER, C. P. (1978). Word discrimination testing. In J. Katz (Ed.), *Handbook of Clinical Audiology* (2nd ed., pp. 149–158). Baltimore: Williams & Wilkins.

GOETZINGER, C. P., & PROUD, G. O. (1955). Speech audiometry by bone conduction. *Archives of Otolaryngology, 62*, 632–635.

GRUBB, P. (1963). Some considerations in the use of half-list speech discrimination tests. *Journal of Speech and Hearing Research, 6*, 294–297.

HAHLBROCK, K. H. (1962). Bone conduction speech audiometry. *International Audiology, 1*, 186–188.

HASKINS, H. (1949). *A phonetically balanced test of speech discrimination for children.* Unpublished master's thesis, Northwestern University.

HIRSH, I., DAVIS, H., SILVERMAN, S. R., REYNOLDS, E., ELDERT, E., & BENSON, R. W. (1952). Development of materials for speech audiometry. *Journal of Speech and Hearing Disorders, 17*, 321–337.

HOSFORD-DUNN, H., RUNGE, C. A., & MONTGOMERY, P. (1983). A shortened rank-ordered word discrimination list. *The Hearing Journal, 36*, 15–19.

HOUSE, A. S., WILLIAMS, C. E., HECKER, M. H. L., & KRYTER, K. D. (1965). Articulation testing methods: Consonantal differentiation with a closed-response set. *Journal of the Acoustical Society of America, 37*, 158–166.

HUDGINS, C. V., HAWKINS, J. E., JR., KARLIN, J. E., & STEVENS, S. S. (1947). The development of recorded auditory tests for measuring hearing loss for speech. *Laryngoscope, 57*–89.

HUFF, S. J., & NERBONNE, M. A. (1982). Comparison of the American Speech-Language-Hearing Association and revised Tillman-Olsen methods for speech threshold measurement. *Ear and Hearing, 3*, 335–339.

JERGER, J., JOHNSON, K., & JERGER, S. (1988). Effect of response criterion on measures of speech understanding in the elderly. *Ear and Hearing, 9*, 49–56.

JERGER, J., SPEAKS, C., & TRAMMELL, J. L. (1968). A new approach to speech audiometry. *Journal of Speech and Hearing Disorders, 33*, 318–328.

KALIKOW, D. M., STEVENS, K. N., & ELLIOTT, L. L. (1977). Development of a test of speech intelligibility in noise using sentence materials with controlled predictability. *Journal of the Acoustical Society of America, 61,* 1337–1351.

KAMM, C., CARTERETTA, E. C., MORGAN, D. E., & DIRKS, D. D. (1980). Use of digital speech materials in audiological research. *Journal of Speech and Hearing Research, 23,* 709–721.

KATZ, D. R., & ELLIOT, L. L. (1980, November). *Development of a new children's speech discrimination test.* Paper presented at the convention of the American Speech-Language-Hearing Association, Chicago.

KONKLE, D. F., & BERRY, G. A. (1983). Masking in speech audiometry. In D. F. Konkle & W. F. Rintelmann (Eds.), *Principles of speech audiometry* (pp. 285–319). Baltimore: University Park Press.

KONKLE, D. F., & RINTELMANN, W. F. (1983). Introduction to speech audiometry. In D. F. Konkle & W. F. Rintelmann (Eds.), *Principles of Speech Audiometry* (pp. 1–10). Baltimore: University Park Press.

KOPRA, L. L., & BLOSSER, D. (1968). Effects of method of measurement on most comfortable loudness for speech. *Journal of Speech and Hearing Research, 11,* 497–508.

KREUL, E. J., NIXON, J. C., KRYTER, K. D., BELL, D. W., LANG, J. S., & SCHUBERT, E. D. (1968). A proposed clinical test of speech discrimination. *Journal of Speech and Hearing Research, 11,* 536–552.

LEHISTE, I., & PETERSON, G. E. (1959). Linguistic considerations in the study of speech intelligibility. *Journal of the Acoustical Society of America, 31,* 280–286.

———. (1962). Revised CNC lists for auditory tests. *Journal of Speech and Hearing Disorders, 27,* 62–70.

LEVITT, H. (1978). Adaptive testing in audiology. *Scandinavian Audiology Supplement, 6,* 241–291.

LEZAK, R. (1962). Determination of an intensity level to obtain PB max. *Laryngoscope, 73,* 267–274.

LYNN, G. (1962). Paired PB-50 discrimination test: A preliminary report. *Journal of Auditory Research, 2,* 34–37.

MARTIN, F. N. (1966). Speech audiometry and clinical masking. *Journal of Auditory Research, 6,* 199–203.

———. (1972). *Clinical Audiometry and Masking.* The Bobbs-Merrill Studies in Communicative Disorders. New York: Bobbs-Merrill.

MARTIN, F. N., BAILEY, H. A. T., & PAPPAS, J. J. (1965). The effect of central masking on threshold for speech. *Journal of Auditory Research, 5,* 293–296.

MARTIN, F. N., & BLYTHE, M. (1977). On the cross-hearing of spondaic words. *Journal of Auditory Research, 17,* 221–224.

MARTIN, F. N., & DIGIOVANNI, D. (1979). Central masking effects on spondee thresholds as a function of masker sensation level and masker sound pressure level. *Journal of the American Audiology Society, 4,* 141–146.

MARTIN, F. N., & DOWDY, L. K. (1986). A modified spondee threshold procedure. *Journal of Auditory Research, 26,* 115–119.

MARTIN, F. N., & FORBIS, N. (1978). The present status of audiometric practice: A follow-up study. *Asha, 20,* 531–541.

MARTIN, F. N., & MORRIS, L. J. (1989). Current audiological practices in the United States. *The Hearing Journal, 42,* 25–42.

MARTIN, F. N., & STAUFFER, M. L. (1975). A modification of the Tillman-Olsen method for obtaining the speech reception threshold. *Journal of Speech and Hearing Disorders, 40,* 25–28.

MERRILL, H. B., WOLFE, D. L., & McLEMORE, D. C. (1973). Air and bone conducted speech reception thresholds. *Laryngoscope, 83,* 1929–1939.

MERRILL, H. B., & ATKINSON, C. J. (1965). The effect of selected variables upon discrimination scores. *Journal of Auditory Research, 5,* 285–292.

OWENS, E., & SCHUBERT, E. D. (1977). Development of the California Consonant Test. *Journal of Speech and Hearing Research, 20,* 463–474.

PASCOE, D. R. (1975). Frequency responses of hearing aids and their effects on the speech perception of hearing impaired subjects.

Annals of Otology, Rhinology and Laryngology, 23 (Supplement), 1–40.

RESNICK, D. (1962). Reliability of the twenty-five word phonetically balanced lists. *Journal of Auditory Research, 2,* 5–12.

ROBINSON, D., & KOENIGE, M. J. (1979). Comparisons of procedures and materials for speech reception thresholds. *Journal of the American Audiology Society, 4,* 223–230.

ROSE, D. E., SCHREURS, K. K., & MILLER, K. E. (1979). A ten-word speech discrimination screening test. *Audiology and Hearing Education, 5,* 15–16.

ROSE, M., & HUNTINGTON, D. A. (1962). Concerning the reliability and equivalency of the CID W–22 auditory tests. *Journal of Auditory Research, 2,* 220–228.

ROSS, M., & LERMAN, J. (1970). A picture identification test for hearing impaired children. *Journal of Speech and Hearing Research, 13,* 44–53.

SANDERSON-LEEPA, M. E., & RINTELMANN, W. F. (1976). Articulation function and test-retest performance of normal-hearing children on three speech discrimination tests: WIPI, PBK 50 and NU Auditory Test No. 6. *Journal of Speech and Hearing Disorders, 41,* 503–519.

SCHWARTZ, D. M., BESS, F. H., & LARSON, V. D. (1977). Split half reliability of two-word discrimination tests as a function of primary to secondary ratio. *Journal of Speech and Hearing Disorders, 42,* 440–445.

SCHWARTZ, D. M., & SURR, R. (1979). Three experiments on the California Consonant Test. *Journal of Speech and Hearing Disorders, 44,* 61–72.

SILVERMAN, S. R., & HIRSH, I. J. (1955). Problems related to the use of speech in clinical audiometry. *Annals of Otology, Rhinology and Laryngology, 64,* 1234–1244.

SPEAKS, C., & JERGER, J. (1965). Method for measurement of speech identification. *Journal of Speech and Hearing Research, 8,* 185–194.

SPEARMAN, C. (1908). The method of "right and wrong cases" ("Constant Stimuli") without Gauss's formulae. *British Journal of Audiology, 2,* 227–242.

SRINIVASSON, K. P. (1974). Bone conducted speech reception threshold: An investigation with the Oticon A20 bone vibrator calibrated on the Bruel and Kjaer artificial mastoid. *Scandinavian Audiology, 3,* 145–148.

STACH, B. A. (1988). Computers and audiologic instrumentation. *Hearing Instruments, 39,* 13–16.

THORNTON, A. R., & RAFFIN, M. J. M. (1978). Speech discrimination scores modified as a binomial variable. *Journal of Speech and Hearing Research, 21,* 507–518.

TILLMAN, T. W., & CARHART, R. (1966). *An expanded test for speech discrimination utilizing CNC monosyllabic words.* Northwestern University Auditory Test No. 6, Technical Report, SAM–TR–66–55. Brooks Air Force Base, TX: USAF School of Aerospace Medicine, Aerospace Medical Division (AFSC).

TILLMAN, T. W., CARHART, R., & WILBER, L. (1963). *A test for speech discrimination composed of CNC monosyllabic words.* Northwestern University Auditory Test No. 4, Technical Report, SAM–TDR–62–135. Brooks Air Force Base, TX: USAF School of Aerospace Medicine, Aerospace Medical Division (AFSC).

TILLMAN, T. W., & JERGER, J. F. (1959). Some factors affecting the spondee threshold in normal-hearing subjects. *Journal of Speech and Hearing Research, 2,* 141–146.

TILLMAN, T. W., & OLSEN, W. O. (1973). Speech audiometry. In J. Jerger (Ed.), *Modern Developments in Audiology* (2nd ed., pp. 37–74). New York: Academic Press.

TOBIAS, J. V. (1964). On phonemic analysis of speech discrimination tests. *Journal of Speech and Hearing Research, 7,* 98–100.

WALL, L. G., DAVIS, L. A., & MYERS, D. K. (1984). Four spondee threshold procedures: A comparison. *Ear and Hearing, 5,* 171–174.

WEBER, S., & REDDELL, R. C. (1976). A sentence test for measuring speech discrimination in children. *Audiology and Hearing Education, 2,* 25–30.

WILSON, R. H., & ANTABLIN, J. K. (1980). A picture identification task as an estimate of the word-recognition performance of non-verbal adults. *Journal of Speech and Hearing Disorders, 45,* 223–238.

WILSON, R. H., & MARGOLIS, R. H. (1983). Measurements of auditory thresholds for speech stimuli. In D. F. Konkle & W. F. Rintelmann (Eds.), *Principles of Speech Audiometry* (pp. 79–126). Baltimore: University Park Press.

WILSON, R. H., MORGAN, D. E., & DIRKS, D. D. (1973). A proposed SRT procedure and its statistical precedent. *Journal of Speech and Hearing Disorders, 38*, 184–191.

WITTICH, W. W., WOOD, T. J., & MAHAFFEY, R. B. (1971). Computerized speech audiometric procedures. *Journal of Auditory Research, 11*, 335–344.

YOUNG, L. L., PARKER, C., & CARHART, R. (1975, November). *Effectiveness of speech and noise maskers on numbers embedded in continuous discourse.* Paper presented to the 90th meeting of the Acoustical Society of America, San Francisco.

SUGGESTED READING

KONKLE, D. F., & RINTELMANN, W. F. EDS.). (1983). *Principles of Speech Audiometry.* Baltimore: University Park Press.

5

AUDITORY TESTS
FOR SITE OF LESION

Chapters 3 and 4 discussed pure-tone thresholds and measurements that can be made with speech audiometers. These procedures provide much quantitative and qualitative information about the type and degree of hearing impairment a patient might have. Through the use of these tests, it is possible to separate hearing disorders into two broad types: conductive and sensorineural. Sophisticated tests have been devised that provide useful clues to the precise areas within the auditory system involved in a hearing loss and, in some cases, some strong indications of the cause of the lesion. The purpose of this chapter is to discuss some of the more popular tests that fall into this category.

In many cases performance of special diagnostic hearing tests requires the use of specially designed equipment. With this equipment audiologists can now accumulate, from a variety of tests, valuable information for diagnostic purposes. Some of these tests measure the growth of loudness in pathological ears as compared to normal ears, the rates at which tones fade away from audibility, different kinds of tracking behavior on automatic audiometers, the ability to detect the presence of brief changes in intensity, measurements of impedance and compliance in the plane of the eardrum membrane, and changes in the ongoing pattern of electrical activity in the brain in response to acoustic stimuli.

The **site of a lesion** producing a hearing loss is of more than casual interest to audiologists. Separating conductive from sensorineural hearing losses is not difficult on the basis of the pure-tone and speech tests described in Chapters 3 and 4, but the distinction between *sensory* and *neural* is more difficult to determine. Lesions of the auditory portions of the inner ear are said to be *cochlear* (sensory), and neural lesions beyond the inner ear are often called *retrocochlear*.

Site of lesion tests are helpful in determining the kinds of medical referrals that need to be made and their urgency. As is discussed in subsequent chapters, some tests for site of lesion uncover disorders that are potentially fatal to the patient. The importance of knowing the underlying concepts and having the ability to perform and interpret these tests cannot be overemphasized.

Although there are now many tests to determine site of auditory lesion, each must be subjected to scrutiny to determine its specific usefulness in a particular situation. There are questions about two factors—reliability and validity. *Reliability* has to do with how well a test score is repeatable. Poor reliability can make a test useless, but good reliability does not necessarily make it valuable unless it is also valid. Questions of *validity* ask whether a test measures what it is supposed to measure—in this case, the power with which a test reveals the locus of the disorder in the auditory system.

Because no diagnostic procedure is infallible, any single test will turn out in one of four ways:

1. *True positive:* The test indicates a lesion site correctly.
2. *True negative:* The test correctly eliminates an anatomical area as causing the problem.
3. *False positive:* The test indicates a lesion site incorrectly.
4. *False negative:* The test incorrectly eliminates an anatomical area as causing the hearing problem.

Jerger and Jerger (1983) and Turner and Nielsen (1984) have suggested that audiological tests for site of lesion can be subjected to a set of mathematical models by means of **clinical decision analysis (CDA)**. CDA asks questions about each test's *sensitivity* (how well it correctly identifies a lesion site—true positive), it's *specificity* (the inverse of sensitivity—how well it rejects an incorrect diagnosis, or true negative), its *predictive value* (the percentage of false positive and false negative results), and its *efficiency* (the percentage of true positive and true negative results). These issues will be discussed with respect to the major tests covered in this chapter. Some tests, which require a greater knowledge of anatomy and physiology than has been provided so far in this book, are discussed in Chapters 6 through 9.

CHAPTER OBJECTIVES

At this point the reader should have a good grasp of the tests described earlier, as well as a general knowledge of how the ear is constructed and how it responds to sound. This chapter reviews a number of site-of-lesion tests available to the audiologist for diagnostic purposes. Completion of this chapter should allow the reader to understand and, with exposure to the proper equipment and a period of supervised practice, perform the tests described herein.

LOUDNESS RECRUITMENT

Loudness increases with intensity in a logical and lawful manner. As the intensity of a sound is increased, so is the experience of loudness. It is useful to measure the manner in which the sensation of loudness increases as the physical intensity of the sound is increased. It is possible to compare this "growth of loudness" in the two ears of an individual with normal hearing by pulsing a tone alternately from one ear to the other. The subject's task consists of matching the loudness of the tone in one ear (the test ear) to that of the other (reference) ear. This loudness-balancing procedure is usually performed at several suprathreshold levels. For purposes of illustration let us create a hypothetical individual with normal hearing sensitivity in both ears. The **laddergram** in Figure 5.1A shows that as the intensity of a tone is increased in one ear, a similar increase in loudness in the opposite ear requires the same increase in intensity. This is the normal increase in loudness with increased intensity.

If a hearing loss is imposed on the right ear of our hypothetical subject, greater intensity is required to reach threshold in that ear, but after the threshold has been reached, increases in intensity (in decibels) above the threshold for the impaired ear result in increases in loudness identical to those in the unimpaired ear (Figure 5.1B). Nothing is very surprising about these statements, for logic tells us that a tone of 40 dB SL in a normal ear should sound as loud as the same tone at 40dB SL in a pathological ear, even though the hearing thresholds are different. There are, however, a number of exceptions to the normal growth of loudness just described.

Recruitment

Figure 5.1C shows a patient with the same degree of hearing loss as that in Figure 5.1B, but note that as intensity increases in the normal ear, the same amount of intensity results in an unusually rapid growth of loudness in the impaired ear. It seems as though a great deal of loudness is compressed into a relatively small amount of intensity increase for this individual. A number of years ago such findings were observed for patients with unilateral hearing losses by using a binaural loudness-balancing procedure. The disproportionate increase in loudness as a function of intensity is called **recruitment**. Recruitment has been shown to be symptomatic of the majority of hearing losses that are caused by damage to the delicate sensory cells of the inner ear. Although loudness recruitment is a very helpful symptom in the differential diagnosis of the site of lesion in the auditory system, it presents a number of difficulties in aural rehabilitation.

Partial Recruitment

Frequently, performance of the loudness-balancing procedure shows that loudness grows more rapidly than normal in the impaired ear, but without

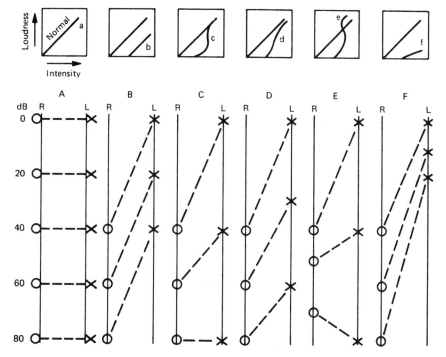

Figure 5.1 Growth of loudness in the left ear relative to the growth of the loudness in the right ear in the following hypothetical cases: (A) The right ear is normal. (B) The right ear has a 40 dB hearing loss without recruitment. (C) The right ear has a 40 dB hearing loss with recruitment. (D) The right ear has a 40 dB hearing loss with partial recruitment. (E) The right ear has a 40 dB hearing loss with hyperrecruitment. (F) The right ear has a 40 dB hearing loss with decruitment.

complete recruitment (Figure 5.1D). Such individuals are said to exhibit **partial recruitment**. Some people believe that partial recruitment has the same diagnostic significance as complete recruitment—that is, damage to the inner ear. Priede and Coles (1974), however, conclude that "incomplete recruitment is a poor indicator of site of lesion."

Hyperrecruitment

In some pathological cases, loudness grows so rapidly with small increases in intensity that a tone may appear to be louder in the impaired ear than it is in a normal ear at the same (high) intensity. People showing this phenomenon are said to exhibit **hyperrecruitment**, or **overrecruitment**. Hyperrecruitment, illustrated in Figure 5.1E, may be a dramatic diagnostic finding, or it may be a variation on recruitment caused by differences in tester performance.

Decruitment

In some hearing losses, nerve units in the auditory system are missing or damaged, and loudness grows more slowly in the impaired ear than it does in a normal ear as intensity is increased. To individuals with this problem, even very intense sounds do not produce much loudness. Such hearing difficulties, illustrated in Figure 5.1F, are called **decruitment** (Davis & Goodman, 1966). Decruitment is frequently associated with lesions of the auditory nerve.

IMPLICATIONS OF LOUDNESS RECRUITMENT

Some examples of the growth of loudness have been illustrated in Figure 5.1. Hearing loss in only one ear was shown so that the normal ear could serve as a reference to which the growth of loudness might be compared at a number of sensation levels. Note that not all patients manifesting different loudness growths have hearing losses in only one ear. In fact, most hearing losses are bilateral. Many different procedures have been developed to test for loudness recruitment since it was first described by Fowler (1936).

The Alternate Binaural Loudness Balance Test

The procedure preferred by most audiologists as a direct test for recruitment in patients with unilateral hearing losses is the **alternate binaural loudness balance (ABLB) test**. There are several versions of this test, and different procedures are favored by different clinicians. It is unlikely that slight variations in procedure produce significantly different results.

A candidate for the ABLB procedure *must* have normal hearing in one ear for the frequencies to be tested. Normal hearing for this purpose is defined as no hearing threshold poorer than 15 dB HL. The test works best if there is at least a 25 dB difference between thresholds of the two ears. The test has been carried out with useful results in cases where hearing is normal in both ears.

The purpose of the ABLB test is to compare the growth of loudness in an impaired ear with the normal growth of loudness in the opposite (normal) ear. In this way the degree of recruitment, if present, can be demonstrated.

Administering the ABLB Test. All that is required to administer the ABLB test is a two-channel audiometer capable of pulsing a tone of one frequency alternately from one ear to the other. The intensity of each tone must be individually controllable from separate attenuators. One tone is directed to the poor ear and the other to the better ear by means of air-conduction receivers.

Usually the duty cycle of the signal is 50% (that is, the tone is on half the time in one ear and half the time in the other ear). Signal durations vary with different audiometers and range from one-half to one second. Hood (1969) has suggested that a silent interval of 600 milliseconds should intervene between tone presentations, but clinical audiometers that allow automatic stimulus introduction do not have this capability.

The patient must be instructed properly before the test. For this reason the ABLB procedure is limited to those adults and older children capable of making relative loudness judgments and appropriate responses. The tone from one channel of the audiometer can be introduced at 10 or 20 dB above the threshold of the poorer ear. This allows the impaired ear to serve as reference for the normal ear. Some audiologists feel that the normal ear should serve as the reference and the matching of loudness should be done in the impaired ear. The probable advantage of using the better ear as the reference ear is slightly greater accuracy; however, using the impaired ear as the reference increases the overall speed of the procedure.

The patient listens to two or three tone presentations in each ear and decides in which ear the tone seems louder. The intensity is then raised or lowered in the better ear several times until an average of the trials results.

It is possible to have a patient respond in a number of different ways during an ABLB test:

1. The patient may have direct control over the attenuator controlling the level of the tone in the test ear. This means that the patient may actually raise and lower the intensity until the loudness is perceived as equal in both ears. Of course, when this method is used the numbers on the hearing-level dial must be masked from the patient's view by placing a ring of some kind over the numbers on the dial.

2. The patient may operate a switch that controls a motor-driven attenuator. This means that the patient presses one button to increase the loudness of the tone in the better ear and another button to decrease the loudness. Another use of pushbuttons is allowed by an automatic audiometer; the patient may bracket equal loudness by pushing the button when the tone in the test ear is just louder than the tone in the reference ear and by releasing the button when the tone is just softer than the tone in the reference ear, and so on. This method results in a write-out that may be seen on an audiogram.

3. Probably the most popular method is to have the patient signal to the examiner when the tone is louder in the right ear or in the left ear, or when the tones are equally loud in both ears. Such signaling may be done by pointing to one ear or the other or by simply telling the examiner the relative loudness of the tones in each ear.

Recording ABLB Test Results. Some clinics record results of the ABLB test directly on an audiogram, placing the symbols for the right and left ears on either side of the ordinate, indicating the test frequency (Figure 5.2). Other clinics develop special forms for this purpose, such as the one shown in Figure 5.2A.

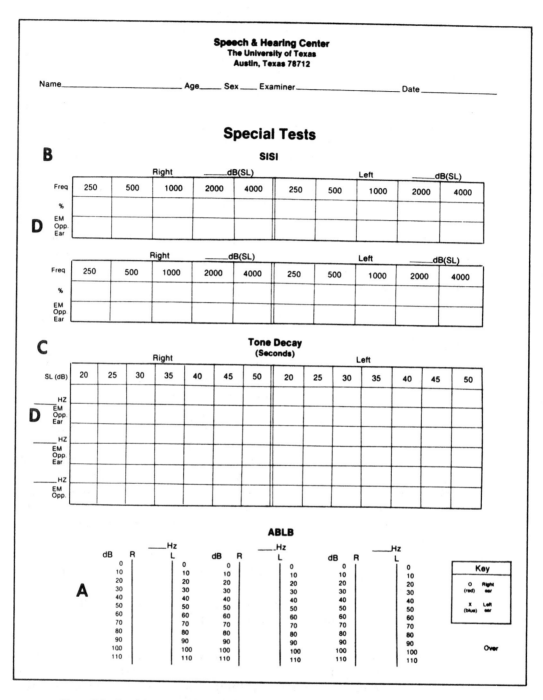

Figure 5.2 Special test worksheet with space allocated to recording results of the following tests: (A) alternate binaural loudness balance: (B) SISI; (C) tone decay. Spaces next to the letter D allow for recording of effective masking levels for the nontest ear.

The Simultaneous Binaural Loudness Balance Test

A procedure that enjoyed brief popularity as a recruitment test, called the **simultaneous binaural loudness balance (SBLB) test**, involves a method patterned after the ABLB. Instead of the tone being pulsed alternately between the ears, however, the tone, fed through separate attenuators to each earphone, is presented simultaneously to both ears. The tones are locked in phase to avoid beats, and the intensity of the tone in the test ear is raised and lowered until the patient reports that the tone is heard in the midline of the head or with equal loudness in both ears. This procedure is somewhat easier for the inexperienced patient than is the ABLB.

Results of the SBLB test were formerly interpreted as in Figure 5.1 for the ABLB. Jerger and Harford (1960) showed that the ABLB and SBLB do not measure the same functions, nor do they yield the same results on some patients. Apparently, **median plane localization** is more dependent on timing between the two cochleas than on the magnitude of the neural activity that is associated with increases in loudness. Although the SBLB test has value in determining lesions that are higher in the auditory system, it should not be used as a test for recruitment.

The Alternate Monaural Loudness Balance Test

Because most hearing-impaired patients do not have one normal ear, Reger (1936) developed a different procedure to test for recruitment. This method, which measures the growth of loudness of two frequencies in the same ear, is called the **alternate monaural loudness balance (AMLB) test**.

The AMLB test is designed to compare the growth of loudness of one frequency (one that demonstrates a hearing loss) to the growth of loudness of another frequency (one at which the patient has normal hearing) in the same ear. The difference between these thresholds should be at least 25 dB.

Administering the AMLB Test. Most two-channel audiometers allow performance of the AMLB test. The inputs must be the two test frequencies, with the output fed to a single earphone.

In administering the AMLB test, the intensity is set 10 to 20 dB above the threshold of the frequency at which hearing sensitivity is poorer. The tones are then pulsed from higher to lower frequency, and the patient is asked to aid in the manipulation of the intensity of the frequency at which hearing is normal. When the patient determines that the "high tone" and the "low tone" are equal in loudness, that portion of the test is complete. Intensity is raised in 10 dB steps for the frequency at which hearing is poorer after each judgment until recruitment is seen or the maximum limit of the audiometer is reached. Methods of response may be identical for the AMLB and the ABLB.

Scoring and Interpreting AMLB Test Results. AMLB test results may be displayed on an audiogram. The phon lines described in Chapter 2 (Figure

2.21) should be superimposed on the audiogram because different frequencies increase in loudness at different rates for people with normal hearing.

The presence of recruitment on the AMLB test is interpreted in the same way as on the ABLB test in terms of the probability of a cochlear disorder. The AMLB test is not very popular among audiologists today, for several reasons. The first is the belief that the test may be too difficult for most patients. Although the task is far from easy, the test can be carried out successfully on many people if both the clinician and the patient persevere. A more cogent argument against the AMLB is that it is more time consuming than other tests that often lead more easily to the same diagnosis. Some of these other tests are discussed later in this chapter.

Value of Recruitment Testing

As a rule, recruitment is more likely to be demonstrated in the higher than in the lower frequencies. Often, only one or two frequencies lend themselves to ABLB or AMLB testing, and decisions regarding the presence of recruitment must be based on these. Even among experts in audiology, disagreement persists regarding the diagnostic value of recruitment tests. This chapter emphasizes that no single procedure or set of procedures in audiology may be relied on completely to determine the site of a hearing disorder.

DIFFERENTIAL INTENSITY DISCRIMINATION

For some time it has been known that as intensity is increased in a normal ear, the ability to detect small changes in intensity in that ear also increases. That is, at low sensation levels a tone might change in intensity several decibels before the listener becomes aware of any change in loudness. When that same tone is very loud, a change in intensity equal to a fraction of a decibel can often be detected. The smallest change in intensity that can be recognized as a change in loudness is the **difference limen for intensity (DLI)**. Because increased loudness of a tone improves the normal listener's ability to tell when the tone has changed in intensity, many clinicians used to believe that the DLI is an indirect measurement of recruitment. That is, if a patient with a hearing loss has a small DLI at low sensation levels, recruitment would be suggested. The conventional wisdom is that although both loudness recruitment and small DLIs near threshold suggest a cochlear lesion, a cause-and-effect relationship does not necessarily exist between the two.

In the 1950s a number of variations on the DLI theme developed. Many audiometers came equipped with separate attenuators for performance of DLI measurements. Audiologists eventually began to despair over the lack of reliability of these tests. A procedure as delicate as the DLI requires, for one thing, a great deal more practice and familiarization on the part of the patient than is practical in most clinical situations. DLI tests are no longer popular, so the individual procedures and interpretations are not discussed here.

The Short Increment Sensitivity Index (SISI)

Clinical experience and experimentation with the DLI procedure suggested that patients with disorders of the cochlea can detect small intensity changes in an otherwise steady-state signal. Patients with normal hearing and those with disorders other than in the cochlea do not possess this ability. Jerger, Shedd, and Harford (1959) developed a test based on this principle, the **short increment sensitivity index (SISI)**. The SISI procedure is designed to test the ability of a patient to detect the presence of a 1 dB increment superimposed on a tone presented at 20 dB SL.

Any subject, with or without a hearing loss, can be tested with the SISI procedure as long as a hearing loss at the frequency tested does not exceed the maximum limit of the audiometer. Because the sensation level for the standard SISI test is 20 dB, the patient's hearing threshold should be at least 20 dB below the audiometer's limit for the frequency tested.

Administering the SISI. The special equipment that is required for this test is built into most diagnostic audiometers. The SISI relies on the addition of a brief increase in intensity over a carrier signal, which is presented as a steady-state pure tone. Every 5 seconds a 200 millisecond tone is superimposed on the carrier tone. This increment may be varied in size, usually from 1 to 5 dB. The test is performed in one ear using an air-conduction earphone, with the other earphone capable of delivering a masking noise if necessary. Unless the equipment performs precisely as designed for this test, the interpretation of results may be entirely erroneous. Figure 5.3 shows a diagram of the stimulus for the SISI.

As with any auditory test, it is important to instruct the patient properly before the test begins. The effects of practice on this test may be great.

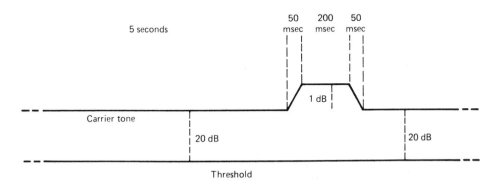

Figure 5.3 Diagram of the stimulus of the short increment sensitivity index. The carrier tone is presented at 20 dB above the patient's threshold for the test frequency. Every 5 seconds an increment is superimposed that rises to maximum in 50 milliseconds, remains at that level for 200 milliseconds, and then returns to the 20 dB SL in 50 milliseconds. The test is performed using a 1 dB increment. In some SISI devices the level of the carrier tone is lowered 1 dB for each decibel that the increment size is increased.

Because the patient will be asked to identify an extremely small increase in the loudness of a steady pure tone, a number of factors such as interest, attention, and intelligence may enter into this test, as well as other conditions over which the audiologist has no control. After the pure-tone audiogram has been completed, the patient is instructed approximately as follows:

> You will hear a steady tone in your right (left) ear. You will occasionally hear a slight increase in the loudness of this tone, a kind of jump. Please signal whenever you hear this jump, even if it is very small. Do not signal unless you are quite certain you have heard the jump in loudness, but signal even if it is a very slight increase. Are there any questions?

The earphones are properly positioned, and a tone is presented at 20 dB above threshold. Any frequency may be tested by the SISI procedure; the more frequencies tested, the greater the diagnostic capability of this test. Some audiologists prefer to test only one or two frequencies in each ear. When the number of test frequencies is limited, it is probably best to test in the high and middle frequencies, such as 4000 and 1000 Hz. If positive findings are absent in the high frequencies, they are not very probable in the lower frequencies.

The SISI apparatus is adjusted so that a 5dB increment is presented every 5 seconds. This increment is large enough so that almost everyone can detect its presence. If no responses are obtained, the patient should be reinstructed. After several responses have been obtained, the increment size should be decreased to 4, 3, and 2 dB. If responses are obtained for the 2 dB increments, the patient is performing properly, and the actual test may be begun using 1 dB increments.

The audiologist should present twenty 1 dB increments for each test. If patients properly identify four or five in a row, several increments should be deleted lest the patients develop response patterns that merely reflect the interincrement interval (5 seconds) and not the actual hearing of the 1 dB increments. On the other hand, if responses are not obtained for several consecutive 1 dB increments, they should be increased to 2 or 3 dB to remind the patients what they are listening for. Then, if responses are obtained, the test may be resumed using the 1 dB increments.

How patients respond to the SISI increments is immaterial to the test results. They may use a signal button, a vocal response such as "Now" or "Yes," or a hand or finger signal whenever they detect the increase in loudness.

Cross-Hearing and Masking during the SISI. Because the SISI is a suprathreshold procedure, the problem of cross-hearing presents itself often. When the HL of the SISI carrier tone is above the bone-conduction threshold of the opposite ear by an amount greater than the patient's interaural attenuation, the nontest ear is involved in the test. This last statement should sound familiar to the reader, for it is based on the same logic as that used in the discussion of cross-hearing for speech discrimination, except that, for purposes of the SISI, the comparison is made to the opposite-ear bone-conduction threshold at the same frequency. Cross-hearing for the SISI is stated as:

$$\text{SISI HL}_{\text{TE}} - \text{IA} \geq \text{BC}_{\text{NTE}}$$

Masking for the SISI test is similar to masking for speech discrimination testing. If the audiometer is calibrated in units of effective masking, the EM level of the masked ear is equal to the HL of the SISI carrier tone, minus interaural attenuation if it is known (if not, use 40 dB), plus any air–bone gap in the masked ear at the test frequency:

$$\text{EM} = \text{SISI HL}_{\text{TE}} - \text{IA} + \text{ABG}_{\text{NTE}}$$

Scoring and Interpreting the SISI Results. The SISI test is scored in terms of the percentage of correctly identified 1 dB increments out of a possible 20. The number correct is simply multiplied by 5%. Although some clinics have specially designed forms or graphs for recording SISI results, any permanent record (Figure 5.2B) is satisfactory.

Scores on the SISI above 70% are usually considered to indicate the presence of a hearing loss produced by damage to the cochlea. This is a positive SISI. Scores below 30%, which are considered negative, are found in patients with disorders elsewhere than in the cochlea and also in persons with normal hearing sensitivity. The literature suggests that the SISI separates most patients at these two extremes of positive and negative. The higher the SISI score, the greater the likelihood that the disorder is in the cochlea. Scores lying between 30% and 70% have only limited diagnostic significance and must be interpreted carefully.

Like responses to the ABLB test, SISI scores tend to be higher for the high frequencies. At frequencies of 1000 Hz and above, 100% SISI scores are common in patients with cochlear hearing losses. Below 500 Hz, scores above 20% are rare even in cochlear disorders. As a general rule, hearing losses of 30 dB (ANSI–1969) or less do not show high SISI scores.

Relationship of SISI to Recruitment. Most patients manifesting recruitment on the ABLB test tend to have high SISI scores. Conversely, most patients without recruitment tend to show low SISI scores. Because the correlations between the two tests are high, many have assumed that they measure the same phenomena. It is probably best, from a clinical viewpoint, to look at each test in terms of the diagnostic information it provides, rather than to regard the SISI as a form of indirect recruitment test.

Modifications of the SISI. Several modifications of the SISI have been suggested on the basis of empirical evidence. One procedure (Koch, Bartels, & Rupp, 1969) involves beginning at 20 dB SL and repeating the SISI test at higher and higher sensation levels until a positive score is obtained. Patients with normal hearing and those with mild inner-ear hearing losses will show higher and higher scores as the levels are raised, whereas those with damage to the higher auditory centers will not show an increase in SISI scores as level is increased. It is probably more common today to perform the high-level SISI at 75 dB HL (Sanders, Josey, & Glasscock, 1974). It has also been suggested that the SISI be performed with increment sizes larger than 1 dB when scores at 20 dB SL are low. In some cases of pathology in the higher centers of the auditory system, even increasing the increment size does not allow the patient to identify the increment.

Discussion of the SISI. Though far less popular today than previously, the SISI fits into the entire battery of diagnostic auditory tests. It may be performed whenever it is felt to be diagnostically useful, but it must be eliminated whenever the hearing loss is too severe or too mild, or when active patient cooperation is precluded. There is enough contradictory evidence in the literature that an attempt to diagnose the site of lesion solely on the basis of the SISI is probably unwise. Exactly why scores on the SISI turn out the way they do has not been completely answered, but this does not mean that the test should not retain a position of importance. The SISI test is sometimes complicated in patients who suffer from severe tone decay.

TONE DECAY

In most cases, even among people with normal and intact auditory systems, listening to sustained signals will bring about a certain amount of shift in an individual's thresholds for those signals. For many years, even predating the audiological era, it has been noted that patients with some forms of hearing disorder find it impossible to hear sustained tones for more than a brief time. To many of these patients, a tone heard clearly at a level 5 dB above threshold fades rapidly to inaudibility. If the level of the tone is increased, the tone may be heard again, only to quickly disappear to silence. Although a number of different names have been ascribed to this phenomenon, perhaps the most popular one among audiologists is **tone decay**.

Since it has been recognized that extreme threshold tone decay may be a powerful symptom of some serious medical conditions, audiologists have become interested in developing tests to quantify its presence. Several methods have been developed, only a few of which are described in this section. Of all the special tests described in this chapter, none requires less esoteric equipment than the tone decay tests; only a standard audiometer and a stopwatch are necessary.

The Carhart Tone Decay Test

Based on some earlier observations of tone decay, Carhart (1957) developed a procedure that is still popular today. A tone is presented to the patient by means of an earphone. The tone level is increased in intensity until it reaches auditory threshold. Patients are asked to listen closely and to signal as soon as they hear a tone at threshold and again when they no longer hear it. As soon as the patient signals that the tone is heard, the stopwatch is started; it is stopped when the patient signals that the tone is no longer heard. The number of seconds that the tone is heard at 0 dB SL is recorded. The stopwatch is reset, and the level of the tone is raised to 5 dB SL *without interrupting the tone.* This procedure is continued until (1) the patient can hear the tone for a full 60 seconds; (2) 30 dB SL has been reached, and the patient fails to hear the tone at that level for at least 60 seconds; or (3) the maximum limit of the audiometer has been reached. The amount of tone decay is expressed as the number of decibels above threshold that the tone can be heard for a full minute.

The Rosenberg Tone Decay Test

Rosenberg (1958, 1969) described a method that he felt provided all the information derived from the Carhart method, but in a much shorter time. In this modification of the Carhart method, the entire test is accomplished in one minute for each frequency. The tone is introduced at 5 dB SL and timing is begun with a stopwatch. When the patient signals that the tone is no longer heard, the level is immediately raised by 5 dB, but the stopwatch is allowed to continue running. If the patient signals silence again, the level is raised another 5 dB, and so forth, until the entire 60 seconds have elapsed. This test is scored as the number of decibels of decay in the 60 second period.

The Green Tone Decay Test

Clinical observation of some patients with disorders of the higher auditory centers (beyond the cochlea) caused Green (1963) to approach tone decay from another viewpoint. Green noticed that, although some patients could continue to hear the tone presented to them, there was a change in the *quality* of that tone. Many patients have remarked that pure tones may be devoid of their tonality shortly after introduction.

The method advocated by Green is similar to the Rosenberg procedure in that it takes a total of one minute's time. In addition to having the patients signal when they no longer hear a tone, they are instructed to notify the examiner if the tone loses its tonal quality. Apparently, many patients do experience loss of tonality much before and even in the absence of threshold shift.

The Olsen-Noffsinger Tone Decay Test

Because some tone decay is usually evident in patients with damage to the inner ear, Olsen and Noffsinger (1974) proposed a modification of the Carhart method in which the test is begun at a level 20 dB above threshold. Olsen and Noffsinger's study found that the same information was obtained with this procedure as with the Carhart method in terms of diagnosis, but with some time savings. When clinical time can be conserved with no loss of test accuracy, the needs of both clinician and patient are better served. Figure 5.2C is useful for recording results of this test.

The Suprathreshold Adaptation Test (STAT)

Many patients with lesions in areas central to the inner ear, such as tumors of the auditory nerve, show greater amounts of tone decay when the presentation of the stimulus is at a high intensity. This is the premise of the **suprathreshold adaptation test (STAT)** (Jerger & Jerger, 1975). Instructions for this test are the same as for all tone decay tests—that the patient continue to signal as long as the tone is audible.

The STAT is done with the tone presented at 110 dB SPL, rounded off to 100 dB HL at 500 and 2000 Hz and to 105 dB HL at 1000 Hz. Timing begins as soon as the patient signals that the tone is heard, and the test is concluded when 60 seconds have elapsed, or when the patient signals that the tone is inaudible. The STAT is interpreted as positive for a neural lesion if complete adaptation occurs within one minute. To check for a false positive response, the test may be repeated using a periodically interrupted tone.

Cross-Hearing and Masking in Tone Decay Tests

Little attention has been paid in the literature to the problems of cross-hearing for tone decay tests. It is logical that as the level of the signal is raised in the test ear, that level, minus the patient's interaural attenuation, may reach the bone-conduction threshold of the nontest ear. As soon as the nontest ear has been stimulated, assuming it has no tone decay, the patient's tone decay in the test ear will appear to have reached a plateau. Cross-hearing for the tone decay test is stated as

$$\text{TDT HL}_{TE} - \text{IA} \geq \text{BC}_{NTE}$$

Because the signal may be initially at a high intensity or constantly increased during a tone decay test, minimum masking is not advocated here. The use of maximum masking seems to be a practical approach for this test and may be stated as the bone-conduction threshold of the test ear plus the patient's interaural attenuation, minus a 5 dB safety factor:

$$\text{EM} = \text{BC}_{TE} + \text{IA} - 5$$

When masking during any tone decay test, the noise should be turned off before the tone to make certain that the patient is signaling the audibility of the tone and not that of the noise.

Interpreting Tone Decay Tests

Interpretation of the Carhart and similar tone decay methods is shown in Table 5.1. Three types of tone decay appear (Owens, 1971), which may be interpreted as follows:

TABLE 5.1 TYPICAL TONE DECAY PATTERNS

SENSATION LEVEL	TYPE I	TYPE II	TYPE III
5 dB	60*	14	3
10 dB		26	12
15 dB		39	9
20 dB		48	16
25 dB		60	11
30 dB			9

*Responses are in seconds.

Type I. No tone decay in 60 seconds at any frequency: This is seen in patients with normal auditory systems, in those with conductive hearing losses, and in some with lesions of the cochlea.

Type II. Progressively slower tone decay as the level is raised in 5 dB steps: Type II tone decay is strongly suggestive of cochlear pathology.

Type III. Type III decay is the most dramatic. Even with increased intensity, the patient is unable to sustain hearing of the tone for increasing periods of time. Type III decay patterns are strongly suggestive of lesions of the auditory nerve.

In addition to rates of decay, tone decay patterns appear with respect to stimulus frequency. In Type I patterns no significant decay is seen at any frequency. In Type II patterns more decay is generally observed for higher than for lower frequencies, suggesting the advisability of testing several different frequencies. Type III patterns show rapid tone decay, even in the low frequencies.

Rosenberg (1958) described some useful criteria in interpreting tone decay tests:

1. Normal—0 to 5 dB in 60 seconds
2. Mild—10 to 15 dB in 60 seconds
3. Moderate—20 to 25 dB in 60 seconds
4. Marked—30 dB or more in 60 seconds

Discussion of Tone Decay Tests

Personal experience with the different kinds of tone decay tests has led to a preference for the Olsen-Noffsinger method. Note that there is space on the form in Figure 5.2D to record the effective masking level used in the opposite ear when testing. The additional information gained from the Carhart and Olsen-Noffsinger methods over the Rosenberg approach, in terms of the rates of decay at succeeding sensation levels, appear to justify the increase time required.

Many patients have difficulty in determining their criteria for loss of tonality, which is necessary for the modified tone decay test described by Green.

Although all the tone decay tests, including some not described in this chapter, are extremely useful, the Olsen-Noffsinger method is used to illustrate typical test results for the different kinds of disorders described in Chapters 6 through 9. It has been suggested (Green, 1978, p. 196) that two or more different tone decay tests should be done on patients whenever time allows.

BÉKÉSY AUDIOMETRY

A modern version of Békésy's automatic audiometer was described in Chapter 2 for use in a procedure that allows patients to track their own auditory thresholds. The patient presses a button when a tone becomes audible in an earphone, keeps the button depressed as long as the tone is heard, and then releases it when the tone becomes inaudible. The tone is allowed to increase in intensity until the button is pressed, which causes the tone to be attenuated. A pen controlled by the attenuator of the audiometer traces the level of the tone on an audiogram as a function of both time and either constantly changing or fixed frequency.

For many years, **Békésy audiometry** has been recognized as a procedure that goes beyond the mere automatic recording of pure-tone thresholds. Extreme narrowing of the swing widths (difference between audibility and inaudibility) was thought at one time to be related to the difference limen for intensity and so, indirectly, to recruitment. Some early studies on pathological ears investigated the very important aspects of attenuation rate, intensity direction (whether the tone was presented above threshold to be decreased in intensity or below threshold to be increased in intensity), frequency direction (sweeping from low frequency to high or from high frequency to low), signal duration, and many other variables.

Békésy Tracing Types

It was undoubtedly the report of Jerger (1960) that led to the widespread acceptance of Békésy audiometry as a clinical tool in the differential diagnosis of site of lesion. Jerger observed the threshold-tracking behavior of 434 subjects with normal hearing and a variety of pathological conditions. Observations were made of responses to continuous and to pulsed tones. The result of these observations was a series of four different kinds of Békésy audiograms. These Békésy types are illustrated in Figure 5.4 and may be described as follows:

Type I Tracing. Patients with normal hearing and those with conductive hearing losses track audiograms in which the pulsed and continuous tracings overlap; that is, the thresholds are the same whether the tone is continuously on or pulsing on and off. This is apparently true whether the tracing is made for the entire frequency range of 100 to 10,000 Hz (sweep frequency) or is restricted to fixed frequencies sampling the low-, middle-, and high-frequency ranges. The width of the trace remains about the same, usually around 10 dB

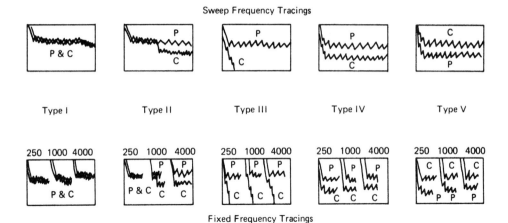

Sweep Frequency Tracings

Type I   Type II   Type III   Type IV   Type V

Fixed Frequency Tracings

Figure 5.4 *Type I* sweep- and fixed-frequency Békésy audiogram showing continuous and pulsed tracings to interweave with swing width about 10 dB.

Type II sweep- and fixed-frequency Békésy audiograms showing continuous and pulsed tracings to interweave in the low frequencies. At about 1000 Hz the continuous-tone tracing drops below the pulsed tracing, suggesting that it is harder to hear a continuous tone. The swing width becomes narrower in the higher frequencies, indicating that the patient can tell sharp distinctions between audibility and inaudibility with very small changes in intensity.

Type III sweep- and fixed-frequency audiograms showing the continuous tone to be difficult to hear even in the low frequencies; the pulsed tone trace follows the pattern of the conventional audiogram.

Type IV sweep- and fixed-frequency audiograms showing the continuous tone to drop below (become harder to hear than) the pulsed tone throughout the frequency range. Unlike the *Type III* tracing, the *Type IV* continuous tracing never completely fades to inaudibility.

Type V sweep- and fixed-frequency Békésy tracings showing the pulsed tone to be more difficult to hear than the continuous tone. This tracing is not explainable on the basis of typical organic pathology.

for both the pulsed and continuous modes. Type I patterns are also observed in some patients with cochlear lesions.

Type II Tracing. In patients with cochlear disorders the pulsed tracing follows generally the audiometric configuration obtained in conventional pure-tone audiometry, as do both the pulsed and continuous Type I tracings. Type II tracings differ sharply, however, in the continuous-tone trace. Although there is often overlap between pulsed and continuous tones for the low frequencies, at about 1000 Hz the continuous tone drops below the interrupted one; that is, the continuous tone appears to be more difficult to hear. At about the point at which the breakaway occurs, the continuous tracing often becomes significantly narrower in its swing width, suggesting that the difference between audibility and inaudibility is much sharper to the patient. For the higher frequencies the continuous trace tends to run not more than 20 dB below the pulsed trace.

Type III Tracing. Undoubtedly the most dramatic but least common of all the Békésy types is the Type III. Again, in this pattern, as in the others, the interrupted trace follows the pattern of manual audiometry. When the continuous mode is used, the patient is observed to exhibit marked adaptation to the signal, finding it difficult or impossible to hear, even with great increases in intensity. This pronounced separation of the continuous from the pulsed tracing occurs at all frequencies. Type III tracings are associated with lesions medial to the inner ear, although not all such lesions manifest Type III tracings.

Type IV Tracing. Type IV tracings appear similar to Type IIs, except for the frequencies at which the continuous tone tends to break away from the pulsed tone. In Type IV tracings, the breakaway often occurs below 500 Hz, with pulsed continuous separation ranging from 5 to 20 dB. Type IV tracings were originally ascribed to lesions medial to the inner ear, although many observations of patients with cochlear disorders exhibiting Type IV tracings have been noted.

Type V Tracing. Jerger and Herer (1961) observed unusual Békésy tracings on a series of patients who were believed to be exaggerating their hearing thresholds for financial gain. In these tracings, called Type V, the hearing for continuous tones appears to be better than for pulsed tones, a phenomenon that defies explanation on the basis of organic pathology. Although Type V tracings might alert the audiologist to a nonorganic disorder, they are by no means evidence of such. Type V tracings are discussed again in the chapter on nonorganic hearing loss.

Cross-Hearing and Masking in Békésy Audiometry

As soon as the level of the tone in the test ear exceeds the bone-conduction threshold of the nontest ear by more than the patient's interaural attenuation, cross-hearing again becomes a problem. Békésy audiometry is no more exempt from this danger than are any of the other audiometric procedures described. Because the continuous tone may be constantly elevated in intensity in some Békésy types, and because this procedure is often most valuable in the poorer ear of patients with unilateral hearing losses, the probability of test contamination is increased in Békésy audiometry.

The amount of contralateral masking to be used in Békésy audiometry is more difficult to define than for other procedures, since the signal is not only changing in intensity but in frequency as well. For these reasons maximum effective masking is recommended (the bone-conduction threshold of the test ear, plus interaural attenuation, minus 5 dB).

Although masking is often necessary during Békésy audiometry, its presence may alter test results. When noise is presented to the opposite ear, some normal-hearing individuals change from Type I to Type II patterns (Blegvad, 1967; Dirks & Norris, 1966). Some patients who normally have Type II tracings show Type IVs when a high-level noise is presented to the opposite ear. At the time of this writing, the masking problem in Békésy audiometry remains unresolved, and interpretation of this procedure requires considerable clinical skill.

Variations on Békésy Audiometry

Several modifications of the standard Békésy procedure described earlier have been suggested. A few of these procedures are briefly described here.

Change in Frequency Direction. Traditionally, during sweep frequency Békésy audiometry, the frequency direction has been from low to high. There is evidence (Jerger, Jerger, & Mauldin 1972; Karja & Palva, 1970; Palva & Jauhiainen, 1976; Palva, Jauhiainen, Sjoblom, & Ylikoski, 1978; Rose, 1962) that, when the frequency direction is reversed, some patients show greater separation between pulsed and continuous tones and narrowing of the continuous-tone swing width. Correct identification of both cochlear and retrocochlear lesions is substantially increased when reversed frequency (high to low) tracings are used over the original procedure (low to high).

Change in Intensity Direction. Instead of increasing the level of the test frequency from below threshold, there may be some value in beginning the test at suprathreshold levels. Although intensity direction does not appear to affect the pulsed or continuous-tone thresholds for normals, Harbert and Young (1968) found some patients with tone decay who exhibited greater adaptation when, at the onset of the test, the continuous tone was presented first at a high level and then decreased in intensity.

Change in Stimulus Duration. It has been known for some time that below a critical duration the ear trades time for intensity in order to achieve audibility. As a tone is decreased in duration below about 200 milliseconds, the intensity must be increased for it to be heard. This is a very simple explanation of what has been called **temporal integration** (Wright, 1968, 1969). Wright (1978, p. 224) suggests that an expeditious way to conduct **brief tone audiometry (BTA)** is to compare Békésy tracings with tonal on-times of 500 milliseconds to those with 20 milliseconds for fixed frequencies. One minute's tracking time is apparently sufficient.

Subjects with normal hearing and patients with conductive hearing loss show lower thresholds for the longer tone than for the shorter one, averaging about 3 dB. Patients with lesions of the cochlea do not show the need for greater intensity to achieve threshold, especially in the higher frequencies. Patients with disorders of the auditory nerve cannot be differentiated from those with conductive hearing loss on the basis of brief tone audiometry.

Tracking at Most Comfortable Loudness. Jerger and Jerger (1974) found that Békésy audiometry increases in its diagnostic sensitivity when the patient is asked to track a level of most comfortable loudness. **Békésy comfortable loudness (BCL)** tracking is accomplished by having the patient press the button when the tone is slightly louder than comfortable (thereby decreasing intensity) and release the button when the tone is slightly softer than comfortable (allowing the tone to increase in intensity). Apparently this suprathreshold tracking mode increases the separation between pulsed and continuous tones and makes for more reliable diagnosis of lesions of the auditory nerve as well as of the brain stem.

Békésy Audiometry and Tone Decay

The separation of continuous and pulsed tones seen in Types II, III, and IV audiograms is strongly reminiscent of results of tone decay tests. Even though they are probably manifestations of the same pathology, tonal adaptation on Békésy audiometry and tone decay tests may not be the same on some patients. The two tests are fundamentally different in that the signal is constantly changing in intensity during Békésy audiometry and remains constant during tone decay tests. Only general inferences may be made from one of these tests to the other.

Interpreting Békésy Audiograms

Not all Békésy audiograms fall neatly into one of the five types described earlier. Some patients find the test extremely difficult to perform because of problems of concentration, boredom, fatigue, reaction time, individual stimulus criteria based on personality, and a host of other causes. Sometimes patients forget to push or release the button, causing the swing widths to be so wide that the audiograms are unclassifiable. Occasionally patients even fall asleep during this procedure, and are awakened either by the clinician or when the tone becomes very loud in the test ear. Reinstruction often alleviates these problems, but occasionally it does not. Therefore, it is sometimes necessary to discard Békésy audiometry as a diagnostic tool.

Even when the patient has cooperated fully, tracings may emerge that do not fit neatly into a single Békésy type. Rather than attempting to force a classification in terms of a numbered type, the experienced clinician looks for aspects of the tracing that suggest appropriate diagnosis. If the Békésy type is clear-cut, it should be noted.

Discussion of Békésy Audiometry

Even though Békésy audiometry is not used routinely with small children, it can be carried out successfully with the majority of patients for whom diagnosis is needed. Experience and research suggest that the slower the attenuation rate, the more information may emerge from a test.

At the usual slow attenuation rate (2.5 dB/second), pulsed and continuous tracings require about 15 minutes per ear. If one adds the fixed-frequency tests and multiplies this times two ears, an hour may easily be spent in Békésy audiometry. Many audiologists feel that as much information is found in fixed-frequency Békésy tracings as in continuous-frequency tracings. Fixed-frequency tracings take less time and are often less confusing to the patient because they eliminate one changing parameter (frequency). Békésy types can be determined by sampling low, middle, and high frequencies and by noting the point and amount of separation of continuous from pulsed tracings and the width of the swings. Although Békésy audiometry appears to be declining in popularity (Martin & Forbis, 1978; Martin & Sides, 1985), Domico (1983) has redemonstrated its usefulness in tracking most comfortable and uncomfortable loudness levels; however, test results must be interpreted very carefully. Brunt (1985, p. 281) feels that reports of improved accuracy of BCL and reversed Békésy tracings over the original methods make the newer techniques more valuable for clinicians inclined to use Békésy audiometry. Clinicians must decide whether they wish to allow sufficient time for each patient to include this procedure, or whether it should be reserved for special cases in which additional site-of-lesion diagnosis is imperative.

ACOUSTIC IMMITTANCE

For a number of years interest has been directed toward the effects of various kinds of pathology on **acoustic impedance** in the plane of the eardrum membrane. Initially most impedance measurements were made with mechanical devices too clumsy and too difficult to use routinely. A variety of electroacoustic impedance meters, which are available commercially (Figure 5.5), are commonly used by audiologists. Some devices attempt to measure the actual impedance of the drum membrane, whereas others measure the inverse of impedance, the admittance of sound energy into the middle ear. Many devices measure **compliance**, which is related to the dimensions of an enclosed volume of air as expressed on a scale of different units of measurement depending on the design of the meter. Examples of the different units are millimhos,[1] cubic centimeters (cm^3) of an equivalent volume of air in the middle ear, and arbitrary units of compliance.

In the short time since acoustic impedance meters have become clinically popular, a number of terms have been used to describe the various measurements made. ASHA (1978) has recommended the word **immittance** as an all-encompassing term to describe measurements made of eardrum membrane impedance, compliance, or admittance. The American National Standards Institute (ANSI, 1987) has recently adopted a set of standards that define both the characteristics of instruments used in the measurement of acoustic immittance and the associated terminology.

---

[1]One millimho (mmho) is one-thousandth of a mho, which is a unit of admittance. Note that *mho* is *ohm* (a unit of impedance) spelled backwards.

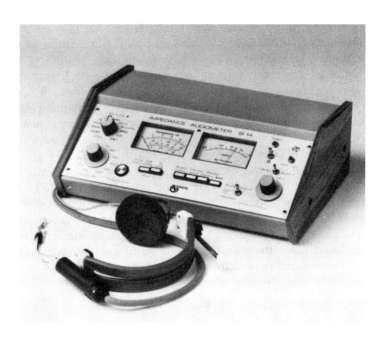

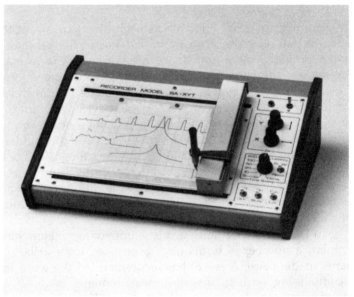

Figure 5.5 An electroacoustic immittance meter with X–Y plotter. (Courtesy of SAICO, Inc.)

Measurements Available on Acoustic Immittance Meters

Basically, three measurements are made in the plane of the eardrum membrane: (1) **static compliance**, which is the mobility of the drum membrane; (2) **tympanometry**, the mobility of the membrane as a function of various amounts of positive and negative air pressure in the external ear canal (which immobilizes or "clamps" the system); and (3) contraction of the middle-ear muscles in response to intense sounds, known as the **acoustic reflex**, which has the effect of stiffening the middle-ear system and decreasing its compliance.

Factors Governing Acoustic Immittance

The reader will recall from Chapter 2 that the impedance (Z) of any object is determined by its frictional resistance (R), mass (M), and stiffness (S). Mass and stiffness are critically dependent on the frequency (f) of the wave being measured. The formula for impedance is stated as

$$Z = \sqrt{R^2 + \left(2\pi fM - \frac{S}{2\pi f}\right)^2}$$

Resistance is obviously independent of the rest of the formula (e.g., frequency), whereas mass and stiffness are inversely related to each other and are critically dependent on frequency. If frequency increases, the total value of the mass factor also increases. Conversely, as frequency goes up, the effect of stiffness diminishes. The combination of mass and stiffness (contained within the parentheses in the formula) is called **reactance**. Mass is the important factor in the high frequencies, and stiffness is the important factor in the low frequencies. As the stiffness of a system increases, it is said to become less compliant; that is, it becomes more difficult to initiate motion in the system. Compliance, therefore, is the inverse of the stiffness factor of the formula.

The anatomy of the ear was described in a cursory fashion in Chapter 1. Details are brought out in Chapters 6 through 9, and the effects of various disorders on immittance are discussed. For the present, however, the following general assignments of values can be made: Resistance is determined primarily by the ligaments of the middle ear that support the three bones within the middle-ear cavity. The mass factor is determined primarily by the weight of these three tiny bones and the eardrum membrane. Stiffness is mostly determined by the load of fluid pressure from the inner ear on the base of the stapes, the most medial bone of the middle ear. The ear, therefore, is largely a stiffness-dominated system, at least in response to low-frequency sounds.

Equipment for Middle-Ear Immittance Measurements

An electroacoustic immittance meter is diagrammed in Figure 5.6. Three small rubber tubes are attached to a metal probe, which is fitted into the external ear canal with an air-tight seal. A plastic or rubber cuff, placed around the

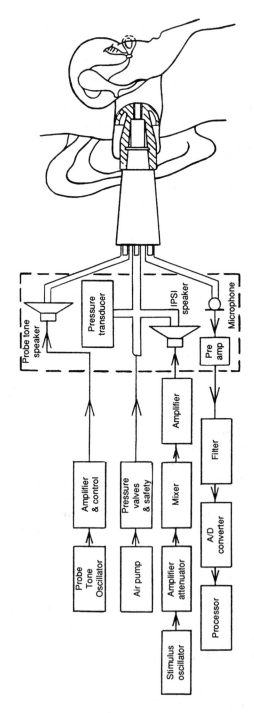

Figure 5.6 Diagram of an electroacoustic immittance meter. (Courtesy of Grason-Stadler, Inc. [A Lucas Co.])

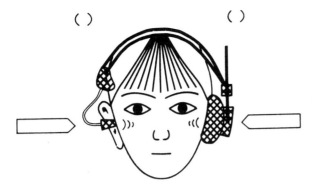

Figure 5.7 Configuration of probe of immittance meter in one ear and audiometer earphone on the other ear.

probe, can be varied in size to accommodate most ears.   The three rubber tubes are connected to (1) a miniature loudspeaker, which emits a pure tone, usually at 220 or 226 Hz (the incident wave); (2) a miniature microphone, which picks up the sound in the ear canal (the sound comprising both the incident wave introduced to the ear from the speaker and the reflected wave as it returns from the eardrum membrane); and (3) an air pump, which can create either positive or negative air pressure within the canal.   The air pump is calibrated either in millimeters of water (mm H_2O) or dekapascals (daPa, or tenths of a Pascal).   The units of measurement are very similar; 1 daPa = 1.02 mm H_2O and 1 mm H_2O = 0.98 daPa when measurements are made at standardized conditions of temperature and pressure.   The devices must be calibrated so that 0 daPa or 0 mm H_2O is equal to atmospheric pressure at the site where measurements are to be made.   The probe is attached to one side of a headset. An earphone connected to an acoustic reflex activator system is attached to the opposite side (see Figure 5.7) and functions as a built-in pure-tone audiometer.

Measurement of Static Compliance

In order for the static compliance of the tympanic membrane to be measured, the ear canal must first be cleared of any occluding ear wax or other debris.   If the canal is obstructed, medical assistance is needed.   Even the smallest amount of material in the ear canal may clog one of the tiny probe tubes and make all measurements impossible or very misleading.   The eartip is pressed into the canal, and the pressure is increased with the air pump. Observation of the meter will indicate whether the necessary air-tight seal has been obtained or whether resealing, perhaps with a different-sized tip, is necessary.   Once the seal is obtained, the pressure is increased to +200 daPa, which can be read directly on the meter.   The intensity of the probe tone is adjusted until the desired SPL is obtained: 85 to 90 dB, depending on the particular instrument.   The clinician can then determine the **equivalent volume** in cubic centimeters.   This measurement, made with the eardrum membrane loaded with +200 mm of pressure, is called c_1.   This first measurement, c_1, therefore, is a measurement made with the eardrum membrane immobilized by positive air pressure, and it represents the compliance of the outer ear.

The second step in determining static compliance is to decrease the pressure in the ear canal gradually until the eardrum membrane achieves maximum compliance—that is, when pressures on both sides of the membrane are approximately equal. A second reading is taken; called c_2, this reading represents the compliance of the outer ear and middle ear together. Many audiologists believe that c_2 should be measured with outer-ear pressure at 0 daPa (the ambient air pressure). The static compliance of the middle ear can then be determined by working through the formula

$$c_x = c_2 - c_1$$

During conditions for measurement of c_1, the drum membrane's relative immobility causes a good deal of energy to be returned to the probe, raising the sound-pressure level in the ear canal. The membrane's increased mobility during the c_2 measurement allows more energy to be admitted to the middle ear, lowering the sound pressure between the membrane and the probe. The static compliance of the middle-ear (ME) mechanism is the difference between these two conditions, which cancels out the compliance of the external auditory canal (EAC). Stated as a formula:

$$c(ME) = c(EAC + ME) - c(EAC)$$

Normal Values for Static Compliance. The research to date suggests a wide range of normal values for static compliance of the middle ear. Most devices available disregard the phase angle of the incident (original) and reflected waves in the ear canal. Differences in compliance are also a natural consequence of the particular measuring instrument used. These factors probably contribute in part to the wide variation in normal values. In addition, as with so many human factors, there is considerable variability for normal ears, overlapping middle-ear conditions that cause high or low compliance. This significantly reduces the value of this test. Values between 0.28 and 2.5 cm^3 may be considered the normal range (Northern & Grimes, 1978). Although this range is broad, a patient's middle-ear compliance values really cannot be considered abnormal unless one of the extremes is clearly exceeded.

The term equivalent volume is used with respect to immittance measures in several different ways, and, according to Popelka (1983), often incorrectly. One common use of the term is to specify an actual volume of air in a closed cavity (such as that in the external ear canal, which can vary with conditions like atmospheric pressure and movement of the eardrum membrane) in terms of a hard-walled cavity that is independent of such variables.

Recording and Interpreting Static Compliance. Results of static-compliance measurements should be recorded on forms specially prepared for this purpose (Figure 5.8A). Such forms should become an integral part of the patient's record.

Compliance values below the normal range suggest some change in the stiffness, mass, or resistance of the middle ear, causing less than normal mobility. This may result from fluid accumulation in the normally air-filled middle

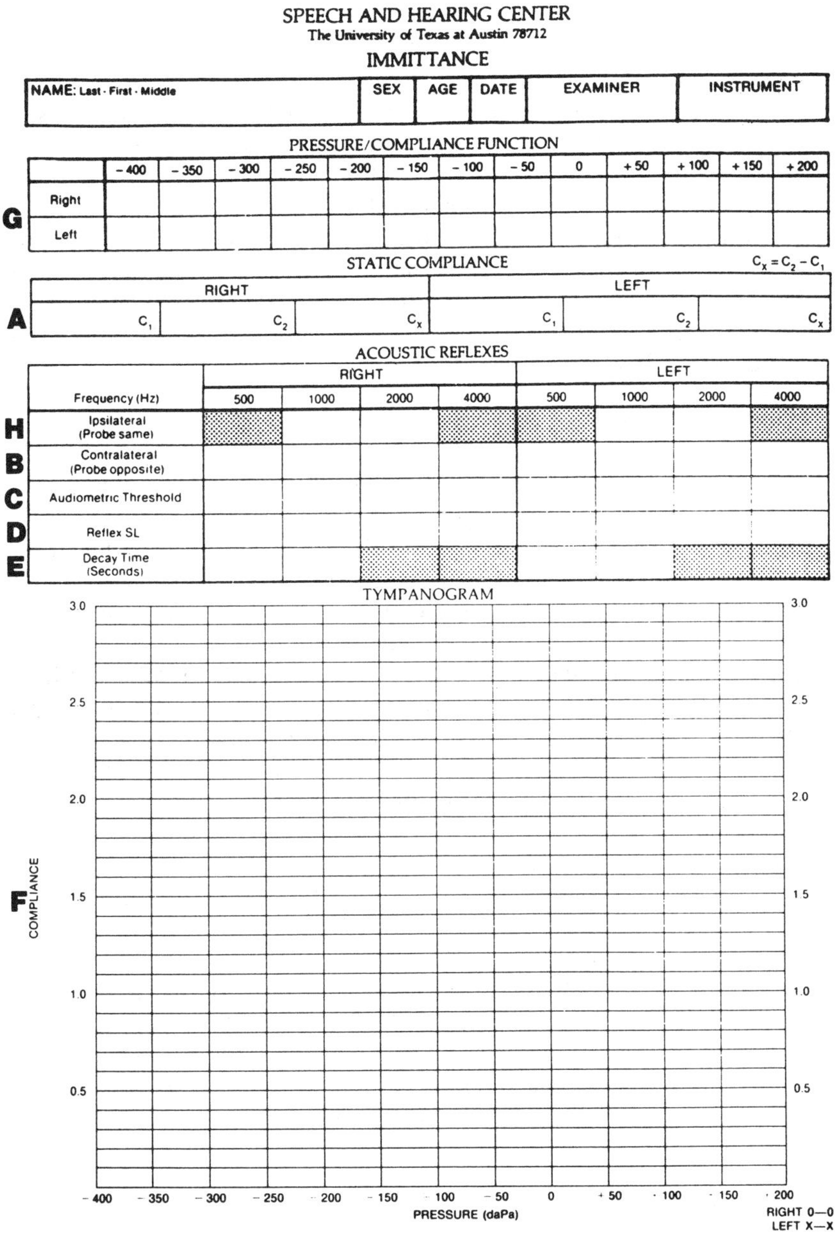

SPEECH AND HEARING CENTER

The University of Texas at Austin 78712

IMMITTANCE

NAME: Last - First - Middle	SEX	AGE	DATE	EXAMINER	INSTRUMENT

PRESSURE/COMPLIANCE FUNCTION

	-400	-350	-300	-250	-200	-150	-100	-50	0	+50	+100	+150	+200
G Right													
Left													

STATIC COMPLIANCE $C_x = C_2 - C_1$

RIGHT			LEFT		
C_1	C_2	C_x	C_1	C_2	C_x
A					

ACOUSTIC REFLEXES

	RIGHT				LEFT			
Frequency (Hz)	500	1000	2000	4000	500	1000	2000	4000
H Ipsilateral (Probe same)								
B Contralateral (Probe opposite)								
C Audiometric Threshold								
D Reflex SL								
E Decay Time (Seconds)								

TYMPANOGRAM

F COMPLIANCE

(vertical axis: 0.5, 1.0, 1.5, 2.0, 2.5, 3.0)

PRESSURE (daPa): -400, -350, -300, -250, -200, -150, -100, -50, 0, +50, +100, +150, +200

RIGHT 0—0
LEFT X—X

Figure 5.8 Form for recording results of immittance measures: (A) static compliance; (B) contralateral acoustic reflex thresholds; (C) behavioral thresholds obtained during standard pure-tone audiometry; (D) sensation levels of the reflex (B minus C); (E) the number of seconds required for the reflex to decay to half of its original amplitude; (F) a graph (the tympanogram) showing the pressure-compliance function; (G) numerical data showing the amount of compliance observed with various amounts of positive and negative air pressure in the external auditory canal; and (H) acoustic reflexes obtained with the probe tone and audiometer tone presented to the same ear.

AUDITORY TESTS FOR SITE OF LESION **183**

ear, immobility of the chain of middle-ear bones, or some blockage of the outer ear. High compliance suggests some interruption in the chain of bones, possibly caused by disease or fracture. Reduced elasticity of the eardrum membrane may be due to age or thinning caused by partial healing of a previous perforation.

Although acoustic compliance measures have grown rapidly in popularity, they, like any other diagnostic test, can be misleading. Remember that these measurements in the plane of the eardrum membrane are indirect indicators of ear disorders. It is possible for different abnormalities of the ear to have opposing effects, resulting in what appear to be essentially normal immittance values (Popelka, 1983).

Tympanometry

As the eardrum membrane is displaced from its resting position by positive or negative pressure in the ear canal, the vibratory efficiency of the membrane is decreased. The membrane vibrates most efficiently when the pressure on both sides is equal. Tympanometry is performed by loading the eardrum membrane with air pressure equal to $+200$ daPa, measuring its compliance, and then making successive measurements of immittance as the pressure in the canal is decreased. Pressure can be varied manually, say in discrete steps of 50 daPa, or can be continuously varied by means of a motor-driven system. After the pressure has reached 0 daPa, negative pressure is created by the pump and additional compliance measurements are made. The purpose of tympanometry is to determine the point and magnitude of greatest compliance of the eardrum membrane. Such measurements give invaluable information regarding the condition of the middle-ear structures. Performing tympanometry immediately after determining c_1 allows determination of both c_2 and the ear canal pressure required for measuring the acoustic reflex thresholds.

Tympanometry is generally conducted using a low-frequency probe tone of 220 or 226 Hz. The use of higher frequency probe tones or a succession of different frequencies can modify results in a variety of ways, making this test much more valuable diagnostically (Shanks, Lilly, Margolis, Wiley, & Wilson, 1988). The difficulties encountered in the use of multifrequency tympanometry are mitigated by the newest generation of devices, which are microprocessor controlled.

Recording and Interpreting Tympanometric Results. The immittance measurements may be recorded directly on a graph called a **tympanogram**, which shows compliance on the Y axis and pressure, in dekapascals, on the X axis (Figure 5.8F). Students often find it useful to record their results numerically (Figure 5.8G) before drawing the graph. If an X–Y plotter is used, the tympanogram is recorded directly and automatically on a graph, showing pressure in dekapascals on the X axis and immittance on the Y axis. The advantage of this recording method is that it provides more accuracy than manually plotting discrete points on the tympanogram. The interpretation of the tympanograms is essentially the same.

Jerger (1970) has categorized typical tympanometric results into different types. To facilitate direct comparison, all five tympanogram types are illustrated on the same form (Figure 5.9).

Type A. Type A curves are seen in patients who have normal middle-ear function. The point of greatest compliance is at 0 daPa (usually ±50 daPa), and the curve is characterized by a rather large inverted V. Some clinics consider values to −100 daPa as representing a Type A.

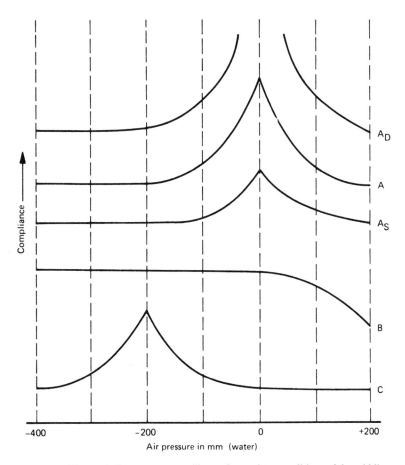

Figure 5.9 Five typical tympanograms illustrating various conditions of the middle ear. Type A shows normal pressure-compliance functions and is typical of normal middle ears. Type A$_S$ curves are like the A curves but are much shallower and are associated with stiffness of the stapes, the smallest of the middle-ear bones. Type A$_D$ curves are much deeper than the normal Type A curves and are symptomatic of interruptions in the chain of bones or flaccidity of the eardrum membrane. Type B shows no pressure setting at which the eardrum membrane becomes most compliant and suggests fluid in the middle-ear space. Type C shows the eardrum membrane to be most compliant when the pressure in the ear canal is negative, suggesting that the pressure within the middle-ear space is below atmospheric pressure.

Type A_s. Type A_S curves show the same characteristic "spike" at or near 0 daPa, suggesting normal middle-ear pressure. However, the dip is much shallower than that of the usual Type A. Type A_S curves are often seen in patients in whom the stapes has become partially immobilized.

Type A_D. In some cases the general Type A pattern is preserved; however, the amplitude of the curve is unusually high, or in some cases the positive and negative sides of the spike do not meet at all in Type A_D curves. Such curves may be associated with flaccidity of the tympanic membrane or separation of the chain of middle-ear bones.

Type B. Type B curves are seen when the middle-ear space is filled with fluid. Because even wide variations of pressure in the ear canal can never match the pressure of fluid behind the tympanic membrane, the point of greatest compliance cannot be found. Type B curves may also be seen when a small amount of ear wax or other debris occludes one of the tiny tubes within the probe, when a wax plug blocks the external ear canal, or when there is a hole in the membrane so that the meter measures the compliance of the rigid walls of the middle ear. Therefore, when Type B curves are evident, the clinician should make certain that these factors are not operating.

Type C. In certain conditions, discussed in Chapter 7, the pressure within the middle ear falls below normal. In such cases the tympanic membrane becomes most compliant when the pressure in the ear canal is negative, thus equaling the middle-ear pressure, which brings the tympanic membrane to its normal position. When maximum membrane compliance occurs at a negative pressure of -100 mm H_2O or greater, middle-ear pressure is considered to be negative.

A number of factors may influence tympanometric results. When pressure is varied from positive to negative, the peak of the wave is lower than when pressure is changed from negative to positive, although this rarely affects interpretation of results. Similarly, there are small changes in the shape of the tympanogram when the rate of pressure change is varied. The width of the tympanogram, sometimes called the gradient as well as the peak pressure, is sometimes useful in diagnosis, but there is little in the way of normative data regarding these measures, probably because of differences observed with different devices and different probe tone frequencies.

Measuring Acoustic Reflexes

Two small muscles, the **tensor tympani muscles** and the **stapedius muscle**, are involved in the operation of the middle-ear mechanism. The anatomy of these muscles is discussed in detail in Chapter 7, but they must be mentioned here. Although there is continuing uncertainty about the role of the tensor tympani in response to sound in humans, it is generally accepted that the stapedius muscles in both middle ears contract reflexively when an intense sound is introduced to either ear. This has been called the acoustic reflex.

Most normal-hearing individuals will effect a bilateral **intra-aural muscle reflex** when pure tones are introduced to the ear at 65 to 90 dB above threshold. The immittance meter enables the clinician to present a tone to one ear and to detect a decrease in tympanic membrane compliance in either that ear or the opposite ear. A pure tone of the desired frequency should be introduced at 70 dB HL. If no immittance change is seen on the meter, the level should be raised to 80 dB, 90 dB, and so on, until a response is seen or the limit of the equipment is reached. If a response is observed, the level should be lowered 10 dB, then raised in 5 dB steps. The tonal duration should be about one second, and measurements should be taken that sample the frequency range— for example, 500, 1000, 2000, and 4000 Hz, although many normal-hearing individuals, for no explainable reason, show no acoustic reflex at 4000 Hz. The lowest level at which an acoustic reflex can be obtained is called the **acoustic reflex threshold (ART)**. Some commercial meters allow intensities up to 125 dB HL to be tested, but great care should be taken in introducing such high levels. It is often inadvisable to exceed 115 dB HL.

Sometimes a very small compliance change is observed, and the audiologist may be uncertain of whether a response has been obtained. In such cases, when the level is raised 5 dB, an unequivocal response is usually observed. Extraneous compliance changes sometimes occur as the patient breathes, or occasionally the very sensitive probe microphone picks up a pulse beat from a blood vessel near the ear canal. Of course, the patient must be completely silent during these measurements lest vocalizations be picked up by the microphone, masking changes in compliance. Proper recording of the intensity required to evoke an acoustic reflex assists in appropriate interpretation of results (Figure 5.8B).

To understand the implications of acoustic reflex testing, it is important to have a basic knowledge of what has been referred to as the *acoustic reflex arc*. This pathway includes centers that are discussed in greater detail in Chapters 6 through 9 of this book, but they are mentioned here and diagrammed in Figure 5.10).

The sound presented to the outer ear passes through the middle ear, is transduced to an electrochemical signal in the inner ear, and is conducted along the VIIIth (auditory) nerve to the brainstem. The impulse is received by the cochlear nucleus in the brain and is transmitted to the superior olivary complex. Here, some very interesting things occur: In addition to transmitting signals to higher centers in the brain, impulses are sent from the superior olivary complex to the VIIth (facial) nerve on the same side of the head, which in turn descends to innervate the stapedius muscle in the middle ear on the same side of the head that received the sound, assuming that all systems are working properly. This is called the *ipsilateral response pathway*.

Almost simultaneously, neural impulses cross the brain stem to the opposite (contralateral) superior olivary complex, which in turn sends impulses by that facial nerve to the opposite middle ear to evoke an acoustic reflex along the *contralateral response pathway*. Although measurement of the acoustic reflex is usually made clinically in one ear at a time, in healthy ears and in some

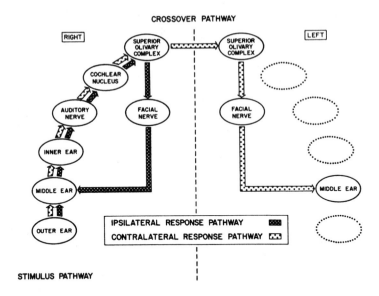

Figure 5.10 Block diagram of the ipsilateral and contralateral acoustic reflex pathways.

pathological cases, responses occur in both ears in response to a stimulus presented to only one ear. It is possible to present a pure tone of the desired frequency from the reflex-activating system of an immittance meter not only through an earphone coupled to the opposite ear (the contralateral reflex), but also through the probe tip itself (the ipsilateral reflex). The presence or absence of ipsilateral or contralateral reflexes is extremely valuable in audiological diagnosis.

Interpreting the Acoustic Reflex. Significance is placed on the intra-aural muscle reflex in terms of its absence or presence and in terms of the level of the tone above the voluntary threshold (Figure 5.8C and 5.8D) required to elicit the response. As stated previously, the reflex is expected in normal hearers at relatively high levels. Different constellations of responses may be attributed to several factors:

1. The middle-ear muscle reflex will be absent if the tone presented to the ear opposite the probe is not sufficiently intense. The intensity of the tone will be attenuated if any of several types of hearing losses are present, especially those caused by middle-ear conductive loss.
2. The contraction of the muscles may not be conducted to the eardrum membrane if the chain of bones in the middle ear is immobile or interrupted.

3. Abnormalities in the muscles themselves will, of course, affect the reflex in the ear to which the probe is affixed.

4. Sometimes the reflex appears in an ear with a hearing loss when the stimulus tone is presented at a fairly low sensation level. Why would a person with a 50 dB hearing loss experience a reflex at 95 dB HL (45 dB SL)? This has been interpreted by some audiologists as a manifestation of loudness recruitment, which occurs because the tone presented at 45 dB SL sounds as though it were very loud (as loud as a 95 dB HL tone to a normal listener). There is no evidence that recruitment per se produces the acoustic reflex at low sensation levels, although both phenomena are often found in the same patients. A precise explanation for low-sensation-level acoustic reflexes, which are associated with cochlear lesions, is lacking at this time.

5. When there is damage to the auditory nerve, acoustic reflexes are often absent or occur at higher-than-normal sensation levels, or the amplitude of the reflex is less than normal (Jerger, Oliver, & Jenkins, 1988).

6. The facial nerve supplies innervation to the stapedius muscle. If the facial nerve is in any way abnormal, the information supplied by the brain that mediates contractions may not be conveyed to the stapedius muscle. When this occurs, the damage is in the ear to which the probe is affixed, regardless of whether the reflex-activating tone is delivered ipsilaterally or contralaterally.

7. Even if the ipsilateral acoustic reflex pathway is normal, if damage occurs in the areas of the brainstem that house portions of the contralateral acoustic reflex pathway, ipsilateral reflexes may be present in both ears, but one or both of the contralateral reflexes may be absent.

8. Lesions in the higher areas of the auditory cortex usually produce no abnormalities in either contralateral or ipsilateral reflexes because these centers are above the acoustic reflex arc.

Figure 5.11 illustrates theoretical findings on acoustic reflex tests with eleven possible conditions of the auditory and related systems. These figures are designed to be illustrative, and there are many other possibilities.

Reflex Decay Test

In normal-hearing individuals, listening to a sustained tone for more than several minutes will result in a small degree of adaptation, during which the loudness of the tone is diminished. If the stapedius muscle is contracted by a loud sound, it will gradually relax as the tone lessens in loudness. This is called **reflex decay**. Reflex decay is checked by sustaining a tone at 10 dB above the reflex threshold and determining the number of seconds required for the amplitude of the reflex to be reduced by 50%. The test is completed when the reflex has decayed to half its original amplitude or at the end of 10 seconds, whichever occurs first.

Figure 5.11 Eleven theoretical examples of the results of ipsilateral and contralateral acoustic reflex testing, given different conditions of the ear. In each (lettered) example the condition is stated and the "patients" appear (facing the reader) as they would with the audiometer earphones over their right ears and with the immittance meter probes in their left, and then configured with the earphones over their left ears and the probes in the right. Four possibilities are illustrated: (1) acoustic reflex present at a normal sensation level; (2) acoustic reflex present at a low sensation level (less than 60 dB sL); (3) acoustic reflex present but at an elevated (higher than normal) sensation level; (4) acoustic reflex absent at the limit of the reflex-activating equipment. During contralateral stimulation in each case the earphone delivers the tone to one ear while the reflex is monitored via the probe in the opposite ear. During ipsilateral stimulation the tone is delivered via the probe and is monitored in the same ear.

(A)

RIGHT (R) - NORMAL HEARING
LEFT (L) - NORMAL HEARING

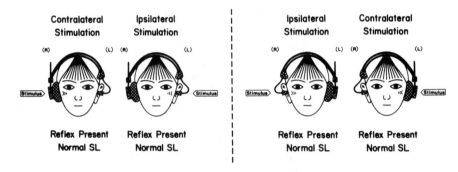

| Contralateral Stimulation | Ipsilateral Stimulation | | Ipsilateral Stimulation | Contralateral Stimulation |
| Reflex Present Normal SL | Reflex Present Normal SL | | Reflex Present Normal SL | Reflex Present Normal SL |

(B)

RIGHT (R) - NORMAL HEARING
LEFT (L) - CONDUCTIVE HEARING LOSS

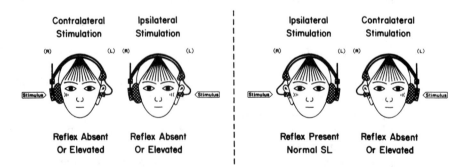

| Contralateral Stimulation | Ipsilateral Stimulation | | Ipsilateral Stimulation | Contralateral Stimulation |
| Reflex Absent Or Elevated | Reflex Absent Or Elevated | | Reflex Present Normal SL | Reflex Absent Or Elevated |

(C)
RIGHT (R) - CONDUCTIVE HEARING LOSS
LEFT (L) - CONDUCTIVE HEARING LOSS

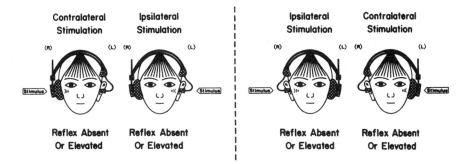

(D)
RIGHT (R) - NORMAL HEARING
LEFT (L) - COCHLEAR HEARING LOSS (MILD to MODERATE)

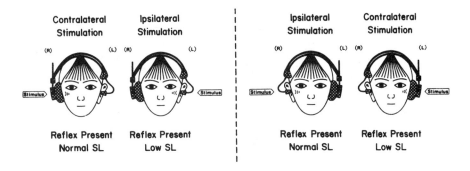

(E)
RIGHT (R) - COCHLEAR HEARING LOSS (MILD to MODERATE)
LEFT (L) - COCHLEAR HEARING LOSS (MILD to MODERATE)

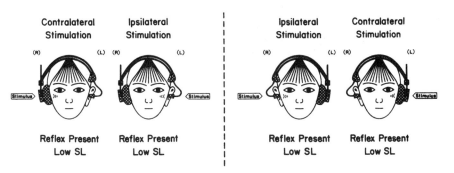

Figure 5.11 (continued)

(F) RIGHT (R) - COCHLEAR HEARING LOSS (SEVERE)
LEFT (L) - COCHLEAR HEARING LOSS (SEVERE)

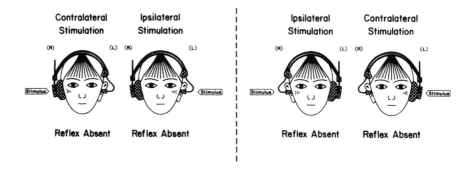

(G) RIGHT (R) - VIIIth NERVE HEARING LOSS
LEFT (L) - NORMAL HEARING

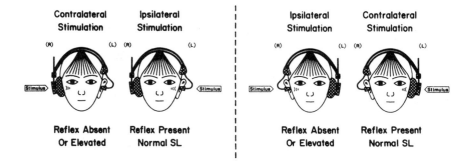

(H) RIGHT (R) - NORMAL HEARING (VIIth NERVE LESION)
LEFT (L) - NORMAL HEARING

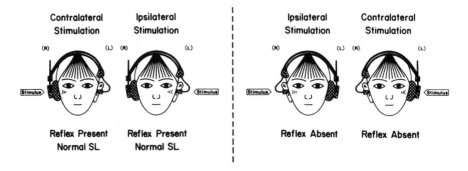

Figure 5.11 (continued)

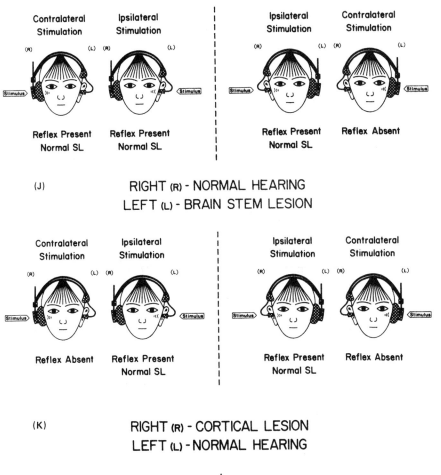

(I)

RIGHT (R) - NORMAL HEARING
LEFT (L) - BRAIN STEM LESION

Contralateral Stimulation — Reflex Present Normal SL
Ipsilateral Stimulation — Reflex Present Normal SL
Ipsilateral Stimulation — Reflex Present Normal SL
Contralateral Stimulation — Reflex Absent

(J)

RIGHT (R) - NORMAL HEARING
LEFT (L) - BRAIN STEM LESION

Contralateral Stimulation — Reflex Absent
Ipsilateral Stimulation — Reflex Present Normal SL
Ipsilateral Stimulation — Reflex Present Normal SL
Contralateral Stimulation — Reflex Absent

(K)

RIGHT (R) - CORTICAL LESION
LEFT (L) - NORMAL HEARING

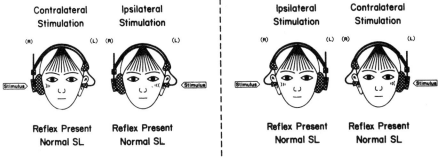

Contralateral Stimulation — Reflex Present Normal SL
Ipsilateral Stimulation — Reflex Present Normal SL
Ipsilateral Stimulation — Reflex Present Normal SL
Contralateral Stimulation — Reflex Present Normal SL

Figure 5.11 (continued)

Recording and Interpreting Reflex Decay Test Results. This test is scored in terms of the number of seconds required for the amplitude of the reflex to decay to half-magnitude. Test results may be recorded on an X–Y plotter, so that changes in the amplitude of the response can be observed as a function of time, or they may be recorded as on the form in Figure 5.8E.

In normal subjects there will be some decay of the reflex at 2000 and 4000 Hz, but not at 500 and 1000 Hz. The slight decay sometimes evident in patients with cochlear hearing losses tends to occur more in the higher frequency range. Rapid reflex decay is interpreted very much like the Type III Békésy pattern and rapid tone decay as representing some neural problem. Lesions in the auditory nerve cause decay to half-magnitude of the reflex, often within 3 to 5 seconds, even at 500 Hz (Anderson, Barr, & Wedenberg, 1970), because the nerve cannot maintain its continuous firing rate. Because the primary innervation of contraction of the middle-ear muscles is by way of the descending tract of the facial nerve (see Chapter 7), damage to that nerve may also cause an absent acoustic reflex or an initial response followed by rapid acoustic reflex decay.

Discussion of Acoustic Immittance Measurements

Both static immittance and tympanometry are measures of the mobility of the middle-ear mechanism. The acoustic reflex and reflex decay give information regarding probable disorders of different areas of the auditory system. These basic tests and their modifications are discussed in the appropriate portions of Chapters 6 to 9. Their inclusion in the test battery is a boon to the audiologist.

Under certain conditions bone-conduction audiometry may be unnecessary when acoustic immittance measures are combined with audiometric procedures. In the presence of normal hearing for pure tones, high speech discrimination scores, Type A tympanograms, and normal acoustic reflex thresholds, normal hearing may be diagnosed without performance of bone conduction. When air-conduction thresholds are depressed, acoustic reflexes are present, and speech-discrimination scores are less than 90%, conductive hearing loss is eliminated as a possible finding and bone-conduction audiometry will not likely produce an air–bone gap, resulting in a diagnosis of sensorineural hearing loss. If any signs of conductive loss do appear, such as absent acoustic reflexes or abnormal tympanograms, bone-conduction audiometry must be carried out. For these reasons many audiologists prefer to do immittance measures as some of the first tests in the battery. The result, of course, is that bone conduction may be eliminated when it is easiest to perform and least complicated (i.e., in patients with normal hearing and sensorineural loss). Bone conduction must be done to determine the amount of air–bone gap when it is most complicated by middle-ear artifacts and masking (in those with conductive and mixed hearing loss).

Static immittance and tympanometric measurements have been called *immittance audiometry*. Because "audiometry" per se is involved only with respect to the acoustic reflex, this term is not strictly accurate. There is no doubt that electroacoustic immittance measurements have reached a point of great importance in diagnostic audiology. New equipment is becoming available with improved design features that will increase the clinical capability and modify interpretation. The acoustic immittance meter has become as indispensable to the audiologist as the audiometer.

AUDITORY EVOKED POTENTIALS

From the time acoustic stimuli reach the inner ear, what is transmitted to the brain is not "sound" but, rather, a series of neuroelectric events (see Chapter 8 for more details). For many years there has been considerable interest in the measurement of the electrical responses generated within the cochlea. To this end, a procedure has evolved called **electrocochleography (ECoG)**. Additionally, because hearing is a phenomenon involving the brain, it is only logical that whenever a sound is heard there must be some change in the ongoing electrical activity of the brain. These electrical responses have been called by a number of names, but when measured today they are commonly known as **auditory evoked potentials (AEPs)**. AEPs can be subdivided on the basis of where and when they occur. They are better understood with the minimum background provided in Chapter 9, which briefly reviews the auditory nervous system. Before attempting to measure AEPs, much more auditory anatomy and physiology, as well as other aspects of neuroscience, should be known than can be presented in an introductory text. No chapter on the subject of auditory tests for site of lesion, however, would be complete without some discussion of AEPs.

In Chapter 1 some mention was made of the connections between the brain stem and the higher centers for audition in the cerebral cortex. These connections occur via a series of waystations, called nuclei, within the central nervous system. When a signal is introduced into the ear, there are immediate electrical responses in the inner ear. As the signal is propagated along the auditory pathway, more time elapses before a response can be recorded. The term *latency* is used to define the time period that elapses between the introduction of a stimulus and the occurrence of the response. Early AEPs that occur in the first 10 milliseconds after the introduction of a signal are believed to originate in the brainstem and are called the **auditory brainstem response (ABR)**. AEPs occurring from 10 to 50 milliseconds in latency are called **auditory middle latency responses (AMLRs)**, and probably originate in the auditory cortex. AEPs called **late evoked responses (LERs)** occur beyond 50 milliseconds and arise in the cortex. Responses recorded at 300 milliseconds or longer have been called *auditory event–related potentials* because they involve association areas in the brain.

AEPs are simply a small part of a multiplicity of electrical events measurable from the scalp. This electrical activity, which originates in the brain, is commonly referred to as *electroencephalic* and is measured on specially designed instruments called *electroencephalographs* (EEGs), which are used to pick up and amplify electrical activity from the brain by way of electrodes placed on the scalp. When changes in activity are observed on a strip chart recorder, waveforms may be seen that aid in the diagnosis of central nervous system disease or abnormality.

In coupling the EEG to a patient to observe responses *evoked* by sounds, the ongoing neural activity is about 100 times greater than the auditory evoked potential and therefore obscures the responses. The measurement of AEP is further complicated by the presence of large electrical potentials from muscles (myogenic potentials). These obstacles were insurmountable until the advent of sophisticated summing computers, devices that allow measurement of event-related potentials even when they are embedded in other electrical activity. A commercial device for measuring AEPs is shown in Figure 5.12.

Equipment for measurement of AEPs can range widely in price. More expensive units tend to provide greater flexibility in terms of the number and variety of tests that can be performed. Ferraro and Ruth (1988) found that relatively inexpensive units (under $10,000) are generally acceptable to users. Calibration and maintenance of equipment is a major factor in the clinical measurement of AEPs. Every device must be calibrated, and normative data should be collected in the audiology clinic where the equipment will be used

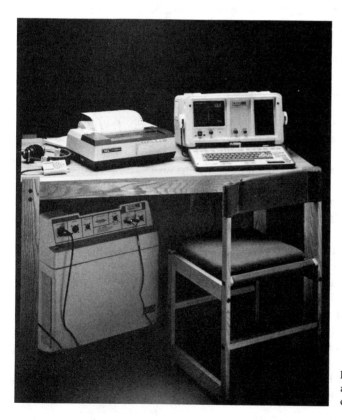

Figure 5.12 Device used for recording auditory evoked potentials. (Courtesy of Nicolet.)

before tests on patients can begin. Periodic recalibration is also necessary. Brey and Robinson (1988) reported problems in calibration among some of the commercially available evoked potential devices. These problems were often due to differences in earphones between devices.

To measure AEPs, a series of auditory stimuli is presented to the subject at a constant rate by means of a transducer (earphone, bone-conduction vibrator, or loudspeaker). Insert earphones are gaining popularity for AEP testing because they are relatively comfortable to wear and help attenuate extraneous room noise. Also, their transducers are 250 millimeters from electrodes placed at the ear and therefore produce fewer electrical artifacts. The EEG equipment picks up the neural response, amplifies it, and stores the information in a series of computer memory time bins. Each bin sums neuroelectric activity that occurs at specific numbers of milliseconds after the onset of the stimulus. Of course, the computer is summing not only the response to the sound in any particular time bin, but also the random brain activity taking place at that precise moment. However, because the random activity consists of positive and negative voltages of varying amplitudes, summing reduces them to a value at or near zero. The polarity of the response is either positive or negative, and summing causes the magnitude of the response to increase in amplitude. It might be said that as the summing or averaging process continues, the signal-to-noise ratio improves. Even though the amplitudes of the responses are extremely small, often on the order of 1 to 5 microvolts (1 μV is equal to one millionth of a volt), they can nevertheless be detected and interpreted.

Electrocochleography (ECoG)

The procedure for measuring electrical responses from the cochlea of the inner ear is called electrocochleography. An active electrode may be placed in one of several positions: (1) on the promontory, the medial wall of the middle ear, which usually necessitates surgery to move the eardrum membrane aside; (2) on the promontory using a needle electrode which is forced through the eardrum membrane; (3) in the skin of the outer ear canal using a needle electrode; (4) in saline-soaked cotton in the space of the outer ear canal; (5) against the eardrum membrane using a very thin electrode; (6) against the skin of the ear canal, using a silver ball electrode held in place by a plastic leaf; (7) using a disposable foam earplug covered by a very thin layer of gold foil, in which case the sound is delivered to the eardrum membrane through a plastic tube extending through the center of the foam.

Less invasive types of electrodes, which are more comfortable and do not require the use of anesthesia, are currently preferred. ECoG, both alone and in combination with other electrophysiological techniques, has been found to be helpful in the diagnosis of some specific disorders of the inner ear, and has been used successfully for monitoring cochlear function during some forms of surgery. The further the active electrode is from the inner ear, the smaller the amplitude of the response, and consequently the greater the number of stimuli that must be summed before the response can be identified with confidence.

Auditory Brainstem Response (ABR) Audiometry

For measuring responses from the brainstem and or the brain, the vertex (top of the skull) is the most common active electrode placement site. A reference electrode is usually placed on the mastoid process behind the outer ear, and a ground electrode on the opposite mastoid or on the forehead. Stimuli with rapid rise times, such as clicks, filtered clicks, or tone pips, must be used to generate these early responses. Using the summing computer, seven small wavelets generally appear in the first 10 milliseconds after signal presentation. Each wave represents neuroelectrical activity at one or more generating sites along the auditory brainstem pathway. Although disagreement persists on the site represented by each wave, Moller (1985) suggests the following simplified scheme of major ABR generators:

Wave Number	Site
I	VIIIth cranial nerve
II	VIIIth cranial nerve
III	Pons
IV	Pons
V	Midbrain
VI and VII	Undetermined

There are several ways in which routine ABR audiometry is performed, only one of which is described here. The patient is first seated in a comfortable chair, often a recliner, which is placed in an acoustically isolated, electrically shielded room. The skin areas to which electrodes will be attached are carefully cleansed, and a conductive paste or gel is applied to the area. An **active electrode** is placed on either the vertex or the forehead, and two other electrodes are attached to either the earlobes or the mastoid processes behind the external ears. The ipsilateral electrode (nearest the ear to be stimulated) is for **reference**, and the contralateral electrode (near the opposite ear) is for **ground**. After the electrodes are taped in place, electrical impedance is checked with an ohmmeter. The impedance between the skin and the electrodes, and between any two electrodes, must be controlled for the test to be performed properly. An earphone is placed over or into the test ear and the patient is asked to relax. The lights are usually dimmed and the chair placed in a reclining position.

In adults, one ear is tested at a time. A series of 1,000 to 1,200 clicks may be presented, at a rate of 33.1 clicks per second. The starting level is often 60 dB nHL (*n* is the reference to the normative group threshold for click stimuli). Clear responses should be seen on the oscilloscope screen in the form of waves I, III, and V. If responses are not present, the intensity is raised 20 dB; if responses are present, the level is lowered in 10 or 20 dB steps until wave V becomes undetectable. With decreased intensity, wave amplitudes become smaller and latencies increase. Since wave V normally has the largest amplitude of the first seven waves and is the most impervious to change, the ABR threshold is considered to be the lowest intensity at which wave V can be observed. Threshold determinations can usually be ascertained to within 10 to 20 dB of behavioral thresholds.

After the test has been completed, a hard copy may be printed out on an $X–Y$ plotter, and these data may be summarized on a special form (see Figure 5.13). A complete ABR test will provide the following information about each ear:

1. Absolute latencies of all identifiable waves I to V at different intensities
2. Interwave latency intervals (i.e., I to V, I to III, III to V)
3. Wave amplitudes
4. Threshold of wave V

Interpreting the ABR. The ABR may be used as a test of audiological or neurological function. If the ABR elicited by click stimuli is used as a test of hearing sensitivity, the auditory threshold in the frequency range from 1000 to 4000 Hz may be inferred from the lowest intensity at which wave V is identified. However, one must also look carefully at the wave V latency-intensity function and the absolute latencies of wave V. The closer the auditory stimulus is to a patient's threshold, the longer the latency of each wave. By plotting the latency of wave V at different intensities (the latency-intensity function), general site-of-lesion information of a hearing loss may be inferred.

If a conductive hearing loss is present, the intensity required to produce the ABR is increased. Threshold is elevated, latencies of all waves are prolonged, but interwave intervals are normal and the slope of the latency-intensity function is similar to one showing normal hearing. If the lesion results in a high-frequency loss in the cochlea, wave V often shows a normal latency at high sensation levels if the intensity of the clicks is above threshold in the 2000 to 4000 Hz region, but is prolonged near threshold, resulting in a steeply sloping latency-intensity function. With every 30 dB of hearing loss at 4000 Hz, there may be an increase of 0.2 milliseconds of wave V latency. When the lesion affects the auditory nerve, as in the case of a tumor, all waves subsequent to wave I are often delayed or absent at all intensities. Wave V and other waves may also be delayed or missing in cases of auditory brain stem tumors.

In addition to serving as a test for threshold and site of lesion, the ABR may be used as a neurological screening test, to assess the integrity of the central auditory pathway. The most significant neurological symptom is an increase in interwave intervals. If wave V can be observed at a slow click rate, for example 11.1 clicks per second (often seen clearly at 60 dB nHL), a higher click rate may be presented, such as 89.1 clicks per second. Under this condition it is normal for the wave V latency to increase up to 0.8 milliseconds. In abnormal central nervous systems, however, such as those with demyelinating diseases like multiple sclerosis, the stress from rapid click rates often causes wave V to disappear entirely. An ABR is considered neurologically abnormal, indicating neuropathology affecting the auditory pathway of the brain stem, when any of the following occur:

1. Interwave intervals are prolonged.
2. Wave V latency is significantly different between ears.

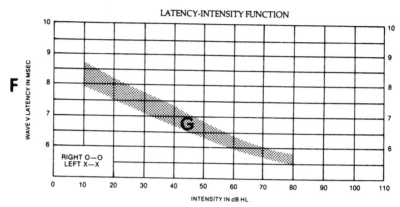

SPEECH AND HEARING CENTER
The University of Texas at Austin 78712

AUDITORY BRAINSTEM RESPONSE
(Adult Form)

NAME: Last - First - Middle	SEX	AGE	DATE	EXAMINER	RELIABILITY	INSTRUMENT

LATENCY-INTENSITY FUNCTION

F

WAVE V LATENCY IN MSEC

RIGHT O—O
LEFT X—X

INTENSITY IN dB HL

SHADED AREA REPRESENTS Normal Wave V Range for patients older than 16 mos. for 30 clicks per second.

G

	STIMULUS			WAVE LATENCY IN MSEC						
EAR	RATE	dB HL	FILTER	I	II	III	IV	V	VI	VII
	A	**B**					**C**			

SUMMARY OF RESULTS   **D**

INTERWAVE INTERVALS. . . . . R _____ L _____
AMPLITUDE RATIO (V SAME OR > I) . . . . R _____ L _____
LATENCY CHANGE WITH INCREASED CLICK RATE. . . . . R _____ L _____
INTERAURAL DIFFERENCES . . . . _____

E

ESTIMATED AIR CONDUCTION THRESHOLD IN dBHL (1-2 kHz) . . . . R _____ L _____
ESTIMATED BONE CONDUCTION THRESHOLD IN dB HL . . . . R _____ L _____

COMMENTS

Figure 5.13 Form used for recording results of auditory brainstem response tests: (A) stimulus click rate; (B) intensity (in dB HL) required to evoke the response; (C) latency (in milliseconds) to each of seven waves; (D) interwave intervals (in milliseconds); (E) estimate of auditory thresholds for each ear, (F) graph showing the latency (in milliseconds) as a function of the intensity of the series of clicks presented to each ear; (G) shaded area showing normal wave V latency values.

3. Amplitude ratios are abnormal (normally wave V is larger than wave I).
4. Wave V is abnormally prolonged or disappears with high click rate stimulation.

Normal ABR results are shown in Figures 5.14 and 5.15.

ABR measurements have been used with increasing frequency in the testing of infants and small children. Improvements in equipment and procedures have also brought ABR testing into the operating room, where it is used to monitor responses from the brain during delicate neurosurgical procedures (Kileny, Niparko, Shepard, & Kemink, 1988). Musiek, Golleghy, Kibbe, and Verkest (1988) find that ABR is often useful in the diagnosis of brain stem lesions when it is used in conjunction with some of the psychophysical procedures described in Chapter 9. In fact, in the past two decades over a thousand papers have been written attesting to the role of the ABR as an important diagnostic tool. The ABR has developed into the most important test in the diagnostic site-of-lesion battery and has proved to be sensitive, specific, and efficient in detecting lesions affecting the auditory pathways through the brain stem.

Auditory Middle Latency Response (AMLR) Audiometry

For some time it was uncertain whether the middle latency responses, which occur between 10 and 50 milliseconds after signal presentation, are *myogenic* (produced by changes in electrical potential generated in muscles on the scalp and behind the ear), or *neurogenic* (produced by electrical potentials in nerve units within the auditory pathways). This controversy is not completely resolved, but it is now generally accepted that the AMLR has a neurogenic component. The generator sites within the brain have not yet been determined, but they may include several areas of the auditory cortex as well as other areas between the auditory brain stem and the cortex.

Patient setup for measurement of the AMLR is essentially the same as for ABR. A major difference lies in the importance of keeping the patient inactive to minimize myogenic (muscle) artifacts. Patients must remain calm but alert. Clicks, filtered clicks, or tone bursts are delivered through an earphone. It may be necessary to deliver 1000 to 2000 stimuli in order to discern a clear AMLR.

Interpreting the AMLR. Because the ABR gives information about hearing primarily in the 1000 to 4000 Hz range, the AMLR is a nice complement in that it can provide information about hearing in the lower frequencies when performed with tone bursts (Fifer & Sierra-Irizarry, 1988). An AMLR response is shown in Figure 5.16. This information can be very helpful, but AMLR is often of least utility in the patients where it is needed most, such as in the diagnosis of infants and other uncooperative individuals. It is affected by state—that is, whether the patient is awake or asleep. Further refinement of

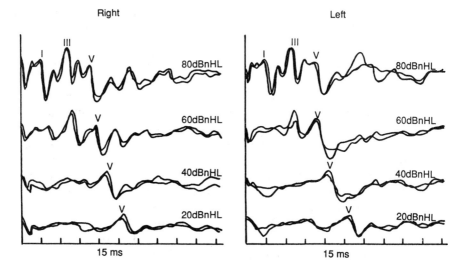

Figure 5.14 Auditory brain stem response testing on a normal hearing individual. Absolute latencies are shown in Figure 5.15.

AMLR measurement techniques will probably increase its use as a neurodiagnostic procedure.

Late Evoked Responses (LER)

The earliest work done on AEPs was on the cortical evoked response, which was involved with those responses that appeared at least 75 milliseconds after signal presentation. Problems in interpreting LER test results, along with improvements in microcomputers and averaging systems, led to a much greater interest in the earlier components of the evoked response (ABR and AMLR), but in recent years renewed interest has been found in the later components. A major advantage of measuring the later responses is that it is possible to use frequency-specific stimuli, such as pure tones, as well as short segments of speech. The responses are considerably larger than the earlier waves and therefore can be tracked closer to the individual's behavioral threshold; however, the responses are affected by patient attention, and therefore the procedure has limitations when used with children. These potentials are dependent on state of consciousness; that is, significant degradation occurs with sleep, whether natural or induced.

The first late response (P1) often occurs at approximately 75 milliseconds latency. P1 is followed by a series of negative (N) and positive (P) waves (N1, P2, N2) occurring between 100 and 250 milliseconds. At approximately 300 milliseconds a large (10 to 20 mv) positive wave, which has become known as P300, is seen in response to rare or novel stimuli that are embedded in more

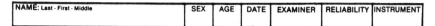

NAME: Last - First - Middle	SEX	AGE	DATE	EXAMINER	RELIABILITY	INSTRUMENT

LATENCY-INTENSITY FUNCTION

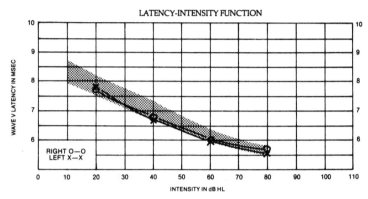

SHADED AREA REPRESENTS Normal Wave V Range for patients older than 16 mos. for 30 clicks per second.

	STIMULUS			WAVE LATENCY IN MSEC						
EAR	RATE	dB HL	FILTER	I	II	III	IV	V	VI	VII
R	33.1	80	150-1500	1.8		3.75		5.7		
L	33.1	80	150-1500	1.6		3.62		5.6		

SUMMARY OF RESULTS

INTERWAVE INTERVALS . . . . R _3.9_ L _4.0_

AMPLITUDE RATIO (V SAME OR > I) . . . . R _NORMAL_ L _NORMAL_

LATENCY CHANGE WITH INCREASED CLICK RATE . . . . R _____ L _____

INTERAURAL DIFFERENCES . . . . _____

ESTIMATED AIR CONDUCTION THRESHOLD IN dBHL (1-2 kHz) . . . . R _≤ 20_ L _≤ 20_

ESTIMATED BONE CONDUCTION THRESHOLD IN dB HL . . . . R _____ L _____

COMMENTS

Figure 5.15 Latency-intensity functions for wave V derived from the auditory brainstem response tracings shown in Figure 5.14 on a normal-hearing individual. All the latencies are normal.

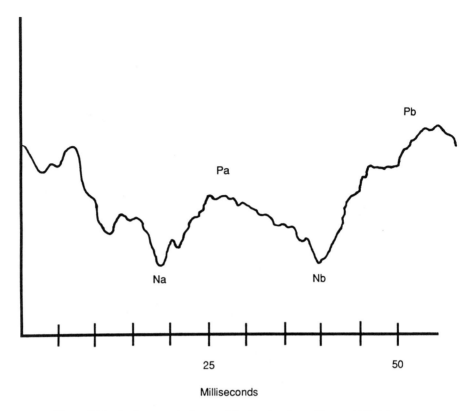

Figure 5.16 Auditory evoked potentials showing the auditory middle latency response.

frequent stimuli. For example, 2000 Hz tones may be presented 15% of the time along with 1000 Hz tones, which are presented 85% of the time (Kibbe-Michal, Verkest, Gollegly, & Musiek, 1986). The subject is instructed to attend only to the higher pitched tones by, for example, counting them or signaling each time one is heard. Also called the **auditory event-related potential**, the P300 is the earliest AEP that requires active participation on the part of the subject to generate the response.

Interpreting the Late Evoked Responses. Late evoked responses (see Figure 5.17) may aid in the estimation of threshold for pure tones over a wide frequency range. Of course, if patients are awake and cooperative enough to allow LERs, they can often be tested voluntarily. The P300 potential is called *event-related* because it depends on discrimination of target stimuli by the listener (Figure 5.18). For this reason the P300 is thought to be related to the perception or processing of stimuli rather than to the mere activation of the auditory nervous system by a stimulus. The late evoked and P300 responses are undergoing intensive research and offer great promise for practical applications in diagnosis of neurological disease and injury.

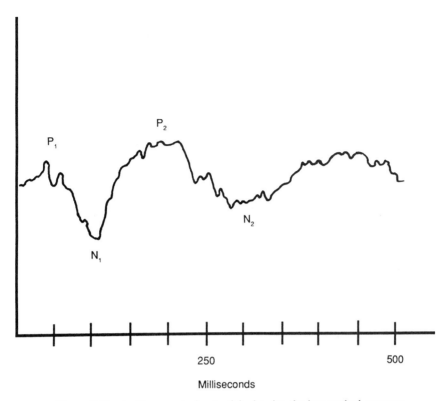

Figure 5.17 Auditory evoked potentials showing the late evoked response.

Discussion of Auditory Evoked Potentials

Using computer averaging techniques and a series of acoustic stimuli, it is possible to evoke responses on the basis of neuroelectric activity within the auditory system. By looking at the kinds of responses obtained during electrocochleography and auditory brain stem response audiometry, along with the later components of electroencephalic audiometry, it is often possible to predict the site of lesion and estimate auditory threshold. Although the ABR is often considered to be more of a test of synchronous neural firings than of hearing per se, its value to diagnostic audiology and to neurological screening is growing rapidly.

SUMMARY

The presence of loudness recruitment is a strong indicator of lesions of the cochlea and may be measured by alternate binaural (ABLB) or monaural (AMLB) loudness balancing procedures. Decruitment is considered to be a strong symptom of neural lesions. The absence of recruitment suggests a lesion elsewhere than the cochlea.

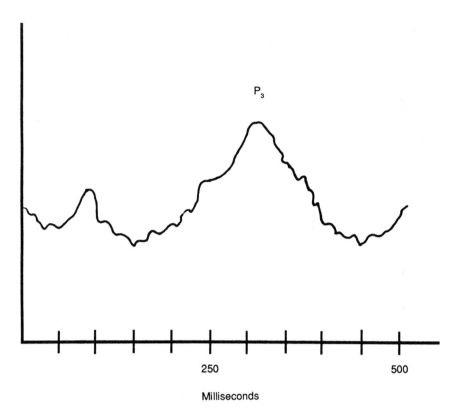

P_3

250   500

Milliseconds

Figure 5.18 Auditory evoked potentials showing the P300 (event-related) response.

High scores on the SISI test at 20 dB SL and acoustic reflexes at low sensation levels are other strong indicators of cochlear disorders. The modified SISI test, performed at high intensities, reveals low scores when retrocochlear lesions are present. Tone decay tests and Békésy audiometry produce patterns suggestive of hearing loss in the conductive, sensory, or neural pathways of

TABLE 5.2 SENSITIVITY, SPECIFICITY, AND EFFICIENCY OF SEVEN POPULAR SITE-OF-LESION AUDITORY TESTS

PROCEDURE	SENSITIVITY	SPECIFICITY	EFFICIENCY
ABR	97%	88%	90%
AR/Decay	85%	86%	86%
PI-PB	93%	98%	97%
Tone decay	75%	91%	88%
SISI	68%	90%	85%
ABLB	51%	88%	64%
Békésy	42%	95%	52%

(From Worthington, 1988)

hearing. Acoustic immittance measurements and tympanometry give remarkably reliable information regarding the function of the middle ear. Auditory brain stem response (ABR) audiometry has become an indispensable part of the site-of-lesion test battery, with the probability that some of the other emerging evoked potential techniques will become valuable as well.

None of the tests described in this chapter is infallible. Roeser (1986), on the basis of the findings of Jerger and Jerger (1983), has pointed out that some tests, like Békésy audiometry and the suprathreshold adaptation test (STAT), have high specificity but low sensitivity (i.e., they rule out the wrong lesion but do not correctly identify the right lesion), whereas others, like performance intensity functions for PB word lists (PI-PB), have high specificity and moderate sensitivity. Still other tests, like ABR, are both highly specific and highly sensitive, and are both efficient and possessive of high predictive value. On the basis of his own clinical observations and the findings of other clinicians, Worthington (1988) prepared a summary of the most popular site-of-lesion tests, comparing their sensitivity, specificity, and efficiency (Table 5.2).

The trends pointed out by Martin and Morris (1989) suggest that the older psychophysical tests are giving way to the newer electrophysiological procedures. No site-of-lesion test is infallible. For any individual case, it might be necessary to use the entire test battery before a diagnosis can be made. All results of special diagnostic tests must be compared to pure-tone and speech results and, above all, to the patient's history.

GLOSSARY

Acoustic impedance The total opposition to the flow of acoustic energy (as in the plane of the eardrum membrane). It consists of mass, stiffness, and frictional resistance and is influenced by frequency.

Acoustic reflex Contraction of one or both of the middle-ear muscles in response to a loud sound.

Acoustic reflex threshold (ART) The lowest intensity at which a stimulus can produce the acoustic reflex.

Active electrode The electrode used in testing auditory evoked potentials in conjunction with a reference electrode. It is placed on an area of the scalp, such as the vertex, where electrical activity is high. The potential difference between these electrodes is amplified, thus canceling out unwanted signals.

Alternate binaural loudness balance (ABLB) test A procedure that tests for recruitment in unilateral hearing losses. The growth of loudness of pure tones in the impaired ear is compared with that of the opposite (normal) ear as a function of increasing intensity.

Alternate monaural loudness balance (AMLB) test A test for recruitment performed in one ear of a patient with normal hearing at one frequency and a hearing loss at a different frequency. The growth of loudness with intensity of the impaired frequency is compared with that of the frequency at which hearing sensitivity is normal.

Auditory brain stem response (ABR) The seven wavelets that appear within 10 milliseconds after signal presentation.

Auditory event related potential AEPs that occur after latencies of about 75 milliseconds with the largest positive wave at about 300 milliseconds. Patients must cooperate by counting "oddball" stimuli.

Auditory evoked potentials (AEP) The use of summing or averaging computers with EEG to observe the very small electrical responses to sound observed from the cochlea, brain stem, and cortex.

Auditory middle latency response (AMLR) Responses that occur 10 to 50 milliseconds after signal onset and are thought to arise from the upper brain stem.

Békésy audiometry A procedure utilizing the Békésy automatic audiometer during which tracings are obtained for both pulsed and continuous tones.

Békésy comfortable loudness (BCL) Comparison of comfort levels for pulsed and continuous tones tracked on a Békésy audiometer.

Brainstem evoked response (BER) See *Auditory brainstem response.*

Brief tone audiometry (BTA) Comparison of thresholds for pure tones with durations of 20 and 500 milliseconds.

Clinical decision analysis (CDA) Procedures by which tests can be assessed in terms of their specificity, efficiency, and predictive value.

Compliance The inverse of stiffness.

Decruitment The less-than-normal growth in loudness of a signal as the intensity is increased. Also called *subtractive hearing loss*, it is suggestive of a loss of nerve units.

Difference limen for intensity (DLI) A test designed to determine a subject's ability to detect small changes in the intensity of a pure tone. In the 1950s a small DLI was considered a symptom of recruitment.

Electrocochleography (ECoG) Response to sound in the form of electrical potentials that occur within the first few milliseconds after signal presentation. The responses that arise from the cochlea are small in amplitude and must be summed on a computer after a number of presentations of clicks or tone pips.

Equivalent volume A method of approximating the compliance component of impedance. The volume (in cm^3) with a physical property equivalent to a similar property of the middle ear.

Ground electrode The third electrode used in testing auditory evoked potentials to ground the subject so that his or her body cannot serve as an antenna.

Hyperrecruitment A condition of some pathological hearing disorders in which a tone of a given intensity produces a sensation of greater loudness than that same intensity would produce for a normal ear.

Immittance A term used to describe measurements made on both impedance and otoadmittance meters.

Intra-aural muscle reflex The contraction of the stapedius muscles produced by introduction of a loud sound to one ear. The reflex is a bilateral phenomenon.

Laddergram The plotting of results on the ABLB or AMLB test. The relative loudness at each ear is shown at several intensities at the test frequency.

Late evoked response (LER) Those auditory evoked potentials evident after about 100 milliseconds. They are usually of larger amplitude than the earlier responses. Pure tones may be used as stimuli, and frequency-specific information may be available.

Median plane localization The sensation that tones of identical frequency and phase introduced to both ears are heard as a single tone in the middle of the head. In normal-hearing subjects, this requires approximately equal intensity in both ears.

Overrecruitment See *hyperrecruitment.*

Partial recruitment The condition in which a given amount of intensity in a pathological ear produces almost as much loudness as the same amount of intensity produces in a normal ear.

Reactance The contribution to total acoustic impedance provided by mass, stiffness, and frequency.

Recruitment A large increase in the perceived loudness of a signal produced by relatively small increases in intensity above threshold. Symptomatic of some hearing losses produced by damage to the inner ear.

Reference electrode An electrode placed on an area of the scalp that is rela-

tively unaffected by electrical activity in the brain.

Reflex decay A change in the dynamic impedance in the plane of the eardrum membrane as the stapedius muscle relaxes during constant acoustic stimulation.

Short increment sensitivity index (SISI) A test designed to determine a patient's ability to detect small changes (1 dB) in intensity of a pure tone presented at 20 dB SL.

Simultaneous binaural loudness balance (SBLB) test A test for median plane localization.

Site of lesion The precise area in the auditory system producing symptoms of abnormal auditory function.

Stapedius muscle A small muscle found in the middle ear. Both stapedius muscles normally contract, causing a change in the resting position of the eardrum membrane, when either ear is stimulated by a loud sound.

Static compliance A measurement of the mobility of the eardrum membrane.

Suprathreshold adaptation test (STAT) A tone decay test that begins at intensities near the limit of the audiometer. If the patient hears the tone for a full 60 seconds, the test result is considered to be negative for a lesion of the auditory nerve.

Temporal integration A time–intensity trading relationship in which the intensity of a tone must be increased to obtain threshold when its duration falls below a critical minimum.

Tensor tympani muscle One of two small muscles in the middle ear that contract in response to loud acoustic stimulation.

Tone decay The loss of audibility of a sound produced when the ear is constantly stimulated by a pure tone.

Tympanogram A graphic representation of a pressure-compliance function.

Tympanometry Measurement of the pressure-compliance function of the eardrum membrane.

STUDY QUESTIONS

1. For each site-of-lesion test described in this chapter, indicate whether it may be performed with (a) unilateral losses, (b) bilateral losses, or (c) both. Explain why.
2. For the tests described in question 1, list the equipment required and consider the performance and interpretation of each test.
3. Draw audiograms for unilateral conductive and sensorineural hearing losses. What are the probable results of the site-of-lesion tests described in this chapter, based on the type of hearing loss and the probable site of lesion?
4. What are the theoretical and practical values of the measures obtained in question 3?
5. Determine the effective masking levels, if needed, for all the tests described in question 3.

REVIEW TABLE 5.1 SUMMARY OF SITE-OF-LESION TESTS

TEST	PURPOSE	UNIT	WHEN TO MASK	HOW TO MASK
ABLB	Test for recruitment	dB		
AMLB	Test for recruitment	dB	When HL at poorer hearing frequency $-$ IA $\geq BC_{NTE}$	Max masking with broad-band noise
SISI	Test for detection of 1 dB increment	%	SISI $HL_{TE} -$ IA $\geq BC_{NTE}$	EM = SISI HL $-$ IA + ABG_{NTE}
Tone decay test	Test for adaptation	Seconds or dB	Routinely	EM = BC_{TE} + IA $-$ 5
Békésy audiometry	Tracking behavior for pulsed and continuous tones	dB	Same as tone decay	Same as tone decay
Tympanometry	Determine compliance of eardrum membrane	Arbitrary, cm³ or mmho		
Static compliance	Determine compliance of middle ear	cm³		
Reflex threshold	Determine SL for acoustic reflex	dB		
ABR	Determine amplitude-latency functions	msec		

REVIEW TABLE 5.2   TYPICAL INTERPRETATION OF SITE-OF-LESION TESTS

	NORMAL HEARING	CONDUCTIVE LOSS	SENSORY LOSS	NEURAL LOSS
Recruitment ABLB or AMLB	No recruitment	No recruitment	Partial recruitment Full recruitment Hyperrecruitment	No recruitment or decruitment
SISI in percentage	0–30	0–30	70–100	0–30
Tone decay type	I	I	II	III
Békésy type	I	I	II or IV	III or IV
Tympanometry type	A	A_D, A_S, B, or C	A	A
Static compliance in cm^3	0.28 to 2.5	More than 2.5 or less than .28	.28 to 2.5	.28 to 2.5
Acoustic reflex threshold	About 85 dB SL	Absent or elevated	Present at low SL	Absent
ABR	Normal wave V and interwave latencies	Normal wave V and interwave latencies	Slightly increased wave V and interwave latencies	Markedly increased wave V and interwave latencies

REFERENCES

AMERICAN NATIONAL STANDARDS INSTITUTE. (1987). *American National standard specifications for instruments to measure aural acoustic impedance and admittance (aural acoustic immittance).* ANSI S3.39–1987. New York: American National Standards Institute.

AMERICAN SPEECH AND HEARING ASSOCIATION. (1978). Guidelines for acoustic immittance screening of middle-ear effusion. *Asha, 20,* 550–555.

ANDERSON, H., BARR, B., & WEDENBERG, E. (1970). Early diagnosis of VIIIth nerve tumors by acoustic reflex tests. *Acta Otolaryngoligica, 263* (Supplement).

BLEGVAD, B. (1967). Contralateral masking and Békésy audiometry in normal listeners. *Acta Otolaryngologica* (Stockholm), *64,* 157–165.

BREY, R. H., & ROBINSON, D. O. (1988). Characteristics of signal stimuli of 19 auditory evoked potential instruments. *Asha, 30,* 30–35.

BRUNT, M. A. (1985). Békésy audiometry and loudness balance testing. In J. Katz (Ed.), *Handbook of clinical audiology* (pp. 273–291). Baltimore: Williams & Wilkins.

CARHART, R. (1957). Clinical determination of abnormal auditory adaptation. *Archives of Otolaryngology, 65,* 32–39.

DAVIS, H., & GOODMAN, A. C. (1966). Subtractive hearing loss, loudness recruitment, and decruitment. *Annals of Otology, Rhinology, and Laryngology, 75,* 87–94.

DIRKS, D. D., & NORRIS, J. D. (1966). Shifts in auditory thresholds produced by ipsilateral and contralateral maskers at low intensity levels. *Journal of the Acoustical Society of America, 40,* 12–19.

DOMICO, W. D. (1983). Békésy-tracked MCL and UCL patterns. *The Hearing Journal, 37,* 18–22.

FERRARO, J. A., & RUTH, R. R. (1988). Comparison of commercial auditory evoked potential units: The economy units. *The American Journal of Otology, 9,* 57–62.

FIFER, R. C., & BENIGNO SIERRA-IRIZARRY, M. A. (1988). Clinical applications of the auditory middle latency response. *The American Journal of Otology, 9,* 47–56.

FOWLER, E. P. (1936). A method for early detection of otosclerosis. *Archives of Otolaryngology, 24,* 731–741.

GREEN, D. S. (1963). The modified tone decay test (MTDT), as a screening procedure for eighth nerve lesions. *Journal of Speech and Hearing Disorders, 28,* 31–36.

––––––. (1978). Tone decay. In J. Katz (Ed.), *Handbook of Clinical Audiology* (2nd ed., pp. 188–200). Baltimore: Williams & Wilkins.

HERBERT, F., & YOUNG, I. M. (1968). Clinical application of Békésy audiometry. *Laryngoscope, 78,* 487–497.

HOOD, J. D. (1969). Basic audiological requirements of neuro-otology. *Journal of Laryngology and Otology, 83,* 695–711.

JERGER, J. F. (1960). Békésy audiometry in analysis of auditory disorders. *Journal of Speech and Hearing Research, 3,* 275–287.

––––––. (1961). Recruitment and allied phenomena in differential diagnosis. *Journal of Auditory Research, 1,* 145–151.

––––––. (1970). Clinical experience with impedance audiometry. *Archives of Otolaryngology, 92,* 311–324.

JERGER, J. F., & HARFORD, E. R. (1960). The alternate and simultaneous balancing of pure tones. *Journal of Speech and Hearing Research, 3,* 17–30.

JERGER, J. F., & HERER, G. (1961). Unexpected dividend in Békésy audiometry. *Journal of Speech and Hearing Disorders, 26,* 390–391.

JERGER, J., & JERGER, S. (1974). Diagnostic value of Békésy comfortable loudness tracings. *Archives of Otolaryngology, 99,* 351–360.

––––––. (1975). A simplified tone decay test. *Archives of Otolaryngology, 101,* 403–407.

JERGER, J., JERGER, S., & MAULDIN, L. (1972). The forward-backward discrepancy in Békésy audiometry. *Archives of Otolaryngology, 96,* 400–406.

JERGER, J., OLIVER, T. A., & JENKINS, H. (1988). Suprathreshold abnormalities of the stapedius reflex in acoustic tumor: A series of case reports. *Ear and Hearing, 8,* 131–139.

JERGER, J. F., SHEDD, J., & HARFORD, E. R. (1959). On the detection of extremely small changes in sound intensity. *Archives of Otolaryngology, 69,* 200–211.

JERGER, S., & JERGER, J. (1983). The evaluation of diagnostic audiometric tests. *Audiology, 22,* 144–161.

KARJA, J., & PALVA, A. (1970). Reverse frequency-sweep Békésy audiometry. *Acta Otolaryngologica* (Stockholm), *263* (Supplement), 225–228.

KIBBE-MICHAL, K., VERKEST, S. B., GOLLEGLY, K. M., & MUSIEK, F. E. (1986). Late auditory potentials and the P300. *Hearing Instruments, 37,* 22–24.

KILENY, P. R., NIPARKO, J. K., SHEPARD, N. T., & KEMINK, J. L. (1988). Neurophysiologic intraoperative monitoring: I. Auditory function. *The American Journal of Otology, 9,* 17–24.

KOCH, L. J., BARTELS, D., & RUPP, R. R. (1969). *The use of a "modified" short increment sensitivity index in assessing site of auditory lesion.* Paper presented at the 45th annual convention of the American Speech and Hearing Association, Chicago.

MARTIN, F. N., & FORBIS, N. K. (1978). The present status of audiometric practice: A follow-up study. *Asha, 20,* 531–541.

MARTIN, F. N., & MORRIS, L. J. (1989). Current audiological practices in the United States. *The Hearing Journal, 42,* 25–42.

MARTIN, F. N., & SIDES, D. (1985). Survey of current audiometric practices. *Asha, 27,* 29–36.

MOLLER, A. R. (1985). Physiology of the ascending auditory pathways with special reference to the auditory brain stem response (ABR). In M. L. Pinheiro & P. E. Musiek (Eds.), *Assessment of central auditory dysfunction: Foundations and clinical correlates* (pp. 23–41). Baltimore: Williams & Wilkins.

MUSIEK, F. E., & BARAN, J. A. (1986). Neuroanatomy, neurophysiology, and central auditory assessment: Part I. Brain stem. *Ear and Hearing, 7,* 207–219.

MUSIEK, F. E., GOLLEGLY, K. M., KIBBE, K. S., & VERKEST, S. B. (1988). Current concepts on the use of ABR and auditory psychophysical tests in the evaluation of brain stem lesions. *The American Journal of Otology, 9,* 25–35.

NORTHERN, J. L., & GRIMES, A. M. (1978). Introduction to acoustic impedance. In J. Katz (Ed.), *Handbook of Clinical Audiology* (pp. 344–355). Baltimore: Williams & Wilkins.

OLSEN, W. O., & NOFFSINGER, D. (1974). Comparison of one new and three old tests of auditory adaptation. *Archives of Otolaryngology, 99,* 94–99.

OWENS, E. (1971). Audiologic evaluation in cochlear versus retrocochlear lesion. *Acta Otolaryngologica, 283* (Supplement), (1971).

PALVA, T., & JAUHIAINEN, T. (1976). Reverse frequency Békésy audiometry in the diagnosis of acoustic neuroma. In S. K. Hirsh, D. H. Eldredge, I. J. Hirsh, & S. R. Silverman (Eds.), *Hearing and Davis: Essays honoring Hallowell Davis* (pp. 353–358). St. Louis: Washington University Press.

PALVA, T., JAUHIAINEN, C., SJOBLOM, J., & YLI-KOSKI, J. (1978). Diagnosis and surgery of acoustic tumors. *Acta Otolaryngologica* (Stockholm) *86,* 233–240.

PICTON, T. W., & FITZGERALD, P. G. (1983). A general description of the human auditory evoked potentials. In E. Moore (Ed.), *Bases of auditory brain-stem evoked responses.* New York: Grune & Stratton. pp. 141–156.

POPELKA, G. R. (1983). Basic acoustic immittance measures. *Audiology: A Journal for Continuing Education, 8,* 1–16.

PRIEDE, V. M., & COLES, R. R. A. (1974). Interpretation of loudness recruitment tests—Some new concepts and criteria. *Journal of Laryngology and Otology, 88,* 641–662.

REGER, S. N. (1936). Differences in loudness response of normal and hard-of-hearing ears at intensity levels slightly above threshold. *Annals of Otology, Rhinology, and Laryngology, 45,* 1029–1039.

ROESER, R. (1986). *Diagnostic audiology.* Austin, TX: Pro-Ed.

ROSE, D. E. (1962). Some effects and case

histories of reversed frequency sweep in Bé-késy audiometry. *Journal of Auditory Research, 2,* 267–278.

ROSENBERG, P. E. (1958, November). *Rapid clinical measurement of tone decay.* Paper presented at the American Speech and Hearing Association convention, New York.

———. (1969). Tone decay. *Maico Audiological Library Series,* Report 6.

SANDERS, J. W., JOSEY, A. F., & GLASSCOCK, M. E. (1974). Audiologic evaluation in cochlear and eighth nerve disorders. *Archives of Otolaryngology, 100,* 283–289.

SHANKS, J. E., LILLY, D. J., MARGOLIS, R. H., WILEY, T. L., & WILSON, R. H. (1988). Tympanometry. *Journal of Speech and Hearing Disorders, 53,* 354–377.

TURNER, R. G., & NIELSEN, D. W. (1984). Application of clinical decision analysis to audiological tests. *Ear and Hearing, 5,* 125–133.

WORTHINGTON, D. W. (1988). *Site of lesion: Special auditory tests.* Presentation at the Scott Haug Audiology Retreat, Kerrville, Texas.

WRIGHT, H. N. (1968). Clinical measurement of temporal auditory summation. *Journal of Speech and Hearing Research, 11,* 109–127.

———. (1969). Békésy audiometry and temporal summation. *Journal of Speech and Hearing Research, 12,* 865–874.

———. (1978). Brief tone audiometry. *Handbook of Clinical Audiology,* ed. J. Katz, Baltimore: Williams & Wilkins. pp. 218–232.

SUGGESTED READINGS

HANNLEY, M. (1984). Immittance audiometry. In J. Jerger (ed.), *Hearing disorders in adults* (pp. 57–83). San Diego: College-Hill Press.

KAPLAN, H., GLADSTONE, V. S., & KATZ, J. (1983). *Site of lesion testing: Audiometric interpretation* (Vol. II). Baltimore: University Park Press.

Part 3: Anatomy and Physiology of the Auditory System: Pathology, Etiology, and Therapy

_____ 6 _____

THE OUTER EAR

The outer ear is responsible for gathering sounds from the acoustical environment and funneling them into the auditory mechanism. Some of the outer-ear structures found in humans are absent in such animals as birds and frogs, whose hearing sensitivity is nevertheless similar to that of humans.

CHAPTER OBJECTIVES

This chapter assumes no previous knowledge of human anatomy, but it does assume an understanding of the physics of sound and the various tests of hearing described earlier. It is not intended that the reader memorize all the miniscule details of the anatomy of the outer ear. These may be obtained readily from books of anatomy.

Upon completion of Chapter 6, the reader should have a basic grasp of outer-ear anatomy and purpose. Knowledge should be acquired about some aspects of genetics, common disorders that affect the outer ear, how they are caused and treated, and how they manifest themselves on a variety of audiometric tests. Although in actual clinical practice, special tests for site of lesion are not usually performed in cases of conductive hearing loss, theoretical findings on these tests are illustrated in chapters 6 and 7 of this book.

ANATOMY OF THE OUTER EAR

The Auricle

The most noticeable portion of the outer-ear mechanism is the **auricle** or **pinna** (Figure 6.1). The auricle varies from person to person in size and shape. Even though it is the first part of the aural anatomy to catch attention, it is the least important as far as hearing is concerned, although its funnel-like action plays a substantial role in gathering sound waves from the environment. The auricle is made entirely of cartilage, with a number of individually characteristic twists, turns, and indentations. The entire cartilage is covered with skin, which is continuous with the face. The bottom-most portion of the auricle is the *lobule* or ear lobe. Extending up from the lobule, the outer rim of the auricle folds over outwardly, forming the *helix*. Above the lobule is the *antitragus*. Another elevation running closer to the center of the auricle is the *antihelix*. A small triangular protrusion, which points slightly backward and forms the anterior portion of the auricle, is called the *tragus*, Greek for "goat's beard"; the tragus is so named because in older men, a number of bristly hairs appear in this region. Depression of the tragus into the opening of the ear canal is an efficient means of blocking out loud sounds. This occlusion provides more efficiency than stopping up the ear with a finger, clasping the hands over the auricle, or even using some ear plugs specifically designed for sound attenuation. Although humans cannot voluntarily close off the tragus as can some animals, vestiges of muscles designed for this purpose remain in the human ear.

The middle-most portion of the ear, just before the opening into the head, is called the *concha* because of its bowllike shape. The concha is divided into two parts, the lower *cavum concha* and the upper *cymba concha*. The concha helps to funnel sounds directed to it from the surrounding air into the opening of the **external auditory canal (EAC)** or *external auditory* **meatus**. The anatomy of the auricle is such that it is more efficient at delivering high-frequency sounds

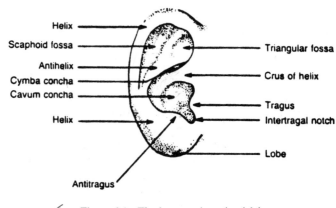

Figure 6.1 The human pinna (auricle).

than low-frequency sounds, and it helps in the localization of sounds delivered to the head.

The External Auditory Canal

In discussing this portion of the ear, it is important not to omit the word *external* in order to avoid confusion with the internal auditory canal, discussed in Chapter 9. The external auditory canal is a tunnel formed in the side of the head, beginning at the concha and extending inward at a slight upward angle for approximately one inch (2.5 cm) in adults. Although it appears round, the EAC is actually elliptical and averages about 9 mm in height and 6.5 mm in width. It is lined entirely with skin (Figure 6.2).

The outer third of the external auditory canal passes through cartilage. The skin in this outer portion supports several sets of glands, including the sebaceous glands, which secrete sebum, an oily, fatty substance. The major product of these secretions is ear wax or **cerumen**. Cerumen exits the ear naturally when the walls of the EAC are distorted by movement of the jawbone during chewing or speaking. The outer third of the external auditory canal contains a number of hair follicles. The combination of hairs and cerumen helps to keep foreign objects, such as insects, from passing into the inner two-thirds of the canal.

The inner two-thirds of the external auditory canal pass through the tympanic portion of the temporal bone. There are no glands and no hair in this area. The two portions of the external auditory canal meet at the **osseo-cartilaginous junction**. One of the protrusions of the mandible (jawbone), the *condyle*, comes to rest just below the osseocartilaginous junction when the jaw is closed. If the mandible overrides its normal position, as in the case of missing or worn molar teeth or a misaligned jaw, the condyle will press into

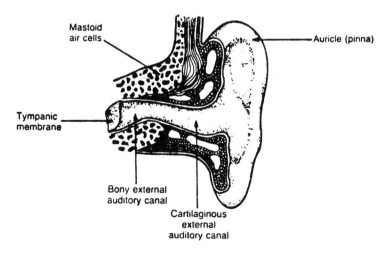

Figure 6.2 Cross section of the external ear.

the junction, causing pain. The term **temporomandibular joint (TMJ) syndrome** has been coined for this neuralgia. The TMJ syndrome produces a referred pain, perceived in the ear, which constitutes a significant amount of **otalgia** (ear pain) in adults.

The term *myofacial pain dysfunction* (MPD) syndrome is sometimes used to include pain in the temporomandibular joint, along with headaches; grating sounds (crepitus); dizziness; and back, neck, and shoulder pain. At times, emotional stress and tension have been associated with MPD syndrome, and treatment has ranged from emotional therapy to biofeedback training to the use of prosthetic devices to major maxillofacial surgery.

In infants and small children the angle of the external auditory canal is quite different from that in adults. The canal angles downward rather than upward and is at a more acute angle. For this reason it is advisable to examine children's ears from above the head rather than from below. When one looks into an ear, the adult pinna is pulled up and back, whereas the child's is pulled down and back.

The external auditory canal serves several important functions. The **tympanic membrane** is situated at the end of the canal, deep inside the head, where it is protected from trauma and where it can be kept at a constant temperature and humidity. The canal also serves as a tube resonator for frequencies between 2000 and 5500 Hz. The pinna and the concha also aid in the human ability to localize the sources of sounds that come from in front of, behind, below, and above the head.

The Tympanic Membrane

The external auditory canal terminates in a concave, disclike structure called the tympanic membrane (Figure 6.3). The term *eardrum* is commonly used to describe this structure, although properly speaking a drum would include the space below a vibrating membrane (in this case the middle ear), and so the term **eardrum membrane** is more accurate. The tympanic membrane is discussed in this book under the heading of the outer ear, because it can be viewed along with the outer-ear structures. Because the tympanic membrane

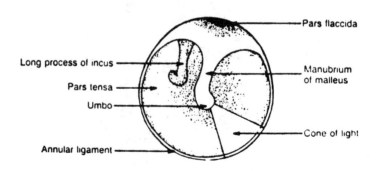

Figure 6.3 A right tympanic membrane.

marks the border between the outer ear and the middle ear, however, it is really a structure of both. In most books the tympanic membrane is considered a part of the middle ear, although obviously what is important is that its structure and function be understood.

The tympanic membrane has a total area of about 63.3 mm² (Harris, 1986, p. 19) and is constructed of three layers. The outer layer is composed of the same skin that is stretched over the osseous meatus. Below the skin is a layer of tough, fibrous connective tissue, which contributes most to the membrane's ability to vibrate with impinging sound waves. Behind the tympanic membrane is the middle-ear space, which is completely lined with **mucous membrane**, including the third layer of the tympanic membrane.

The tympanic membrane is extremely thin, averaging about 0.07 mm. Harris (1986, p. 18) describes the tympanic membrane as "a little conical loudspeaker." The entire area of the tympanic membrane is very rich in blood supply, which is why it appears so red when infection is present and blood comes to the area. The tympanic membrane is an extremely efficient vibrating surface. Movement of one billionth of a centimeter is sufficient to produce a threshold response in normal-hearing individuals in the 800 to 6000 Hz range (Harris, 1986, p. 21).

Embedded in the fibrous portion of the tympanic membrane is the *malleus*, the largest bone of the middle ear (described in Chapter 7). The tip of the malleus ends in the approximate center of the tympanic membrane and angles downward and backward slightly (see Figure 6.3). If you draw an imaginary line through the tympanic membrane at a 180° angle to the handle of the malleus, and bisect this line through the center of the tympanic membrane at right angles, the two intersecting imaginary lines thus drawn conveniently divide the tympanic membrane into four quadrants, called *anterior-superior, posterior-superior, anterior-inferior,* and *posterior-inferior*.

The tip of the handle of the malleus is so poised as to cause the center of the tympanic membrane to be pulled inward, resulting in its concave configuration. The point of greatest retraction is called the **umbo**. In order to visualize the tympanic membrane, it is necessary to direct a light, as from an **otoscope**, into the external auditory canal. Because the tympanic membrane is semitransparent, such a light allows some of the structures of the middle ear to become visible. However, some of the light rays directed against the membrane are reflected and refracted away. The concavity of the tympanic membrane causes the light reflex to appear in a cone shape directed inferiorly and anteriorly.

The tympanic membrane is held in position at the end of the external auditory canal by a ring of tissue called the tympanic **annulus**. The tympanic membrane's being stretched slightly into the middle ear results in its tension and conical appearance. The greatest surface area of the tympanic membrane is taut and has been called the **pars tensa**. At the top of the tympanic membrane, above the malleus, the tissues are looser, resulting in the term **pars flaccida**. The pars flaccida is also called **Shrapnell's membrane**, for the English anatomist who described it.

The auricle and external auditory canal provide a resonant tube through which sound waves may pass, and the tympanic membrane is the first mobile link in the chain of auditory events. Pressure waves, which impinge upon the tympanic membrane, cause it to vibrate, reproducing the same spectrum of sounds that enters the external auditory canal. Movement of the tympanic membrane causes identical vibration of the malleus to which it is attached. The further transmission of these sound waves is discussed in ensuing chapters.

DEVELOPMENT OF THE OUTER EAR

About 28 days after conception of the human embryo, bulges begin to appear on either side of the tissue that will develop into the head and neck. These are the **pharyngeal arches**. Although there may be as many as six arches, separated by grooves or clefts, significant information is only available about the first three: the mandibular arch, the hyoid arch, and the glossopharyngeal arch. These arches are known to have three layers, the **ectoderm** or outer layer, the **entoderm** or inner surface, and the **mesoderm** or inner core. Each arch contains four components: an artery, muscle and cartilage that come from the mesoderm, and a nerve that forms from the ectoderm.

The auricle develops from the first two pharyngeal arches. The tragus forms from the first arch and the helix and antitragus from the second arch. Development of the auricle begins before the second fetal month.

The external auditory canal forms from the first pharyngeal groove and is very shallow until after birth. A primitive meatus forms in about the fourth week, and a solid core forms near the tympanic membrane in the eighth week. The solid core canalizes (forms a tube or canal) by the twenty-eighth gestational week, although the entire osseous meatus is not complete until about the time of puberty. Pneumatization of the temporal bone surrounding the external auditory canal begins in the thirty-fifth fetal week, accelerates at the time of birth, and is not complete until puberty.

The tympanic membrane annulus forms in the third fetal month. The outer layer of the membrane itself forms from ectoderm, the inner layer from entoderm, and the middle layer from **mesenchymal** tissue, which is a network of embryonic tissue that later forms the connective tissues of the body as well as the blood vessels and the lymphatic vessels. The tympanic membrane has begun formation by the beginning of the second embryonic month.

HEARING LOSS AND THE OUTER EAR

When conditions occur that interfere with or block the normal sound vibrations transmitted through the outer ear, conductive hearing loss results. Except in isolated cases, the loss of hearing is rarely severe and never exceeds approximately a 60 dB air–bone gap. Because some of the disorders alter the normal resonance frequency of the outer ear or otherwise interfere with the osseotympanic mode of bone conduction, the bone-conduction audiogram may be slightly altered; however, this does not in itself suggest abnormality of the sensorineural system.

DISORDERS OF THE EXTERNAL EAR AND THEIR TREATMENT

As is shown next, some abnormalities of the external ear do not result in hearing loss. They are mentioned nonetheless because of the audiologist's usual curiosity about disorders of the ear in general and because abnormalities in one part of the body, specifically congenital ones, are frequently related to other abnormalities.

Disorders of the Auricle

Since hearing tests performed with earphones ignore the auricle, they do not reveal any effects it may have on hearing sensitivity, discrimination, and localization. For example, people who have had a portion or an entire auricle removed by accident or surgery, as in the case of cancer, appear to have no apparent hearing loss.

At times, one or both ears may be near-perfectly formed but of very small size (**microtia**), or the pinna may be entirely absent (**anotia**). Congenital malformations of the auricle have also been associated with other disorders, such as **Down's syndrome**.

When the auricle protrudes markedly from the head or when it is pressed tightly against the head, a simple surgical procedure called **otoplasty** may be performed. Otoplasties improve the patient's appearance, which often has a beneficial psychological effect. In cases of missing auricles in children, plastic surgery is often inadvisable because the scar tissue formed from the grafts does not grow as normal tissue. Plastic auricles can be made that are affixed to the head with adhesive and are amazingly realistic. Hairstyles can sometimes be arranged to conceal malformed auricles entirely.

Disorders of the External Auditory Canal

Atresia of the External Auditory Canal. In some patients, either the cartilaginous portion, the bony portion, or the entirety of the external auditory canal has never formed at all. Such congenital abnormalities may occur in one or both ears. This condition, called **atresia**, occurs in the external auditory canal either in isolation or in combination with other anomalies. One condition, Treacher Collins syndrome, which is hereditary and sex-linked, involves the facial bones, especially the cheek and lower jaw, the auricle, and congenital atresia of the external auditory canal.

Not all atresias are congenital; some may occur as the result of trauma or burns. Sometimes when an ear is malformed in a small child, it is difficult for the physician to determine whether the condition is one of congenital atresia or a marked **stenosis** (narrowing) of the canal.

Surgical procedures for correction of atresia of the external auditory canal have improved in recent years, and surgeons have been assisted greatly by the advent of modern imaging techniques. Chances for success are better when only the cartilaginous canal is involved and when the middle ear and tympanic membrane are normal. Drillouts of the bony canal have led to some serious aftercare problems. Although in some cases it may appear that it is better to treat a child with a congenital external ear canal atresia with a hearing aid rather than with surgery, the ultimate decision on such matters is always left to the physician.

Stenotic external auditory canals do not produce hearing loss as does atresia, although the very narrow lumen can easily be clogged by ear wax or other debris and thus cause a conductive problem. In cases of atresia of the canal, the hearing loss is directly related to the involved area and the amount of occlusion. The loss may be mild if only the cartilaginous area is involved and certainly will be more severe if the bony canal is occluded. As stated earlier, the presence of a congenital anomaly in one part of the body increases the likelihood of another anomaly elsewhere. For this reason, when an atresia is seen, it must be suspected that the tympanic membrane and middle ear may likewise be involved. Figures 6.4 and 6.5 show the test results for a theoretical patient with atresia of the external ear canals. Notice that the conductive loss reaches near maximum. Conductive hearing losses in excess of 60 dB are rare because intensities beyond this level result in mechanical vibrations of the air-conduction headband and earphone and cause bone-conduction vibrations to be sent to the inner ear. In cases of atresia, the valuable information from measurements of acoustic immittance is unobtainable because the probe cannot be inserted into the external auditory canal.

Foreign Bodies in the External Ear Canal. For unexplained reasons, children are fond of putting foreign objects, such as paper, pins, and crayons, into their mouths and ears. If the object is pushed past the osseocartilaginous junction of the external ear canal, swelling at the isthmus formed by this junction may result. Although hearing loss may result from such an incident, it is of secondary importance to prompt and careful removal of the object, which may be a formidable task and may require surgery in some cases.

External Otitis. An infection that occurs in the skin of the external auditory canal is called **external otitis**. The condition is often called "swimmer's ear" because it frequently develops in people who have been swimming and have had water trapped in their ears. External ear infections are often called *fungus* infections, although bacterial infections are more common than are fungal infections. External otitis is quite common in tropical areas.

The use of systemic antibiotics or ear drops is frequently unsuccessful in the treatment of external otitis because the pocket of infection may be inaccessible, either topically or through the bloodstream. Itching is a common complaint in early or mild infections. Patients are sometimes in extreme pain,

SPEECH AND HEARING CENTER
The University of Texas at Austin 78712
AUDIOMETRIC EXAMINATION

NAME: Last - First - Middle	SEX	AGE	DATE	EXAMINER	RELIABILITY	AUDIOMETER

AIR CONDUCTION

MASKING Type	RIGHT 250	500	1000	1500	2000	3000	4000	6000	8000	LEFT 250	500	1000	1500	2000	3000	4000	6000	8000
NB	55	60	60/60	60	55	60	65	65	70	60	55	55/55	60	60	60	65	65	60
	55*	60*	60*	60*	60*	60*	65*	65*	70*	60*	55*	55*	60*	60*	60*	65*	65*	60*
EM Level in Opp. Ear	60	55	55	60	60	60	60	65	60	55	60	60	60	55	60	65	65	70

BONE CONDUCTION

MASKING Type	RIGHT 250	500	1000	2000	3000	4000	FOREHEAD 250	500	1000	2000	3000	4000	LEFT 250	500	1000	2000	3000	4000
NB	10*	10*	15*	20*	20*	20*	10	10	15	20	20	20	10*	10*	15*	20*	20*	25*
EM Level in Opp. Ear	60	55	55	60	60	65							70	60	60	55	60	80

Pure Tone Average	2 Frequency	3 Frequency	WEBER						Pure Tone Average	2 Frequency	3 Frequency
	60	60	M	M	M	M	M	M		55	57

SPEECH AUDIOMETRY

MASKING Type	RIGHT SRT 1	SRT 2	Discrimination 1	Discrimination 2	LEFT SRT 1	SRT 2	Discrimination 1	Discrimination 2
WB	60	60*	List 1A 30 SL 100%*	List SL %	60	60*	List 2A 30 SL 96%*	List SL %
EM Level in Opp. Ear		60	95			60	95	

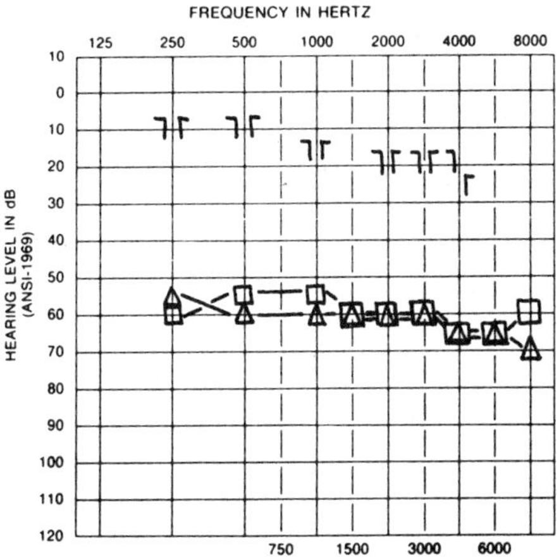

FREQUENCY IN HERTZ

COMMENTS

AUDIOGRAM KEY

(handwritten margin notes: "hearing loss", "sensori neural Okay")

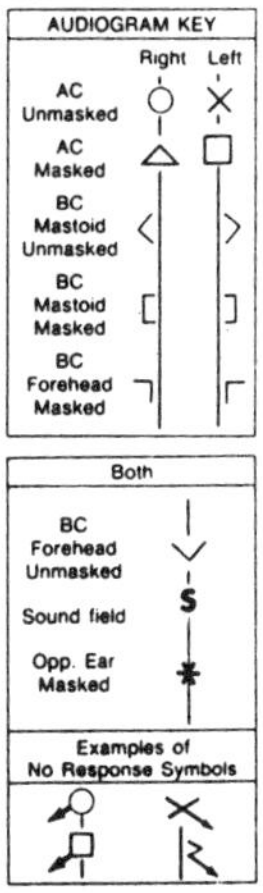

Figure 6.4 Audiogram showing a moderately severe conductive hearing loss consistent with Treacher-Collins syndrome. Note the large air–bone gaps with essentially normal bone conduction. The SRTs and pure-tone average are in close agreement, and the speech discrimination scores are normal.

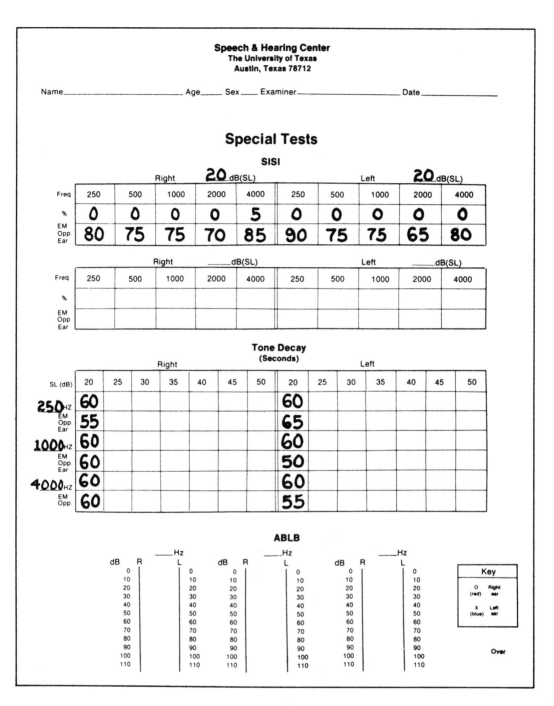

Figure 6.5 Theoretical results on the SISI and tone decay tests for a patient with bilateral external ear canal atresia (Figure 6.4). Note the low SISI scores and absence of tone decay. Masking was required for both tests for both ears.

especially upon touch to the infected area, which may become red and swollen. Often body temperature elevates. The condition may be successfully treated by an otologist by irrigating the canal with warm salt water, drying it carefully, and applying antibiotic drops. Sometimes a cotton wick is inserted into the canal and is saturated with antibiotic drops. The skin may be treated topically with steroids to curtail the inflammation.

Hearing tests often cannot be performed on patients with external otitis because the ear is too painful to allow the pressure of the earphones. It is suspected that if the lumen of the canal is closed, either by the piling up of infectious debris or by the swelling of the canal walls, a mild conductive loss is likely, as shown in figures 6.6 and 6.7. Some concern has been expressed by audiologists regarding the contamination by bacteria of earphones and their rubber cushions. Talbott (1969) found large colonies of certain organisms on earphone cushions used in routine practice, and he recommended using ultra-violet light to prevent the spread of infection. A commercial version of a device designed for this purpose is shown in Figure 6.8.

Sometimes the tympanic membrane itself becomes inflamed, often in response to systemic viral infection. The patient may develop blood blisters on the surface of the tympanic membrane, which in turn produce fever and pain. Often these blebs must be carefully lanced to relieve the pain. Inflammations of the tympanic membrane are called **myringitis**.

Several forms of external otitis are considered particularly dangerous to the patient and require rather aggressive therapy. One *necrotizing*, or *malignant external otitis*, is often initially simply a routine skin infection of the external auditory canal. The condition is particularly threatening to diabetic and elderly patients and may result in massive bone destruction in the external, middle, and inner ears. It can also result in osteitis and in osteomyelitis of the temporal bone. Patients suffering from this condition, which is often fatal, may be hospitalized and treated with systemic antibiotics. Surgery is sometimes required to stop the spread of infection through the bone.

Tumors of the External Auditory Canal. Tumors, both benign and malignant, have been found in the external auditory canal. Bony tumors, called *osteomas,* are sometimes seen in the ears of people who have done a great deal of swimming in very cold water. In any case, tumors do not present hearing problems unless their size is such that the lumen of the canal is occluded and produces conductive hearing loss.

Ear Wax in the External Auditory Canal. In some cases the glands in the external auditory canals are extremely active, producing copious amounts of cerumen. When the canal is small, it may become blocked and produce a hearing loss. Even when a large amount of wax is found in the ear, hearing may remain normal as long as a tiny opening is present between the tympanic membrane and the outside environment. Overzealous cleaning of the external ears, however, may result in cerumen being pushed from the cartilaginous canal into the bony canal, from which natural cleansing cannot take place. Cotton swabs and wadded tissues are often used for such purposes, frequently

NAME: Last - First - Middle	SEX	AGE	DATE	EXAMINER	RELIABILITY	AUDIOMETER

AIR CONDUCTION

MASKING Type	RIGHT									LEFT								
	250	500	1000	1500	2000	3000	4000	6000	8000	250	500	1000	1500	2000	3000	4000	6000	8000
	0	0	0/0	0	5	10	5	10	10	20	25	25/25	25	30	25	30	30	35
EM Level in Opp. Ear																		

BONE CONDUCTION

MASKING Type	RIGHT						FOREHEAD						LEFT					
	250	500	1000	2000	3000	4000	250	500	1000	2000	3000	4000	250	500	1000	2000	3000	4000
NB							0	0	0	5	5	10	0*	0*	0*	5*	5*	10*
EM Level in Opp. Ear													25	25	10	5	10	5

		2 Frequency	3 Frequency	WEBER							2 Frequency	3 Frequency
Pure Tone Average		0	3	L	L	L	L	L	L	Pure Tone Average	25	27

SPEECH AUDIOMETRY

MASKING Type	RIGHT				LEFT			
	SRT 1	SRT 2	Discrimination 1	Discrimination 2	SRT 1	SRT 2	Discrimination 1	Discrimination 2
WB	5		1A List 30 SL 100 %	List SL %	30		2A List 30 SL 100* %	List SL %
EM Level in Opp. Ear							25	

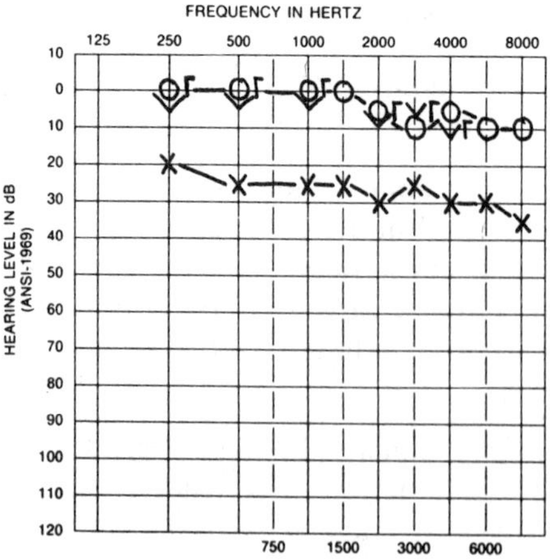

FREQUENCY IN HERTZ   COMMENTS

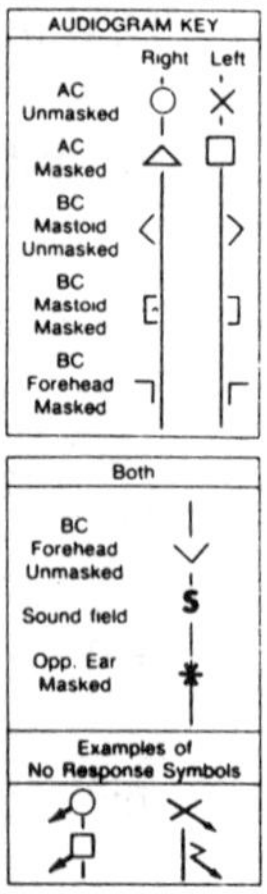

Figure 6.6 A mild unilateral (left) conductive hearing loss occurring with external otitis. SRT and pure-tone findings are in close agreement, and speech discrimination is normal. The Weber results show lateralization to the left ear.

SPEECH AND HEARING CENTER
THE UNIVERSITY OF TEXAS AT AUSTIN 78712

Name: Last-First-Middle	Sex	Age	Examiner	Reliability	Date

	AUDIOMETRIC BING TEST					
	RIGHT			LEFT		
Frequency (Hertz)	250	500	1000	250	500	1000
1) Unoccluded	0	0	0	0	0	0
2) Occluded	-25	-15	-10	0	0	0
3) Occlusion Effect (1-2)	25	15	10	0	0	0

Figure 6.7 Results on the Bing test for a patient with unilateral conductive hearing loss caused by external otitis (see Figure 6.6). Note the absence of the occlusion effect in the left ear on the Bing test.

by well-meaning parents on the ears of their children. Once the wax is deposited in the bony canal, it must remain there until it is removed by a physician. Wax deposited in the bony canal becomes dry, causing an itch which encourages the individual to push still more wax down from the cartilaginous canal. Sometimes water pressure forces wax deep into the canal during diving. If cerumen is deposited on the tympanic membrane, it may impede vibration.

The usual method for removing ear wax is water irrigation. This may be dangerous unless properly carried out with appropriate visualization of the area and controlled water pressure. When the canal is filled with wax, it is impossible to know whether or not the patient has an intact tympanic membrane. If the membrane is not intact, wax or other materials may be washed into the middle ear through the perforation. If too much water pressure is used, a thin or even a healthy tympanic membrane may become ruptured. Proper removal of ear wax is a simple matter in the hands of a competent otologist.

As in the case of external otitis, the amount of hearing loss produced by impacted ear wax is directly related to the amount of ear canal occlusion. Losses range from very mild to moderately severe. Audiologists must be careful when using electroacoustic impedance bridges lest they occlude the external ear canal of the patient with ear wax while they attempt to diagnose the problem.

Perforations of the Tympanic Membrane. The tympanic membrane may become perforated in several ways. Excessive pressure buildup during a middle-ear disorder may cause rupturing of the membrane. Sometimes, in

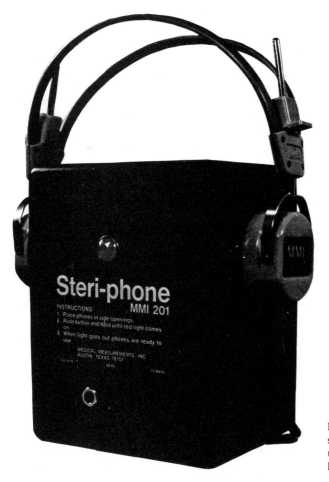

Figure 6.8 A commercial device for sterilization of audiometer earphones using ultraviolet light. (Courtesy of Allison Laboratories.)

response to infection, usually in the middle ear, the membrane may become necrosed (dead) and perforate.

A frequent cause of perforation is direct trauma with a pointed object such as a cotton swab or hairpin. This may happen if patients are attempting to clear their own ears and either misjudge the length of the external auditory canal or are jarred while probing in the canal. Such accidents are extremely painful as well as embarrassing. The tympanic membrane may also be perforated from sudden pressure in the external ear canal, as from a hand clapped over the ear or an explosion.

Because traumatic perforations alter what is essentially normal tissue, they tend to close spontaneously better than do perforations resulting from disease. Perforations in the inferior portion of the tympanic membrane heal more rapidly than those in the superior portion because the normal epithelium migration is more active inferiorly. The migration of tissue has been encouraged by placing a thin piece of cigarette paper over the perforation. Often when a perforation is thus healed, the mucosal and skin layers close off the opening, but a thin area remains in the fibrous layer, which does not migrate as well. Such thin areas in the tympanic membrane lend themselves to easy reperforation, as with water irrigation of the external canal or even a strong sneeze.

Surgical repair of a perforated tympanic membrane is called **myringoplasty.** In early versions of myringoplasty, skin grafts, usually taken from the inner aspect of the arm, were placed over the perforation. Even though the grafts often "took" initially, they tended to desquamate (flake off) with consequent reperforation. Skin grafts were later replaced by vein grafts. For the vein-graft technique, a piece of vein was taken from the patient's hand or arm. Vein worked well because its elasticity is similar to that of the fibrous layer of the tympanic membrane. Narrow veins proved inadequate for large perforations. Most middle-ear surgeons today prefer to use fascia, the tough fibrous protective covering over muscle. Results with myringoplasty have been very gratifying.

The amount of hearing loss produced by a perforated tympanic membrane depends on several variables. The exact size and place of the perforation can cause variations not only in the amount of hearing loss but in the audiometric configuration as well. Measurements on acoustic immittance meters are impossible because an air-tight seal cannot be formed as a consequence of leakage of pressure from the air pump of the bridge through the perforation into the middle ear. Sometimes perforations, not readily visible with the naked eye because of their small size, are detected by use of the immittance meter.

Thickening of the Tympanic Membrane. Often, in response to infection, usually of the middle ear, the tympanic membrane becomes thickened and scarred. At times calcium plaques appear, adding to the mass of the tympanic membrane and interfering with its vibration. Such conditions are called *tympanosclerosis*, and they do not respond well to medical or surgical treatment.

Often the tympanic membrane can become quite thickened, but little or no effect on auditory sensitivity will result. The thickening can be coincidental with disorders of the middle ear, thus making it impossible to determine the amount of hearing loss each disorder contributes.

SUMMARY

The outer ear, including the auricle, external auditory canal, and tympanic membrane, is the channel by which sounds from the environment are first introduced to the hearing mechanism. The auricle helps gather the sound, the canal directs it, and the tympanic membrane vibrates in sympathy with the airborne vibrations that strike it. When portions of the outer ear are abnormal or diseased, hearing may or may not become impaired, depending on which structures are involved and the nature of their involvement.

Abnormalities of the external ear do not affect the sensorineural mechanism. However, alterations in the canal may cause a change in the osseotympanic mode of bone conduction, which may slightly alter the bone-conduction curve. Audiometric findings on speech discrimination, tone decay, Békésy audiometry, and the SISI are the same as expected for persons with normal hearing. Measurements on the acoustic immittance bridge are frequently impossible in external-ear anomalies by virtue of the disorder itself.

Whenever an audiologist sees a patient with an external-ear disorder, an otological consultation should be recommended. If hearing is impaired and no medical therapy is available, other habilitative or rehabilitative avenues should be investigated, depending on the extent of hearing loss and the needs of the patient.

GLOSSARY

Anotia Absence of the pinna.

Annulus The ring of tissue around the periphery of the tympanic membrane that holds it in position at the end of the external auditory canal.

Atresia Closure of a normally open body orifice, such as the external auditory canal.

Auricle The cartilaginous appendage of the external ear.

Cerumen Ear wax.

Down's syndrome Sometimes called "trisomy 21 syndrome," this syndrome is characterized by mental retardation; a small, slightly flattened skull; abnormal digits; and other unusual facial and body characteristics.

Eardrum membrane The tympanic membrane.

Ectoderm The outermost of the three primary embryonic germ layers.

Entoderm The innermost of the three primary embryonic germ layers.

External auditory canal (EAC) The channel in the external ear from the concha of the auricle to the tympanic membrane.

External otitis Infection of the outer ear. Also called *otitis externa*.

Meatus A passage, such as the external auditory canal.

Mesenchymal tissue A network of embryonic connective tissue in the mesoderm, which forms the connective tissue, blood vessels, and lymph vessels of the body.

Mesoderm The middle-most of the three primary embryonic germ layers, lying between the ectoderm and the entoderm.

Microtia A congenitally, abnormally small external ear.

Mucous membrane The moist lining of cavities of the body, such as the middle ear.

Myringitis Any inflammation of the tympanic membrane. red blisters

Myringoplasty Surgery for restoration or repair of the tympanic membrane.

Osseocartilaginous junction The union between the bony and cartilaginous portions of the external auditory canal.

Otalgia Pain in the ear.

Otoplasty Any plastic surgery of the outer ear.

Otoscope A flashlight-like device with a funnel-like speculum on the end, designed to visualize the tympanic membrane.

Pars flaccida The loose folds of epithelium of the tympanic membrane above the malleus.

Pars tensa All of the remaining (taut) portion of the tympanic membrane besides the pars flaccida.

Pharyngeal arches Paired embryonic arches that modify, in humans, into structures of the ear and neck. In lower animals they modify into gills.

Pinna The auricle of the external ear.

Shrapnell's membrane The pars flaccida of the tympanic membrane.

Stenosis An abnormal narrowing, as of the external auditory canal.

Temporomandibular joint (TMJ) syndrome Pain felt in the ear but referred from a neuralgia of the temporomandibular joint.

Tympanic membrane The separation between the outer and middle ears, located at the end of the external auditory canal. It comprises an outer layer of skin, a middle layer of connective tissue, and an inner layer of mucous membrane.

Umbo The point at the approximate center of the tympanic membrane at which it is most retracted.

STUDY QUESTIONS

1. Make sketches of the outer ear and tympanic membrane. Label from memory as many parts as you can. Compare your drawings with the ones shown in Figures 6.1, 6.2, and 6.3.

2. List as many disorders of the outer ear as you can remember. Divide them into two columns, those that produce hearing loss and those that do not.

3. For each of the disorders you listed that produce hearing loss, draw a pure-tone audiogram. Predict the probable SRT speech discrimination scores, and results on the following tests: recruitment, Békésy audiometry, SISI, and the tone decay test.

REVIEW TABLE 6.1 THE OUTER EAR

ANATOMICAL AREA	DISORDER	TREATMENT	PRODUCES HEARING LOSS
Auricle	Missing, small, or malformed	Plastic surgery	No
External auditory canal	Wax	Removal	Sometimes
	Infection	Medical treatment	Sometimes
	Atresia	Occasionally surgery Hearing aid	Yes
Tympanic membrane	Foreign bodies	Removal	Sometimes
	Perforation	Surgery	Yes
	Thickening	None	Sometimes

REFERENCES

HARRIS, J. D. (1986). Anatomy and physiology of the peripheral auditory mechanism. In *The Pro-Ed Studies in Communication Disorders*. Austin, TX: Pro-Ed.

TALBOTT, R. E. (1969). Bacteriology of earphone contamination. *Journal of Speech and Hearing Research, 12,* 326–329.

SUGGESTED READINGS

MAUE-DICKSON, W. (1981). The outer ear—Prenatal development. In F. N. Martin (Ed.), *Medical Audiology* (pp. 15–35), Englewood Cliffs, NJ: Prentice-Hall.

SENTURIA, B. H., MARCUS, M. D. & LUCENTE, F. E. (1980). *Diseases of the external ear.* New York: Grune & Stratton.

7

THE MIDDLE EAR

The development of the middle ear must have been one of evolution's most splendid engineering feats. The middle ear carries sound vibrations from the outer ear to the inner ear by transferring the sound energy from the air in the outer ear to the fluids of the inner ear. The middle ear overcomes the loss of energy that results when sound passes from one medium (in this case, air) to another medium (fluid).

Fish have an organ called the *lateral line* that is similar in some ways to an unrolled version of a portion of the inner ear of humans. This fluid-containing structure runs along the sides of the fish's body. The water in which the fish swims conducts waves that distort the membranes covering the lateral lines, setting the fluids within them into motion. Distortion of the membranes causes wave motion within the fluids of the lateral line.

CHAPTER OBJECTIVES

This chapter assumes a basic understanding of hearing loss as introduced in Chapter 1, the physics of sound discussed in Chapter 2, and the details of hearing tests and their interpretation provided in Chapters 3, 4, and 5. Oversimplifications of the anatomy of the middle ear and its function provided as an introduction earlier in this book should be cleared up.

At the completion of this chapter, readers should understand the middle ear in terms of its anatomy and physiology, and they should be familiar with the etiologies and treatments for common disorders which produce hearing loss. In addition, they should be able to predict what the typical audiometric results for each of the pathologies might be, and they should be able to make a reasonable attempt at diagnosing the etiology of the hearing loss based on audiometric and other findings.

ANATOMY OF THE MIDDLE EAR

An average adult middle ear is an almost oval, air-filled space (roughly 2 cm³, about one-half inch high, one-half inch wide, and one-quarter inch deep). The roof of the middle ear is a thin layer of bone, separating the middle-ear cavity from the brain. Below the floor of the middle ear is the **jugular bulb**, and behind the anterior wall is the **carotid artery**. The labyrinth of the inner ear lies behind the medial wall, and the mastoid process is beyond the posterior wall. The lateral portion of the middle ear is sometimes called the *membranous wall*, as it contains the tympanic membrane. The space in the middle ear above the tympanic membrane is called the **epitympanic recess**.

As is shown in Figure 7.1, the middle ear is separated from the external auditory canal by the tympanic membrane. The middle ear is connected to the **nasopharynx** via the **eustachian tube**, a channel that enters the middle ear anteriorly at a 30 degree angle. The eustachian tube and middle ear form the **middle-ear cleft**. The entire middle-ear cleft, including the portion of the tympanic membrane that is within the middle ear, is lined with **mucous membrane**, the same lining found in the nose and paranasal sinuses. Much of this mucous membrane is ciliated; that is, the top-most cells contain **cilia**, small

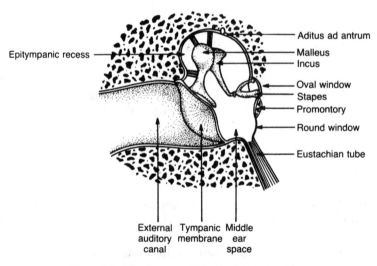

Figure 7.1 The human middle ear in cross-section.

hairlike projections that provide a motion similar to that of a wheat field in the wind. The motion of the cilia creates a wiping action that tends to cleanse the middle ear by moving particles down and out of the eustachian tube.

The Eustachian Tube

The eustachian tube passes down into the nasopharynx, that area where the back of the throat and the nose communicate. In adults the tube is normally kept closed by the spring action of cartilage. Opening is accomplished by the action of three sets of muscles at the orifice of the tube in the nasopharynx. This opening occurs during yawning, sneezing, or swallowing, or when excessive air pressure is applied from the nose. While we are awake our eustachian tubes open about once per minute, during sleep on an average of once every five minutes. In infants the eustachian tube is shorter, wider, and in a more horizontal plane than it is in adults. The orifice of the eustachian tube in the nasopharynx tends to remain open in infants up until the age of about six months.

The air pressure of the middle ear must match that of the external auditory canal in order to keep the pressure equal on both sides of the membrane and maximize its mobility. The absorption of air by middle-ear tissues is the major reason for the need for a pressure equalization system. The only way for this pressure equalization to be maintained is through the eustachian tube. At one time or another most people have had the experience of fullness in the ear— for example, when flying or driving to a higher or lower elevation. During ascension this fullness results from the air in the external ear canal's becoming rarefied (thin) while the middle ear remains at ground-level pressure. The full sensation results from the tympanic membrane's being pushed outward by the greater pressure from within the middle ear. Upon descent, the pressure in the middle ear may be less than in the external ear canal, resulting in the tympanic membrane's being pushed in. The sensations are the same whether the tympanic membrane is pushed in or out. The simple solution is to swallow, yawn, or otherwise open the eustachian tube so that the pressure may be equalized. Because the normal function of the tube is for release, moving from lesser to greater air pressure is more traumatic. At extreme pressures the eustachian tube will lock shut, making pressure equalization impossible and great pain and tympanic membrane rupture likely.

The Mastoid

Figure 7.1 shows that some of the bones of the skull that surround the ear are not solid but, rather, are honeycombed with hundreds of air cells. Each of these cells is lined with mucous membrane, which, though nonciliated, is similar to that of the middle-ear cleft. These cells form the pneumatic mastoid of the temporal bone. The middle ear opens up, back, and outward in an area called the **aditus ad antrum** to communicate with the mastoid. The bony protuberance behind the auricle is called the **mastoid process**.

Windows of the Middle Ear

A section of the bony portion of the inner ear extends into the middle-ear space. This is caused by the basal turn of the cochlea, which is described in Chapter 8. This protrusion is the **promontory** and separates two connections between the middle and inner ears. Above the promontory is the **oval window**, and below it the **round window**, both of whose names were determined from their shapes. The round window is covered by a very thin but tough and elastic membrane. The oval window is filled by the base of the stapes, the tiniest bone of the human body.

Bones in the Middle Ear

In order to accomplish its intended function of carrying sound waves from the air-filled external auditory canal to the fluid-filled inner ear, the middle ear contains a set of three very small bones called **ossicles**. Each of these bones bears a Greek name descriptive of its shape: the **malleus, incus,** and **stapes**.

The **manubrium** of the malleus is embedded in the middle (fibrous) layer of the tympanic membrane; it extends from the upper portion of the tympanic membrane to its approximate center (the umbo). The head of the malleus is connected to the incus, and this area of connection extends upward into the aditus ad antrum (or epitympanic recess). Details of the anatomy of the malleus are shown in Figure 7.2. The incus (Figure 7.3) has a long process, or **crus**, which turns abrupty to a very short crus, the lenticular process. The end of the lenticular process sits squarely on the head of the stapes. As is shown in Figure 7.4, the stapes is comprised of a head, neck and two **crura** (plural of crus). The posterior crus is longer and thinner than the anterior crus. The base, or **footplate**, of the stapes occupies the space in the oval window.

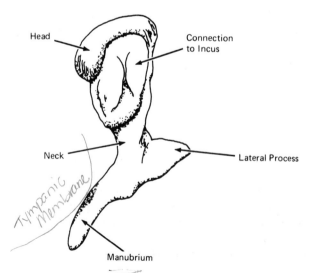

Head

Connection to Incus

Neck

Lateral Process

Tympanic Membrane

Manubrium

Figure 7.2 Anatomy of the human malleus.

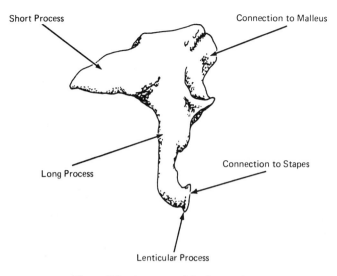

Figure 7.3 Anatomy of the human incus.

Because the malleus and incus are connected rather rigidly, inward and outward movement of the umbo of the tympanic membrane causes these two bones to rotate, which transfers this force to the stapes, which in turn results in the inward and outward motion of the oval window. Each of the ossicles is so delicately poised by its ligamental connections within the middle ear that their collective function is unaltered by gravity when the head changes in position. The photograph in Figure 7.5 illustrates the very small size of the ossicles.

Vibrations of the tympanic membrane are conducted along the ossicular chain to the oval window. The chain (2 to 6 mm in length) acts much like a single unit when transmitting sounds above about 800 Hz. It is the action of these ossicles that provides the energy transformation for which the middle ear was designed.

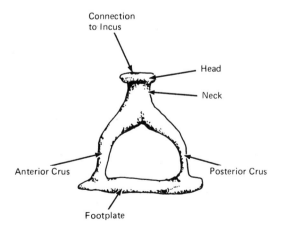

Figure 7.4 Anatomy of the human stapes.

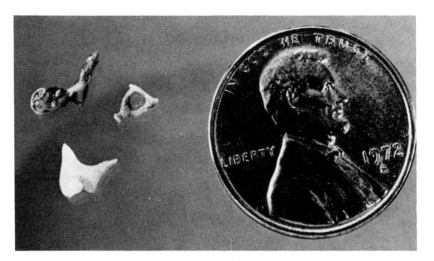

Figure 7.5 Three human ossicles shown against a penny to illustrate their size.

The Middle-Ear Impedance Matcher

The average adult tympanic membrane is 85 to 90 mm^2 but the effective vibrating area is only about 55 mm^2. This vibrating area is 17 times that of the oval window. Therefore, the sound pressure collected over the entire area of the tympanic membrane is concentrated on the oval window. This concentration increases the sound pressure in the same way that a hose increases water pressure when a thumb or a finger is placed over the opening. What results is not a greater volume of water but greater pressure. The drawing in Figure 7.6 illustrates this action. Despite the exquisite engineering of the middle ear, all sound pressure delivered to the tympanic membrane is not made available to the inner ear; the middle-ear mechanism as an impedance-matching device is not 100% efficient.

The mass of the ossicular chain (malleus = 25 mg, incus = 25 mg, stapes = 2.5 mg) is poised in such a way as to take advantage of the physical laws of leverage. Figure 7.7 illustrates this simple principle. Through the use of leverage, the force received at the footplate of the stapes is greater than that applied at the malleus. In this way the ratio of tympanic membrane displacement to oval window displacement is increased by about 1.3:1. The ossicular chain actually rocks back and forth on an imaginary axis, and the action of the stapes in the oval window is not that of a piston but, rather, like a pivot.

The combined effects of increased pressure and the lever action of the malleus result in a pressure increase at the oval window 23 times what it would be if air-borne sound impinged upon it directly. This value is equivalent to approximately 30 dB, remarkably close to the 28 dB loss that would be caused by the air-to-fluid impedance mismatch without the ossicular chain. The fact

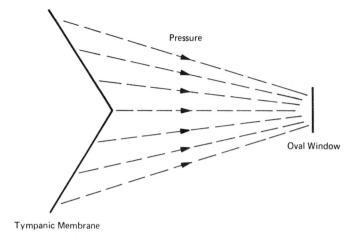

Figure 7.6 Sound pressure collected over the surface area of the tympanic membrane is concentrated on the (smaller) surface area of the oval window, thus increasing the pressure.

that the tympanic membrane is conical rather than flat assists slightly in the process of impedance matching by increasing the force and decreasing the velocity, because the handle of the malleus does not move with the same amplitude as the tympanic membrane.

Nonauditory Structures in the Middle Ear

The middle ear contains several structures that are unrelated to hearing. The **fallopian canal**, containing the **facial** (VIIth cranial) **nerve**, passes through the middle ear as a protrusion on its medial wall. The fallopian canal is a

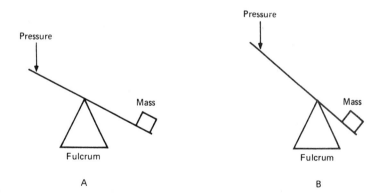

Figure 7.7 Demonstration of the advantage of the level action. Note that the advantage is increased in (B) when the fulcrum is moved closer to the mass to be lifted.

bony channel covered with mucous membrane. The facial nerve runs beside the auditory (VIIIth cranial) nerve as the two travel to the brain stem, about which more is said in Chapter 9.

The **chorda tympani nerve** is a branch of the facial nerve that passes through the middle-ear space. This nerve carries information about the sensation of taste from the anterior two-thirds of one side of the tongue. Unfortunately, the chorda tympani frequently acts as an obstruction during middle-ear surgery. Sometimes the nerve is accidentally or intentionally sacrificed to increase visibility of the operative field. Taste changes caused by surgical severance of the chorda tympani nerve frequently disappear after several months.

The Middle-Ear Muscles

Two muscles, whose primary functions continue to be debated, are active in each middle ear. It has been thought that contractions of these muscles may serve a protective function for the inner ear by stiffening the ossicular chain and attenuating loud and therefore potentially damaging sounds from entering it. It is known, however, that the latency of the reflex is too long to protect the inner ear from impulsive sounds such as gunshots. Contraction of these muscles may additionally serve to decrease the loudness of sounds generated within the head, for example by chewing or speaking.

The **stapedius muscle** (length 7 mm, cross-section 5 mm^2), originates in the posterior (mastoid) wall of the middle ear. The stapedius tendon emerges through a tiny hole in a pyramidal eminence, but the muscle itself is in a canal beside the facial canal. The tendon attaches to the posterior portion of the neck of the stapes. When the stapedius muscle is contracted, the stapes moves to the side and tenses the oval window, reducing the amplitude of vibration. It is possible that contraction of the stapedius muscle may help to improve speech discrimination in noise by attenuating the low-frequency components of the noise. The stapedius muscle is innervated by a branch of the facial (VIIth cranial) nerve. In addition to its function of attaching the stapedius muscle to the stapes, the stapedius tendon also supplies blood to the lenticular process of the incus.

The **tensor tympani** muscle (length 25 mm, cross-section 5 mm^2) is also encased in a small bony cavity. The tendon from this muscle inserts into the manubrium of the malleus and, upon contraction, moves the malleus in such a way as to tense the tympanic membrane. The innervation of the tensor tympani is from the **trigeminal (Vth cranial) nerve.**

Both the stapedius and tensor tympani muscles respond reflexively and bilaterally, but in humans only the stapedius is thought to respond to sound. For example, introduction of a loud sound into the right ear will cause both stapedius muscles to contract. The tensor tympani can be caused to contract by a jet of air in the external auditory canal or the eye, and by changes in temperature or touch in the external auditory canal.

DEVELOPMENT OF THE MIDDLE EAR

During embryonic or fetal develoment, specific anatomical areas form or differentiate. Like the outer ear, the middle ear and eustachian tube form from the pharyngeal arch system, limited to the first two arches. As in the outer ear and all areas of the body, developmental milestones are somewhat variant and times should be viewed as approximate.

Both the middle-ear space and the eustachian tube form the first pharyngeal pouch, which is lined with entoderm. During gestation, the middle-ear space is filled with mesenchyme as the ossicles are developing. The ciliated epithelium which lines these spaces also arises from the entoderm. The oval window is formed by about the 47th gestational day.

The middle-ear ossicles first form as cartilage of the first and second pharyngeal arches. The superior portions of the incus and malleus, which form the incudo-malleal joint, come from the first arch. The lower parts of the incus and malleus and the superstructure of the stapes come from the second arch. The base of the stapes forms from the otic capsule.

At about 29 to 32 days tissue forms which will become the malleus and incus. By the 12th fetal week the ossicles differentiate and are fully formed by the 16th week as cartilaginous structures that have begun to ossify. Almost total ossification of the malleus and incus has taken place by the 21st week. The 24th week shows rapid ossification of the incus and stapes. The middle-ear muscles derive from mesenchyme, the tensor tympani from the first arch, and the stapedius from the second arch.

HEARING LOSS AND THE MIDDLE EAR

Abnormalities of the middle ear produce conductive hearing losses. The air-conduction level drops in direct relationship with the amount of attenuation produced by the disorder. Theoretically, bone conduction should be unchanged from normal unless the inner ear becomes involved; however, our knowledge of middle-ear anatomy and physiology should make our understanding of the effects of inertial bone conduction even clearer. Conductive hearing losses produced by middle-ear disorders may show alteration in the bone-conduction thresholds even without the presence of sensorineural involvement. The amount of sensorineural impairment in mixed hearing losses may be exaggerated by artifacts of bone conduction.

DISORDERS OF THE MIDDLE EAR AND THEIR TREATMENT

Suppurative Otitis Media

One of the most common disorders of the middle ear, which causes conductive hearing loss, is infection of the middle-ear space, or **otitis media**. Otitis media is any infection of the mucous-membrane lining of the middle-ear cleft.

Factors that predispose an individual to <u>otitis media</u> include poorly functioning eustachian tubes, **barotrauma** (sudden changes in air pressure, as when flying or diving), abnormalities in the action of the cilia of the mucous membranes, anatomical deformities of the middle ear and <u>eustachian tube</u>, age, race, socioeconomic factors, and the integrity of the individual's immune system. This last fact suggests that the growing epidemic of acquired immune deficiency syndrome (AIDS) will probably increase the incidence of otitis media. External factors associated with otitis media include exposure to cigarette smoke or other fumes. The incidence of otitis media, along with that of upper respiratory infections, is much higher in children whose parents smoke in the household.

Although otitis media is primarily a disease of childhood, it can occur at any age. Meyerhoff (1986, p. 37) states that otitis media will affect 75% to 95% of all children before the age of six years. There are clear seasonal effects (otitis media is most common in the winter months), but it is less clear why the disease is more common in males than in females. Also difficult to explain is the difference in incidence among racial groups; otitis <u>media is most</u> common <u>in Eskimos and Native Americans,</u> less common in whites, and least common in blacks (Giebink, 1984, pp. 5–9). The interrelationships between socioeconomic and anatomical (genetic) differences is unclear.

As a rule, organisms gain access to the middle ear through the eustachian tube from the nasopharynx. They travel as a subepithelial extension of a sinusitis or pharyngitis, spreading the infection up through the tube. Often the infection is literally blown through the lumen of the tube by a stifled sneeze or by too-hard blowing of the nose. In general, it is probably a good idea not to teach small children to blow their noses at all. They should also be encouraged to minimize pressure through the eustachian tube when sneezing by keeping their mouths open. Infection may also enter the middle ear through the external auditory canal if a perforation exists in the tympanic membrane. Blood-borne infection from another site in the body may occur, but this source of middle-ear infection is unusual.

As stated earlier, infection usually begins at the orifice of the eustachian tube and spreads throughout the middle-ear cavity. When the tube is infected it becomes swollen, interfering with its middle-ear pressure equalization function. Also, when the tubal lining becomes swollen, the cleansing action of the cilia is interfered with and the infection is spread to adjacent tissues. A major contributing cause of otitis media, especially in children, is exposure to tobacco smoke. One study shows that in households in which more than three packages of cigarettes are smoked in a day, the risk to children of otitis media and other respiratory infections is four times what it would be without such exposure (Kraemer et al., 1983).

Patients often report that as little as several hours may elapse between the appearance of initial symptoms and a full-blown infection. In such rapidly progressing cases, it is probable that fluids that functioned as a culture medium for pus-producing (**purulent**) organisms had previously been deposited in the middle ear, perhaps from an earlier bacterial or viral infection. The rate of spread is also related to the infectiousness of the organisms.

In cases of otitis media, otologic treatment is imperative. Proper diagnosis of the several usual stages can result in appropriate therapy. In the initial stage of eustachian-tube swelling causing occlusion of the tube, negative middle-ear pressure may be set up. The tympanic membrane may appear to be retracted (sucked in). Often audiometric examination reveals normal hearing on all tests. The tympanometric function may appear as a Type C, suggesting that the pressure within the middle ear is lower than that of the external auditory canal.

Before the actual accumulation of pus in the middle ear, the tympanic membrane and middle-ear mucosa may become very vascular. This inflammation produces the so-called red ear described by many physicians. If the condition is allowed to continue beyond this stage, suppuration (production of pus) may result. Enzymes are usually produced by bacterial infections, some of which have a dissolving effect on middle-ear structures.

In **suppurative** otitis media, the mucosa becomes filled with excessive amounts of blood, the superficial cells break down, and pus accumulates. Patients complain of pain in the ear, their pulse rates and body temperatures become elevated, and they are visibly ill. If pressure from the pus goes up, there will be compression of the small veins and capillaries within the middle ear, resulting in **necrosis** (death) of the mucosa, submucosa, and tympanic membrane. If the condition continues even further, the tympanic membrane may eventually rupture. Pus that cannot find its way out of the middle ear may invade the mastoid. The resulting **mastoiditis** causes a breakdown of the walls separating the air cells. Untreated mastoiditis can result in meningitis and sometimes death.

The general category of suppurative otitis media is frequently dichotomized by the terms **chronic** and **acute**. As a rule, the chronic form implies a condition of long standing. Symptoms of acute otitis media generally develop rapidly and include swelling, redness, and bleeding. Bleeding within the middle ear may also be caused by barotrauma, when there is a sudden pressure change, causing the blood vessels in the lining of the middle ear to rupture. Bleeding in the middle ear from any cause is called **hemotympanum**.

Audiometric Findings in Suppurative Otitis Media.

Otitis media results in the typical audiogram of the conductive hearing loss (see Figure 7.8). Generally, the amount of hearing loss is directly related to the accumulation of fluid in the middle ear. The audiometric contour is usually rather flat, showing approximately equal amounts of hearing loss across frequencies. Speech discrimination scores are generally excellent, although proper masking must often be instituted to ensure against cross-hearing. Bone-conduction results are usually normal. SISI scores are generally low, and there is little or no tone decay (see Figure 7.9).

Figure 7.10 shows the Type I Békésy tracing for both continuous and pulsed tones typical of conductive hearing losses. Measurements of static compliance show lower than normal values. The tympanometric function is a Type B (Figure 7.11), suggesting the presence of fluid behind the tympanic

Short Increment Sensitivity Index (SISI)

SPEECH AND HEARING CENTER
The University of Texas at Austin 78712
AUDIOMETRIC EXAMINATION

NAME: Last - First - Middle	SEX	AGE	DATE	EXAMINER	RELIABILITY	AUDIOMETER

AIR CONDUCTION

MASKING Type	RIGHT									LEFT								
	250	500	1000	1500	2000	3000	4000	6000	8000	250	500	1000	1500	2000	3000	4000	6000	8000
NB	55	60	55/50	55	55	65	60	70	80	60	60	55/55	60	65	60	65	75	NR
	55*	60*								60*	60*	55*	60*	65*	60*	65*	75*	
EM Level in Opp. Ear	60	60								55	60	55	55	55	65	60	70	

BONE CONDUCTION

MASKING Type	RIGHT						FOREHEAD						LEFT					
	250	500	1000	2000	3000	4000	250	500	1000	2000	3000	4000	250	500	1000	2000	3000	4000
NB	10*	15*	15*	20*	20*	25*	5	10	15	20	20	25	5*	10*	15*	20*	20*	25*
EM Level in Opp. Ear	75	75	55	65	60	65							55	60	55	55	65	60

	2 Frequency	3 Frequency	WEBER							2 Frequency	3 Frequency
Pure Tone Average	53	55	M	M	M	M	M	M	Pure Tone Average	58	60

SPEECH AUDIOMETRY

MASKING Type	RIGHT				LEFT			
	SRT 1	SRT 2	Discrimination 1	Discrimination 2	SRT 1	SRT 2	Discrimination 1	Discrimination 2
WB	55	55*	List 1A 30 SL · 100 %*	List SL · %	55	55*	List 2A 30 SL · 96 %*	List SL · %
EM Level in Opp. Ear		55	95			55	85	

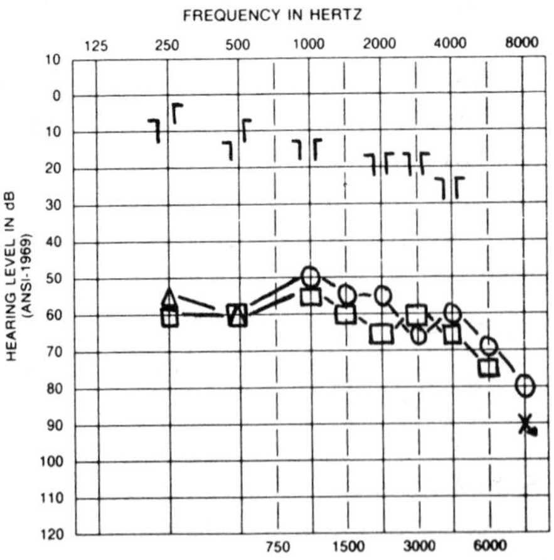

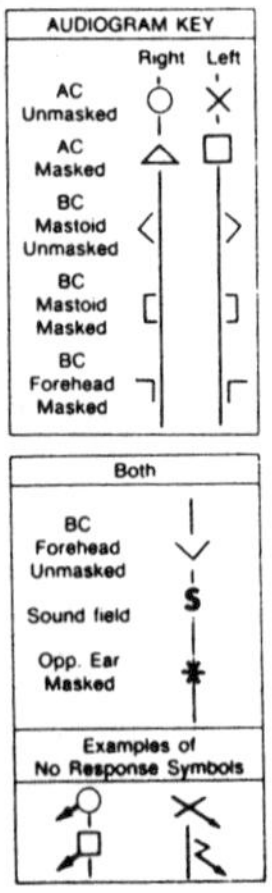

Figure 7.8 Audiogram illustrating a moderate conductive hearing loss in both ears. The contour of the audiogram is relatively flat and fairly typical of otitis media. Speech discrimination scores are excellent. Note that masking is used for all tests. Because no cross-hearing was shown, interaural attenuation must exceed 50 dB for this case.

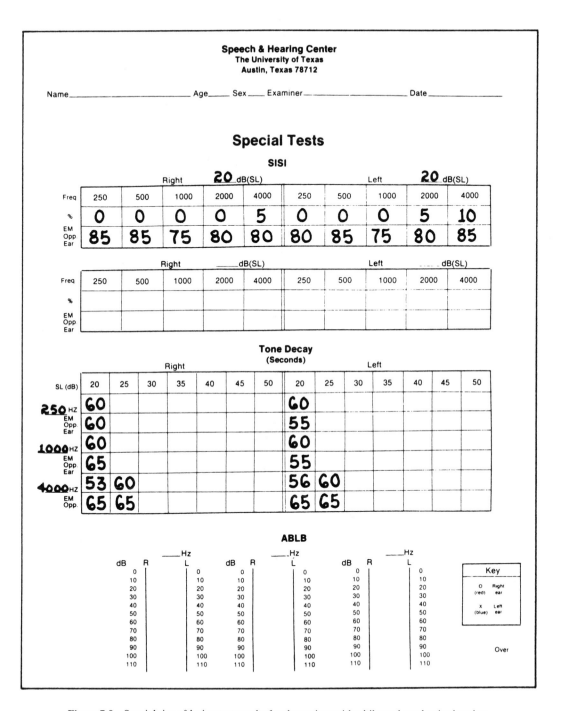

Figure 7.9 Special site-of-lesion test results for the patient with a bilateral conductive hearing loss shown in Figure 7.8. Note the low SISI scores and absence of tone decay.

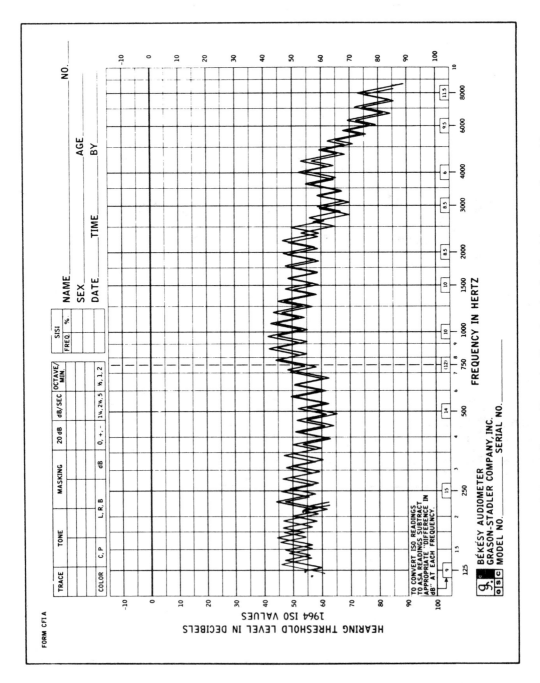

Figure 7.10 Békésy audiogram illustrating Type I tracing for the right ear consistent with the conductive hearing loss shown in Figure 7.8.

SPEECH AND HEARING CENTER
The University of Texas at Austin 78712
IMMITTANCE

NAME: Last · First · Middle	SEX	AGE	DATE	EXAMINER	INSTRUMENT

PRESSURE/COMPLIANCE FUNCTION

	−400	−350	−300	−250	−200	−150	−100	−50	0	+50	+100	+150	+200
Right			.90	.90	.85	.85	.85	.80	.74	.72	.70	.61	.61
Left			.91	.91	.89	.84	.80	.76	.70	.68	.62	.58	.53

STATIC COMPLIANCE $C_x = C_2 - C_1$

RIGHT			LEFT		
.61 C_1	.80 C_2	.19 C_x	.53 C_1	.70 C_2	.17 C_x

ACOUSTIC REFLEXES

	RIGHT				LEFT			
Frequency (Hz)	500	1000	2000	4000	500	1000	2000	4000
Ipsilateral (Probe same)		NR	NR			NR	NR	
Contralateral (Probe opposite)	NR	NR	NR	NR	NR	NR	NR	NR
Audiometric Threshold								
Reflex SL								
Decay Time (Seconds)								

TYMPANOGRAM

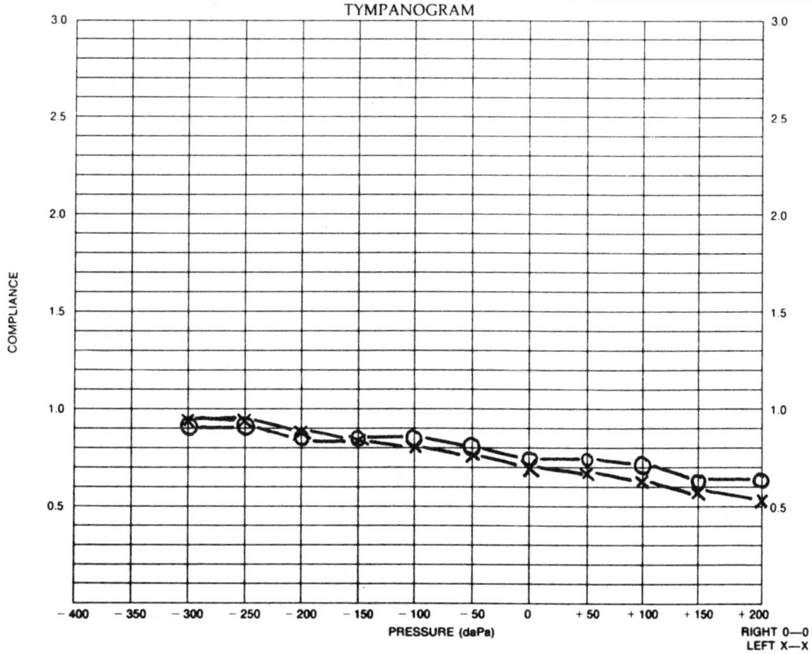

Figure 7.11 Typical results on immittance tests performed on a patient with right otitis media or serous effusion (see Figures 7.8, 7.9, and 7.10). Note that the tympanogram is Type B, the static compliance is low, and reflex thresholds are absent in both ears.

membrane. The acoustic reflexes cannot be elicited in either ear, because the intensity of each tone delivered, even at maximum levels of the audiometer, is below the reflex threshold; additionally, abnormalities of the middle ear cause increased impedance of the ossicular chain, which resists movement in response to contraction of the stapedius muscle. Figures 7.12 and 7.13 show that the latencies of all the waves resulting from ABR testing are increased at all sensation levels.

Many or all of the audiometric results that point so clearly to otitis media as the cause of the conductive hearing loss shown in Figures 7.8 through 7.13 may be absent in the infant or small child. However, with a minimal amount of patient cooperation, measurements of static compliance and tympanometry can be obtained and may suggest the presence of middle-ear infection.

Cholesteatoma

Whenever skin is introduced to the middle-ear cleft, the result may be a pseudotumor called **cholesteatoma**. Cholesteatomas form as a sac with onion-like concentric rings made up of keratin (a very insoluble protein) mixed with squamous (scaly) epithelium and with fats such as cholesterol. In patients with perforated tympanic membranes, the skin may enter the middle ear through the perforations. This invasion produces a secondary acquired cholesteatoma. A primary acquired cholesteatoma may result without history of otitis media if the epithelium of the attic of the middle ear becomes modified. This alteration may occur if the pars flaccida of the tympanic membrane becomes sucked into

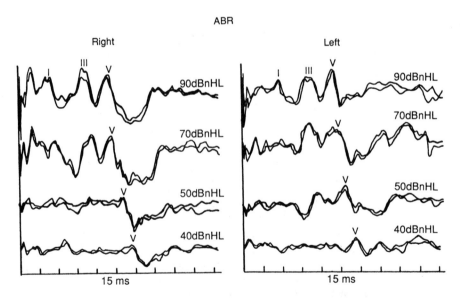

Figure 7.12 Results of auditory brain stem response testing on the patient with a bilateral conductive hearing loss, caused by otitis media (see Figure 7.6).

AUDITORY BRAINSTEM RESPONSE
(Adult Form)

NAME: Last · First · Middle	SEX	AGE	DATE	EXAMINER	RELIABILITY	INSTRUMENT

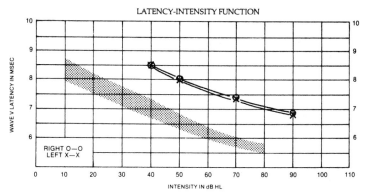

LATENCY-INTENSITY FUNCTION

RIGHT O—O
LEFT X—X

SHADED AREA REPRESENTS Normal Wave V Range for patients older than 16 mos. for 30 clicks per second.

	STIMULUS			WAVE LATENCY IN MSEC						
EAR	RATE	dB HL	FILTER	I	II	III	IV	V	VI	VII
R	33.1	90	150 · 1500	2.7		5.1		6.85		
L	33.1	90	150 · 1500	2.8		5.0		6.8		

SUMMARY OF RESULTS

INTERWAVE INTERVALS . . . . R __4.15__ L __4.0__

AMPLITUDE RATIO (V SAME OR > I) . . . . R __NORMAL__ L __NORMAL__

LATENCY CHANGE WITH INCREASED CLICK RATE . . . . R _____ L _____

INTERAURAL DIFFERENCES . . . . _____

ESTIMATED AIR CONDUCTION THRESHOLD IN dBHL (1-2 kHz) . . . . R __≤ 40__ L __≤ 40__

ESTIMATED BONE CONDUCTION THRESHOLD IN dB HL . . . . R _____ L _____

COMMENTS

Figure 7.13 Latency-intensity functions for wave V derived from the auditory brain stem response tracings shown in Figure 7.12 on the patient with bilateral conductive hearing loss (see Figure 7.8). The latencies of all waves are increased at all levels tested.

the middle ear through negative pressure and then opens, revealing the skin from the outer portion of the tympanic membrane to the middle ear.

Cholesteatomas may also enter the middle ear in several other ways. In any case cholesteatomas are extremely dangerous and have been known to occupy the entire middle ear and even pass down through the opening of the eustachian tube into the nasopharynx or up into the brain cavity. They are highly erosive and may cause destruction of bone and other tissue.

Although antibiotics may arrest otitis media and even mastoiditis, the best treatment for cholesteatoma is still surgery. The condition spreads rapidly, and the surgeon must be absolutely certain that all of the cholesteatomatous material has been removed, for if even a small amount remains the entire condition may flare up again in a short period of time. Most ears with cholesteatomas are secondarily infected and produce foul-smelling discharges that drain from the ears (**otorrhea**).

Facial Palsy

In some cases of chronic otitis media, the bony covering of the fallopian canal becomes eroded, exposing the facial nerve to the disease process. Damage to the facial nerve may result in a flaccid paralysis of one side of the face. Appropriate treatment, often involving middle-ear surgery, is required.

At times unilateral facial paralysis results when no other clinically demonstrable disease is present. Although there are several theories as to why the paralysis, called **Bell's palsy**, occurs, the reason is probably related to the blood supply to the nerve or to viral infection. A diagnosis of Bell's palsy is made by ruling out any other causative lesion in a patient with a flaccid facial paralysis. Bell's palsy resolves spontaneously in the majority of cases.

Antibiotic Treatment of Otitis Media

Bacterial infections, like those found in otitis media, survive by multiplication. Each bacterial cell forms a protective capsule around itself to ensure its survival. Some antibiotics kill the bacteria directly. Other antibiotics serve to inhibit the formation of the protective covering, thereby limiting the growth within the bacterial colony and allowing the white blood cells to surround and carry off the bacteria. When a substantial pocket of infection exists, as in suppurative otitis media, the mass of bacteria, by virtue of numbers alone, may resist a complete bacteria-killing action. Different drugs are specific to different organisms, and unless the appropriate drug is prescribed, the action may be less than useful. Modern laboratory facilities allow for culturing the organism causing the infection, so that the physician may take advantage of the specificity of a given antibiotic.

When the middle ear is filled with pus, produced by the body to carry cells to the area to ingest the bacteria, frequently the best procedure is to remove the pus rather than to rely completely on the effects of antibiotics. As long as the tympanic membrane remains intact, using drops in the ear canal can have no therapeutic effect in cases of otitis media because the drops cannot reach the infection. Prescription of such medications may result from poor understanding of the problem.

Dormant Otitis Media. The introduction of antibiotics at the close of World War II drastically altered the treatment of otitis media. Although antibiotics have dramatically decreased the number of serious effects of otitis media, they have also had some undesirable side effects. Unless the proper type and dosage of antibiotics are used, the disease may go not to resolution but, rather, to a state of quiescence. Because the overt symptoms may disappear, both the physician and patient may assume complete cure. Several weeks later the patient may experience what seems like a whole new attack of otitis media, which is in reality an exacerbation of the same condition experienced earlier but allowed to lie dormant. Many patients discontinue their own antibiotic treatments when their symptoms abate, leaving some of the hardier bacteria alive. Then, when the condition flares up again, it is as a result of a stronger strain, less susceptible to medication. Antibiotics, therefore, may lead to a false sense of security in the treatment of otitis media and mastoiditis.

Surgical Treatment for Otitis Media

In the days predating antibiotics, therapy for otitis media was primarily surgical. Today surgery is still required in many cases. The primary purpose of surgery for patients with infection or destruction in the middle ear is to eliminate disease. Reconstructing a damaged hearing apparatus is an important but secondary goal.

Myringotomy. When disease-laden fluids are present in the middle ear and must be removed, the surgical procedure is called **myringotomy**. Myringotomy is frequently performed as a simple office operation but at times, especially in the case of some small children, it requires brief hospitalization. An incision is made using a special knife, generally in the inferior-posterior quadrant of the tympanic membrane. The fluids are removed by suction, using a suction tip placed through the incision. If myringotomy is performed on small children while they are awake, care must be taken to immobilize them sufficiently so that any sudden movement does not redirect the action of the myringotomy knife, which could possibly cause damage within the middle ear.

Mastoidectomy. Even with modern drug therapy, often the only treatment for mastoiditis is **mastoidectomy**, usually done under a general anesthetic. In earlier days the incision was made behind the auricle and the bone in the mastoid process was scraped until all the infection was removed. This technique frequently resulted in a large concavity behind the ear. In addition, the surgically created mastoid bowl required cleaning for the rest of the patient's life and was in itself a breeding ground for infection.

The modern surgical approach to mastoidectomy is to avoid creating a mastoid cavity whenever possible. When a mastoid cavity does exist, it can often be obliterated using portions of the temporalis muscle and/or bone chips taken from the patient. The obliteration of the mastoid cavity may be done at the time of initial surgery, or it may be staged at a later date, depending on the disease process found in the mastoid. This procedure has been found to be very gratifying in recent years.

Tympanoplasty. Surgical reconstruction of the middle-ear auditory apparatus is called **tympanoplasty**. The simplest form of tympanoplasty is myringoplasty, repair of the tympanic membrane described in Chapter 6. Many surgical approaches have been attempted to substitute metal or plastic prosthetic devices for damaged or missing ossicles. These attempts have met with limited success because the body tends to reject such foreign materials. In recent years tympanoplasties have been performed by attaching existing middle-ear structures together. This attachment may mean the loss of the function of one or more ossicles. The surgeon may place the tympanic membrane directly on the head of the stapes in order to restore a remnant of ossicular chain function.

Hearing improvement following tympanoplasty varies considerably, depending on the preoperative condition of the middle ear and, to a great extent, on the function of the eustachian tube. If the tube fails to function properly and the middle ear is not normally pressurized, the surgical procedure is almost certainly doomed to failure.

Sometimes, though rarely, a patient's hearing may be poorer following surgery. The surgeon may have found, for example, that the long process of the incus is necrosed, but instead of there being a hiatus between the main portion of the incus and the stapes, the gap has been closed by a bit of cholesteatoma. Removal of the cholesteatoma is a must even though the result is interruption of the ossicular chain and increased hearing loss. Patients to whom this has happened may be very difficult to console.

Audiograms of patients with interrupted ossicular chains show all the expected findings consistent with conductive hearing loss. The compliance of the tympanic membrane in such cases is unusually high because it has been decoupled from the stapes. The expected pressure-compliance function is a Type A_D (see Figure 7.14).

Although static compliance values may not in themselves determine the presence of a conductive problem in the middle ear, comparison of c_x in the right and left ears of the same patient may be extremely useful. De Jonge and Valente (1979) suggest that when the static-compliance difference between ears exceeds 0.22 cm³, a conductive problem may exist in one ear, even if both values fall within the normal range.

Anderson and Barr (1971) reported on high-frequency conductive hearing losses that may result from **subluxations** (partial dislocations) in the ossicular chain. When a portion of one of the ossicles is replaced by soft connective tissue, the elasticity of this connection, acting as an insulator against vibrations, transmits low frequencies more easily than high frequencies. Hearing losses caused by this condition are usually mild and result in an elevated acoustic reflex threshold.

IMMITTANCE

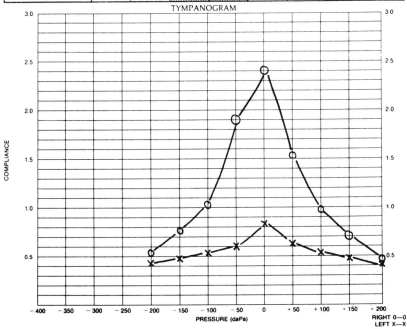

NAME: Last - First - Middle		SEX	AGE	DATE	EXAMINER	INSTRUMENT

PRESSURE/COMPLIANCE FUNCTION

	-400	-350	-300	-250	-200	-150	-100	-50	0	+50	+100	+150	+200
Right					.52	.77	1.01	1.90	2.40	1.51	.99	.70	.48
Left					.42	.49	.52	.60	.82	.61	.53	.49	.41

STATIC COMPLIANCE

$c_x = c_2 - c_1$

RIGHT			LEFT		
.48 c_1	2.40 c_2	1.92 c_x	.41 c_1	.82 c_2	.41 c_x

ACOUSTIC REFLEXES

	RIGHT				LEFT			
Frequency (Hz)	500	1000	2000	4000	500	1000	2000	4000
Ipsilateral (Probe same)		NR	NR			95	85	
Contralateral (Probe opposite)	NR	NR	NR	NR	NR	NR	NR	NR
Audiometric Threshold								
Reflex SL								
Decay Time (Seconds)								

TYMPANOGRAM

COMPLIANCE

PRESSURE (daPa)

RIGHT 0—0
LEFT X—X

Figure 7.14 Typical results on immittance tests performed on a patient with right ossicular chain discontinuity. Note that the tympanogram is Type A_D (normal middle-ear pressure but extremely compliant tympanic membrane), the static compliance is high, and reflex thresholds are absent in both ears. The left ear is normal in this case.

Negative Middle-Ear Pressure

Eustachian tube function may fail for a number of reasons. Two of the more common causes are edema of the eustachian tube secondary to infection or to allergy, and blockage of the orifice of the eustachian tube by hypertrophied (overgrown) adenoids. Either infection or allergy may affect the adenoids, which adds further to the problem. Structural abnormalities of the mechanism responsible for opening the tube are sometimes also present.

Any condition that interferes with the eustachian tube's function of equating air pressure between the middle ear and outer ear may cause the air trapped within the middle ear to become absorbed by the tissues that line it, resulting in a drop in pressure. When this absorption occurs, the greater pressure in the external auditory canal causes the tympanic membrane to be retracted (see Figure 7.15). The retraction interferes with the normal vibration of the tympanic membrane and may or may not produce a slight conductive hearing loss.

Immittance meters may be used to determine the very important matter of eustachian tube function. The tests are rapid and objective, and they take considerably less time than more elaborate methods. The patient is instructed to prevent eustachian tube opening during the test by not swallowing and by remaining as motionless as possible. The test is designed for patients with tympanic membrane perforations or with patent pressure equalization tubes in place.

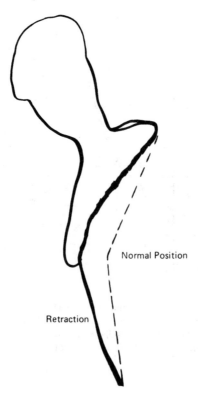

Normal Position

Retraction

Figure 7.15 Retracted tympanic membrane secondary to negative middle-ear pressure.

The first step is to establish a pressure of +200 daPa and to have the patient open the tube by swallowing or yawning. If the tube opens, pressure equalization will take place in the middle ear and the manometer will indicate a shift toward 0 daPa. Eustachian tube function has been qualified by Rock (1974) as "good," "fair," or "poor," depending on the degree to which the pressure is reduced by this maneuver. According to Gladstone (1984) the eustachian tube function test must be performed with positive air pressure in the external auditory canal because negative pressure could cause the tube to "lock" shut rather than be forced open.

Another method has been developed to use the immittance meter to test eustachian tube function, if the eardrum membrane is intact, by using a pressure-swallow technique (Williams, 1975). The patient is asked to swallow normally, after which a tympanogram is run. Then +400 daPa is applied to the membrane, and the patient is asked to swallow four times; a second tympanogram is then run on the same graph. Pressure is returned to 0 daPa and the patient swallows again to equalize middle-ear pressure. Finally the patient is asked to swallow four times with −400 daPa in the external auditory canal, and a third tympanogram is run. If the eustachian tube is normal, the peaks of the three tympanograms will differ by at least 15 daPa. Differences smaller than this suggest dysfunction because the tube cannot equalize the middle-ear pressure.

If otoscopic examination reveals a retracted tympanic membrane, and no infectious fluids are visible in the nose, then the otologist may elect to pressurize the middle ear through a process called **politzerization**. One nostril is held closed while an olive tip, connected to a tube or nebulizer, is held tightly in the other nostril. The patient elevates the soft palate by saying "k-k-k" and then swallows; the otologist, meanwhile, observes the movement of the tympanic membrane during this process. In this fashion, tympanic membrane perforation or eustachian tube failure may be diagnosed. The patient may autoinflate the eustachian tube by means of increased pressure on forced expiration with the nostrils held shut, a maneuver called **valsalva**, which must be performed by divers as they descend or surface. Patients are often taught the valsalva maneuver following middle-ear surgery. The **Toynbee maneuver** accomplishes eustachian tube opening when the patient closes the jaw, holds the nose, and swallows.

Figure 7.16 illustrates a mild conductive hearing loss in the left ear. The bone-conduction results are essentially normal, as are word discrimination scores. Results on all site-of-lesion tests suggest conductive hearing loss. Acoustic compliance measurements show normal compliance in both ears, with a Type C tympanometric function in the left ear typical of negative middle-ear pressure (Figure 7.17). All of these findings are produced by the partial vacuum set up within the left middle-ear space.

Pregnant women sometimes report feeling pressure in their ears. The hormones that alter the mucosal lining of the uterus during pregnancy also may cause changes in the nasal and tubal mucosa. Schiff (1968) has reported the same symptoms of aural pressure among women taking oral contraceptives.

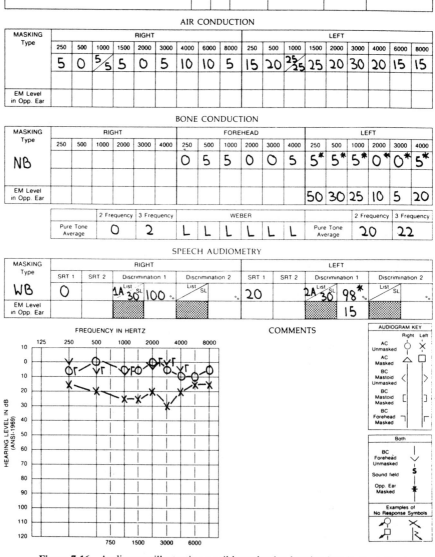

Figure 7.16 Audiogram illustrating a mild conductive hearing loss in the left ear produced by a retracted tympanic membrane. The right ear is normal. Masking was required for bone-conduction and speech discrimination tests for the left ear. The Weber lateralizes to the left ear at all frequencies.

SPEECH AND HEARING CENTER
The University of Texas at Austin 78712

IMMITTANCE

NAME: Last - First - Middle	SEX	AGE	DATE	EXAMINER	INSTRUMENT

PRESSURE/COMPLIANCE FUNCTION

	−400	−350	−300	−250	−200	−150	−100	−50	0	+50	+100	+150	+200
Right					.65	.71	.77	.80	.99	.81	.70	.62	.55
Left			.75	.80	1.05	.87	.77	.72	.68	.64	.62	.60	.58

STATIC COMPLIANCE

$C_x = C_2 - C_1$

RIGHT			LEFT		
.55 C_1	.99 C_2	.44 C_x	.58 C_1	1.05 C_2	.47 C_x

ACOUSTIC REFLEXES

	RIGHT				LEFT			
Frequency (Hz)	500	1000	2000	4000	500	1000	2000	4000
Ipsilateral (Probe same)		90	85			NR	NR	
Contralateral (Probe opposite)	80	85	80	85	NR	NR	NR	NR
Audiometric Threshold	5	0	0	10				
Reflex SL	75	85	80	75				
Decay Time (Seconds)	10⁺	10⁺						

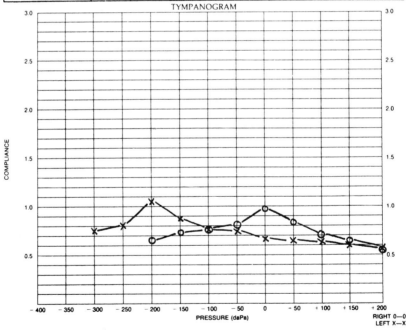

TYMPANOGRAM

COMPLIANCE

PRESSURE (daPa)

RIGHT 0—0
LEFT X—X

Figure 7.17 Typical results on immittance tests performed on a patient with a normal right ear and left negative middle-ear pressure. Note that the tympanogram is Type A for the right ear and Type C for the left. Static compliance is within the normal range for both ears. The acoustic reflex threshold is normal when the tone is introduced to the (normal) right ear and absent when introduced to the (impaired) left ear.

Patulous Eustachian Tubes

There are some individuals in whom the eustachian tube is chronically patent (open). These individuals are bothered by the sensation of **autophony**, the head-in-a-barrel feeling, as a result of which their own voices are subjectively loud. Another annoying effect of the condition is that the sound of breathing is heard loudly in the affected ear. A number of different procedures have been tried to alleviate these unpleasant symptoms, none with great success. Hearing is usually unaffected in chronic patulous eustachian tubes.

If the patient suffers from a chronically patent eustachian tube and exhibits a Type A tympanogram, a simple test can verify the problem. Tympanic membrane compliance is observed during nasal breathing, oral breathing, and momentary cessation of breathing. If the tube is open, the compliance will increase during inhalation and decrease during exhalation. Interruption in breathing stops the changes in compliance.

Serous Effusion of the Middle Ear

If a partial vacuum in the middle ear is allowed to continue, the fluids normally secreted by the mucous membrane lining of the middle ear may literally be sucked into the middle-ear space, resulting in **serous effusion**. As the fluid level rises, otoscopic examination reveals the presence of a fluid line, called the **meniscus**, visible through the tympanic membrane. As the fluid pressure continues to increase and the level rises, the tympanic membrane may return to its normal position when the meniscus rises above the superior margin of the tympanic membrane. At this stage the condition is sometimes difficult to diagnose visually.

When fluid fills the middle-ear space, a Type B tympanometric function results (Figure 7.11). This function occurs because no amount of air pressure delivered to the tympanic membrane from the pump of the immittance meter can match the pressure on the middle-ear side of the tympanic membrane. Because a serous accumulation in the middle ear affects the mass of the system, it is expected that the audiogram will show a greater loss for higher than for lower frequency sounds (Figure 7.18). It is likely that the slightly depressed bone-conduction thresholds in Figure 7.18 are artifacts produced by the fluid in the middle ear. Posttreatment audiograms would probably show a disappearance of the air–bone gap and some improvement in the bone-conduction thresholds.

Because serous effusion is often secondary to a poorly functioning eustachian tube, drug therapy, including the use of decongestants or decongestant–antihistamine combinations, has long been used to restore normal middle-ear pressure and to help clear the tube of secretions. Now, however, decongestants are believed to be virtually useless for this purpose in infants and small children, whose eustachian tubes are less efficient than those of adults. As the middle ear may not be actively infected during serous effusion, antibiotics frequently are not indicated. However, some physicians prescribe an-

NAME: Last - First - Middle	SEX	AGE	DATE	EXAMINER	RELIABILITY	AUDIOMETER

AIR CONDUCTION

MASKING Type	RIGHT									LEFT								
	250	500	1000	1500	2000	3000	4000	6000	8000	250	500	1000	1500	2000	3000	4000	6000	8000
NB	25	35	40/40	40	45	55	60	60	60	15	25	35/35	40	45	55	65	60	60
							60*									65*		
EM Level in Opp. Ear							75									70		

BONE CONDUCTION

MASKING Type	RIGHT						FOREHEAD						LEFT					
	250	500	1000	2000	3000	4000	250	500	1000	2000	3000	4000	250	500	1000	2000	3000	4000
NB	0*	0*	10*	15*	20*	35*	0	-5	5	15	20	25	0*	-5*	5*	15*	20*	35*
EM Level in Opp. Ear	25	40	55	45	55	80							25	35	40	45	55	75

	2 Frequency	3 Frequency	WEBER							2 Frequency	3 Frequency
Pure Tone Average	38	40	M	M	M	M	M	M	Pure Tone Average	30	35

SPEECH AUDIOMETRY

MASKING Type	RIGHT				LEFT			
	SRT 1	SRT 2	Discrimination 1	Discrimination 2	SRT 1	SRT 2	Discrimination 1	Discrimination 2
WB	40	40*	List 38 SL 30 96* %	List SL %	40	40*	List 40 SL 30 98* %	List SL %
EM Level in Opp. Ear		50	65			50	70	

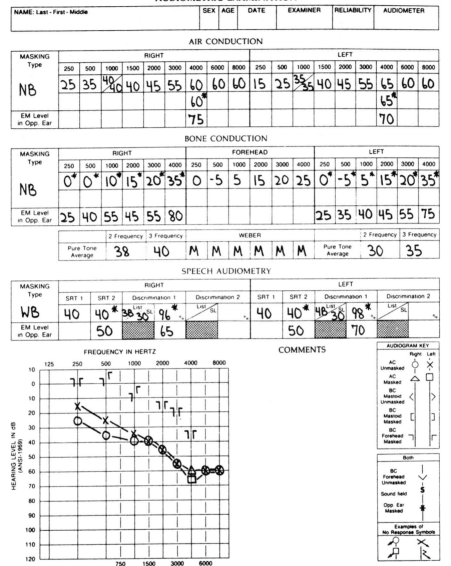

Figure 7.18 Audiogram illustrating conductive hearing loss in both ears produced by serous effusion. Note that masking was indicated for air-conduction tests in both ears only at 4000 Hz, but that it was needed at all frequencies for bone conduction and speech discrimination. Speech discrimination is normal. The Weber does not lateralize. The audiogram falls slightly in the higher frequencies.

tibiotics prophylactically because the fluid, though sterile, may serve as a culture base for bacterial infection. The prescription of antibiotics is a matter of individual medical philosophy.

If the fluid pressure continues to build within the middle ear, perforation of the tympanic membrane becomes a threat. If perforation appears imminent, the otologist may elect to perform a myringotomy to relieve the fluid pressure, suction out the remaining fluid, and place a plastic **pressure-equalizing (P.E.) tube** through the tympanic membrane. The tube allows for direct ventilation of the middle ear and functions as a sort of artificial eustachian tube to equalize air pressure within the middle ear. The plastic tube provides a second vent to the middle ear, which acts much in the same way as the second hole punched in the top of a beer can. Air may enter the middle ear via the tube, allowing drainage down the eustachian tube. Figures 7.19A and B show a myringotomy incision and a P.E. tube in position. A photograph of one kind of P.E. tube is shown in Figure 7.20. The tubes may remain in position from several weeks

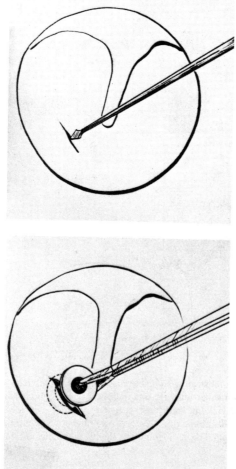

Figure 7.19 (A) A myringotomy incision. (B) A pressure-equalizing tube positioned through the tympanic membrane to allow for adequate middle-ear ventilation. (Courtesy of the Ear and Nose-Throat Clinic, P.A., Little Rock, Arkansas.)

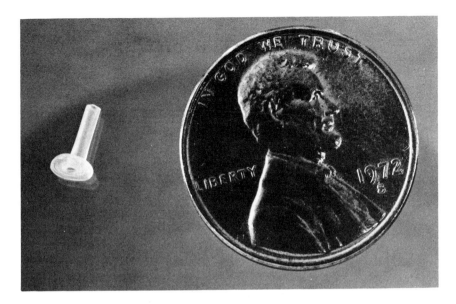

Figure 7.20 A pressure-equalizing tube for insertion through a myringotomy incision in a tympanic membrane to allow middle-ear drainage and ventilation.

to several months, after which time some types extrude naturally and fall into the external auditory canal. In the interim, the eustachian tube problem should be appropriately handled through adenoidectomy, allergic desensitization, or whatever medical means seem to be indicated.

Some otologists have found that tubes remain in position longer if they are placed in the superior-anterior quadrant of the tympanic membrane because there is less migration of epithelium in this area than in the larger inferior quadrants. Positioning the tube in this superior area requires the use of a surgical microscope. Failure to resolve the eustachian tube difficulty will frequently lead to a recurrent attack of serous effusion.

Acoustic immittance meters can be very useful in diagnosing perforations of the tympanic membrane, even those too small to be seen with an ordinary otoscope or by experienced examiners. The **physical-volume test (PVT)** can be used in the same way to test the patency of pressure-equalizing tubes placed through the tympanic membrane. If the clinician observes that c_1 is an unusually large value, in excess of 4 cm^3, he or she may assume that this measurement is of a cavity that includes both the outer ear canal and the middle ear. Of course, many patients, especially children, have tympanic membrane perforations or open P.E. tubes and show less than 4 cm^3 as the c_1 value.

Mucous Otitis Media

At times, thick mucoid secretions, often blown through the eustachian tube, accumulate in the middle ear. If these secretions are allowed to remain, they may become dense and darken in color. This condition, which has been referred to as *glue ear*, produces the same kind of audiometric results as sup-purative otitis media. After some period of time, however, the hearing loss is not reversible by simple myringotomy. Even after the inflammatory process has been removed, imperfect healing of the tissue may leave scars. The tissues forming these scars may be fibrous in nature, resulting in a network or web of adhesions. These adhesions cause particular difficulty because they may bind any or all of the ossicles. Besides adhesions in the middle ear, calcium deposits sometimes form on the tympanic membrane, resulting in a condition called **tympanosclerosis**. Surgical dissection of adhesions in the middle ear may be fruitless because they tend to recur, causing conductive hearing loss. According to Meyerhoff (1986, p. 40), mucous otitis media is more common in younger children, whereas serous effusion is more common in older children.

Otosclerosis

Otosclerosis is a common cause of hearing loss in adults. The condition originates in the bony labyrinth of the inner ear and is recognized clinically when it affects the middle ear, causing conductive hearing loss. Otosclerosis is a progressive disorder whose age of onset varies from mid-childhood to late middle-adult life. The great majority of patients begin to notice some loss of hearing soon after puberty up to the age of 30. Otosclerosis is rare among children. It occurs primarily among members of the white race, with the incidence in women approximately twice that in men. Women frequently report increased hearing loss due to otosclerosis at times of pregnancy or menopause.

Otosclerosis appears as the formation of a new growth of spongy bone, usually over the stapedial footplate of one or both ears. Because the bone is not really sclerotic (hard), some clinicians call this condition (more appropri-ately) **ostospongiosis**. When this happens, the footplate becomes partially fixed in the oval window, limiting the amplitudes of vibrations transmitted to the inner ear. At times the growth appears on the stapedial crura or over the round window. Very rarely does it occur on other ossicles or occupy consid-erable space in the middle ear. Sometimes the sclerotic bone, which replaces the normal bone of the middle ear, may completely obliterate the margins of the oval window.

Patients with otosclerosis often exhibit a bluish cast to the whites of their eyes, similar to that present in certain other bone diseases. They complain of difficulty hearing while chewing, probably a result of the increased loudness of the chewing sounds delivered to their inner ears by bone conduction. Fre-quently they are also bothered by hissing sounds called **tinnitus** in the affected ear (or ears). The hearing loss itself is usually slowly progressive. Physical examination of the ear shows normal structures and tympanic membrane land-marks. Occasionally the promontory becomes very vascular, resulting in a rosy glow that can be seen through the tympanic membrane. This glow is the so-called **Schwartze sign**.

One interesting and peculiar symptom of otosclerosis is **paracusis willisii**.

Most hard-of-hearing patients claim they hear and understand speech better in quiet surroundings. Otosclerotic patients (and often patients with other forms of conductive hearing loss) may find that speech is easier to understand in the presence of background noise. This phenomenon results from the fact that normal-hearing persons speak louder in noisy environments. The increase in vocal loudness, something we have all experienced, is called the **Lombard voice reflex**. Because otosclerotic patients' hearing losses attenuate the background noise to some degree, such people are able to enjoy the increased loudness of speakers' voices with less distracting noise. Paracusis willisii is illustrated in Figure 7.21.

Audiometric Findings in Otosclerosis. Carhart (1964) has shown that the first symptom of otosclerosis is the appearance of a low-frequency air–bone gap. He also found that alterations in the inertia of the ossicular chain produced by even partial fixation alter the normal bone-conduction response. This artifact varies significantly from patient to patient, but on the average it causes the bone-conduction readings to appear poorer than the true sensorineural sensitivity by 5 dB at 500 Hz, 10 dB at 1000 Hz, 15 dB at 2000 Hz, and 5 dB at 4000 Hz. This anomaly of bone conduction is called the **Carhart notch** and probably occurs as a mechanical artifact because of a shift in the normal resonant frequency of the middle ear (about 2500 Hz) produced by the immobility of the oval window. The Carhart notch is also seen in some cases of middle-ear fluid.

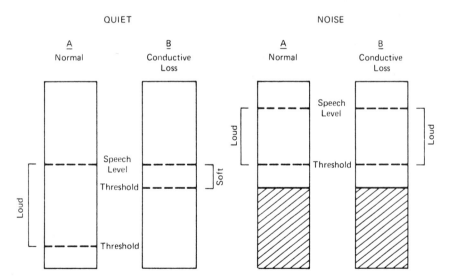

Figure 7.21 Illustration of paracusis willisii. The normal listener (A) has an advantage over the hard-of-hearing listerner (B) in the quiet situation, because the speech is received for A at a higher sensation level and is therefore louder. In the noisy situation, the threshold is raised by the noise much more for A than for B. The speaker's voice is raised by the noise (the Lombard effect). Therefore, A and B both enjoy the same speech level above threshold (equal loudness), but B is much less aware of the background noise.

Figure 7.22 illustrates an audiogram typical of early otosclerosis. Contrary to the typical audiometric contour in serous effusion, the otosclerotic shows a drop in sensitivity in the low-frequency areas first, which is consistent with what is known of the effects of stiffness on impedance. As the principal place of otosclerosis increases in size, the hearing loss becomes greater (Figure 7.23). Later in the disease, when the stapes has become completely fixed, the mass effect becomes apparent, causing a reduction of sensitivity in the high frequencies, thus flattening the audiogram. With complete fixation, the entire mass of the skull is in fact added to the stapes. All auditory tests for site of lesion remain consistent with conductive hearing loss.

The pressure-compliance function remains normal in otosclerosis, except that the point of greatest compliance is not as great as normal on the tympanogram. Jerger (1970) has called this type of tympanogram (Figure 7.24) a Type A_S (stiffness). The A_S tympanogram appears in many, but not all, cases of otosclerosis. The acoustic reflex disappears early in otosclerosis, even in unilateral cases. When the tone is delivered to the involved ear, the hearing loss attenuates the loudness of even a very intense sound so that the reflex is not triggered. When a tone is delivered to a normal ear opposite one with otosclerosis, the reflex does not register because the stapes is incapable of movement even though it is pulled by the stapedius tendon. In otosclerosis the acoustic impedance may be expected to be high and the compliance low.

Treatment of Otosclerosis. Interest in the surgical correction of otosclerosis dates back many years. Even in fairly recent times surgical relief of otosclerotic hearing loss met with failure, primarily for two reasons. First, before the introduction of antibiotics, postoperative infection caused severe complications. Second, until the development of the operating microscope, middle-ear surgeons did not have proper visualization of the very small operative field of the middle ear.

Because attempts to free the immobilized stapes resulted in failure, often in the form of fractured crura, attention was turned to bypassing the ossicular chain. A new window was created in the lateral semicircular (balance) canal of the inner ear so that sound waves could pass directly from the ear canal to the new window. This procedure was conducted as a two-stage operation until the one-stage **fenestration** was developed by Lempert (1938).

Fenestration surgery resulted in considerable hearing improvements for many patients with otosclerosis. It was recognized early that complete closure of the preoperative air–bone gap was impossible, as a result of loss of the tympanic membrane and the ossicular chain. Approximately 25 dB residual conductive hearing loss remained following even the best fenestration. The proper selection of candidates for surgery, based on their bone-conduction thresholds, was critical. Careful comparisons of preoperative bone-conduction audiograms with the postoperative bone-conduction audiograms led to the discovery of the Carhart notch (1952).

Although many people were helped dramatically by fenestration surgery, numbers of others were less than satisfied with the results. Many people

SPEECH AND HEARING CENTER
The University of Texas at Austin 78712
AUDIOMETRIC EXAMINATION

NAME: Last - First - Middle	SEX	AGE	DATE	EXAMINER	RELIABILITY	AUDIOMETER

AIR CONDUCTION

MASKING Type	RIGHT									LEFT								
	250	500	1000	1500	2000	3000	4000	6000	8000	250	500	1000	1500	2000	3000	4000	6000	8000
	25	20	20/20	15	5	10	0	0	0	30	20	15/15	10	5	0	0	5	5
EM Level in Opp. Ear																		

BONE CONDUCTION

MASKING Type	RIGHT						FOREHEAD						LEFT					
	250	500	1000	2000	3000	4000	250	500	1000	2000	3000	4000	250	500	1000	2000	3000	4000
NB	0*	5*					-5	5	10	15	10	5	-5	5*				
EM Level in Opp. Ear	60	50											60	55				

	2 Frequency	3 Frequency	WEBER						2 Frequency	3 Frequency
Pure Tone Average	13	15	M	M	M	M	M	Pure Tone Average	10	13

SPEECH AUDIOMETRY

MASKING Type	RIGHT				LEFT			
	SRT 1	SRT 2	Discrimination 1	Discrimination 2	SRT 1	SRT 2	Discrimination 1	Discrimination 2
WB	20		1C 30 List/SL 96* %	List/SL 50 %	15		2C 30 List/SL 94 %	List/SL %
EM Level in Opp. Ear								

FREQUENCY IN HERTZ

COMMENTS

AUDIOGRAM KEY

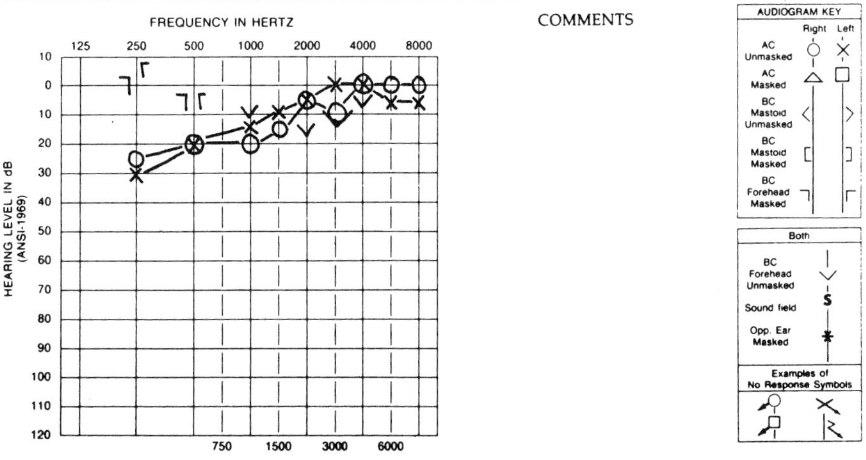

Figure 7.22 Audiogram illustrating early otosclerosis in both ears. The loss appears first in the low frequencies, owing to the increased stiffness of the ossicular chain. A small air–bone gap is present. Speech discrimination scores are normal, and the Weber does not lateralize. Masking was used for bone conduction only at 250 and 500 Hz and for speech discrimination testing. Note the early appearance of the Carhart notch.

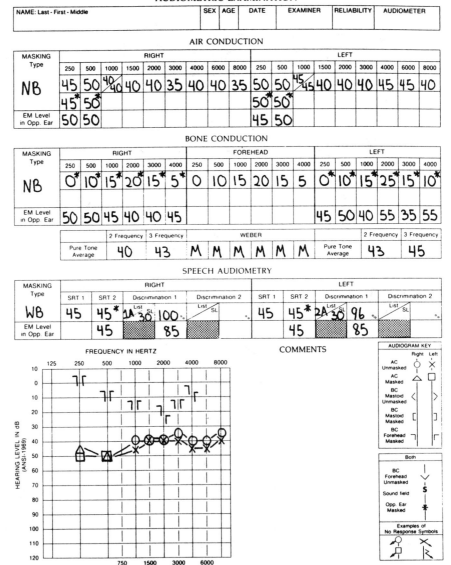

SPEECH AND HEARING CENTER
The University of Texas at Austin 78712
AUDIOMETRIC EXAMINATION

NAME: Last - First - Middle	SEX	AGE	DATE	EXAMINER	RELIABILITY	AUDIOMETER

AIR CONDUCTION

MASKING Type	RIGHT									LEFT								
	250	500	1000	1500	2000	3000	4000	6000	8000	250	500	1000	1500	2000	3000	4000	6000	8000
NB	45	50	40/40	40	40	35	40	40	35	50	50	45/45	40	40	40	45	45	40
	45*	50*								50*	50*							
EM Level in Opp. Ear	50	50								45	50							

BONE CONDUCTION

MASKING Type	RIGHT						FOREHEAD						LEFT					
	250	500	1000	2000	3000	4000	250	500	1000	2000	3000	4000	250	500	1000	2000	3000	4000
NB	0*	10*	15*	20*	15*	5*	0	10	15	20	15	5	0*	10*	15*	25*	15*	10*
EM Level in Opp. Ear	50	50	45	40	40	45							45	50	40	55	35	55

	2 Frequency	3 Frequency	WEBER						2 Frequency	3 Frequency
Pure Tone Average	40	43	M	M	M	M	M	M	Pure Tone Average 43	45

SPEECH AUDIOMETRY

MASKING Type	RIGHT				LEFT			
	SRT 1	SRT 2	Discrimination 1	Discrimination 2	SRT 1	SRT 2	Discrimination 1	Discrimination 2
WB	45	45*	1A List 30 SL 100 %	List SL %	45	45*	2A List 30 SL 96 %	List SL %
EM Level in Opp. Ear		45	85			45	85	

FREQUENCY IN HERTZ   COMMENTS

Figure 7.23 Audiogram showing a moderate loss of hearing in both ears caused by otosclerosis. The audiometric configuration is fairly flat, showing the combined effects of stiffness and mass. Bone conduction is normal except for the Carhart notch. Masking is required for all tests.

SPEECH AND HEARING CENTER
The University of Texas at Austin 78712

IMMITTANCE

NAME: Last - First - Middle	SEX	AGE	DATE	EXAMINER	INSTRUMENT

PRESSURE/COMPLIANCE FUNCTION

	– 400	– 350	– 300	– 250	– 200	– 150	– 100	– 50	0	+ 50	+ 100	+ 150	+ 200
Right					.60	.62	.65	.75	.84	.71	.76	.64	.62
Left					.76	.77	.79	.85	.95	.85	.80	.79	.77

STATIC COMPLIANCE

$C_x = C_2 - C_1$

RIGHT						LEFT					
.60	c_1	.84	c_2	.24	c_x	.76	c_1	.95	c_2	.19	c_x

ACOUSTIC REFLEXES

	RIGHT				LEFT			
Frequency (Hz)	500	1000	2000	4000	500	1000	2000	4000
Ipsilateral (Probe same)		NR	NR			NR	NR	
Contralateral (Probe opposite)	NR	NR	NR	NR	NR	NR	NR	NR
Audiometric Threshold								
Reflex SL								
Decay Time (Seconds)								

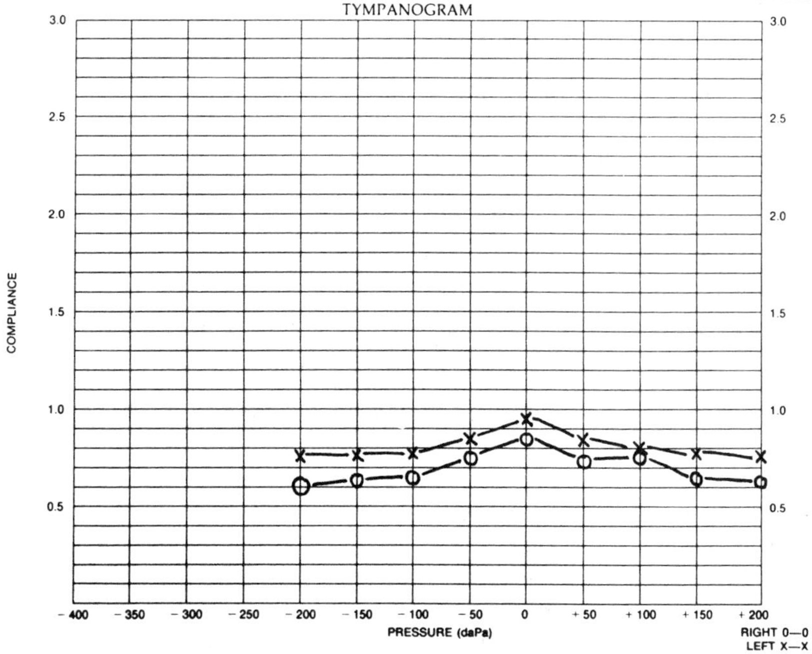

TYMPANOGRAM

RIGHT 0—0
LEFT X—X

Figure 7.24 Results on immittance tests performed on a patient with bilateral otosclerosis (Figure 7.21). The tympanogram is Type A_S, the static compliance is low, and the acoustic reflexes are absent in both ears.

found no improvement in their hearing, and a number showed considerable drops in their sensorineural sensitivity. Some individuals had total loss of hearing. Using Figure 7.23 as an example of a preoperative audiogram, Figure 7.25 shows the maximum improvement possible with fenestration surgery, and Figure 7.26 shows a poor result. Often, patients with poor fenestration results were bothered by vertigo and increased tinnitus, as well as by poorer speech discrimination and occasional facial paralysis. Hearing-aid use was sometimes obviated in the operated ear by a combination of poor speech discrimination and the large ear cavity created during surgery. Even if some patients were happy with the hearing results of their surgery, they were bothered by the constant aftercare required to clean the cavity.

While palpating a stapes on a patient preparatory to performing a fenestration, Rosen (1953) managed to mobilize the stapes, breaking it free and restoring the sound vibrations into the inner ear. This happenstance led to a completely new introduction, the **stapes mobilization** procedure.

Advantages of the mobilization over the fenestration were manifold. Patients could be operated on under local anesthesia, eliminating some of the serious side effects of general anesthesia. Because the ossicular chain remained intact, the patient's potential for postoperative hearing could be fairly well predicted by the preoperative bone conduction. Of great importance was the fact that no aftercare was required for mobilizations because no mastoid cavity was created during surgery.

In stapes mobilization the ear canal is carefully cleansed and dried. The skin near the tympanic membrane is then injected (several times) to deaden the area. (The anesthetic works so rapidly that many patients only notice one injection.) A triangular incision is made in the skin and the tympanic membrane reflected, exposing the middle ear. The surgeon then places a right-angle hook against the neck of the stapes, determines that it is fixed, and then rocks it until it is freed.

A number of variations of Rosen's operation were introduced, and although many patients were initially helped, it was found that a great number of those patients whose hearing originally improved failed to retain this improvement after one year. The regression in hearing resulted from refixation of the stapes as new otosclerotic bone was laid down over the footplate. Refixation appears to be a greater problem for young patients, in whom the otosclerosis is more active, and for males.

Refixation following stapes mobilization led Shea (1958) to revive an operative procedure that had been described more than a half century earlier. This technique is called **stapedectomy**, which means "removal of the stapes." Stapedectomy is undoubtedly the procedure of choice for otosclerosis today.

The approaches to the middle ear for stapedectomy and mobilization are identical. After fixation has been determined, the incudo-stapedial joint is interrupted, the stapedius tendon is cut, and the superstructure of the stapes and remainder of the footplate are removed. In the original procedure a vein graft, taken from the patient's hand or arm, was placed over the open oval window and draped upon the promontory and over the facial ridge to obtain

SPEECH AND HEARING CENTER
The University of Texas at Austin 78712
AUDIOMETRIC EXAMINATION

NAME: Last - First - Middle	SEX	AGE	DATE	EXAMINER	RELIABILITY	AUDIOMETER

AIR CONDUCTION

MASKING Type	RIGHT									LEFT								
	250	500	1000	1500	2000	3000	4000	6000	8000	250	500	1000	1500	2000	3000	4000	6000	8000
NB	45	50	50/50	50	50	45	55	60	65	30	25	25/25	20	20	20	25	25	30
	45*	50*	50*	50*	50*	45*	55*	60*	65*									
EM Level in Opp. Ear	30	25	25	20	20	20	25	25	30									

BONE CONDUCTION

MASKING Type	RIGHT						FOREHEAD						LEFT					
	250	500	1000	2000	3000	4000	250	500	1000	2000	3000	4000	250	500	1000	2000	3000	4000
NB	5*	10*	15*	20*	10*	10*	0	0	5	5	5	5	0*	0*	5*	5*	5*	5*
EM Level in Opp. Ear	65	60	45	40	40	45							75	70	60	50	45	55

	2 Frequency	3 Frequency	WEBER								2 Frequency	3 Frequency
Pure Tone Average	50	50	R	R	R	R	R	R	Pure Tone Average	22	23

SPEECH AUDIOMETRY

MASKING Type	RIGHT				LEFT			
	SRT 1	SRT 2	Discrimination 1	Discrimination 2	SRT 1	SRT 2	Discrimination 1	Discrimination 2
WB	50	50*	1A List 30 SL 96 * %	List SL %	25	2A List 30 SL	94 * %	List SL %
EM Level in Opp. Ear		25	65				50	

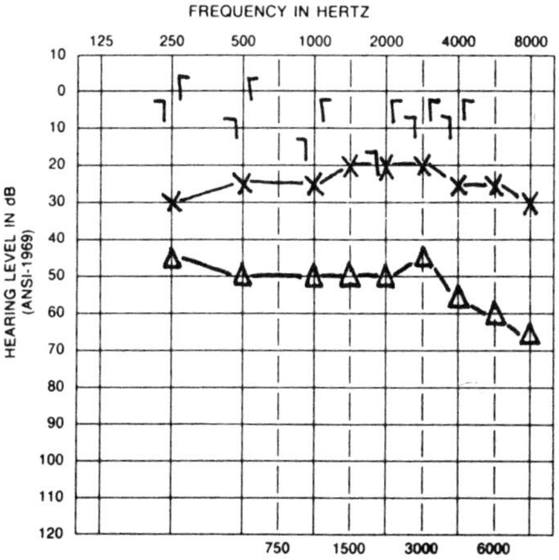

FREQUENCY IN HERTZ   COMMENTS

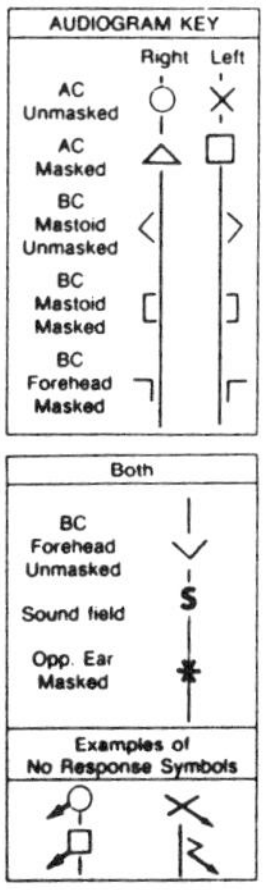

Figure 7.25 Audiogram showing a conductive hearing loss in both ears. The right ear shows a moderate loss owing to otosclerosis, and the left ear, a postoperative fenestration. Note the presence of the Carhart notch in the right ear and its absence in the left. The left ear shows the maximum obtainable result with fenestration surgery. All special hearing tests are as would be expected with conductive hearing loss.

SPEECH AND HEARING CENTER
The University of Texas at Austin 78712
AUDIOMETRIC EXAMINATION

NAME: Last - First - Middle	SEX	AGE	DATE	EXAMINER	RELIABILITY	AUDIOMETER

AIR CONDUCTION

MASKING Type	RIGHT									LEFT							
	250	500	1000	1500	2000	3000	4000	6000	8000	250	500	1000	1500	2000	3000	4000	6000	8000
NB	60	65	65	65	70	80	75	85	90	55	55	60/60	60	55	50	55	60	65
	70*	75*	75*	75*	80*	90*	85*	90*	NR*	55	55*	60*	60*	55*	50*	55*	60*	65*
EM Level in Opp. Ear	75	75	75	80	80	75	75	80	80	70	75	75	80	80	90	85	90	90

BONE CONDUCTION

MASKING Type	RIGHT						FOREHEAD						LEFT					
	250	500	1000	2000	3000	4000	250	500	1000	2000	3000	4000	250	500	1000	2000	3000	4000
NB	NR*	65*	NR*	NR*	NR*	NR*	5	10	15	25	30	20	15*	15*	25*	35*	35*	20*
EM Level in Opp. Ear	80	90	90	90	85	90							80	90	90	80	95	85

	2 Frequency	3 Frequency	WEBER							2 Frequency	3 Frequency
Pure Tone Average	75	77	L	L	L	L	L	L	Pure Tone Average	55	57

SPEECH AUDIOMETRY

MASKING Type	RIGHT				LEFT			
	SRT 1	SRT 2	Discrimination 1	Discrimination 2	SRT 1	SRT 2	Discrimination 1	Discrimination 2
WB	65	80*	4A List 30 SL 66* %	List SL %	55		4B List 30 SL 96 %	List SL %
EM Level in Opp. Ear		75	105					

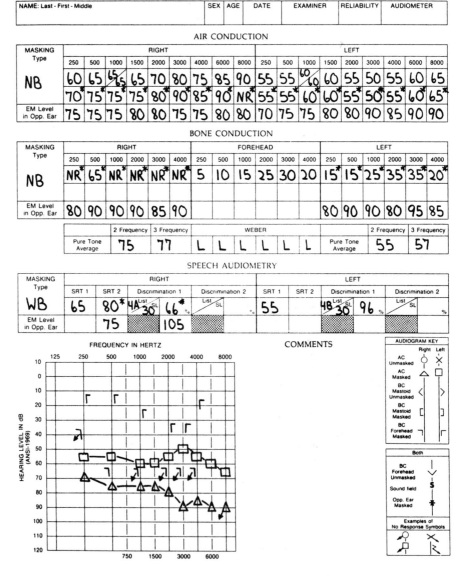

COMMENTS

Figure 7.26 Audiogram illustrating conductive hearing loss in the left ear owing to otosclerosis. The right ear shows a sensorineural hearing loss produced by unsuccessful middle-ear surgery to correct for otosclerosis. Note that masking is required to show the true bone-conduction thresholds for the right ear. Masked speech discrimination tests show the right ear to be impaired. The Weber is lateralized to the left ear.

adequate blood supply. A hollow polyethylene strut was pulled onto the lenticular process of the incus, and the opposite end, which was beveled for better fit, was placed in the oval window niche on the vein graft. In this way the polyethylene tube replaced the stapes.

In some cases, the polyethylene with vein procedure, though very popular, resulted in **fistulas** (leaks of inner-ear fluids into the middle ear), perhaps as a result of the sharp end of the strut resting on the vein. Testing for a fistula can be accomplished with the pressure portion of an immittance meter and an electronystagmograph (ENG) (see Chapter 8). Positive pressure is delivered to the middle ear by increasing the output of air pressure from the meter to 300 or 400 mm H_2O. This may be accomplished whether a perforation of the tympanic membrane exists or not. If a fistula is present, the increased pressure within the middle ear may result in the patient's experiencing vertigo and an increase in the rapid eye movement, called *nystagmus*, which can be monitored on the ENG.

In recent years a number of modifications of the original Shea stapedectomy have been introduced. Different materials have been used as the prosthesis: stainless steel wire, stainless steel pistons, Teflon pistons, combinations of steel and plastic, and so on. Some surgeons have used fat plugs from the tragus of the pinna, or **fascia** (the tough, protective cover over muscle) to cover the oval window and support the prosthesis. Although the success of stapedectomy has been substantial and many patients with unsuccessful mobilizations have been reoperated on with great improvements in hearing, some adverse reactions can and do occur, including further loss of hearing and prolonged vertigo.

To reduce risk in stapedectomy, many middle-ear surgeons today prefer to use a small fenestra and avoid the trauma to the inner ear of complete removal of the stapedial footplate. Small fenestra stapedectomies have been referred to as *stapedotomies*. One such procedure is illustrated in Figures 7.27 to 7.32. After the ear has been locally anesthetized and the tympanic membrane elevated from its sulcus exposing the middle ear, the stapedectomy is begun.

First, the proper length for the piston prosthesis is determined (Figure 7.27). A small perforation is made in the center of the footplate with a pick or small drill; the hole is then enlarged to a diameter of .8 mm (Figure 7.28). The crura are weakened and fractured away from the footplate with a pick. Then the incudo-stapedial joint is separated and the stapedial tendon cut (Figure 7.29), after which the entire superstructure is removed (Figure 7.30). The prosthesis is placed in the small fenestra (Figure 7.31), and the wire hook is crimped over the long process of the incus. Fascia from the temporalis muscle is packed around the prosthesis, where it enters the fenestra, to create an immediate seal of the inner ear (Figure 7.32).

As further modifications of the stapedectomy procedure continue to be perfected, such as the use of an argon laser, some form of stapedectomy will surely remain popular.

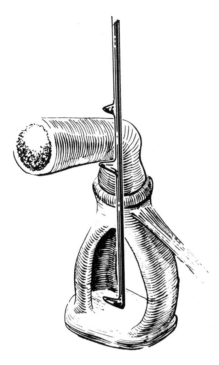

Figure 7.27 The proper length for the prosthesis is determined by measuring the distance from the undersurface of the incus to the footplate. A special measuring rod is used.

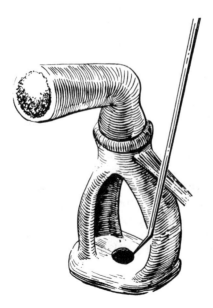

Figure 7.28 A small "control hole" is made in the center of the footplate; the hole is then enlarged with a pick or hand drill.

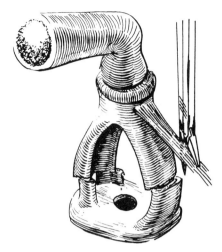

Figure 7.29 The crura are weakened and fractured, the incudo-stapedial joint is separated, and the stapedial tendon is severed with microscissors.

OTHER CAUSES OF MIDDLE-EAR HEARING LOSS

A variety of middle-ear abnormalities occur in isolation or in association with other congenital anomalies. Some cases of stapedial fixation appear purely on a genetic basis. A number of congenital middle-ear disorders were found in the offspring of mothers who took the drug thalidomide during pregnancy. Such conditions as fixation of the incudo-malleal joint have been associated with atresias of the external auditory canal and microtias of the auricle. Other ossicular abnormalities have been associated with syndromes of the cheek, jaw, and face. Congenital malformations of the middle and outer ears are often seen together because these areas arise from the same embryonic tissue. Meyerhoff (1986, p. 23) recommends delaying surgical repair in these situations

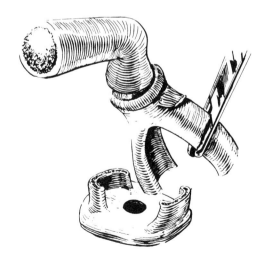

Figure 7.30 The superstructure of the stapes is removed.

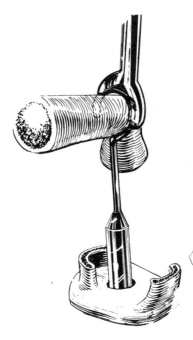

Figure 7.31 The prosthesis is carefully positioned, the wire hook is placed over the long process of the incus just above the lenticular process, and the hook is crimped snugly into position with a special crimping instrument.

until the child is 4 to 6 years old to permit the mastoid air cell system to enlarge, allowing better surgical access.

Skull fractures have been known to result coincidentally in fractures or interruptions of the ossicular chain. Ossicular interruption has been reported in cases of skull trauma, even without fracture. An ossicle may also be damaged by a foreign object during traumatic perforation of the tympanic membrane, as with a cotton swab or bobby pin.

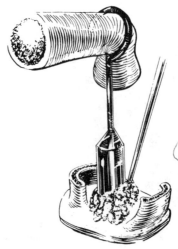

Figure 7.32 Superficial fascia from the temporalis muscle is placed around the end of the prosthesis, where it enters the footplate, to seal the inner ear.

(Figures 7.27–7.32 courtesy of the Ear and Nose-Throat Clinic, P.A., Little Rock, Arkansas.)

Tumors, both benign and malignant, may form in the middle ear. They may take the form of polyps, granulomas in response to middle-ear infections, or in rare cases cancer of the squamous cells of the middle ear.

SUMMARY

The middle ear is an air-filled space separating the external auditory canal from the inner ear. Its function is to increase sound energy through the use of leverage, the step-down size ratio provided by the ossicular chain, and the area ratio between the tympanic membrane and the oval window.

Abnormalities of the structure or function of the middle ear result in conductive hearing losses, wherein the air-conduction thresholds are depressed in direct relationship with the amount of disease. Bone-conduction thresholds are only slightly deviated from normal in conductive hearing losses, not because of abnormality of the sensorineural mechanism, but because of alterations in the middle ear's normal (inertial) contribution to bone-conduction hearing. In middle-ear conductive hearing losses, results on such tests as word discrimination, SISI, tone decay, and Békésy audiometry are identical to those of normal hearers. Alterations in the pressure-compliance functions give general information regarding the presence of fluid or negative air pressure in the middle ear, stiffness or interruption of the ossicular chain. Measurements of static compliance may be higher or lower than normal, and acoustic reflex thresholds are either elevated or absent. Auditory brain stem responses show increased latencies for all waves.

Patients with conductive hearing losses are excellent candidates for hearing aids because of their relatively flat audiometric contours, good word discrimination, and tolerance for loud sounds. Remediation should first be concerned with medical or surgical reversal of the problems. When this fails, must be postponed, or is not available, careful audiological counseling should be undertaken and therapeutic avenues, such as the use of hearing aids, investigated.

GLOSSARY

Acute A condition characterized by rapid onset, frequently of short duration.

Aditus ad antrum A space in the middle ear containing the head of the malleus and the greater part of the incus. It communicates upward and backward with the mastoid antrum.

Autophony A condition produced by some middle-ear or eustachian tube abnormalities in which individuals' voices seem louder than normal to themselves.

Barotrauma Damage to the ear by sudden changes in pressure, as in flying or diving.

Bell's palsy Paralysis of the peripheral branch of the facial nerve.

Carhart notch An artifactual depression in the bone-conduction audiogram of patients with otosclerosis. It disappears following corrective surgery.

Carotid artery   The main large artery on either side of the neck. It passes beneath the anterior wall of the middle ear.

Cholesteatoma   A tumor, usually occurring in the middle ear and mastoid, that combines fats and epithelium from outside the middle-ear space.

Chorda tympani nerve   A branch of the facial nerve that passes through the middle ear. It conveys information about taste from the anterior two-thirds of one side of the tongue.

Chronic   A condition characterized by long duration.

Cilia   Eyelash-like projections of some cells that beat rhythmically to move certain substances over their surfaces.

Crura   Legs, as of the stapes.

Crus   Singular of *crura*.

Epitympanic recess   That part of the middle ear above the upper level of the tympanic membrane. Also called the *attic* of the middle ear.

Eustachian tube   The channel connecting the middle ear with the nasopharynx on each side. It is lined with mucous membrane. Sometimes called the auditory tube.

Facial nerve   The VIIth cranial nerve. It innervates the muscles of the face and the stapedius muscle.

Fallopian canal   A bony channel, on the medial wall of the middle ear, through which the facial nerve passes. It is covered with mucous membrane.

Fascia   Layers of tissue that form the sheaths of muscles.

Fenestration   An operation designed to correct hearing loss from otosclerosis. A new window is created in the lateral balance canal of the inner ear and the ossicular chain is bypassed.

Fistula   An abnormal opening, as by incomplete closure of a wound, which allows fluid to leak out.

Footplate   The base of the stapes, which occupies the oval window.

Hemotympanum   Bleeding in the middle ear.

Incus   The second bone in the ossicular chain, connecting the malleus to the stapes. It is named for its resemblance to an anvil.

Jugular bulb   The bulbous protrusion of the jugular vein in the floor of the middle ear.

Lombard voice reflex   The normal elevation of vocal intensity when the speaker listens to a loud noise.

Malleus   The first and largest bone in the ossicular chain of the middle ear, connected to the tympanic membrane and the incus; so named because of its resemblance to a hammer.

Manubrium   A process of the malleus embedded in the fibrous layer of the tympanic membrane.

Mastoidectomy   An operation to remove infected cells of the mastoid. Mastoidectomies are divided into simple, radical and modified radical, depending on the extent of surgery.

Mastoiditis   Infection of the mastoid.

Mastoid process   A protrusion of the temporal bone, one portion of which is pneumatized (filled with air cells).

Meniscus The curved surface of a column of fluid. A meniscus is sometimes seen through the tympanic membrane when fluids are present in the middle ear.

Middle-ear cleft The space composed of the middle ear and the eustachian tube.

Mucous membrane A form of epithelium found in many parts of the body, including the mouth, nose, paranasal sinuses, eustachian tube, and middle ear. Its cells contain fluid-producing glands.

Myringotomy Incision of the tympanic membrane. *fluids removed*

Nasopharynx The area where the back of the nose and the throat communicate.

Necrosis The death of living cells.

Ossicles The chain of three tiny bones found in each middle ear (malleus, incus, and stapes).

Otitis media Any infection of the middle ear.

Otorrhea Any discharge from the external auditory canal or from the middle ear.

Otosclerosis The laying down of new bone in the middle ear, usually around the footplate of the stapes. When it interferes with stapedial vibration, it produces a progressive conductive hearing loss.

Otospongiosis See *otosclerosis*.

Oval window A tiny oval-shaped aperture beneath the footplate of the stapes. The oval window separates the middle ear from the inner ear.

Paracusis willisii A condition found among patients with conductive hearing loss in which the patient understands speech better in noisy than in quiet surroundings.

Physical-volume test (PVT) A high sound intensity, suggesting a large volume of air (greater than 4 cm^3), may be observed on c_1 during immittance measures. This suggests that a patent P.E. tube or tympanic membrane perforation is present.

Politzerization Inflation of the middle ear via the eustachian tube by forcing air through the nose.

Pressure-equalizing (P.E.) tube A short tube or grommet placed through a myringotomy incision in a tympanic membrane to allow for middle-ear ventilation.

Promontory A protrusion into the middle ear, at its labyrinthine wall, produced by the basal turn of the cochlea.

Purulent Related to the formation of pus.

Round window A small round aperture containing a thin but tough membrane. The round window separates the middle ear from the inner ear.

Schwartze sign A red glow seen through the tympanic membrane and produced by increased vascularity of the promontory in some cases of otosclerosis.

Serous effusion The collection of fluid in the middle-ear space, with possible drainage into the external ear canal. Often called *serous otitis media*.

Stapedectomy An operation designed to improve hearing in cases of otosclerosis by removing the affected stapes and replacing it with a prosthesis.

Stapedius muscle   A tiny muscle, innervated by the facial nerve and connected to the stapes in the middle ear by means of the stapedius tendon.

Stapes   The third and smallest bone in the ossicular chain of the middle ear, connected to the incus and standing in the oval window. Named because of its resemblance to a stirrup.

Stapes mobilization   An operation to improve hearing in cases of otosclerosis by breaking the stapes free of its fixation in the oval window and allowing normal vibration.

Subluxation   An incomplete dislocation or sprain.

Suppurative   Producing pus.

Tensor tympani muscle   A small muscle, innervated by the trigeminal nerve and inserted into the malleus in the middle ear.

Tinnitus   Ear noises, usually described as ringing, roaring, or hissing.

Toynbee maneuver   A method for forcing the eustachian tube open by swallowing with the nostrils and jaw closed.

Trigeminal nerve   The Vth cranial nerve, which innervates the tensor tympani and also some of the palatal muscles.

Tympanoplasty   A surgical procedure designed to restore the hearing function to a middle ear that has been partially destroyed (as by otitis media).

Tympanosclerosis   New calcium formations in the middle ear or on the tympanic membrane secondary to otitis media. The result is loss of mobility of the conductive mechanism.

Valsalva   Autoinflation of the middle ear by closing off the mouth and nose and forcing air up the eustachian tube.

STUDY QUESTIONS

1. List as many parts of the middle ear as you can. Consider their functions. Compare your list to the diagram of the ear shown in Figure 7.1.
2. Make a list of disorders of the middle ear that produce conductive hearing loss. Next to each item, name an appropriate treatment.
3. For each of the disorders just listed, sketch a pure-tone audiogram. What would the probable results be on the following tests: SRT, speech discrimination, ABLB, SISI, Békésy audiometry, tone decay test, immittance measures and ABR?

REVIEW TABLE 7.1 Conductive Hearing Loss in the Middle Ear

ETIOLOGY	DEGREE OF LOSS	AUDIOMETRIC CONFIGURATION	STATIC COMPLIANCE	TYMPANOGRAM TYPE	ACOUSTIC-REFLEX THRESHOLD
Suppurative otitis media	Mild to moderately severe	Flat	Normal to low	B	Elevated to absent
Tympanic membrane perforation	Mild	Flat	Not testable	Not testable	Not testable
Ossicular chain discontinuity	Moderate	Flat	High	A_D	Absent
Serous effusion	Mild to moderate	Flat or poorer in high frequencies	Normal to low	B	Elevated to absent
Negative middle-ear pressure	Mild	Flat	Normal	C	Elevated to absent
Otosclerosis	Mild to moderately severe	Flat or poorer in low frequencies	Low	A_S	Absent
Congenital disorders	Mild to moderately severe	Varies	Varies	Varies	Absent

REFERENCES

ANDERSON, E. E. & BARR, B. (1971). Conductive high-tone hearing loss. *Archives of Otolaryngology, 93,* 599–605.

BAILEY, H. A. T. & GRAHAM, S. S. (1984). Reducing risk in stapedectomy: The small fenestra stapedectomy technique. *Audiology: A Journal for Continuing Education, 9,* 1–13.

CARHART, R. (1952). Bone conduction advances following fenestration surgery. *Transactions of the American Academy of Ophthalmology and Otolaryngology, 56,* 621–629.

————. (1964). Audiometric manifestations of preclinical stapes fixation. *Annals of Otology, Rhinology and Laryngology, 73,* 740–755.

DE JONGE, R. R. & VALENTE, M. (1979). Interpreting ear differences in static compliance measurements. *Journal of Speech and Hearing Disorders, 44,* 209–213.

GIEBINK, G. S. (1984). Epidemiology and natural history of otitis media. In D. Lim, C. Bluestone, J. Klein, & J. Nelson (Eds.), *Recent advances in otitis media,* Philadelphia: B. C. Decker.

GLADSTONE, V. S. (1984). Advanced acoustic immittance considerations. In H. Kaplan, V. S. Gladstone, & J. Katz (Eds.), *Site of Lesion Testing: Audiometric Interpretation,* (Vol. 2, pp. 59–79). Baltimore: University Park Press.

JERGER, J. (1970). Clinical experience with impedance audiometry. *Archives of Otolaryngology, 92,* 311–324.

KRAEMER, M. J. RICHARDSON, M. A., WEISS, N. S., FURUKAWA, C. T., SHAPIRO, G. G., PIERSON, W. E., & BIERMAN, C. W. (1983). Risk factors for persistent middle-ear effusions. *Journal of the American Medical Association, 249,* 1022–1025.

LEMPERT, J. (1938). Improvement of hearing in cases of otosclerosis: A new one-stage surgical technique. *Archives of Otolaryngology, 28,* 42–97.

MEYERHOFF, W. L. (1986). *Disorders of hearing.* Austin, TX: Pro-Ed.

ROCK, E. H. (1974). Practical otologic applications and considerations in impedance audiometry. *Impedance Newsletter Supplement,* Vol. 3. New York: American Electromedics Corporation.

ROSEN, S. (1953). Mobilization of the stapes to restore hearing in otosclerosis. *New York Journal of Medicine, 53,* 2650–2653.

SCHIFF, M. (1968). The "pill" in otolaryngology. *Transactions of the American Academy of Ophthalmology and Otolaryngology, 72,* 76–83.

SHEA, J. J. (1958). Fenestration of the oval window. *Annals of Otology, Rhinology and Laryngology, 67,* 932–951.

WILLIAMS, P. S. (1975). A tympanometry pressure swallow test for assessment of eustachian tube function. *Annals of Otology, Rhinology and Laryngology, 84,* 339–343.

SUGGESTED READINGS

LIPSCOMB, D. M. (1976). Mechanisms of the middle ear. In J. L. Northern (Ed.), *Hearing Disorders* (pp. 78–88). Boston: Little, Brown.

MAUE-DICKSON, W. (1981). The middle ear—prenatal development. In F. N. Martin (Ed.), *Medical Audiology* (pp. 109–122). Englewood Cliffs, NJ: Prentice-Hall.

8

THE INNER EAR

Because of its similarity to an intricately winding cave, the inner ear has been called a **labyrinth**. The inner ear is extremely complicated, with literally thousands of moving parts; it is responsible for sending information to the brain regarding both hearing and balance. Nevertheless, it is so tiny that its size has been compared to that of a small pea.

Because the animal brain cannot make use of sound vibrations in the form described in Chapter 2, the function of the inner ear is to **transduce** the mechanical energy delivered from the middle ear into a form of energy that can be interpreted by the brain. In addition to hearing information, the inner ear also converts information regarding the body's position and movement into a biolectrical code.

CHAPTER OBJECTIVES

This chapter describes the inner ear as a device providing the brain with information regarding sound and the body's position in space. The reader is exposed first to the anatomy and physiology of the inner ear, along with a number of disorders that affect it and their causes. Probable results on the auditory tests, described earlier in this volume, should be understood in terms of inner-ear disorders.

perilymph in:
vestibule   bony labyrinth
scala vestibuli
scala tympani

endolymph in:
membranous
labyrinth
saccule   cochlea
utricle   duct

THE INNER EAR

The oval window beneath the stapedial footplate allows entry from the middle ear into the inner ear. The immediate entryway, called the **vestibule**, is a space through which access may be gained to various chambers of the inner ear, just as a vestibule of a house is a space that may communicate with several different rooms. Rather than being filled with air, as in a room, the vestibule is filled with a fluid called **perilymph**. It is within the vestibular portion of the inner ear that the organs of equilibrium are housed, and even though they are intricately connected both anatomically and physiologically with the organs of hearing, they are considered separately here.

The Vestibular Mechanism

2 canal systems / bony labyrinth – filled w/ perilymph
membranous labyrinth – filled w/ endolymph

A significant part of the balance portion of the inner ear is housed within the vestibule. Within the vestibule are membranous sacs called the **utricle** and **saccule**. Both sacs are surrounded by perilymph and contain another fluid, very similar in constitution, called **endolymph**. The saccule is slightly smaller than the utricle. The end-organ for balance within the utricle (*macula acoustica utriculi*) is located on the bottom and within the saccule (*macula acoustica sacculi*) on the side.

Arising from the utricle are the three **semicircular canals**, which are also membranous, containing endolymph and surrounded, in a larger bony cavern, by perilymph. Each of the canals returns to the utricle through enlarged areas called *ampullae*. Each **ampulla** contains an end-organ (*crista*) for the sense of equilibrium. The semicircular canals are arranged perpendicular to each other so as to cover all dimensions in space. With any angular acceleration, at least one semicircular canal is simulated.

When the head is moved, the fluids within the vestibule tend to lag behind because of their inertia. In this way the fluids are set into motion, which stimulates the vestibular mechanism. It is generally agreed that the utriculo-saccular mechanism is responsible for interpreting linear acceleration. It is through this mechanism that we perceive when an elevator or automobile has begun or stopped. The utricle and saccule are stimulated by the rate of change of linear velocity, which can be measured in centimeters per second squared. The semicircular canals provide for the perception of motion and turning. Therefore, the semicircular canals are the receptors for angular acceleration, or the rate of change of angular velocity. These receptors report, for example, the increase or decrease in the number of revolutions per minute that the body is turning. Thus, angular acceleration can be measured in degrees per second squared.

When the vestibular mechanisms of equilibrium become damaged or diseased, a common symptom results called **vertigo**. Patients with vertigo are truly ill, because they experience the sensation of whirling or spinning. Because of connections in the brain between the vestibular portion of the auditory nerve and the oculomotor nerve, a rapid rocking movement of the eyes, called

in vestibule w/ (filled w/ perilymph)
utricle
saccule
filled w/ endolymph
contains organ of balance

nystagmus, sometimes occurs. Nystagmus always occurs with vertigo whether one can see it or not. Nystagmus may occur spontaneously in cases of vestibular upset. It is important to differentiate true vertigo from dizziness, lightheadedness, or falling tendencies, which do not result in the sensation of true turning.

Tests for Vestibular Abnormality. For some time, attempts to determine the normality of the vestibular system have centered around artificial stimulation. In one test the patient is placed in a chair capable of mechanically controlled rotation. Following a period of rotation, the eyes are examined for nystagmus. The presence, degree, and type of nystagmus are compared to the examiner's concept of "normal."

A considerably easier test to administer in the otologist's office is the **caloric test**. Stimulation of the labyrinth is accomplished by washing 5 to 10 cm³ of cold or warm water against the tympanic membrane. In patients with normal vestibular systems, the result when cold water is used is a nystagmus with rapid movement away from the irrigated ear and slow movement back. When warm water is used, the direction of nystagmus is reversed. Interpretations of responses as normal, hyperactive, or hypoactive are highly subjective and vary considerably among administrators of this test.

A difference in electrical potential exists between the cornea (positive charge) and the retina (negative charge) of the eye. Knowledge of this fact led to the development of a device called the **electronystagmograph (ENG)** to measure the changes in potential produced by nystagmus and to markedly increase the objectivity of caloric testing. Electrodes are placed one each on the bony ridge of the outer canthus of each eye, and a ground electrode is placed on the bony ridge of the outer canthus of each eye, and a ground electrode is placed on the bony ridge of the center of the forehead above the eyes. Using this equipment allows for measurement of the rate and direction of nystagmus, which can be displayed on a paper chart as a permanent recording. Most commercial ENGs heat and cool the water for irrigation to precise temperatures (30° and 44°C) and eject the proper amount (250 milliliters) over a prescribed period of time (40 seconds). All this automaticity has considerable advantage over manual methods of testing, but most important is the fact that a permanent and accurate result is available. A photograph of an electronystagmograph is shown in Figure 8.1. A patient with electrodes placed for ENG seated in a torsion swing chair is shown in Figure 8.2.

Until recently, vestibulography was limited to the vestibulo-ocular reflexes, the connections between the balance and visual systems in the brain. New frontiers exist in pursuit of other central nervous system interactions, including posturography, the assessment of the ability to coordinate movement by measuring vestibulospinal reflexes. Many of the tests now available are directly related to the introduction of computers to the measurement of vestibular function.

The use of microcomputers in vestibulography allows for better quantification of the eyebeats resulting from caloric testing through better control of the stimuli and resolution of the responses. A variety of tests is currently

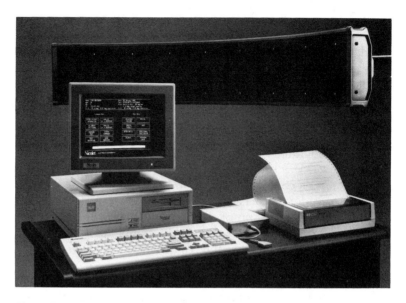

Figure 8.1 A commercial electronystagmograph. (Courtesy of Nicolet Instrument Corporation.)

available, and software to control the hardware is constantly being upgraded. Also significant are the ways in which data can be stored and retrieved without the need for searching, cutting, and pasting long paper readouts. Computers have allowed for the reintroduction of rotary chairs as a means of assessing the functions of the vestibular system, including measurements on children.

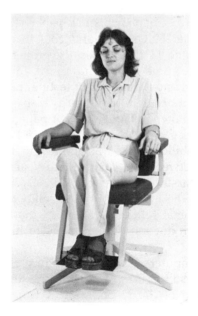

Figure 8.2 Proper placement of electrodes for ENG testing. (Courtesy of Tracoustics.)

Before the advent of computerized vestibulography, ENG testing on infants and small children was difficult, if not impossible. Cyr and Moller (1988) recommend that children be tested for vestibular dysfunction if: (1) they evidence delayed or abnormal motor function, (2) they take ototoxic drugs, (3) they have a spontaneous nystagmus, or (4) there is suspected neurological disease. It would probably be advisable to carry out vestibular testing on children with sensorineural hearing loss whenever possible, because many of them apparently suffer from significant vestibular abnormalities (Brookhouser, Cyr, & Beauchaine, 1982).

Although computerized vestibulography is lending innovative and exciting aspects to diagnosis of disease of the inner ear and central nervous system, it should be regarded as just one of many tools to be used. Vestibular function tests must be considered along with the medical history, medical examination, and audiometric findings.

The Auditory Mechanism

The vestibular portions of the inner ear are shown in Figure 8.3, along with the auditory portions. Notice that the vestibule also looks into a snail-like shell called the **cochlea.** For purposes of clarification, teachers are fond of "unrolling" the cochlea, an act that is graphically advantageous but physically impossible because the cochlea is composed of a twisting bony shell about 1 cm wide and 5 mm from base to apex (in humans). This temptation is yielded to nonetheless, as is shown in Figure 8.4.

Beyond the oval window within the cochlea lies the **scala vestibuli**, so named because of its proximity to the vestibule and its resemblance to a long hall. At the bottom of the cochlea, the **scala tympani** is visible, beginning at the round window. Both of these canals contain perilymph, which is continuous through a small passageway at the apex of the cochlea called the **helicotrema**. In this way, when the oval window moves in, the perilymph flows through the helicotrema and pushes the round window out. In fact, for frequencies above about 60 Hz, there is little fluid movement through the heli-

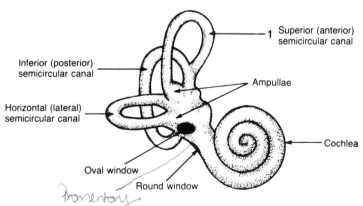

Figure 8.3 Anatomy of the human inner ear.

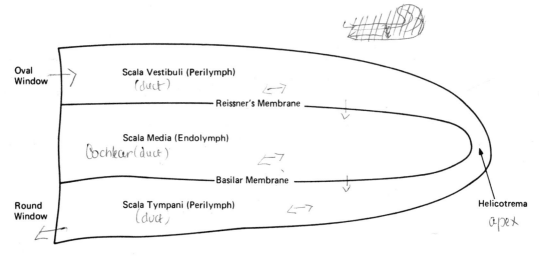

Figure 8.4 Diagram of an "unrolled" cochlea, showing the relationships among the three scalae. *Know these names↑*

cotrema, as energy is transmitted through the fluid levels of the cochlea by means of the membranes.

Between the two canals just described lies the **scala media** or **cochlear duct**. This third canal is filled with endolymph, which is continuous through the **ductus reuniens** with the endolymph contained in the saccule, utricle, and semicircular canals. The scala media is separated from the scala vestibuli by **Reissner's membrane** and from the scala tympani by the **basilar membrane**. When the cochlea, which curls about two and a half turns, is seen from the middle ear, the large turn at the base forms the protrusion into the middle ear called the promontory.

Along the full length of the scala media lies the end-organ of hearing — the **organ of Corti**, so named for the nineteenth-century anatomist who described it. The organ of Corti resides on the basilar membrane, one of the three walls of the scala media. The other two walls are comprised of Reissner's membrane and a bony shelf formed by a portion of the bony labyrinth. From this shelf extends the **spiral ligament**, thought to support the scala media, and also the **stria vascularis**, which produces the endolymph and supplies oxygen and other nutrients to the cochlea. The blood supply and nerve supply enter the organ of Corti by way of the **modiolus**, the central core of the cochlea around which it is wound.

A cross section of the cochlea is shown in Figure 8.5. Much of what is known of the anatomy and physiology of the inner ear has been advanced in recent years with the introduction of electron microscopy.

Basilar Membrane The basilar membrane is about 35 mm long and varies in width from less than 0.1 mm at the basal turn to about 0.5 mm at the apical turn, quite the reverse of the cochlear duct, which is broad at the basal end and narrow at the apex. Situated on the fibrous basilar membrane are three to five parallel rows of 12,000 to 15,000 outer hair cells and one row of 3,000

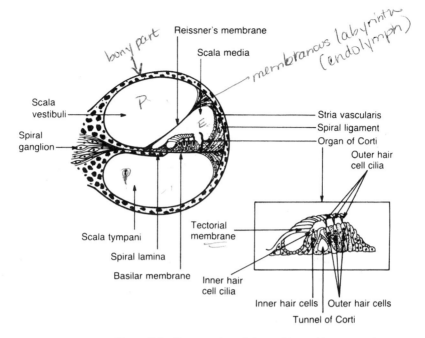

bony part
membranous labyrinth (endolymph)

Figure 8.5 Cross-section of the cochlea. *Know this crap !*

inner hair cells. The outer and inner hair cells are separated from each other by **Corti's arch.** The auditory nerve endings are located on the basilar membrane; these nerve fibers either connect to the hair cells in a one-to-one relationship, or they may make contact with many hair cells. The hair cells themselves are about 0.01 mm long and 0.001 mm in diameter. The direction in which they are bent during stimulation is of great importance. If the cilia bend in one direction, the nerve cells are stimulated; if they bend the other way, the nerve impulses are inhibited; and if they bend to the side, there is no stimulation at all. A flow diagram showing a model of cochlear function is shown in Figure 8.6.

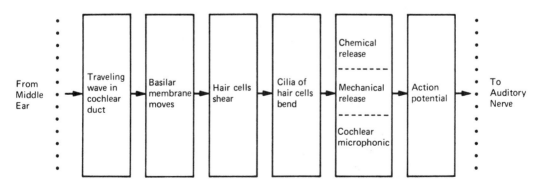

Figure 8.6 The functions of the cochlea.

high frequency at basal end
low   "   apex

Physiology of the Cochlea

When the oval window is moved in by the stapes, the annular ligament around the footplate stretches and displaces the perilymph at the basal end of the cochlea, propagating a wave toward the apex of the cochlea. Because the fluids of the inner ear are noncompressible, when they are displaced inward the round window membrane must yield, moving into the middle ear. It may be said, therefore, that the two windows are out of phase: One moves in when the other moves out. It is obvious that if they were in phase, a great deal of cancellation of sound waves would take place within the cochlea, just the opposite of the desired effect.

Sound vibrations that are introduced to the scala vestibuli are conducted into the cochlear duct by the yielding of Reissner's membrane. The endolymph is thereby disturbed, and so the vibrations continue and the basilar membrane is similarly displaced, resulting in the release of the round window membrane. Therefore, sounds introduced to the inner ear cause a wavelike motion, which always moves from the base of the cochlea to the apex. This is true of either air- or bone-conducted sounds. Given areas along the basilar membrane show greater displacement for some frequencies than for others. Tones of low frequency with longer wavelengths show maximum displacement near the apical end, whereas tones of high frequency with shorter wavelengths show maximum displacement near the basal end.

The basilar membrane reacts more to vibrations of the inner ear than do most of the other structures. Because the organ of Corti resides on this membrane, the vibrations are readily transmitted to it. The **stereocilia** (hairs) on the tips of the outer hair cells are embedded in the **tectorial membrane**, a gelatinous flap which is fixed on its inner edge and, according to some researchers, on its outer edge as well. When the basilar membrane moves up and down in response to fluid displacement caused by the in-and-out movement of the stapes, the hair cells are sheared (twisted) in a complex manner. Part of this shearing is facilitated by the fact that the basilar membrane and the tectorial membrane have slightly different axes of rotation and slide in opposite directions as they are moved up and down. The cilia atop the inner hair cells are not connected to the tectorial membrane, leaving uncertain the precise manner in which they are stimulated. It appears likely that although stimulation of outer hair cells takes place because of the magnitude of basilar membrane *displacement*, stimulation of the inner hair cells is due to the *velocity* of the membrane's movement—that is, the rate at which the membrane's displacements change.

The disturbances of the organ of Corti are very complex, resulting from motion of the basilar membrane in directions up and down, side to side, and lengthwise. The size of electrical response of the cochlea is directly related to the extent to which the hair cells, or the ciliary projections at their tops, are sheared. The source of the electrical charge is derived from within the hair cell. When the hair cell cilia are sheared, a chemical is released at the base of the hair cell.

The Auditory Neuron

The human cochlea contains about 30,000 afferent (sensory) **neurons** and about 1800 efferent neurons. A neuron is a specialized cell designed as a conductor of nerve impulses. It is composed of a **cell body**, an **axon**, and **dendrites** (Figure 8.7). The axon and dendrites are branching systems. The dendrites, which consist of many small branches, receive nerve impulses from other nerve cells. The axon transmits the impulses along the neurons, which vary dramatically in length. The afferent neurons carry impulses from the cochlea to the central auditory nervous system and have their cell bodies in the spiral ganglion in the modiolus. As Figure 8.7 shows, auditory neurons are bipolar, in this case having one axon projecting to the hair cells and the other axon projecting to the sensory cells in the brain stem. The efferent axons project from the superior olivary complex in the brain stem and contact the hair cells both directly and indirectly, as well as in a variety of proportions.

Electrical impulses travel along the entire length of the axon. The stimulus is received by the dendrites, which conduct it to the cell body and then to the axon. The electrical power of the neuron is derived from the axon, which generates its voltage chemically from its surroundings. Connections between neurons are called **synapses**. Since the turn of the century it has been recognized that a nerve fiber, once its threshold has been reached, always responds with its maximum charge regardless of the stimulus intensity. This has been called the all-or-none principle.

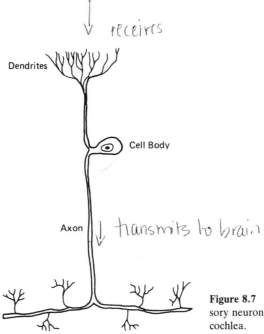

receives

Dendrites

Cell Body

Axon | transmits to brain

Figure 8.7 Diagram of a bipolar sensory neuron, such as are seen in the cochlea.

The Fluids of the Cochlea

Though similar, the constituents of the perilymph and endolymph are different in ways essential to the physiology of hearing. Endolymph is high in its concentration of potassium ions, and low in sodium, whereas the reverse is true of perilymph. Another way in which the two fluids are dissimilar is in their DC potentials (voltages). Endolymph exhibits a strong positive potential, averaging about 80 millivolts (mV), caused by its high potassium concentration with respect to the perilymph of the scala tympani. The perilymph in the scala vestibuli demonstrates a positive, but much smaller, potential of about 3 mV when compared to the perilymph of the scala tympani. The remainder of the cochlear structures exhibit a negative DC potential. All of these potentials fluctuate.

The Cochlear Microphonic

The cochlea is the transducer that converts sound waves into an energy form useful to the auditory nerve. Because of this resemblance to the action of a microphone, which converts the pressure waves issuing from a speaker's mouth into an alternating electrical current, this action has been named the **cochlear microphonic (CM)**. The cochlear microphonic is probably the result of changes in polarization caused by the bending back and forth of the hair cells. For every up-and-down cycle of the basilar membrane, there is one in-and-out cycle of the stereocilia of the outer hair cells, causing them to become alternately depolarized and hyperpolarized. The size of the cochlear microphonic has been measured in experimental animals and in humans by placing pickup electrodes over the round window, and, in some cases, within the cochlea.

air wave → electrical signal

The Action Potential

At the moment that auditory neurons are stimulated by the hair cells that rest on them, a change in the electrical potential occurs on the surface of each neuron. This is called the **action potential (AP)**. Increases in the intensity of the auditory input signal to the cochlea result in increased electrical output from the hair cells. This stimulation causes increased electrical activity in the neuron, although each individual neuron continues to follow the all-or-none rule.

The Efferent System of the Cochlea

We tend to think of all our sensory systems as being entirely **afferent**, carrying messages only from the sense organs, like the ear, to the brain for analysis. It is clear that the cochlea contains an efficient **efferent** system, receiving impulses from the brain. The relationship between afferent and efferent fibers is delicately balanced to provide a feedback or monitoring system for the cochlea.

Theories of Hearing

The precise means by which we hear remains unknown. Most of the theories that attempt to explain how the ear utilizes the mechanical energy delivered to the cochlea from the middle ear are largely theories of how we perceive pitch.

Helmholtz's **resonance theory of hearing** dates back to 1857. Helmholtz believed that the structures within the cochlea consisted of many tiny resonators, each tuned to a specific frequency. He postulated that, when a complex tone is introduced to the cochlea, each resonator responds to the frequency at which it is tuned and that the ear performs a Fourier analysis, breaking the complex sound into its components. It is probable that Helmholtz mistook the transverse fibers of the basilar membrane for these small resonators. He believed that each resonator responded most vigorously to its tuned frequency and with less amplitude to adjacent frequencies. It was Helmholtz who described the placement of the higher frequency fibers at the basal end of the cochlea and the lower frequencies near the apex.

A logical early belief was that every tone that could be heard was assigned to its own specific place within the cochlea, much as the keys of a piano are laid out with specific representation. Therefore, the **place theory of hearing** is largely mechanical in nature; it assumes that there is neural representation for every place on the basilar membrane. Place theories are handy for explaining some hearing phenomena, such as masking and the sharp pitch discriminations the human ear can make. The theory begins to break down in an attempt to explain why pitch discrimination is so poor close to auditory threshold. The place theory, therefore, is unacceptable as a theory of hearing, although its consideration as an incomplete theory of pitch perception may be viable.

Békésy (1960) described what he called the **traveling wave theory**. For each inward and outward movement of the footplate of the stapes, there is a downward and upward movement of the basilar membrane, produced by disturbance of the endolymph. The wave moves down the cochlear duct from base to apex, with the maximum amplitude for high-frequency tones occurring at the basal end and that for the low frequencies at the apical end. Although high frequencies excite only the fibers in the basal turn of the cochlea, the low frequencies excite fibers all along the length of the basilar membrane. The input frequency, then, determines not only the *distance* the traveling wave moves before it peaks, but also the *rate* of basilar membrane vibration. The frequency of basilar membrane vibration is directly related to frequency and inversely related to period.

The place theories attributed analysis of pitch to the cochlea, but the **frequency theories of hearing**, of which there were several, considered that this analysis was accomplished in a retrocochlear area. The frequency theories had in common the belief that the auditory nerve transmits a pattern that corresponds directly with the input signal—that is, if a 100 Hz tone is introduced, the auditory nerve would fire 100 times in a second.

Because the auditory nerve is only capable of firing up to about 400 times per second, the frequency theory leaves without explanation perception of tones above this frequency. It was suggested by Wever (1949) that a series of impulses is sent along the auditory nerve and that the sum of these impulses represents a reproduction of the vibrations of the basilar membrane. Basically, the **volley theory of hearing** suggests that during the refractory (rest) period of one set of neurons, another set is actively firing. Experimental evidence suggests that only frequencies up to 4000 Hz may be accounted for by volley theory alone.

The **resonance-volley theory of hearing** combines the spatial representation suggested by the place theories plus the temporal dimension of the volley theories. In this way, place explains high-frequency perception, and volley explains low-frequency interpretation, with some overlapping no doubt taking place.

The place theories explain loudness in terms of the amplitude of movement of the basilar membrane; that is, a louder sound creates a greater amplitude than a softer sound. This greater amplitude increases the number of impulses transmitted by the nerve fibers. The frequency theories explain loudness in terms of the amount of spread along the basilar membrane. The greater the amplitude of the input signal, the larger the surface area of the basilar membrane stimulated and the greater the number of nerve fibers firing, both at the peak of the traveling wave and on both sides of it. Although intensity coding is extremely complicated and poorly understood, it is generally agreed that as the intensity of a signal is increased, neurons in the brain stem fire at higher rates (Musiek & Baran, 1986), resulting in greater loudness of the signal.

Hypotheses for Hair Cell Transduction

It is still not entirely understood how the mechanical motion of the hair cells (shearing) converts a sound source into a form of energy that can be transmitted by the auditory nerve. The *mechanical hypothesis* assumes that the pressure that moves the hair cells stimulates the nerve endings directly. The *chemical hypothesis* assumes that when the hair cells are deformed, a neurotransmitter substance is released that stimulates the nerve endings. The *electrical hypothesis* assumes that the cochlear potential stimulates the nerve endings.

Cochlear Emission

One of the most remarkable discoveries in recent years with respect to cochlear function was the report by Kemp (1978) that the cochlea, always believed to be a purely passive organ, in fact generates sounds of its own. These acoustic emissions, although observed in previous research, had been ignored and considered to be artifacts of the experiments. What Kemp discovered, through the use of miniature microphones sealed in the external ear canals of human subjects, was a weak acoustical signal emanating from the cochlea about 6 milliseconds after the presentation of a click introduced into the ear. This signal grows in amplitude and then declines, and the entire **evoked otoacoustic emission** disappears within about 60 milliseconds (although the emission may last longer than the stimulus). These so-called Kemp echoes are generally described as being in the frequency range between 500 and 4000 Hz, and when pure tones are used as stimuli, the emissions are close in frequency to the stimulus.

Spontaneous otoacoustic emissions, present in the absence of specific external stimulation, have also been observed in human subjects and, to a lesser extent, in animals. Frick and Matthies (1988) observed spontaneous otoacoustic emissions in 30% of 62 normal ears tested. In some cases these emissions are audible to the subjects themselves at very low sensation levels. The precise source for these emissions is unknown at present and is under study by auditory researchers, but it is generally accepted that the source is within the cochlea. It is thought to be conducted through the intracochlear fluids via the ossicular chain to the tympanic membrane, which acts as a poor loudspeaker in delivering a weak sound to the external auditory canal. It is known that the emissions are present in one or both ears of some humans but not of others, and that they are often absent in people with cochlear hearing losses.

Explanations that the phenomenon of acoustic emission arises from something other than a cochlear event (such as a muscular contraction or a sound generated in the middle ear) have been systematically eliminated. The relationship between these emissions and cochlear tinnitus (ringing noises in the ears) has been studied (e.g., Kemp, 1981), but at present cannot be used to explain loud tinnitus or even the soft tinnitus observed by many subjects.

The excitement generated by the discovery of acoustic emissions promises to provide what may be an entirely new way of understanding how the auditory system functions. To call it a breakthrough is an understatement, for as the understanding of these phenomena unfolds, insights will be gained into both the normal and abnormal processes of hearing. Cochlear emissions are being used today to screen the hearing of newborn babies.

Frequency Analysis in the Cochlea

The frequency response of the nerve cells of the cochlea is laid out in an orderly fashion, with the lowest frequencies to which the ear responds (about 20 Hz) at the apical end near the helicotrema, and the highest frequencies (about 20,000 Hz) at the basal end near the oval window. The spacing between the nerve fibers is not equal all along the basilar membrane. Fibers for the frequencies between 2000 and 20,000 Hz lie from the midpoint of the basilar membrane to the basal end of the cochlea. Fibers for frequencies below 2000 Hz are contained on the other half of the basilar membrane.

Humans are capable of excellent frequency discrimination, apparently due in part to the fact that auditory nerve fibers are sharply tuned to specific frequencies. The frequency that can increase the firing rate of a neuron above its spontaneous firing rate is called its *characteristic frequency* or *best frequency*. Békésy (1960), who was among the first to study the tuning mechanism of the cochlea, observed that the tuning becomes sharper (narrower band width) as frequency is increased (traveling wave peak closer to the basal end of the cochlea), although it is less sharply tuned than the auditory nerve. The slope of the tuning curve is much steeper above the stimulating frequency than below it.

The concept of the **psychophysical tuning curve (PTC)** (e.g., Pick, 1980) has been used to attempt measurements of the cochlea's frequency-resolving abilities. It seems apparent that when the cochlea becomes damaged, its frequency-resolving power may become poorer, but this is not evident in all cases. Preservation of the normal psychophysical tuning curve contributes to the ear's ability to resolve complex auditory signals, such as speech. Conversely, widening of the PTC in damaged ears may help to explain the kinds of speech discrimination difficulties characteristic of patients with cochlear impairment.

Development of the Inner Ear

Differentiation of the inner ear begins during the third week of gestation, and it reaches adult size and configuration by the sixth month. Placodes form early in embryonic life as thickened epidermal plates. The **auditory placode** invaginates to form a pit, which closes off to form a capsule. This capsule divides to form a saccular division, from which the cochlea arises, and a utricular division, which forms the semicircular canals and probably the endolymphatic duct and sac. The vestibular portions of the inner ear develop earlier than the auditory portions. The fact that development takes place so rapidly probably accounts for the observation that interruption of normal development, as by a maternal disease in early pregnancy, can have such dire consequences on the inner ear.

Development of the inner ear springs primarily from entoderm although the membranous labyrinth is ectodermal in origin. The structure forms initially as cartilage and then changes to bone, usually by the 23rd gestational week. The cochlea and vestibule reach full size in their primitive form by the 20th week.

The cochlear turns begin to develop at about the sixth week and are complete by the ninth or tenth week. This is a particularly active time of embryogenesis of the inner ear because the endolymphatic sac and duct and the semicircular canals are also forming, and the utricle and saccule are clearly separated. The utricle, saccule, and endolymphatic duct form from the **otocyst**, the auditory vesicle, or sac, that begins its formation at the end of the first month of gestational age.

By the middle of the eighth week the scalae are forming, and the semicircular canals reach adult configuration, including the ampullae with the cristae forming inside. The maculae are also forming within the utricle and saccule, as are the ducts that connect the saccule with the utricle and cochlear duct.

Between the 10th and 12th weeks the organ of Corti has begun to form. By the 18th week adult configuration of the membranous labyrinth has been reached, and by 25 weeks the inner ear is at full size.

HEARING LOSS AND THE INNER EAR

Because the inner ear contains both sensory cells and nerve cells, **sensorineural hearing loss** is the expected result of abnormality of the cochlea. In such cases air and bone conduction sensitivity should be equally depressed in direct relationship to the severity of the disorder. The reasons that air-conduction and bone-conduction results may not be identical in cases of pure sensorineural hearing loss were discussed in Chapter 3, and some variations should be expected even though the inner ear theoretically contributes the pure distortional mode of bone conduction.

DISORDERS OF THE COCHLEA

Disorders of hearing produced by abnormality or disease of the cochlea probably constitute the largest group of hearing losses called sensorineural.

One fact generally agreed on is that, as damage or abnormality occurs in the cochlea, loss of hearing sensitivity is not the only symptom. Indeed, a common complaint of patients with sensorineural hearing loss is not that they cannot hear but that they have difficulty understanding speech. This speech discrimination problem has been called **dysacusis** to differentiate it from **hypacusis**, which suggests merely a loss of sensitivity to sound. Dysacusis probably results from a combination of frequency and harmonic distortion in the cochlea. As a general rule, patients with greater cochlear hearing losses have more dysacusis.

Many patients with unilateral losses of hearing indicate that a pure tone of a given frequency has a different pitch in each ear. This is often noted during performance of the alternate binaural loudness balance test and is called **diplacusis** binauralis. At times patients perceive that a pure tone lacks the musical quality we associate with it, and that it sounds like a musical chord or a noise instead. One patient described a pure tone as sounding like "bacon frying." Such a lack of perception of tonal quality for a pure tone is called diplacusis monauralis.

CAUSES OF INNER-EAR DISORDERS

Alterations in the structure and function of the cochlea produce more hearing losses than do abnormalities in other areas of the sensorineural auditory system. Hearing losses may result from either endogenous or exogenous causes. For purely arbitrary reasons, this chapter examines cochlear hearing losses as they relate generally to the patient's age at onset.

Prenatal Causes

Prenatal causes are those that have an adverse effect on the normal development of the cochlea.

It is difficult to know, in cases of congenital hearing loss, the extent of genetic versus environmental factors or their possible interrelationships in a given patient. For some time it has been known that some forms of hearing loss tend to "run in families." Some patients are born with the hearing affliction, and others inherit the tendency for abnormalities to occur later in life. This latter form has been called **hereditodegenerative hearing loss**.

Cases of hereditary hearing loss have been documented in patients with no associated abnormalities, as well as in association with external ear, skull, and facial deformities; eye disease; cleft palate; changes in eye, hair, and skin pigmentation; thyroid disease; disorders of the heart; musculoskeletal anomalies; mental retardation; difficulty with balance and coordination; and other sensory and motor deficits. Whenever a group of symptoms is considered together for the diagnosis of a particular disease, such a combination of signs is called a **syndrome**.

A number of different audiometric configurations have been suggested as *typical* of a given cause. There is, however, no unanimity on hereditary hearing loss, and clearly some cases may be moderate to severe bilateral losses with flat audiograms (Figure 8.8) or predominantly high-frequency or low-frequency patterns. Some losses have been described as typically unilateral.

Problems associated with the Rh baby have become fewer in recent years as physicians have learned to predict and prevent the disorders with maternal immunization and infant blood transfusion immediately after birth. The danger presents itself when a fetus whose blood contains the protein molecule called the **Rh factor** is conceived by a mother in whom the factor is absent. The mother's body produces antibodies for protection against the harmful effects of the Rh factor, and this antibody count is increased with succeeding pregnancies. Usually by the third pregnancy a sufficient number of antibodies is present so that the developing red blood cells of the fetus are damaged to the extent that they cannot properly carry oxygen to essential body parts, including the cochlea. In addition, the blood of the newborn child may carry bilirubin (a component of liver bile) in increased concentration such that it may become deposited in the cochlea and produce a sensorineural hearing loss.

In addition to hearing loss, Rh incompatibility can result in a number of abnormalities in the newborn, including cerebral palsy. **Cerebral palsy** may be defined as damage to the brain, usually congenital, which affects the motor and frequently the sensory systems of the body. There are a number of causes of cerebral palsy, including the Rh factor, many of which are associated with sensorineural hearing loss. Athetotic cerebral palsy, or **athetosis**, wherein the patient exhibits an uncontrolled writhing or squirming motion, has long been associated with hearing loss. Until fairly recently it was assumed that because cerebral palsy is the result of brain damage, the hearing loss is also produced by damage within the central auditory nervous system. There is evidence that

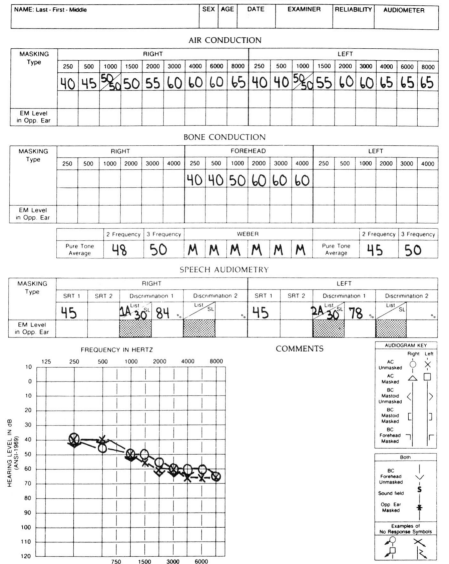

SPEECH AND HEARING CENTER
The University of Texas at Austin 78712
AUDIOMETRIC EXAMINATION

NAME: Last - First - Middle	SEX	AGE	DATE	EXAMINER	RELIABILITY	AUDIOMETER

AIR CONDUCTION

MASKING Type	RIGHT									LEFT								
	250	500	1000	1500	2000	3000	4000	6000	8000	250	500	1000	1500	2000	3000	4000	6000	8000
	40	45	50/50	50	55	60	60	60	65	40	40	50/50	55	60	60	65	65	65
EM Level in Opp. Ear																		

BONE CONDUCTION

MASKING Type	RIGHT						FOREHEAD						LEFT					
	250	500	1000	2000	3000	4000	250	500	1000	2000	3000	4000	250	500	1000	2000	3000	4000
							40	40	50	60	60	60						
EM Level in Opp. Ear																		

	2 Frequency	3 Frequency	WEBER							2 Frequency	3 Frequency
Pure Tone Average	48	50	M	M	M	M	M	Pure Tone Average	45	50

SPEECH AUDIOMETRY

MASKING Type	RIGHT				LEFT			
	SRT 1	SRT 2	Discrimination 1	Discrimination 2	SRT 1	SRT 2	Discrimination 1	Discrimination 2
	45		1A List 30/SL 84 %	List /SL %	45		2A List 30/SL 78 %	List /SL %
EM Level in Opp. Ear								

FREQUENCY IN HERTZ   COMMENTS

Figure 8.8 Audiogram showing a moderate sensorineural hearing loss in both ears. The contour of the audiogram is relatively "flat," which suggests approximately equal hearing loss at all frequencies. This configuration is typical of some congenital losses, plus a number of other causes. The SRT and pure-tone average are in close agreement, and the word discrimination scores show some difficulty in understanding speech. Masking is not required for any of the tests.

in some cases the damage may be cochlear. Because the hearing loss that accompanies athetotic cerebral palsy is often in the high frequencies, it may escape detection for years because of the more dramatic motor symptoms.

In the 1960s, thalidomide, a tranquilizing drug first used in Europe, was introduced to pregnant women. The drug was allegedly free from unwanted side effects, but this lack of side effects was more apparent than real, as evidenced over time by the number of children born with horrible birth deformities to mothers who had taken the drug. The most dramatic symptom was missing or malformed arms and legs; in addition, although it was not generally known, disorders of hearing also afflicted a large number of the thalidomide babies. Because large quantities of drugs, both legal and illegal, are being consumed by women of child-bearing age, it is probable that future research will disclose that many of these also contribute to congenital hearing loss.

Although a pregnant woman must always be fearful of contracting a viral disease, the fear is greatest during the first trimester (three months) of pregnancy, when the cells of the ear and central nervous system are differentiating most rapidly.

Probably the most dreaded viral infection is rubella, or German measles. Rubella is especially fearsome, as it is one of the few viruses that cross the placental barrier. Although this disease is frequently very mild in the patient, in fact sometimes asymptomatic, the effects on the fetus may be devastating. Increased use of the rubella vaccine has cut down to some extent on the incidence of hearing loss from maternal rubella.

Rubella babies tend to be smaller at birth and to develop more slowly than normal infants. They are shorter, weigh less, and have head circumferences that are less than normal. Common results of maternal rubella are brain damage, blindness, heart defects, mental retardation, and sensorineural hearing loss. The rubella hearing-impaired child presents special difficulties in habilitation and education because of the probability of multiple handicaps. The combination of symptoms from maternal rubella has led to the term *maternal rubella syndrome* (Anderson, Barr, & Wedenberg, 1970).

Contrary to popular belief, the danger of damage to the infant from maternal rubella continues past the first trimester of pregnancy. Even though the number of defects and their severity tend to decrease, the virus remains the causative factor in a number of abnormalities, possibly produced by chronic infection after birth (Hardy, McCracken, Gilkerson, & Sever, 1969). Estimates show the likelihood of abnormality of the newborn to be 30% to 100% if infection occurs in the first gestational month, 20% to 50% in the second month, and 13% to 40% in the third month (Borton & Stark, 1970).

Viral infections may actually kill or destroy cells, or they may slow down the rate at which each cell can divide and reproduce by mitosis. The rubella baby has normal-sized cells but fewer of them. It is not always clear whether the virus has affected the fetus by crossing the placental barrier or by contagion during the birth process. As the maternal body temperature increases in response to a viral or other infection, the oxygen requirement of the fetus increases dramatically. Oxygen deprivation is called **anoxia** and may result in damage to the specific and important cells of the cochlea.

Of all the congenital abnormalities produced by maternal rubella in the first trimester of pregnancy, hearing loss is the most common (Karmody, 1969). The main development of the cochlea occurs during the 6th fetal week and of the organ of Corti at the 12th week, making these critically susceptible times.

It is highly likely that the virus enters the inner ear through the stria vascularis, which would explain why the cochlea, rather than the vestibular apparatus, is usually affected. Alford (1968) has suggested that the rubella virus remains in the tissues of the cochlea even after birth. If destruction of cochlear tissue continues, the child may experience a form of progressive hearing loss that might not be associated with a prenatal cause.

In recent years there has been a major focus on the **acquired immune deficiency syndrome (AIDS)** and on the **human immunodeficiency virus (HIV)** found in those with AIDS. Mothers with HIV have a 50% chance of delivering a baby with the disease (Lawrence, 1987). How the HIV affects the cochlea and the incidence with which this occurs are not known. Viral infections in the unborn are far more likely to occur when the mother suffers from a disease causing deficiency in her immune system.

Probably a major cause of prenatal sensorineural hearing loss is **cytomegalovirus (CMV),** a seemingly harmless and often asymptomatic illness, which is a member of the herpes group of viruses. The cause of the problem is an infection called cytomegalic inclusion disease (CID). When the developing fetus is infected, a variety of physical symptoms may be present in addition to hearing loss. About 31% of infants infected with CMV have a serious hearing loss (Johnson, Hosford-Dunn, Paryani, Yeager, & Malachowski, 1986).

Cytomegalovirus may be transmitted from mother to child in several ways:

1. It may be transmitted by means of the placenta (prenatally) to the developing fetus.
2. The infant may contract the virus from the cervix of an infected mother during the birth process (perinatally).
3. The virus may be transmitted in infected mother's milk (postnatally).

When CMV is acquired perinatally or postnatally, there are usually no serious side effects in the child. Unlike rubella, CMV does not warn an expectant mother with a telltale rash or other symptoms. Another difference is that at present there is no vaccine to prevent CMV.

Perinatal Causes

Perinatal causes of hearing loss are those that occur during the process of birth itself. Such causes frequently produce multiple handicaps.

A common cause of damage both to the cochlea and to the central nervous system is **anoxia**, deprivation of oxygen to important cells, which alters their metabolism and results in damage or destruction. In the newborn, anoxia may result from prolapse of the umbilical cord, which cuts off the blood supply to the head, from premature separation of the placenta, or from a wide variety of other factors.

Accumulations of toxic substances in the mother's bloodstream may reduce the passage of oxygen across the placenta, which also results in anoxia. The fetus may also suffer from damage produced by the toxic substances themselves. For this reason, pregnant women should cautiously avoid exposure to contagious diseases, such as hepatitis.

Prematurity is determined by the weight of the child at the time of birth and not necessarily by the length of the pregnancy, as the word itself suggests. When infants weigh less than 5 pounds at birth, they are considered premature. Prematurity is often associated with multiple births, and both are associated with sensorineural hearing loss.

It is common practice to place premature infants in incubators so that, at least for the early days of life, their environments can be carefully controlled. Care must be taken not to overadminister oxygen because this produces retinal defects. Some motors operating incubators were found to be producing extremely high noise levels (up to 95 dB SPL). Hearing losses in children thus treated may have been produced by noise rather than, or in addition to, the results and causes of prematurity.

Trauma to the fetal head either by violent uterine contractions or by the use of so-called high forceps during delivery may also result in damage to the brain and to the cochlea. It is possible that the head trauma itself does not produce the damage; instead, the initial cause of the difficulty in delivery may be the cause of the hearing loss.

Postnatal Causes

Postnatal causes of cochlear hearing loss are any factors occurring after birth.

An often-named cause of cochlear hearing loss is otitis media. The toxins from the bacteria in the middle ear may enter the inner ear by way of the round or oval window, or pus may enter the labyrinth from the middle ear or from the meninges, the protective covers of the brain and spinal cord. **Meningitis**, inflammation of the meninges, may cause total deafness, for if the labyrinth fills with pus, as healing takes place the membranes and other loosely attached structures of the labyrinth are replaced by bone. If the enzymes produced by the infectious process enter the cochlea by diffusion through the round window, a hearing loss may surely result. Often, patients with primarily conductive hearing losses produced by otitis media begin to show additional cochlear degeneration, resulting in **mixed hearing loss** (see Figure 8.9).

Some viral infections have definitely been identified as the causative factors in cochlear hearing loss. These infections include measles, mumps, chicken pox, influenza, and viral pneumonia, among others. The two most common hearing-loss-producing viruses are measles and mumps. Rubeola, the 10-day variety of measles, carries a significantly greater threat to the patient than does

SPEECH AND HEARING CENTER
The University of Texas at Austin 78712
AUDIOMETRIC EXAMINATION

NAME: Last - First - Middle	SEX	AGE	DATE	EXAMINER	RELIABILITY	AUDIOMETER

AIR CONDUCTION

MASKING Type	RIGHT									LEFT								
	250	500	1000	1500	2000	3000	4000	6000	8000	250	500	1000	1500	2000	3000	4000	6000	8000
NB	60	65	70/70	70	75	80	80	85	85	55	55	60/60	60	60	70	75	75	70
	60*									55*								
EM Level in Opp. Ear	55									60								

BONE CONDUCTION

MASKING Type	RIGHT						FOREHEAD						LEFT					
	250	500	1000	2000	3000	4000	250	500	1000	2000	3000	4000	250	500	1000	2000	3000	4000
NB	15*	25*	35*	50*	55*	55*	15	25	35	50	55	55	20*	35*	45*	50*	55*	55*
EM Level in Opp. Ear	55	55	60	60	70	75							75	85	90	75	80	80

	2 Frequency	3 Frequency	WEBER		2 Frequency	3 Frequency
Pure Tone Average	68	70		Pure Tone Average	57	58

SPEECH AUDIOMETRY

MASKING Type	RIGHT						LEFT					
	SRT 1	SRT 2	Discrimination 1		Discrimination 2		SRT 1	SRT 2	Discrimination 1		Discrimination 2	
WB	70	70*	List 1A SL 30	80*%	List SL	%	60	60*	List 2A SL 30	76*%	List SL	%
EM Level in Opp. Ear		60		90				70		90		

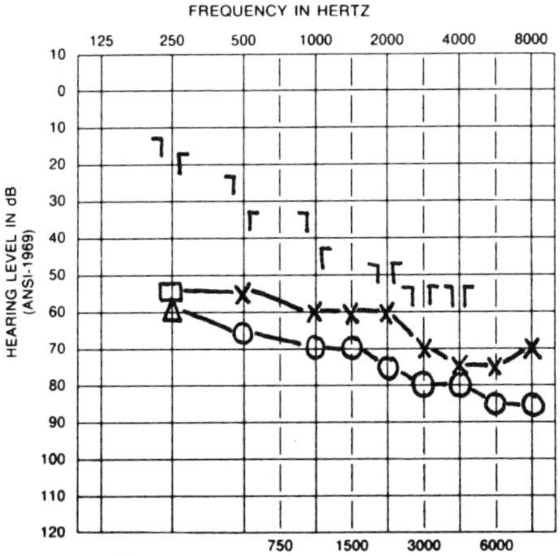

COMMENTS

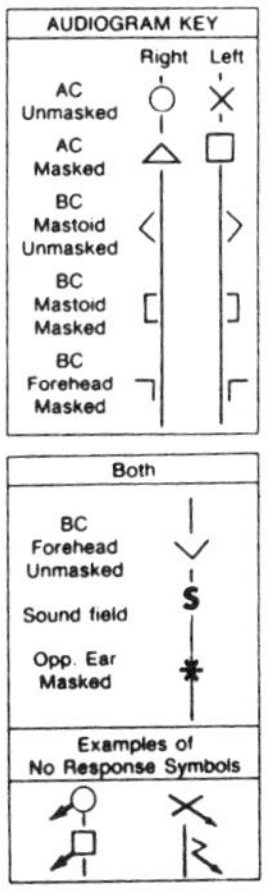

Figure 8.9 Audiogram showing a mixed hearing loss in both ears. Repeating bone conduction with masking was indicated because of the air–bone gaps. The sensorineural component of the loss is reflected by the impaired speech discrimination.

rubella. Measles may cause a sudden hearing loss that may not begin until some time after the other symptoms disappear.

Most virus-produced hearing losses are bilateral, but some viral infections, notably mumps, are associated with unilateral losses as well. Everberg (1957) estimates an incidence of hearing loss from mumps at 0.05 per 1000 in the general population.   Although the precise mechanism producing hearing loss from mumps is not clear, it seems likely that the probable route of infection is the bloodstream.   Other theories, such as general infection of the labyrinth, would not explain why vestibular symptoms are frequently absent.

A disease once thought to be on the decrease, but now recognized as quite the opposite, is syphilis.   This disease may be prenatal or acquired, and often goes through three distinct but overlapping stages.   Because its symptoms may resemble those of a number of different systemic diseases, it has been called the great imitator.   Brain damage is a frequent sequela of syphilis, but the cochlea may also be involved.   A number of bizarre audiometric patterns have been associated with syphilis, and the variations are so great that a typical pattern does not emerge.

Infections of the labyrinth are called **labyrinthitis** and may affect both the auditory and vestibular mechanisms, producing symptoms of hearing loss and vertigo.   The causes of labyrinthitis are not always known, and the condition is frequently confused with other causes of hearing loss; however, tuberculosis, syphilis, cholesteatoma, or viral infection may be the cause.

The body's natural response to infection is elevation of temperature.   When the fevers become excessive, however, cells, including those of the cochlea, may become damaged.   Sometimes children run high fevers with no apparent cause, but with ensuing hearing loss.   When such histories are clear-cut, it is tempting to blame the fever even when it would be logical to suspect the initial cause of the fever, such as a viral infection, as the real cause.   In many cases, diagnosis of the primary cause of a hearing loss is mere speculation.

A number of illnesses have been associated with cochlear hearing loss.   Chief among them are infections of the kidneys, which result in the deposit of toxic substances in the inner ear.   Kidney disease keeps medications from being excreted, thereby raising their levels in the blood abnormally high and introducing ototoxicity.   Other illnesses, including diabetes, have also been directly linked to cochlear damage.

Toxic Causes of Cochlear Hearing Loss

It has been said that progress has its side effects.   This is notably true of the side effects of antibiotics, the wonder drugs that have saved many lives in the last five decades.   Most noted among the drugs that are cochleotoxic (i.e., cause hearing loss) are dihydrostreptomycin, viomycin, neomycin, and kanamycin.   Because hearing losses ranging from mild to profound may result from the use of these drugs, it is hoped that they will not be prescribed unless it is fairly certain that other drugs, with fewer or less severe side effects, will not be just as efficacious.   Vestibulotoxic drugs (those that are known to affect the vestibular organs) include streptomycin and gentamycin.

In situations where the prolonged use of **ototoxic** drugs is mandatory, such as in tuberculosis sanitaria, the patient's hearing should be monitored frequently so that any loss of hearing or its progression may be noted.   In such cases, decisions regarding continued use of the medication must be made on the basis of the specific needs of the patient. Although the final decision on drug use is always made by a physician, it is within the purview of audiologists to make their concerns over hearing loss known.

Quinine is a drug that has long been used to combat malaria and to fight fever and reduce the pain of the common cold. Many patients who have taken this drug have complained of annoying tinnitus and hearing loss. Quinine is still prescribed for certain disorders, but far less than in past years.

Other drugs that have been associated with hearing loss include aspirin, certain diuretics, nicotine, and alcohol. It is usually expected that these drugs will not affect hearing unless they are taken in large amounts and over prolonged periods of time. Certainly there are many individuals who appear to consume these substances in what might be considered excess with no side effects. The individual's own constitutional predispositions must surely be a factor here, as in many disorders.

Otosclerosis

As mentioned in Chapter 7, otosclerosis is a disease of the bony labyrinth that manifests as a conductive hearing loss when the new bone growth affects either the oval window or the round window. If the otosclerosis involves the cochlea, sensorineural hearing loss results and may be either bilateral or unilateral. Although there are no binding rules, the audiometric configuration is generally flat, and speech discrimination is not severely affected. Attempts have been made to arrest the progression of cochlear otosclerosis with the use of sodium fluoride, but the effectiveness of this treatment has not been proved.

Barotrauma

Barotrauma was mentioned as a cause of conductive hearing loss. In addition, sudden changes in middle-ear pressure, as from diving, flying, or even violent sneezing, may cause a rupture in the round window or a tearing of the annulus of the oval window. The resulting fistula (perilymph leak) can often be surgically repaired and may reverse a cochlear hearing loss and/or vertigo. Barotrauma may produce a mild to profound hearing loss.

Noise-Induced Hearing Loss

The Industrial Revolution's introduction of high levels of noise brought a greater threat to the human auditory system than evolution had prepared for. Documented cases of noise-induced hearing loss go back two hundred years. Hearing losses from intense noise may be associated with brief exposure to high-level sounds, with subsequent partial or complete hearing recovery, or with repeated exposure to high-level sounds, with permanent impairment. Cases in which hearing thresholds improve after an initial impairment following noise are said to be the result of **temporary threshold shift (TTS)**; irreversible losses are called **permanent threshold shift (PTS)**. A number of agents may interact with noise to increase the danger to hearing sensitivity. Research has shown that aspirin, which has been known to produce reversible hearing loss after ingestion, synergizes with noise to produce a greater temporary threshold shift than would otherwise be observed (McFadden & Plattsmier, 1983). Although the effects of aspirin on permanent hearing loss have not been demonstrated, it certainly seems prudent for audiologists to advise that people who must be exposed to high levels of noise should refrain from taking this drug, at least at times closely related to exposure.

Although controversy continues over many aspects of noise-induced hearing loss, certain facts are generally agreed on. Men appear to have a higher incidence of hearing loss from noise than do women (Ewertson, 1973; Surjan, Devald, & Palfavi, 1973), perhaps because as a group they have greater noise exposure, both on the job and during leisure activities. Post-mortem electron microscope studies have shown loss of hair cells and their supporting structures in the basal end of the cochlea, and nerve degeneration in the osseous lamina (Johnson & Hawkins, 1976). The hearing loss may be due to biological changes in the sensory cells, physical dislodging of hair cells during hyperacoustic stimulation, changes in the cochlear blood supply with consequent alterations in the function of the stria vascularis, loss of the outer hair cells, rupture of Reissner's membrane, detachment of the organ of Corti from the basilar membrane, or a variety of other causes.

Acoustic trauma is the term often used to describe noise-induced hearing loss from impulsive sounds, such as explosions. A typical audiometric configuration has emerged, shown in Figure 8.10, depicting the so-called **acoustic trauma notch**. Characteristically, the hearing is poorest in the range between 3000 and 6000 Hz, with recovery at 8000 Hz, suggesting damage to the portion of the basal turn of the cochlea related to that frequency range (Igarashi, Schuknecht, & Myers, 1964). As a rule, the amounts of hearing loss are similar in both ears when individuals acquire noise-induced hearing losses in the workplace. Rifle shooters generally show more hearing loss in the ear opposite the shoulder to which the rifle stock is held; that is, right-handed shooters will have more hearing loss in the left ear. A survey in Canada on noise-induced hearing loss in truck drivers revealed greater loss in the left ear, probably produced by the rush of air past the open window on the driver's side (Dufresne, Alleyne, & Reesal, 1988).

The audiometric pattern shown in Figure 8.10 is not found in all cases of acoustic trauma, nor is it restricted to this cause. It is, however, strongly suggestive of noise and should be corroborated with supporting evidence, such as the clinical history. If noise-induced hearing loss is suspected, hearing should always be tested at 3000 and 6000 Hz, even if sensitivity at adjacent octave and midoctave frequencies is normal.

Industrial noise is a factor long recognized as a cause of hearing loss. The term *boilermaker's disease* was coined many years ago to describe the hearing losses sustained by men working in the noisy environs of that industry. Although boilermakers may be fewer in number today, modern technology has produced new and even noisier industries. Exposure to such devices as jet

SPEECH AND HEARING CENTER
The University of Texas at Austin 78712
AUDIOMETRIC EXAMINATION

NAME: Last - First - Middle	SEX	AGE	DATE	EXAMINER	RELIABILITY	AUDIOMETER

AIR CONDUCTION

MASKING Type	RIGHT									LEFT								
	250	500	1000	1500	2000	3000	4000	6000	8000	250	500	1000	1500	2000	3000	4000	6000	8000
	5	0	5/5	5	10	25	60	35	20	0	0	5/5	10	20	40	70	55	25
EM Level in Opp. Ear																		

BONE CONDUCTION

MASKING Type	RIGHT						FOREHEAD						LEFT					
	250	500	1000	2000	3000	4000	250	500	1000	2000	3000	4000	250	500	1000	2000	3000	4000
							0	5	5	15	35	65						
EM Level in Opp. Ear																		

	2 Frequency	3 Frequency	WEBER		2 Frequency	3 Frequency
Pure Tone Average	3	5		Pure Tone Average	3	8

SPEECH AUDIOMETRY

MASKING Type	RIGHT				LEFT			
	SRT 1	SRT 2	Discrimination 1	Discrimination 2	SRT 1	SRT 2	Discrimination 1	Discrimination 2
	5		List 4C / SL 30 — 96 %	List / SL — %	5		List 5C / SL 30 — 94 %	List / SL — %
EM Level in Opp. Ear								

FREQUENCY IN HERTZ

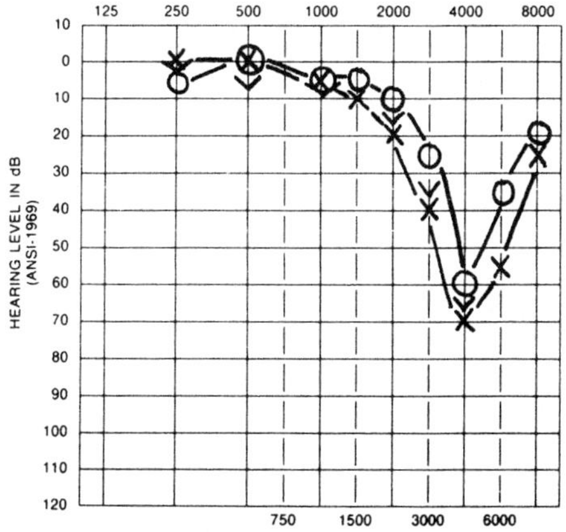

COMMENTS

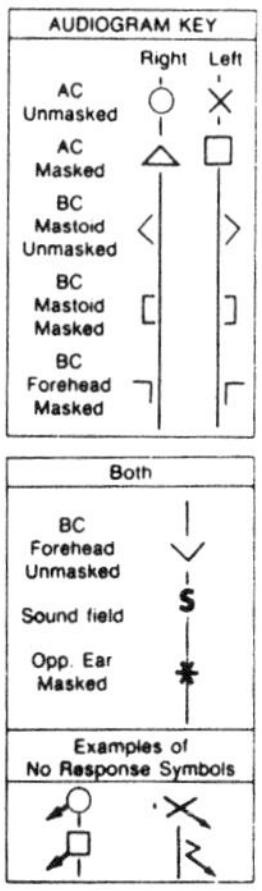

Figure 8.10 Audiogram showing a typical acoustic trauma notch at 4000 Hz. SRTs and SDSs are normal because the hearing loss is primarily above the critical frequency range for hearing and understanding speech.

engines, drop forges, pneumatic hammers, subways, rock music, and even computers has been documented as causing hearing loss. A study of the effects of noise on hearing (Rosen, Bergman, Plester, El-Mofty, & Hammed, 1962) has shown that older populations in societies that have lower noise exposure levels exhibit better hearing sensitivity than do those populations in other societies. Of course, differences in diet, lifestyle, and so on, that exist in different cultures may also account for the improved hearing sensitivity of the older members of more primitive societies.

Noise in society is an ever-increasing problem. Millions of dollars are paid monthly to military veterans in compensation for hearing loss. Insurance companies whose coverage includes noisy industries have been forced to become increasingly concerned with the effects of noise on hearing. Aside from the psychological, social, and vocational handicaps imposed on patients with noise-induced hearing loss, the financial figures have led to concern on the part of government and industry alike.

After a number of proposals, lawsuits, and reversals, the Occupational Safety and Health Administration (OSHA) (1983) has recommended a scale on which the time that a worker may be safely exposed to intense sounds is decreased as the intensity of the noise is increased. Under this rule, the maximum exposure level is 85 dBA for an eight-hour work day. For every 5 dB increase in noise, half the time is allowed—for example, four hours for 90 dBA, two hours for 95 dBA, one hour for 100 dBA, 30 minutes for 105 dBA, and so on.

Sound-level meters or individually worn noise dosimeters are used to measure the intensity of sound in noisy areas, such as in factories and around jet aircraft. Such measurements are made to determine whether the noise levels fall within or exceed the **damage-risk criteria** set up by OSHA. Workers

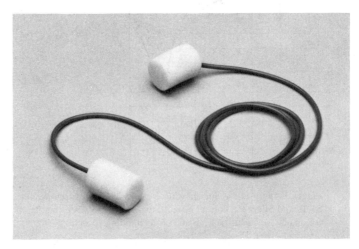

Figure 8.11 Commercial ear plugs designed to attenuate high noise levels. (Courtesy of E.A.R. Division of Cabot Corp.)

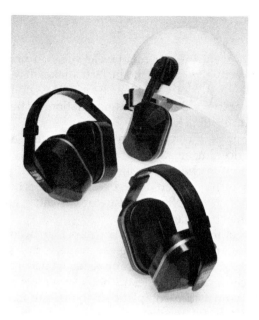

Figure 8.12 Commercial ear muffs designed for use in areas of intense noise. (Courtesy of E.A.R. Division of Cabot Corp.)

are being advised about the dangers of noise and are being encouraged to wear ear protectors, such as those shown in Figures 8.11 and 8.12. Earplugs are an interim measure. The law requires noise reduction where feasible. Preemployment physicals in some areas now include pure-tone audiometry, and in some cases periodic hearing examinations are required for noise-exposed workers. Important inroads are being made in the area of noise pollution.

A patient with apparent noise-induced hearing loss should be advised to limit exposure to loud noise and to use protective earplugs or muffs whenever exposure is necessary. Periodic hearing examinations to monitor progression should also be encouraged. Hunters, target shooters, and snowmobile drivers are often a particularly difficult group to work with because of their reluctance either to wear hearing protectors or to limit their sport. Music enthusiasts who use stereo headphones or portable stereo systems are often at risk for hearing loss because of the high levels of sound delivered directly to their ears.

Often, initial examination of hearing is made on the basis of a complaint of tinnitus alone. In patients with an acoustic trauma notch, the tinnitus is often described as a pure tone and can be matched to frequencies in the 3000 to 6000 Hz range. Many such patients are unaware of the existence of hearing loss at all and may even deny it. By the time progression of the hearing impairment has been demonstrated to patients, their communicative difficulties have often worsened considerably. The persuasiveness and tact of the audiologist in counseling such patients is of paramount importance.

There is increasing evidence that, in addition to hearing loss, noise has other adverse effects upon us. It may play a role in increased anxiety levels, loss of the ability to concentrate, and loss of sleep.

Surgical Complications

There are times when even the best middle-ear surgeon not only fails to improve hearing with corrective surgery but, in fact, makes it worse. Many otologists estimate that the chance of a cochlear hearing loss following stapedectomy is probable in 1% or 2% of the operated population. The odds appear very good except for the unfortunate few.

Postoperative infections as a complication are rare today, although they may occur. An early practice during stapedectomy was to move the ossicular chain following stapedectomy to check for a light reflex on the round window to ensure mobility. This is no longer done because it has been found to generate traveling waves of an amplitude greater than most environmental sounds and can cause cochlear damage.

Excessive bleeding or other surgical complications may account for some cases of cochlear hearing loss following middle-ear surgery, but some cases of even total hearing loss in the operated ear cannot be related to any specific cause. In one case a piece of a metal fenestra hook broke off and remained in the vestibule of a man who had a complete air–bone gap closure postoperatively and otherwise successful results. A number of technically perfect operations are also followed by total deafness of the operated ear. Evidently, for specific physiological reasons, some patients do not tolerate the surgery well. It is to this group that the term *fragile ears* has been assigned, and it is unfortunate that these cases cannot be predicted preoperatively. Common complications of middle-ear surgery include transitory vertigo and alterations in the sense of taste.

Vasospasm of the Internal Auditory Artery

The nutrition of the cochlea is supplied by the stria vascularis, which is fed by the internal auditory artery with no collateral blood supply. If a spasm occurs in that artery, total unilateral deafness may result. For this reason, sudden loss of hearing in one ear should be treated as a medical emergency, with therapy directed at vasodilation. Naturally, the sooner therapy is instituted following onset of symptoms, the better is the prognosis for complete recovery. Such treatment of **vasospasm** often includes hospitalization, with intravenous administration of the appropriate medications. Often hearing recovery is complete. Vestibular symptoms, such as vertigo and nausea as well as the often-accompanying tinnitus, may also abate. In some patients symptoms disappear spontaneously, whereas in others symptoms persist in the form of severe or total unilateral hearing loss.

Ménière's Disease

Another cause of sudden unilateral hearing loss is **Ménière's disease**, named for the nineteenth-century French physician who described it. The seat of the difficulty lies within the labyrinth. The disorder is characterized by sudden attacks of vertigo, tinnitus, vomiting, and unilateral hearing loss. Bilateral Ménière's disease has been observed in 5% to 10% of the cases of aural vertigo studied.

The onset of symptoms is described by many patients in the same way. The difficulty may begin with a sensation of fullness in one ear, followed by a low-frequency roaring tinnitus, hearing loss with great difficulty in speech discrimination, the sensation of violent turning or whirling in space, and vomiting.

Many authorities believe that Ménière's disease is caused by endolymphatic hydrops, the oversecretion or underabsorption of endolymph. As the fluid pressure builds in the cochlear duct, the pressure on the hair cells produces the tinnitus and hearing loss. If the pressure builds sufficiently, the vestibular apparatus becomes overstimulated and vertigo ensues. One excellent procedure for diagnosing Ménière's disease is the **glycerol test**. Pure-tone thresholds and speech discrimination scores are measured, after which the patient is asked to drink six ounces of a mixture of 50% glucose and water. These audiometric procedures are repeated after a three-hour wait. Because glycerol acts as a diuretic, increasing urinary output, the fluid pressure in the labyrinth is expected to drop temporarily, resulting in improved pure-tone thresholds of at least 10 dB at three frequencies in the 250 to 4000 Hz range, and an improvement of at least 12% in speech discrimination scores (Klockhoff, 1976).

According to Lawrence (1969) excessive endolymphatic pressure alone could not alter the function of the inner ear unless the metabolic or ionic balances were disturbed, as by a rupture of Reissner's membrane. Treatment is usually designed to limit fluid retention through the use of diuretic drugs and the decrease of sodium intake in the diet. Sedatives, tranquilizers, and vestibular suppressants have all been used. Reports on the success rates of different therapies vary in the medical literature; some have even been ascribed as placebo effects. Anxiety and allergic factors have been considered as causes of Ménière's disease, which affects more men than women and rarely affects children. Other causes may be trauma, surgery, syphilis, hypothyroidism, and low blood sugar.

Ménière's disease may be extremely handicapping. The paroxysmal attacks of vertigo may interfere with driving an automobile or even with performing one's job. Cases of bilateral hearing loss due to Ménière's disease rarely respond well to amplification from hearing aids. The disease has been called the "labyrinthine storm" because of the sudden and dramatic appearance of symptoms; it is characterized by remissions and exacerbations.

Surgical approaches to Ménière's disease are often aimed at decompressing the endolymphatic sac or draining the excessive endolymph by inserting a shunt into spaces in the skull so that the fluid can be excreted along with cerebrospinal fluid. Ultrasonic and freezing procedures have also been used. In extreme cases, the entire labyrinth has been surgically destroyed or the auditory nerve cut to alleviate the vertigo and tinnitus. Even such dramatic steps as these are not always entirely successful. Audiometric findings in Ménière's disease are shown in Figures 8.13 through 8.17.

NAME: Last - First - Middle	SEX	AGE	DATE	EXAMINER	RELIABILITY	AUDIOMETER

AIR CONDUCTION

MASKING Type	RIGHT									LEFT								
	250	500	1000	1500	2000	3000	4000	6000	8000	250	500	1000	1500	2000	3000	4000	6000	8000
NB	45	50	45/45	50	55	55	60	65	60	10	5	5/5	5	0	5	10	10	5
	45*	50*	45*	50*	55*	55*	60*	65*	60*									
EM Level in Opp. Ear	30	25	20	20	20	20	25	25	25									

BONE CONDUCTION

MASKING Type	RIGHT						FOREHEAD						LEFT					
	250	500	1000	2000	3000	4000	250	500	1000	2000	3000	4000	250	500	1000	2000	3000	4000
NB	5	10	0	0	5	15							10	5	0	0	5	10
	45*	45*	45*	55*	55*	60*												
EM Level in Opp. Ear	55	40	30	15	20	25												

	2 Frequency	3 Frequency	WEBER							2 Frequency	3 Frequency
Pure Tone Average	47	50	L	L	L	L	L	L	Pure Tone Average	2	3

SPEECH AUDIOMETRY

MASKING Type	RIGHT				LEFT			
	SRT 1	SRT 2	Discrimination 1	Discrimination 2	SRT 1	SRT 2	Discrimination 1	Discrimination 2
WB	50	50*	1A List/30 SL 70*	List/SL %	5		2A List/30 SL 100%	List/SL %
EM Level in Opp. Ear		5	35					

FREQUENCY IN HERTZ

COMMENTS

AUDIOGRAM KEY

	Right	Left
AC Unmasked	O	X
AC Masked	△	□
BC Mastoid Unmasked	<	>
BC Mastoid Masked	[	]
BC Forehead Masked	⌐	⌐

Both
BC Forehead Unmasked
Sound field   S
Opp. Ear Masked   *
Examples of No Response Symbols

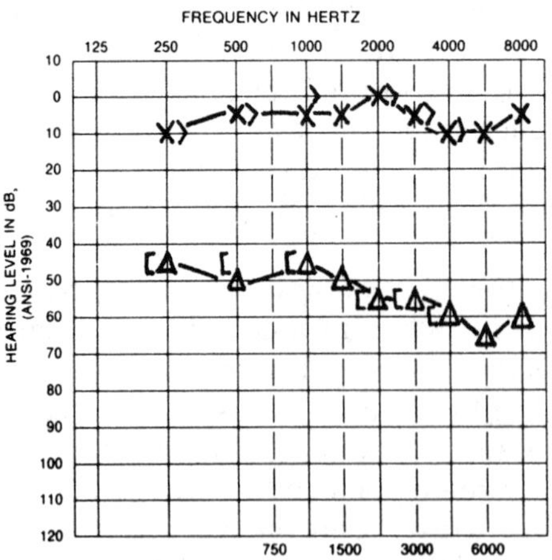

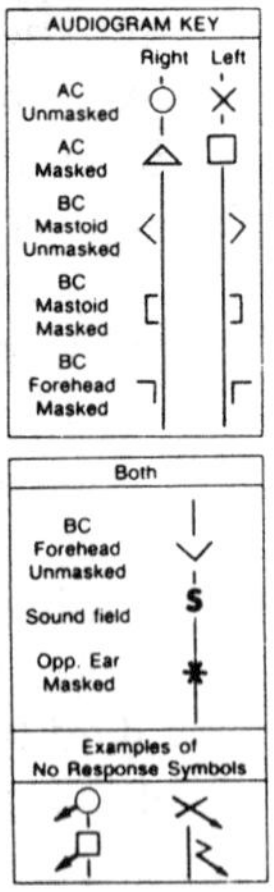

Figure 8.13 Audiogram showing a unilateral (right) sensorineural hearing loss observed in a patient with Ménière's disease. Speech discrimination is impaired in the right ear. This case points up the great need for proper masking on all tests.

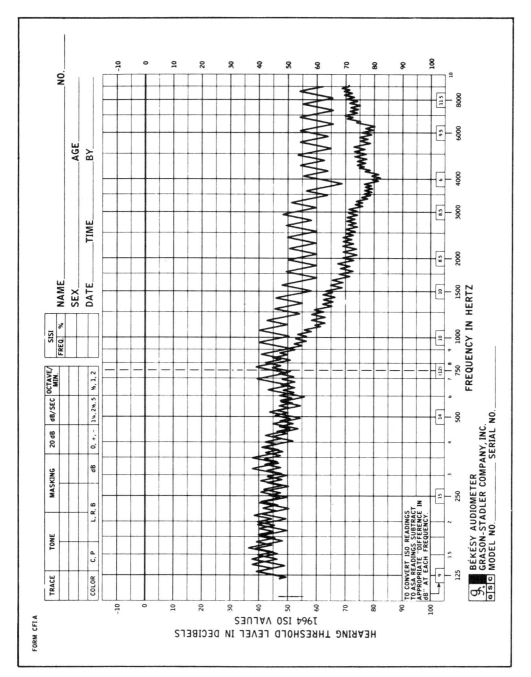

Figure 8.14 Békésy tracing obtained from the right ear of the patient described in Figure 8.13. Note the extremely narrow swing excursions for the continuous traces, even in the low frequencies.

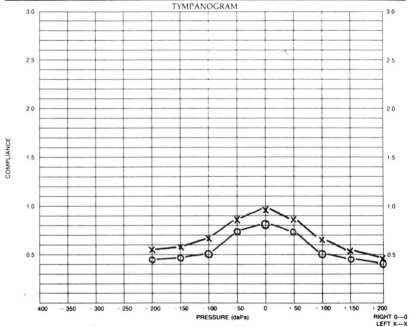

SPEECH AND HEARING CENTER
The University of Texas at Austin 78712

IMMITTANCE

NAME: Last - First - Middle		SEX	AGE	DATE	EXAMINER	INSTRUMENT

PRESSURE/COMPLIANCE FUNCTION

	− 400	− 350	− 300	− 250	− 200	− 150	− 100	− 50	0	+ 50	+ 100	+ 150	+ 200
Right					.44	.48	.50	.72	.80	.71	.50	.44	.40
Left					.55	.59	.68	.87	.96	.86	.64	.52	.45

STATIC COMPLIANCE
$C_x = C_2 - C_1$

RIGHT						LEFT					
.40	C_1	.80	C_2	.40	C_x	.45	C_1	.96	C_2	.51	C_x

ACOUSTIC REFLEXES

	RIGHT				LEFT			
Frequency (Hz)	500	1000	2000	4000	500	1000	2000	4000
Ipsilateral (Probe same)		90	90			95	100	
Contralateral (Probe opposite)	95	90	100	100	85	85	90	95
Audiometric Threshold	50	45	55	60	5	5	0	10
Reflex SL	45	45	45	40	80	80	90	85
Decay Time (Seconds)	10⁺	10⁺			10⁺	10⁺		

Figure 8.15 Results on immittance measures for the patient with Ménière's disease illustrated in Figure 8.13. The tympanogram in the left ear is normal but shows a lower point of maximum compliance on the right ear due to increased pressure in the inner ear. Static compliance is lower in the right ear than in the left. The sensation level of the acoustic reflex is reduced in the right ear, suggesting a lesion of the cochlea.

Presbycusis

The case load of any audiology clinic will evidence the large number of patients who have no contributing etiological factors to hearing loss except advancing age. It would be inaccurate to assume that lesions in **presbycusis** (hearing loss due to aging) are restricted to the cochlea, regardless of the relationship to noise exposure mentioned earlier. The aging process undoubtedly produces alterations in many areas of the auditory system, including the tympanic membrane, ossicular chain, cochlear windows, and central auditory nervous system. There is probably some relationship to general oxygen deficiency due to arteriosclerosis. A definition of the age at which presbycusis begins is lacking in the literature, but it should be expected in men by the early sixties and women by the late sixties, all other factors being equal. It is possible that the hearing mechanism begins to deteriorate slowly at birth.

A common characteristic of presbycusis is significant difficulty in speech discrimination, which Gaeth (1948) has called **phonemic regression**. Many older people report that they often understand speech better when people speak slowly than when they speak loudly. A number of "typical" presbycusic audiometric contours have been suggested.

The classical work on presbycusis is by Schuknecht (1974), who defined four different, but overlapping, causes of this hearing loss:

1. *Sensory presbycusis.* This sensory loss is produced by a loss of outer hair cells and supporting cells in the basal turn of the cochlea. The audiogram shows a greater hearing loss in the higher frequencies.
2. *Neural presbycusis.* Loss of neurons in the cochlea causes poor speech discrimination. The audiogram may be generally flat or slightly poorer in the higher frequencies.
3. *Strial presbycusis.* Atrophy of the stria vascularis in the middle and apical turns of the cochlea produces a fairly flat audiogram. Speech discrimination is reasonably good.
4. *Cochlear conductive presbycusis.* Impaired mobility of the cochlear partitions produces a sensorineural hearing loss which is primarily mechanical in nature.

Head Trauma

In cases in which a hearing loss may be directly related to injury to the head, the audiogram is frequently similar to that for acoustic trauma. Proctor, Gurdjian, and Webster (1956) have shown that, in addition to damage to the tympanic membrane and middle-ear mechanism, the structures of the inner ear may be torn, stretched, or deteriorated from the loss of oxygen following hemorrhage. If a fracture line runs through the cochlea, the resulting hearing loss will be severe to profound. External and/or internal hair cells may be lost, and the organ of Corti may be flattened or destroyed. Trauma to the skull may also result in complications, such as otitis media or meningitis, which may

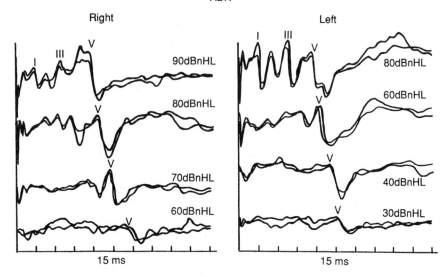

Figure 8.16 Results of auditory brain stem response testing on the patient with a cochlear hearing loss (Ménière's disease) in the right ear (see Figure 8.13). Absolute latencies are shown in Figure 8.17 (facing page).

themselves be the cause of the hearing loss. Cochlear hearing loss may result from head trauma, even without fracture, if a contusion in the cochlea results. This may be ipsilateral or contralateral to the skull insult.

Head injuries, acoustic trauma, diving accidents, or overexertion may cause rupture of the round-window membrane or a fistula of the oval window with a perilymph leak into the middle ear. When there is the possibility of a fluid leak, the fistula test using an immittance meter, described in Chapter 7, can be of great assistance in medical diagnosis.

SUMMARY

The inner ear is a fluid-filled space interfaced between the middle ear and the auditory nerve. It acts as a device to convert sound into a form of electro-chemical energy that transmits information to the brain about sound waves in terms of their frequency, intensity, and phase. The vestibular portion of the inner ear provides the brain with data concerning the position and movement of the body.

When the cochlear portion of the inner ear becomes abnormal, the result is a combination of sensorineural hearing loss and dysacusis. Bone-conduction and air-conduction results essentially interweave on the audiogram, and speech discrimination generally becomes poorer in direct relation to the amount of hearing loss. As a general rule, patients with cochlear hearing loss show high SISI scores and moderate amounts of tone decay (especially in the higher

AUDITORY BRAINSTEM RESPONSE
(Adult Form)

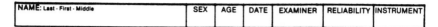

NAME: Last - First - Middle	SEX	AGE	DATE	EXAMINER	RELIABILITY	INSTRUMENT

LATENCY-INTENSITY FUNCTION

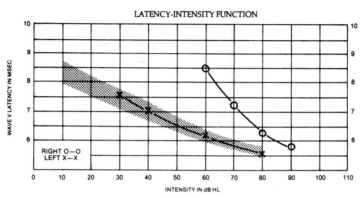

RIGHT O—O
LEFT X—X

SHADED AREA REPRESENTS Normal Wave V Range for patients older than 16 mos. for 30 clicks per second.

	STIMULUS				WAVE LATENCY IN MSEC						
EAR	RATE	dB HL	FILTER	I	II	III	IV	V	VI	VII
R	33.1	90	150-1500	1.6		3.75		5.8		
L	33.1	80	150-1500	1.52		3.7		5.6		

SUMMARY OF RESULTS

INTERWAVE INTERVALS .... R __4.2__ L __4.08__
AMPLITUDE RATIO (V SAME OR > I) .... R __NORMAL__ L __NORMAL__
LATENCY CHANGE WITH INCREASED CLICK RATE .... R _____ L _____
INTERAURAL DIFFERENCES .... _____

ESTIMATED AIR CONDUCTION THRESHOLD IN dBHL (1-2 kHz) .... R __≤60__ L __≤30__
ESTIMATED BONE CONDUCTION THRESHOLD IN dB HL .... R _____ L _____

COMMENTS

_____
_____
_____
_____
_____

Figure 8.17 Latency-intensity functions for wave V derived from the auditory brain stem response tracings shown in Figure 8.16 on the patient with a unilateral (right) cochlear hearing loss (see Figure 8.13). The latencies are normal for the left ear and increased for the right ear, primarily at lower intensities.

frequencies). Békésy audiometry usually results in Type II tracings, although Type I and IV tracings are sometimes seen. Recruitment can usually be demonstrated on binaural loudness balance tests. Acoustic reflex thresholds are obtained at low sensation levels. Results on tympanometry and static compliance in the plane of the tympanic membrane are usually within normal limits unless the sensorineural loss has a superimposed conductive component, resulting in a mixed hearing loss. In pure cochlear hearing losses the latency-intensity functions obtained from ABR testing are rather steep, showing longer latencies close to threshold.

Habilitation or rehabilitation of patients with sensorineural hearing losses of cochlear origin is considerably more difficult than that of patients with conductive lesions. Medical or surgical correction is usually obviated by the very nature of the disorder. Combinations of harmonic and frequency distortion and loudness recruitment often make the use of a hearing aid difficult, but not impossible. Auditory rehabilitation of patients with cochlear disorders is of special concern to audiologists.

GLOSSARY

Acoustic trauma notch A precipitous increase in hearing loss in the 3000 to 6000 Hz range, with recovery of hearing function at higher frequencies. Especially, but not exclusively, associated with patients with noise-induced hearing loss.

Acquired immune deficiency disease (AIDS) See human immunodeficiency virus.

Action potential (AP) A change in voltage measured on the surface of a neuron when it fires.

Afferent Nerves that carry impulses from the periphery toward the brain.

Ampulla The cilated end of each of the three semicircular canals where they return to the utricle. Each ampulla contains an end organ for the sense of equilibrium.

Anoxia Deprivation of oxygen to specific cells of the body affecting their normal metabolism.

Athetosis One of the three major categories of cerebral palsy, characterized by squirming or writhing movements.

Auditory placode A thickened plate, near the hindbrain in the human embryo, that develops into the inner ear.

Axon The efferent portion of a neuron.

Basilar membrane A membrane extending the entire length of the cochlea, separating the scala tympani from the scala media and supporting the organ of Corti.

Caloric test Irrigation of the external auditory canal with warm or cold water to stimulate the vestibular labyrinth. In normal patients the result is nystagmus with some sensation of vertigo.

Cell body The central portion of a nerve cell.

Cerebral palsy A motor disorder produced by damage to the brain; it usually occurs prenatally, perinatally, or in early infant life.

Cochlea A cavity in the inner ear resembling a snail shell and containing the essential end organs for hearing.

Cochlear duct See *scala media*.

Cochlear microphonic (CM) The measurable electrical response of the hair cells of the cochlea

Corti, organ of The end organ of hearing found within the scala media of the cochlea.

Corti's arch A series of arches made up of the rods of Corti in the cochlear duct.

Cytomegalovirus (CMV) A common virus that is a member of the herpes family of viruses and can cause congenital hearing loss when contracted by a pregnant woman.

Damage-risk criteria The maximum safe allowable noise levels for different band widths.

Dendrite The branched portion of a neuron that carries the nerve impulse to the cell body.

Diplacusis Hearing a tone of single frequency as different pitches in the two ears (*diplacusis binauralis*) or hearing a single frequency in one ear as a chord or noise (*diplacusis monauralis*).

Ductus reuniens A tube connecting the saccule with the scala media that carries endolymph to the cochlea.

Dysacusis Distortion of an auditory signal that is associated with loss of auditory sensitivity. Evidenced by poor speech discrimination.

Efferent Nerves that carry impulses from the brain toward the periphery.

Electronystagmograph (ENG) A device used to monitor electrically the amount of nystagmus occurring spontaneously or from caloric stimulation.

Endolymph The fluid contained within the membranous labyrinth of the inner ear in both the auditory and vestibular portions.

Evoked otoacoustic emissions A weak but measurable sound, in the frequency range from 500 to 4000 Hz, apparently produced within the cochlea in response to external acoustic stimulation, such as a click.

Frequency theory of hearing The explanation for pitch perception based on the frequency of neural impulses in the auditory nerve.

Glycerol test An auditory test for Ménière's disease in which pure-tone thresholds and word discrimination scores are measured before, and several hours after, patient ingestion of concentrated glucose and water. Improvements in threshold and word discrimination suggest that the diuretic action of the glucose solution results in decreased endolymphatic pressure, making the test positive for Ménière's disease.

Helicotrema A passage at the apical end of the cochlea connecting the scala vestibuli with the scala tympani.

Hereditodegenerative hearing loss Hearing loss that has its onset after birth but is nonetheless hereditary.

Human immunodeficiency virus (HIV) A sexually transmitted virus that first appeared in the United States in the early 1980s. The virus affects the immune system and creates the possibilities of conductive, sensory, and neural hearing loss.

Hypacusis   Loss of hearing sensitivity.

Labyrinth   The system of interconnecting canals of the inner ear, composed of the bony labyrinth (filled with perilymph), that contains the membranous labyrinth (filled with endolymph).

Labyrinthitis   Inflammation of the labyrinth, resulting in hearing loss and vertigo.

Ménière's disease   A disease of the inner ear, the symptoms of which are tinnitus, vertigo, and hearing loss (usually unilateral).

Meningitis   Inflammation of the meninges, the three protective coverings of the brain and spinal cord.

Mixed hearing loss   A sensorineural hearing loss with superimposed conductive hearing loss. The air-conduction level shows the entire loss; the bone-conduction level, the sensorineural portion; and the air–bone gap, the conductive portion.

Modiolus   The central pillar of the cochlea.

Neuron   A cell specialized as a conductor of nerve impulses.

Nystagmus   An oscillatory motion of the eyes.

Organ of Corti   See *Corti, organ of.*

Otocyst   The auditory vesicle (sac) of the human embryo.

Ototoxic   Poisonous to the ear.

Perilymph   The fluid contained in both the auditory and vestibular portions

with the bony labyrinth of the inner ear.

Permanent threshold shift (PTS)   Permanent sensorineural loss of hearing, usually associated with exposure to intense noise.

Phonemic regression   A slowness in auditory comprehension associated with advanced age.

Place theory of hearing   The explanation for pitch perception based on a precise place on the organ of Corti, which, when stimulated, results in the perception of a specific pitch.

Presbycusis   Hearing loss associated with old age.

Psychophysical tuning curve (PTC)   The measurable response in the cochlea to specific frequencies introduced into the ear.

Reissner's membrane   A membrane extending the entire length of the cochlea, separating the scala media from the scala vestibuli.

Resonance theory of hearing   A nineteenth-century theory of pitch perception that suggested that the cochlea consisted of a series of resonating tubes, each tuned to a specific frequency.

Resonance-volley theory of hearing   A combination of the place and frequency theories of hearing, which suggests that nerve units in the auditory nerve fire in volleys, allowing pitch perception up to about 4000 Hz. Perception of pitch above 4000 Hz is determined by the point of greatest excitation on the basilar membrane.

Rh factor   Pertaining to the protein factor found on the surface of the red blood cells in most humans. Named for the Rhesus monkey, in which it was first observed.

Saccule The smaller of the two sacs found in the membranous vestibular labyrinth; it contains an end organ of equilibrium.

Scala media The duct in the cochlea separating the scala vestibuli from the scala tympani. It is filled with endolymph and contains the organ of Corti. *Cochlear duct*

Scala tympani The duct in the cochlea below the scala media, filled with perilymph.

Scala vestibuli The duct in the cochlea above the scala media, filled with perilymph.

Semicircular canals Three loops within the vestibular portion of the inner ear responsible for perception of the sensation of turning.

Sensorineural hearing loss Formerly called *perceptive loss* or *nerve loss*, this term refers to loss of hearing sensitivity produced by damage or alteration of the sensory mechanism of the cochlea or the neural structures that lie beyond.

Spiral ligament The thickened outer portion of the periosteum of the cochlear duct which forms a spiral band and attaches to the basilar membrane.

Spontaneous otoacoustic emissions A still unexplained phenomenon in which a sound, apparently generated within the cochlea, may be produced without external stimulation. This sound is measurable with a tiny microphone sealed in the external auditory canal.

Stereocilia A protoplasmic filament on the surface of a cell (e.g., a hair cell).

Stria vascularis A vascular strip that lies along the outer wall of the scala media. It is responsible for the secretion and absorption of endolymph, it supplies oxygen and nutrients to the organ of Corti, and it affects the positive DC potential of the endolymph.

Synapse The area of communication between neurons where a nerve impulse passes from an axon of one neuron to the cell body or dendrite of another.

Syndrome A set of symptoms that appear together to indicate a specific pathological condition.

Tectorial membrane A gossamer membrane above the organ of Corti within the scala media in which the tips of the cilia of the hair cells are imbedded.

Temporary threshold shift (TTS) Temporary sensorineural hearing loss, usually associated with exposure to intense noise.

Transduce To convert one form of power to another (e.g., pressure waves to electricity, as in a microphone).

Traveling wave theory The theory that sound waves move in the cochlea from its base to its apex along the basilar membrane. The crest of the wave resonates at a particular point on the basilar membrane, resulting in the perception of a specific pitch.

Utricle The larger of the two sacs found in the membranous vestibular labyrinth; it contains an end-organ of equilibrium.

Vasospasm The violent constriction of a blood vessel, usually an artery.

Vertigo The sensation that a person (or his or her surroundings) is whirling or spinning.

Vestibule The cavity of the inner ear containing the organs of equilibrium and giving access to the cochlea.

Volley theory of hearing A variation of the frequency theory in which some neurons fire during the refractory periods of other neurons.

STUDY QUESTIONS

1. List from memory as many parts of the inner ear as you can, separating them into auditory and vestibular categories.
2. List some disorders of the inner ear. Break them down according to age of onset.
3. Draw typical audiograms from the preceding list. Hypothesize the results on tests of speech reception and discrimination, recruitment tests, SISI test, Békésy audiometry, tone decay test, ABR, and immittance measures.

REVIEW TABLE 8.1 USUAL CAUSES OF COCHLEAR HEARING LOSS ACCORDING TO AGE AT ONSET

PRENATAL	CHILDHOOD	ADULTHOOD
Anoxia	Birth trauma	(All of column 2 plus)
Heredity	Drugs	Labyrinthitis
Prematurity	Head trauma	Otosclerosis
Rh factor	High fevers	Ménière's disease
Toxemia of pregnancy	Kidney infection	Presbycusis
Trauma	Noise	Vasospasm
Viral infection (maternal)	Otitis media	
	Surgery (middle ear)	
	Systemic illnesses	
	Venereal disease	
	Viral infections	

REFERENCES

ALFORD, B. (1968). Rubella: A challenge for modern medical science. *Archives of Otolaryngology, 88,* 27–28.

ANDERSON, H. BARR, B., & WEDENBERG, E. (1970). Genetic disposition: A prerequisite for maternal rubella deafness. *Archives of Otolaryngology, 91,* 141–147.

BÉKÉSY, G.V. (1960). *Experiments in Hearing* (E. G. Wever, Ed.). New York: McGraw-Hill.

BORTON, T., & STARK, E. (1970). Audiological findings in hearing loss secondary to maternal rubella. *Pediatrics, 45,* 225–229.

BROOKHOUSER, P. E., CYR, D. G., & BEAU-

CHAINE, K. (1982). Vestibular findings in the deaf and hard of hearing. *Otolaryngology, Head and Neck Surgery, 90,* 773–777.

CYR, D. G., & MOLLER, C. G. (1988). Rationale for the assessment of vestibular function in children. *The Hearing Journal, 41,* 38–39, 45–46, 48–49.

DUFRESNE, R. M., ALLEYNE, B. C., & REESAL, M. R. (1988). Asymmetric hearing loss in truck drivers. *Ear and Hearing, 9,* 41–42.

EVERBERG, G. (1957). Deafness following mumps. *Acta Otolaryngologica, 48,* 397–403.

EWERTSON, H. W. (1973). Epidemiology of professional noise-induced hearing loss. *Audiology, 12,* 453–458.

FRICK, L. R., & MATTHIES, M. L. (1988). Effects of external stimuli on spontaneous otoacoustic emissions. *Ear and Hearing, 9,* 190–197.

GAETH, J. H. (1948). *A study of phonemic regression in relation to hearing loss.* Unpublished doctoral dissertation, Northwestern University.

HARDY, J. G., McCRACKEN, G. H., GILKERSON, M. R., SEVER, J. L. (1969). Adverse fetal outcome following maternal rubella after the first trimester of pregnancy. *Journal of the American Medical Association, 207,* 2414–2420.

IGARASHI, M., SCHUKNECHT, H. F., & MYERS, E. N. (1964). Cochlear pathology in humans with stimulation deafness. *Journal of Laryngology and Otology, 78,* 115–123.

JOHNSON, L. G., & HAWKINS, J. E. (1976). Degeneration patterns in human ears exposed to noise. *Annals of Otology, 85,* 725–739.

JOHNSON, S. J., HOSFORD-DUNN, H., PARYANI, S., YEAGER, A. S., & MALACHOWSKI, N. (1986). Prevalence of sensorineural hearing loss in premature and sick term infants with perinatally acquired cytomegalovirus infection. *Ear and Hearing, 7,* 325–327.

KARMODY, C. (1969). Asymptomatic maternal rubella and congenital deafness. *Archives of Otolaryngology, 89,* 720–726.

KEMP, D. T. (1978). Stimulated acoustic emissions from within the human auditory system. *Journal of the Acoustical Society of America, 65,* 1386–1391.

———. (1981). Physiologically active cochlear micromechanics—One source of tinnitus. In D. Evered & G. Lawrenson (Eds.), *Tinnitus, Ciba Foundation Symposium* (Vol. 85, pp. 54–81). Bath, England: Pittman Books.

KLOCKHOFF, I. (1976). Diagnosis of Ménière's disease. *Archives of Otolarngology, 212,* 309–312.

LAWRENCE, J. (1987). HIV infections in infants and children. *Infections in Surgery, 8,* 249–255.

LAWRENCE, M. (1969). Labyrinthine fluids. *Archives of Otolaryngology, 89,* 85–89.

McFADDEN, D., PLATTSMIER, H. S. Aspirin can potentiate the temporary hearing loss induced by noise. *Hearing Research, 9,* 295–316.

MUSIEK, F. E., & BARAN, J. A. (1986). Neuroanatomy, neurophysiology, and central auditory assessment: Part I. Brain stem. *Ear and Hearing, 7,* 207–219.

OCCUPATIONAL SAFETY AND HEALTH ADMINISTRATION (OSHA). (1983). Occupational noise exposure: Hearing conservation amendment: Final rule. *Federal Register, 48,* 9737–9785.

PICK, G. F. (1980). Level dependence of psychological frequency resolution and auditory filter shape. *Journal of the Acoustical Society of America, 68,* 1085–1095.

PROCTOR, B., GURDJIAN, E. S., & WEBSTER, J. E. (1956). The ear in head trauma. *Laryngoscope, 66,* 16–59.

ROSEN, S., BERGMAN, M., PLESTER, D., EL-MOFTY, A., & HAMMED, H. (1962). Presbycusis study of a relatively noise-free population in the Sudan. *Annals of Otology, Rhinology and Laryngology, 71,* 727–743.

SCHUKNECHT, H. F. (1974). *Pathology of the Ear.* Cambridge, MA: Harvard University Press, pp. 389–403.

SURJAN, L., DEVALD, J., & PALFAVI, L. (1973). Epidemiology of hearing loss. *Audiology, 12,* 396–398.

WEVER, G. (1949). *Theory of Hearing.* New York: Wiley.

SUGGESTED READINGS

Evans, E. F. (1983). Pathophysiology of the peripheral hearing mechanism. In M. E. Lutman & M. P. Haggard (Eds.), *Hearing Science and Hearing Disorders* (pp. 61–80). New York: Academic Press.

Maue-Dickson, W. (1981). The inner ear— Prenatal development. In F. N. Martin (Ed.), *Medical Audiology* (pp. 220–235). Englewood Cliffs, NJ: Prentice-Hall.

Miller, M. H. (1986). *Occupational hearing conservation*. Austin, TX: Pro-Ed.

Moore, B. C. J. (1982). *An introduction to the psychology of hearing*. New York: Academic Press.

Pickles, J. O. (1982). *An introduction to the physiology of hearing*. New York: Academic Press.

9

THE AUDITORY NERVE AND CENTRAL AUDITORY PATHWAYS

The previous three chapters have been concerned with the propagation and conduction of sound waves through the outer and middle ears and the transduction in the cochlea of these pressure waves into neural activity to be processed by the central auditory system. Because sound is meaningful only if it is perceived, an understanding of its transmission to and perception by the brain is essential to the audiologist.

In recent years a great deal has been learned about auditory neuroanatomy, largely through experiments performed on animals. However, much remains to be learned about how the nervous system receives, processes, and transmits information related to sound. This chapter's treatment of the anatomy and physiology of the central auditory system is designed mainly to introduce the reader to these processes, and is therefore far from complete.

Diagnosis of disorders of the auditory system from the outer ear through the auditory nerve is best made through the use of the test battery approach. This battery includes pure-tone and speech audiometry, measurements of acoustic immittance at the tympanic membrane, SISI, tone decay, loudness balance tests, Békésy audiometry, and ABR. The special tests described in this chapter for site-of-lesion diagnosis in the brain have met with varying degrees of clinical acceptance and are offered to the new student in diagnostic audiology because they seem to be the most appropriate ones at the time of this writing.

CHAPTER OBJECTIVES

Like the previous chapter, this presentation relies heavily on what has been learned in the foregoing sections of this book. The reader should gain an appreciation of the complexity of the central auditory system and the difficulties of diagnosing disorders within the brain. It is intended that the concepts of central hearing disorders be developed so that the reader will be able to institute and interpret test procedures for proper diagnosis. For deeper understanding, reading of some of the suggested references is encouraged.

THE AUDITORY NERVE AND ASCENDING AUDITORY PATHWAYS

Each inner hair cell of the cochlea is supplied by about 20 nerve fibers, with each nerve fiber contacting only one hair cell. This is not true of the outer hair cells, where the neurons/hair cell ratio is 1:10. Each hair cell may be innervated by many different nerve fibers, and a given nerve fiber goes to several outer hair cells. The nerve fibers exit the cochlea and extend centrally toward the modiolus, where their cell bodies group together to form the spiral ganglion. The nerve fibers pass from the modiolus to form the cochlear branch of the VIIIth cranial nerve, the **auditory nerve**.

Although this is not always repeated with each explanation, the reader should remember that each anatomical structure on one side of the brain has an identical structure on the opposite side of the brain. For purposes of clarity, a block diagram (Figure 9.1), rather than a realistic drawing, is shown to illustrate the auditory pathways. This diagram bears only slight resemblance to the actual anatomical arrangement within the system and merely illustrates the directions of neural impulses and the primary waystations from cochlea to auditory cortex.

The Auditory Nerve

The nerve fibers pass from the modiolus of the cochlea through the **internal auditory canal**, which begins at the base of the modiolus and terminates at the base of the brain. The internal auditory canal also carries the vestibular portion of the VIIIth nerve, whose fibers innervate the utricle, saccule, and semicircular canals. There are approximately 30,000 nerve fibers in the cochlear portion and 20,000 in the vestibular portion. The auditory portion of the VIIIth nerve actually spirals through the internal auditory canal. The nerve fibers form a cylindrically arranged bundle or "cable," with fibers that arise from the basal turn of the cochlea forming the outer portion and fibers from the apical area forming the center, together creating the nerve trunk. Responses to high-frequency sounds are carried by the fibers on the outer part of the nerve trunk, and responses to low-frequency sounds are carried by fibers on the inner part of the trunk. In addition to the VIIIth nerve, the internal auditory canal, which

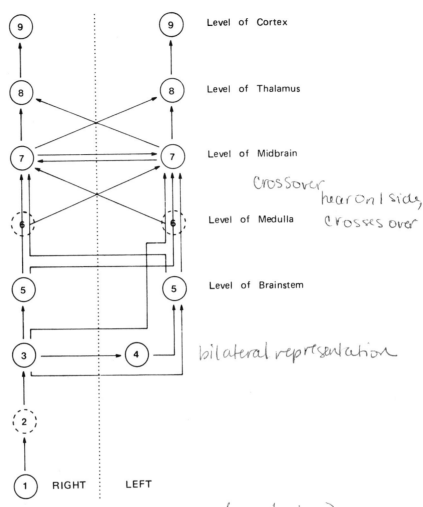

Figure 9.1 Block diagram of the auditory pathways. *(way stations)*

1. Cochlea (hair cells)
2. Auditory nerve fibers *(20 for each hair cell)*
3. Cochlear nucleus
4. Trapezoid body
5. Superior olivary complex
6. Lateral lemniscus
7. Inferior colliculus
8. Medial geniculate body *(in thalamus)*
9. Auditory cortex

Crossover — hear on 1 side, crosses over

bilateral representation

signals spread out then radiates to temporal lobe of cerebral cortex — called Heschl's gyrus

Listing?

Know! for test!

name them, not the pic!

runs a distance of approximately 10 mm in adults, also carries fibers of the VIIth (facial) nerve and the internal auditory artery.

The auditory nerve extends 17 to 19 mm beyond the internal auditory canal, where it attaches to the brain stem where the **cerebellum, medulla oblongata**, and **pons** join to form the **cerebellopontine angle (CPA)**. At this level the auditory and vestibular portions of the VIIIth nerve separate. One part of the cochlear bundle descends to the **dorsal cochlear nucleus**, and the other ascends to the **ventral cochlear nucleus**.

The Cochlear Nucleus

As previously mentioned, neurons from the cochlea are arranged in an orderly fashion in the cochlear bundle according to frequency. The orderly arrangement of fibers in the cochlea and auditory nerve is repeated in the cochlear nuclei and is said to represent **tonotopic** organization. The auditory nerve fibers terminate in the cochlear nuclei—basal turn fibers in one area, apical turn fibers in other areas, and so on.

Each cochlear nucleus is divided into three portions: the anteroventral, posteroventral, and dorsal. Each division is organized tonotopically. The cochlear nucleus is composed of a variety of different cell types. These different cells react differently to the incoming auditory nerve impulses, thus modifying input to the brain. It is probable that the cochlear nucleus preserves, but does not necessarily enhance, acoustical information it receives from the auditory nerve.

The brain is characterized by many **decussations**, or crossover points, that unite symmetrical portions of the two halves of the brain. Specialized nerve fiber bundles called **commissures** unite similar structures on both sides of the brain or spinal cord. The first decussation in the auditory pathways occurs after the cochlear nucleus at the level of the **trapezoid body** of the pons.

Some fibers terminate in the contralateral trapezoid body, but other fibers begin their ascent in the brain on both the ipsilateral and contralateral sides. This is the beginning of bilateral representation of sound from a signal presented to just one ear. The fibers from the ventral cochlear nucleus proceed to the ipsilateral and contralateral **superior olivary complexes (SOC)**. Some fibers from the dorsal cochlear nucleus extend to the contralateral **inferior colliculus**. The ascending pathway is along the **lateral lemniscus**, which is an extension of the olivary complex on both sides of the brain. Fibers also pass from the ventral cochlear nucleus to the **reticular formation**.

The Reticular Formation

The reticular formation resides within the center of the brain stem and communicates with virtually all areas of the brain, including the cortex and the spinal cord. It plays a major role in auditory alertness, reflexes, and habit-uation. Sometimes called the reticular activating system, the reticular formation may be the primary control center for the central nervous system.

The Superior Olivary Complex

Most of the fibers from the cochlear nucleus project to the superior olivary complex. The lateral superior olivary nucleus, the largest area, and the medial superior olivary complex receive input from both the ipsilateral and contralateral cochlear nuclei. The large number of ipsilateral and contralateral neural inputs gives the superior olivary complex the capability to sense the direction of a sound source by analyzing small differences in the time or intensity of sounds arriving at the two ears.

In addition to its major function as a relay station for neural activity on the way to the cerebral cortex, the superior olivary complex also mediates the reflex activity of the tensor tympani and stapedius muscles of the middle ear. Some of the cells of the superior olive interact with some neurons of the facial nerve. By a system not completely understood, loud sounds produce activation of certain motor fibers of the facial nerve, which innervate the stapedial branch of the nerve. The decussations at this anatomical point explain the contraction of the stapedius muscles in both middle ears when sound is presented to just one ear.

Neural connections in the superior olives also supply innervation to branches of the abducens (VIth cranial) nerve, which supplies fibers to the extraocular muscles of the eyes. This provides an explanation of why the muscles around the eyes contract at a sudden presentation of a loud sound. This is known as the *auropalpebral reflex*.

The Lateral Lemniscus

Little is known about the precise function of the lateral lemniscus except that it provides a major pathway for the transmission of impulses from the lower brain stem on the ipsilateral side. Some fibers terminate in the nucleus of the lateral lemniscus, others course to the contralateral lateral lemniscus, and still others continue to the inferior colliculus.

The Inferior Colliculus

The inferior colliculus receives afferent stimulation from both superior olivary complexes. This is the first waystation at which a 1:1 ratio of entering and departing fibers is found. Most fibers from the lower centers at each cochlear nucleus and superior olive reach the higher centers by way of the inferior colliculus of the midbrain. Neurons that connect the inferior colliculus with the next relay station, the **medial geniculate body**, represent the third or fourth link in the ascending auditory system. A few fibers bypass the inferior colliculus to reach the medial geniculate body directly from the lateral lemniscus.

The Medial Geniculate Body

The medial geniculate body, located in the **thalamus**, is the last subcortical relay station for auditory impulses. Only one of its three main areas, the ventral division, is responsible specifically for auditory information. There is some spiral organization in this area, but tonotopicity is uncertain. Most of the fibers come from the ipsilateral inferior colliculus, and a few fibers come from the lateral lemniscus. After this point, nerve fibers fan out as the **auditory**

radiations and then ascend to the auditory cortex. Because there are no commissural neurons at the level of the medial geniculate body, no decussations exist there.

The Auditory Cortex

The areas of auditory reception are in the **temporal lobes** on both sides of the cerebral cortex in an area called the **superior temporal gyrus** or **Heschl's gyrus**. Because there are many interconnections among parts of the cortex through association areas, a part of the cortex is involved in the process of hearing.

There is evidence that the selective representation of frequency, observed at specific places in the cochlea, is repeated in the auditory cortex, though to a lesser degree. Research evidence suggests that the temporal area is concerned primarily with the frequency characteristics of sound; the insular area with temporal aspects of sound, the parietal area with association of sound with past experiences (and, because this area has inputs from all sensory modalities, the auditory stimulus is compared or matched with input from other senses), and the frontal area with memory of sounds.

At one time it was believed that the auditory cortex was the only center of auditory discrimination. It is now known that many of the discriminations previously ascribed to the auditory cortex may be mediated subcortically. Perceptions of pitch and loudness can be maintained in animals whose cortices have been surgically removed. Although discrimination of some simple sounds may be retained, the understanding of speech requires at least minimal integrity of the auditory cortex.

THE DESCENDING AUDITORY PATHWAYS

The auditory system is generally considered to be a sensory system (like the skin or the eyes) that provides the brain with information conducted to the cochlea in the form of pressure waves, and transduced by the cochlea into neural activity. Rasmussen (1960, 1964) has proved that, in addition to the afferent pathways, the auditory system contains a complex efferent system of descending fibers. These descending fibers correspond closely with the ascending fibers and connect the auditory cortex with lower centers and with the cochlea. One purpose of this descending system is to provide inhibitory feedback by elevating the thresholds of neurons at lower stations in the auditory tract. It is true, however, that some descending connections have an excitatory function, but its purpose is unknown.

The Descending (Efferent) Tract

The descending fibers appear to originate in all auditory areas of the cerebral cortex and descend first in the auditory radiations. Some of these fibers terminate in the medial geniculate body, and some continue to the inferior colliculus and lateral lemniscus. These fibers terminate on both sides of the brain in the **olivocochlear bundle (OCB)**, which consists almost entirely of efferent neurons. The olivocochlear bundle originates in the superior olivary complex and terminates in both the ipsilateral and contralateral cochleas.

A second efferent pathway also arises from the auditory cortex. Although some fibers terminate in various areas of the brain, most continue down to the inferior colliculus. Fibers from this area pass to the ipsilateral dorsal cochlear nucleus. Other fibers pass from the superior olive to the ventral cochlear nucleus. The ventral cochlear nucleus also receives fibers from the olivocochlear bundle.

DEVELOPMENT OF THE AUDITORY NERVE AND CENTRAL AUDITORY NERVOUS SYSTEM

There is relatively little information available on the prenatal development of the outer, middle, and inner ear; even less is available about the VIIIth nerve and central auditory nervous system. Development of the nervous system (neurogenesis) in general is still poorly understood.

In humans, the VIIIth nerve begins to form at about the 25th gestational day and appears almost complete at about 45 days. It is probable that the efferent fibers develop later than the afferent fibers. The cochlear and vestibular ganglia appear by the fifth week.

Improved understanding of the embryogenesis and fetogenesis of the central auditory pathways would undoubtedly provide insights into the causes of some types of lesions of the auditory nervous system. It is generally agreed that the entire nervous system forms from the ectoderm.

SUMMARY OF THE AUDITORY PATHWAYS

Even the oversimplified descriptions just presented should make it apparent that the auditory nerve and central pathways are tremendously complex. The ascending (afferent) system provides stimulation from one ear to both sides of the brain, including the temporal cortex. Descending fibers from each side of the brain provide inhibition to both cochleas.

The waystations in the auditory system probably perform the complex processing of the incoming nerve impulses. The series of cochlear nucleus, superior olivary complex, lateral lemniscus, inferior colliculus, and medial geniculate body are not simply parts of an elaborate transmission line, whereby the coded information of the VIIIth nerve is relayed to the cortex. Recoding and processing of information undoubtedly takes place all the way up through the system.

HEARING LOSS AND THE AUDITORY NERVE AND CENTRAL AUDITORY PATHWAYS

Because there are many collateral nerve fibers and so much analysis and re-analysis of an acoustic message as it travels to the higher brain centers, it is said that the auditory pathways provide considerable *intrinsic redundancy*. There are also many forms of *extrinsic redundancy* in speech messages themselves, such as the usual inclusion of more words than necessary to round out acceptable grammar and syntax. Also, the acoustics of speech offer more frequency information than is absolutely essential for understanding. People with normal auditory systems rarely appreciate the ease these factors provide in understanding. Those who are deprived of some intrinsic redundancy may not show difficulty in discrimination until the speech message has been degraded by noise, distortion, or distraction.

Lesions in the conductive portions of the outer and middle ears and the sensory cells of the cochlea result in loss of hearing sensitivity. The extent of the hearing loss is in direct proportion to the degree of damage. Loss of hearing sensitivity, such as for pure tones, becomes less obvious as disorders occur in the higher centers of the brain. For these reasons, even though site-of-lesion tests may be extremely useful in diagnosing disorders in the more peripheral areas of the central auditory pathways, such as the auditory nerve and cochlear nuclei, these tests frequently fail to identify disease in the higher centers.

DISORDERS OF THE AUDITORY NERVE

Disorders of the auditory nerve result in hearing losses that are classified as sensorineural. Bone conduction and air conduction interweave, and there is usually nothing in the general audiometric configuration that differentiates cochlear from VIIIth nerve disorders. Johnson (1977) points out that in more than 50% of a series of patients with acoustic tumors, consistent audiometric configurations appeared but could not be differentiated according to audiometric pattern from cochlear lesions. Two common early symptons of auditory nerve disorders are tinnitus and high-frequency sensorineural hearing loss. Whenever cases of unilateral or bilateral sensorineural hearing loss with different degrees of impairment in each ear occur, alert audiologists suspect the possibility of neural lesions. The philosophy that all unilateral sensorineural hearing losses are of neural origin until proved otherwise is a good one to adopt.

A second symptom of auditory nerve disorders is apparent when a discrepancy exists between the amount of hearing loss and the scores on speech discrimination tests. In most cochlear disorders, as the hearing loss increases, the amount of dysacusis also increases. When difficulties in speech discrimination are excessive for the amount of hearing loss for pure tones, a neural lesion is suggested. In some cases of VIIIth nerve disorder, hearing for pure tones is normal in the presence of a speech discrimination loss. Despite these statements, it must be remembered that even in cases of neural lesions, patients' speech discrimination scores may be perfectly normal.

Causes of Auditory Nerve Disorders

There are fewer causes of VIIIth nerve than of cochlear disorders. Lesions of the VIIIth nerve may occur as a result of disease, irritation, or pressure on the nerve trunk. Because the cochlear nerve extends into the brain for a short distance beyond the end of the internal auditory canal, some lesions of the nerve may occur within the canal and some in the cerebellopontine angle of the brain.

Tumor of the Auditory Nerve. Most tumors of the auditory nerve are benign and vary in size depending on the age of the patient and the growth characteristics of the **neoplasm**. Usually these tumors arise from sheaths that cover the vestibular branch of the VIIIth nerve (Pool, Pava, & Greenfield, 1970). The term usually applied to these tumors is **acoustic neuroma**, although some neuro-otologists believe that the term *acoustic neurinoma* is more descriptive of some growths that arise from the peripheral cells of the nerve.

An acoustic neuroma is considered small if it is contained within the internal auditory canal; medium-sized if it extends up to one centimeter into the cerebellopontine angle; and large if it extends any further (Pool et al., 1970). The larger the tumor within the canal, the greater the probability that pressure will cause alterations in the functions of the cochlear, vestibular, and facial nerves, and in the internal auditory artery. The larger the tumor extending into the cerebellopontine angle, the greater the likelihood of the pressure involving other cranial nerves and the cerebellum, which is the seat of balance and equilibrium in the brain.

Most cases of acoustic neuroma occur in adults over the age of 30, although naturally there are exceptions to this. Most of these tumors are unilateral, but they have been known to occur in both ears, either simultaneously or successively. One disease, **neurofibromatosis (NF)** or von Recklinghausen's disease, may cause dozens or even hundreds of neuromas in different parts of the body.

The earlier in their development acoustic neuromas are discovered, the better the chance for successful surgical removal. Audiological examination is very helpful in making an early diagnosis. Most hearing clinics, however, do not see patients with early acoustic neuromas, because hearing loss is not a primary concern in the early stages. As the tumor increases in size, VIIIth nerve symptoms such as tinnitus, hearing loss, and speech discrimination difficulties become apparent. Although these tumors usually result in gradually progressive hearing loss, pressure on the internal auditory artery may result in interference with the blood supply to the cochlea and cause sudden hearing loss and/or progressive sensory hearing loss as a result of damage within the cochlea. Changes in blood supply to the cochlea may cause cochlear symptoms to appear, such as recruitment of loudness and high SISI scores, and may possibly result in the misdiagnosis of cochlear disease as the primary disorder.

Cranial nerves other than the VIIIth nerve may be affected as an acoustic tumor increases in size. Symptoms of Vth nerve involvement include pain and numbness in the face. VIIth nerve symptoms include the formation of tears in the eyes, alterations in the sense of taste, and development of facial paralysis. Abnormalities in this nerve often result in the loss of the corneal reflex; that is, the patient's eyes may not show the expected reflexive blink when a wisp of cotton is touched to the cornea. Dizziness and blurred vision may also occur. The loss of both ipsilateral and contralateral acoustic reflexes may result when measurement is taken in the ear on the same side as an impaired facial nerve (see Figure 5.11h). As the IXth (glossopharyngeal) and Xth (vagus) cranial nerves become involved, difficulty in swallowing (dysphagia) may ensue.

Figure 9.2 shows an audiogram illustrating a high-frequency hearing loss. The findings on special tests for the patient illustrated are typical of acoustic neuroma, but in any given case one or more of these results may differ from what is expected. Remember that auditory nerve lesions cannot be diagnosed on the basis of a "typical" audiometric configuration.

Proper audiological diagnosis naturally consists of applying the entire test battery. As shown in Figure 9.2, speech discrimination scores are poor in the impaired ear. Low SISI scores occur (Figure 9.3), often even when the test is modified by presenting the carrier tone at high sensation levels or by using large increments (e.g., 5 dB). The alternate binaural loudness balance test will generally show either no recruitment or decruitment of loudness, and tone decay may be dramatic at all frequencies (Figure 9.3). Békésy audiometry will show a Type III (Figure 9.4) or IV (Figure 9.5) pattern, but many reports appear in the literature of Type IIs in the early stages of the tumor. Acoustic reflexes are absent in many cases (see Figure 9.6) even at very high stimulus levels (Anderson, Barr, & Wedenberg, 1969). If an acoustic reflex can be obtained, the time required for its amplitude to decay 50% is markedly reduced in the low frequencies (less than 10 seconds). In 10 cases of acoustic neuroma described by Anderson and colleagues (1969), the acoustic reflex half-life was less than 3 seconds for frequencies at and below 1000 Hz. Jerger, Oliver, and Jenkins (1987) reported on several cases of acoustic tumors in which the most dramatic finding was the decrease in acoustic reflex amplitude when the eliciting stimulus was presented to the ear on the affected side. ABR latencies in the affected ear are markedly increased (Figures 9.7 and 9.8).

Confirmation of acoustic neuroma is made through an interdisciplinary approach. Vestibular tests often show a number of abnormal signs, including spontaneous nystagmus with the eyes closed and generally decreased vestibular function on the affected side. An increase in the amount of protein found in cerebrospinal fluid is helpful in determining the presence of tumors. X-ray techniques have been somewhat useful in diagnosing acoustic neuromas, but new advances in the specialty of medical imaging have vastly improved this diagnostic tool.

AUDIOMETRIC EXAMINATION

NAME: Last - First - Middle	SEX	AGE	DATE	EXAMINER	RELIABILITY	AUDIOMETER

AIR CONDUCTION

MASKING Type	RIGHT									LEFT								
	250	500	1000	1500	2000	3000	4000	6000	8000	250	500	1000	1500	2000	3000	4000	6000	8000
NB	O	5	10/10	5	5	10	5	5	5	10	15	15/15	20	30	35	50	55	60
																50*	55*	60*
EM Level in Opp. Ear																5	5	5

BONE CONDUCTION

MASKING Type	RIGHT						FOREHEAD						LEFT					
	250	500	1000	2000	3000	4000	250	500	1000	2000	3000	4000	250	500	1000	2000	3000	4000
NB	O	5	10	10	10	10							5	10	10	10	10	15
																30*	40*	50*
EM Level in Opp. Ear																35	35	40

		2 Frequency	3 Frequency	WEBER				2 Frequency	3 Frequency
Pure Tone Average		5	7				Pure Tone Average	15	20

SPEECH AUDIOMETRY

MASKING Type	RIGHT				LEFT			
	SRT 1	SRT 2	Discrimination 1	Discrimination 2	SRT 1	SRT 2	Discrimination 1	Discrimination 2
WB	5		1A List 30 SL 100 %	List SL %	20		2A List 30 SL 60* %	List SL %
EM Level in Opp. Ear							15	

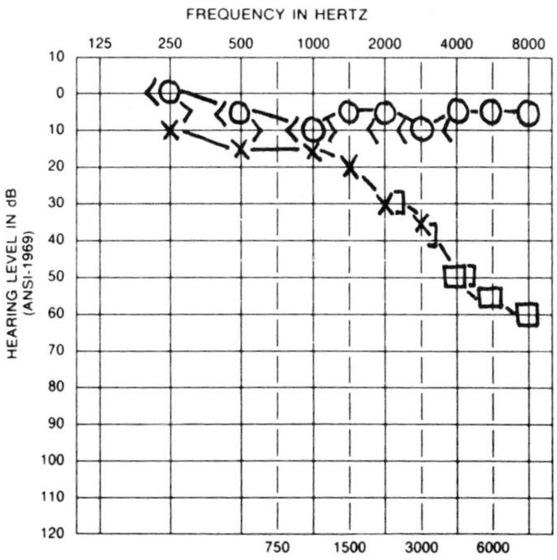

FREQUENCY IN HERTZ

COMMENTS

AUDIOGRAM KEY

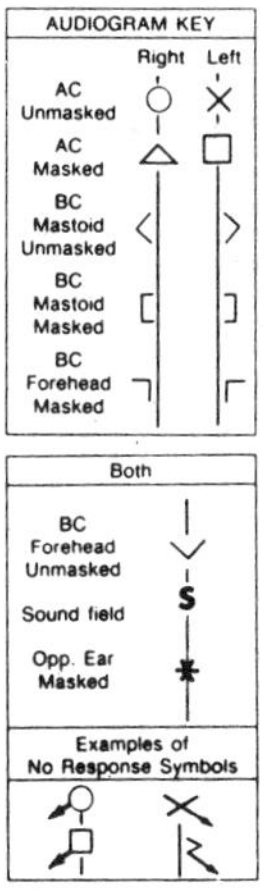

Figure 9.2 Audiogram exemplifying a left acoustic neuroma. Although the hearing loss in the left ear is mild, the speech-discrimination score is poor. Naturally, proper masking is essential in this case, especially for bone-conduction and speech discrimination testing.

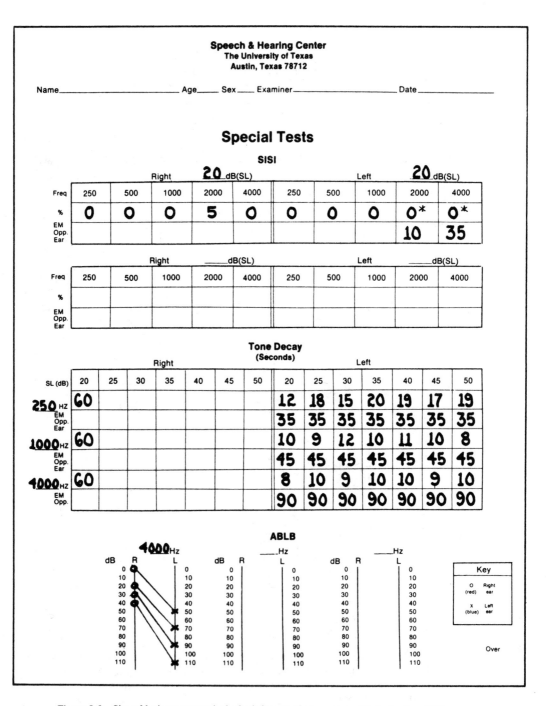

Figure 9.3 Site-of-lesion tests typical of a left acoustic neuroma. Note the low SISI scores in the left ear at 2000 and 4000 Hz, the marked tone decay at all frequencies, and the decruitment at 4000 Hz.

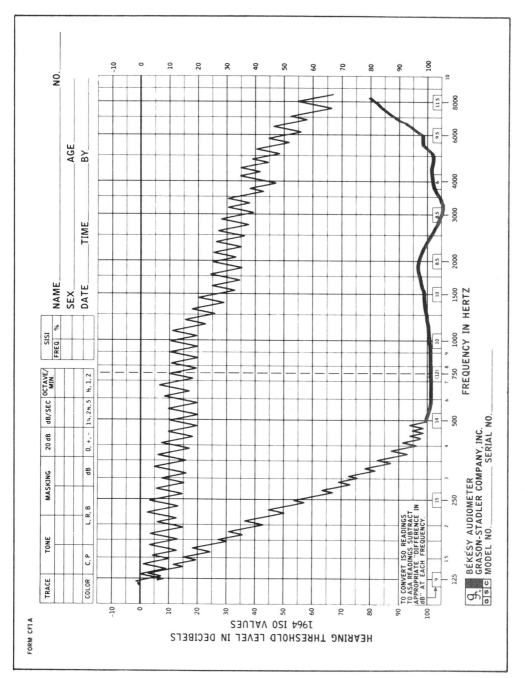

Figure 9.4 Theoretical Type III Békésy tracing for the patient with a left acoustic neuroma (Figure 9.2). Note how the continuous tone fades rapidly to inaudibility, even in the low frequencies.

335

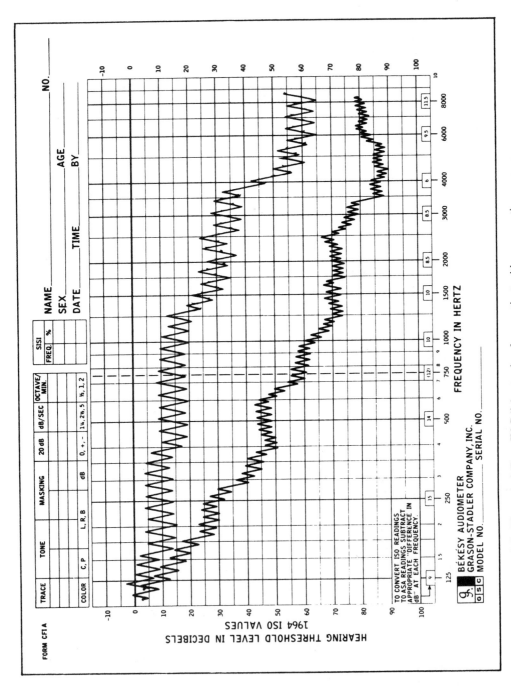

Figure 9.5 Theoretical Type IV Békésy tracing for a patient with an acoustic neuroma (Figure 9.2). Note that the continuous tone becomes more difficult to hear than the interrupted tone, even in the low frequencies. This adaptation to continuous tones is evident throughout the test frequency range, although it is not as dramatic as the Type III tracing shown in Figure 9.4.

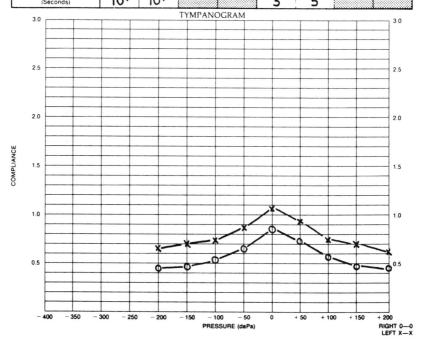

SPEECH AND HEARING CENTER
The University of Texas at Austin 78712

IMMITTANCE

NAME: Last - First - Middle		SEX	AGE	DATE	EXAMINER		INSTRUMENT	

PRESSURE/COMPLIANCE FUNCTION

	−400	−350	−300	−250	−200	−150	−100	−50	0	+50	+100	+150	+200
Right					.44	.47	.53	.65	.85	.71	.57	.49	.46
Left					.66	.70	.73	.88	1.08	.91	.74	.70	.61

STATIC COMPLIANCE

$C_x = C_2 − C_1$

RIGHT						LEFT					
.46	c_1	.85	c_2	.39	c_x	.61	c_1	1.08	c_2	.47	c_x

ACOUSTIC REFLEXES

	RIGHT				LEFT			
Frequency (Hz)	500	1000	2000	4000	500	1000	2000	4000
Ipsilateral (Probe same)		80	85			NR	NR	
Contralateral (Probe opposite)	75	75	80	80	100	105	NR	NR
Audiometric Threshold	5	10	5	5	10	15		
Reflex SL	70	65	75	75	90	90		
Decay Time (Seconds)	10+	10+			3	5		

TYMPANOGRAM

Figure 9.6 Results on immittance measures for the theoretical patient illustrated in Figure 9.2. Tympanograms and static compliance are normal for both ears. The acoustic reflexes are normal when the tone is presented to the right (normal) ear. Reflex thresholds are elevated when tones are presented to the left ear (acoustic neuroma) in the low frequencies and absent for the higher frequencies. Reflex decay time is very rapid in the left ear in the low frequencies, with no decay in the right ear.

THE AUDITORY NERVE AND CENTRAL AUDITORY PATHWAYS 337

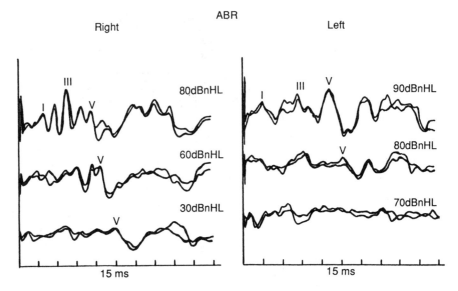

Figure 9.7 Results of auditory brain stem response testing on the patient with an VIIIth nerve hearing loss (acoustic neuroma) in the left ear (see Figure 9.2).

Medical Imaging. During the last two decades remarkable new technologies have been introduced to the science of medical imaging. The revolutionary development of **computed tomography (CT)** has permitted the viewing of numerous anatomical abnormalities in the body with a sensitivity unrivaled by previous techniques. In this procedure, often called *computerized axial tomography (CAT)*, an X-ray transmitter scans around a transverse plane (at right angles to the long axis) of the head or body along a 180 degree arc, while an electronic detector simultaneously measures the intensity of the beam emerging from the other side of the patient. With the aid of a computer, the detector's information is converted to a picture, or "slice," of the patient. CT technology has permitted the noninvasive detection of intracranial hemorrhages, tumors, and deformities with sensitivity that was heretofore impossible. A CT scan of an acoustic neuroma is shown in Figure 9.9.

CT is now an integral part of most major medical facilities. In addition, **magnetic resonance imaging (MRI)**, also referred to as *nuclear magnetic resonance (NMR) imaging*, is rapidly emerging as an exciting adjunct to CT scanning. CT uses ionizing radiation to obtain images; MRI employs magnetic fields and radio waves to produce images in the different planes of the body. One of the most satisfying aspects of this technology is that the waves presented to the body are believed to be virtually harmless. Furthermore, the technique is excellent for seeing many soft-tissue masses, such as acoustic neuromas.

Prior to the implementation of CT and MRI, more invasive and potentially dangerous procedures were necessary to obtain images of the brain and its surrounding structures. In **pneumoencephalography**, air is introduced into

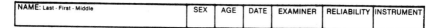

SPEECH AND HEARING CENTER
The University of Texas at Austin 78712

AUDITORY BRAINSTEM RESPONSE
(Adult Form)

NAME: Last · First · Middle	SEX	AGE	DATE	EXAMINER	RELIABILITY	INSTRUMENT

LATENCY-INTENSITY FUNCTION

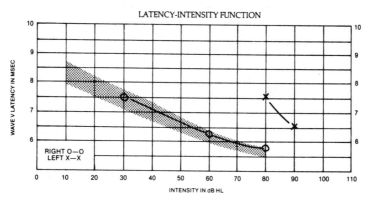

SHADED AREA REPRESENTS Normal Wave V Range for patients older than 16 mos. for 30 clicks per second.

EAR	STIMULUS RATE	dB HL	FILTER	I	II	III	IV	V	VI	VII
R	13.1	80	150-1500	1.9		3.8		5.8		
L	13.1	90	150-1500	1.68		4.0		6.6		

SUMMARY OF RESULTS

INTERWAVE INTERVALS.. R __3.9__ L __4.92__
AMPLITUDE RATIO (V SAME OR > I).............................. R __NORMAL__ L __NORMAL__
LATENCY CHANGE WITH INCREASED CLICK RATE.................. R _____ L _____
INTERAURAL DIFFERENCES..................................... _____

ESTIMATED AIR CONDUCTION THRESHOLD IN dBHL (1-2 kHz)....... R _____ L _____
ESTIMATED BONE CONDUCTION THRESHOLD IN dB HL .... R _____ L _____

COMMENTS

Figure 9.8 Latency-intensity functions for wave V derived from the auditory brain stem response tracings shown in Figure 9.7, based on the patient with a unilateral retrocochlear hearing loss caused by an acoustic neuroma in the left ear (see Figure 9.2). Wave V latencies are normal for the right ear and markedly increased for the left ear at all the sensation levels tested.

THE AUDITORY NERVE AND CENTRAL AUDITORY PATHWAYS   339

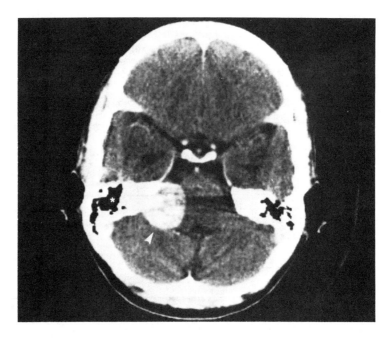

Figure 9.9 CT scan showing a tumor in the right cerebellopontine angle (arrow). Asterisk shows right mastoid air cells (Courtesy David C. Martin, M.D.)

the space around the brain by means of spinal puncture. The air acts as a contrast substance to allow X-ray examination of such areas as the internal auditory canal and cerebellopontine angle. In *positive-contrast encephalography*, dyes are injected in a manner similar to air injection in pneumoencephalography. Because X-ray studies are frequently more accurate in outlining the region of the internal auditory canal when such contrasts are used, these procedures are still necessary in some cases.

In a series of 100 patients with acoustic neuromas reported by Josey, Glasscock, and Musiek (1988), 93 had sufficient hearing to allow ABR testing, and 97% of that group showed abnormal ABR results reflecting the disorder. By contrast, 69% of the lesions were correctly identified by medical imaging alone. This further emphasizes the need to use both procedures in diagnosis.

Telian and Kileny (1988) reported three case histories in which ABR, ENG, CT, and MRI at times suggested different problems. In other words, some of the tests resulted in both false positive and false negative results. Telian and Kileny also concluded that false normal ABR responses are more likely when an acoustic tumor is in the cerebellopontine angle than when it is in the internal auditory canal.

Other Causes of VIIIth Nerve Hearing Loss

Because of their dramatic symptoms and the danger they pose to the life of the patient, acoustic neuromas come to the audiologist's mind first when VIIIth nerve signs appear. This is a safe and prudent attitude, but other conditions of the auditory nerve can produce identical audiological symptoms. These conditions include **acoustic neuritis** (inflammation of the vestibular or cochlear nerve) and **multiple sclerosis (MS)**.

DISORDERS OF THE COCHLEAR NUCLEI

The cochlear nuclei represent the first of the relay stations in the central auditory nervous system but the last point at which entirely ipsilateral representation is maintained. As mentioned earlier, the cochlear nuclei serve as more than waystations for the transmission of auditory information. Because the tonotopic layout of these nuclei allows for frequency analysis, lesions in these areas may produce clinical loss of hearing sensitivity. Beyond the cochlear nuclei, the stimulus presented to one ear is processed and transmitted along fibers on both sides of the brain.

Audiologists work under the assumption that on special diagnostic tests lesions central to the cochlea will produce results specific to retrocochlear disorders. Such results are usually observed with VIIIth nerve lesions but are not always the case in the cochlear nuclei. Carhart (1967) has pointed out that place and volley information, coded by the cochlea and transmitted by the auditory nerve, are processed separately in the cochlear nuclei. In certain situations in which the cochlear nuclei are damaged, a hearing loss will result, which means that site-of-lesion tests must be performed at relatively high stimulation levels. In such cases special tests, such as the SISI, ABLB, and Békésy audiometry, may give rise to results that are similar to the results of tests performed on normal-hearing individuals at high sound-pressure levels. For patients with cochlear pathology, the sensation levels for these tests are low, but the sound-pressure levels are high.

There is often uncertainty as to whether site-of-lesion test results in cases of damage to the cochlear nuclei will suggest a cochlear disorder, as in Ménière's disease, or retrocochlear lesions, as in acoustic neuroma. The tests that are now available cannot completely solve this dilemma. Therefore, audiologists must proceed cautiously in cases of unilateral sensorineural hearing loss.

Causes of Cochlear-Nuclei Disorders

Damage to the cochlear nuclei are difficult to diagnose with certainty without post-mortem study. Lesions in the nuclei, like those in the auditory nerve, may result from disease, toxicity, irritation, pressure, or trauma.

Rh incompatibility was discussed briefly in Chapter 8 as a prenatal cause of cochlear hearing loss. Reports in the literature, such as by Blakely (1959) and Matkin (1965), show positive indications of cochlear pathology on site-of-lesion tests. Post-mortem studies have shown deposits of bilirubin in the cochlea as well as in different areas of the brain, including the cochlear nuclei. Goodhill (1950) coined the term *nuclear deafness* to describe the site of lesion in hearing-impaired children with cerebral palsy secondary to Rh incompatibility.

The term **kernicterus** has been used for some time to describe the condition characterized by bile deposits (often neonatal) in the central nervous system. Kernicterus often results in degeneration of the nerve cells that come into contact with bile. Carhart (1967) poses a number of compelling arguments to suggest that hearing losses in Rh babies are caused by damage in the cochlear nuclei rather than in the cochlea, even though site-of-lesion tests may imply the opposite. Until these matters are resolved, the precise locus of the disorder in these cases will be difficult to determine.

Disorders that interfere with or alter the blood supply to the cochlear nuclei may result in hearing loss. Such disorders, called *vascular accidents*, include the rupturing of blood vessels, as well as clots that obstruct the arterial space. These clots may either be thromboses that form and remain in a specific area of the vessel, or they may be embolisms that are formed by bits of debris that circulate through the system until they reach a narrow passageway through which they cannot pass. Either one may obstruct the blood vessel or cause it to burst. Arteries have also been known to rupture where aneurysms (dilations in the blood vessels) form, because aneurysms usually cause the walls to become stretched and thin. Cases of obstruction or rupture of blood vessels within the brain are called **cerebrovascular accidents (CVAs)**, or strokes.

An increasingly common condition today is arteriosclerosis, or hardening of the arteries. In addition, the narrowing of the lumen within an artery may be associated with accumulations of fatty debris due to improper diet, insufficient exercise, or metabolic problems. When blood supply to critical nerve cells is diminished, the result is anoxia, which alters cell metabolism and may cause destruction of nerve tissue.

A number of congenital defects of the brain, including the central auditory pathways, have been described in the literature. These defects may be the result of birth trauma or agenesis of parts of the brain.

Pressure within the brain stem may also produce hearing loss. This pressure may be caused by tumors (either benign or malignant), by increased cerebrospinal fluid pressure produced secondary to trauma, or by direct insult to the head. Hemorrhage produced by vascular or other accidents may also cause pressure and damage.

Syphilis (lues) can produce damage anywhere in the auditory system, from the outer ear to the cortex. Cells are damaged or destroyed either by direct degeneration of the nerve units or, secondarily, by CVAs associated with the infection.

Degeneration of nerve fibers in the brain is expected with advancing age. Although presbycusis was listed as one of the causes of cochlear hearing loss, it has become accepted that, with aging, changes occur virtually everywhere in the auditory system, including the brain stem. Such diseases as multiple sclerosis can produce degeneration of nerve fibers in younger people as well.

DISORDERS OF THE HIGHER AUDITORY PATHWAYS

The types of disorders that affect the cochlear nucleus may also affect higher neural structures. Tumors, for example, are not limited to specific sites. Head injury, the major cause of death or serious brain damage among young people in the United States, can produce lesions in a variety of sites. Lesions may encompass large portions of the brain or be localized to small areas.

Factors influencing audiometric results include not only the sizes of the lesions, but also their locations. Lesions of the temporal cortex, such as CVA or epilepsy, usually lead to abnormal results on special tests in the ear contra-lateral to the lesion. Lesions in the brain stem are not so predictable.

Jerger and Jerger (1975) point out that when a lesion is **extra-axial** (on the outside of the brain stem), audiometric symptoms appear on the same side of the head. Such patients often show considerable loss of sensitivity for pure tones, especially in the high frequencies. When the lesion is **intra-axial** (within the brainstem), central auditory tests may show either contralateral or bilateral effects. Often, hearing sensitivity for pure tones is normal or near normal at all frequencies.

Minimal Auditory Deficiency Syndrome

The mild hearing loss that is often associated with otitis media may go undetected in very young children. Even when it is correctly diagnosed, parents and physicians alike are relieved when symptoms abate and the child appears normal in all respects. Experts have recognized that even these transient and very mild conductive hearing losses may affect the development of skills essential to the learning of language. The term ascribed to this set of circumstances is the **minimal auditory deficiency syndrome**.

What may be happening in the young human brain has been demonstrated in the laboratory on experimental animals (see, for example, Webster & Webster, 1977). Within 45 days, mice with conductive hearing loss surgically induced shortly after birth showed smaller neurons in the cochlear nuclei, superior olivary complex, and trapezoid body than did mice in the control group. Katz (1978) reported that the attenuation of sound may produce similar effects in children and contribute to the development of learning disabilities.

Concern over the relationship between language disorders and otitis media was demonstrated by Rentschler and Rupp (1984). These researchers found that 70% of a group of speech- and language-impaired children also had histories of hearing problems, and suggested persistent monitoring of children with middle-ear disorders. They also reported tympanometry to be superior to pure-tone audiometry in finding these disorders.

The relationship between otitis media in children and subsequent language-learning disorders is not without controversy. In a study of 602 preschool children, Allen and Robinson (1984) could not demonstrate a statistical relationship between the two. However, like Ventry (1980), they recommended continued research because such a link may have profound effects if proved to exist. A commonsense approach dictates that audiologists should recognize the potential for language disorders secondary to early otitis media, and should monitor hearing losses and counsel families of affected children.

As many as eight parameters may affect language learning when acoustic input is inconsistent to the young child (Skinner, 1978). The magnitude of the problems caused by early acoustic deprivation is not completely known, but it is a matter that should be recognized by physicians, teachers, parents, and audiologists. Prevention and early cure of otitis media are the obvious avenues to follow. Failing this, early diagnosis of associated problems must be made to provide appropriate remediation to children suffering from the effects of minimal auditory deficiency syndrome.

TESTS FOR CENTRAL AUDITORY DISORDERS

Lesions in the auditory nerve and cochlear nuclei produce obvious and dramatic hearing symptoms in the ears ipsilateral to the lesions. As stated earlier in this chapter, once the level of the olivary complex is reached, both sides of the brain are involved in the transmission of auditory information. Even massive lesions in the brain may produce either no audiological symptoms or symptoms that are very subtle. For this reason, emphasis must be placed on developing tests that are specifically sensitive to lesions in the central auditory system.

For the most part, tests using pure tones have been unsuccessful in identifying central auditory lesions. Newer insights into diagnosis of this type of disorder have included manipulation of the temporal aspects of the signal, which has been largely ignored in traditional audiometric procedures. Because pure-tone tests have been disappointing, much of the emphasis in diagnosing central auditory disorders has been placed on speech tests. As Keith (1981) points out, tests to evaluate these disorders in children share certain characteristics, including language-dependent administration and scoring.

Performance-Intensity Function Using PB Word Lists

Jerger and Jerger (1971) described the use of the *performance-intensity function for PB words* (PI-PB) as a method of screening for central auditory disorders. Patients with normal hearing sensitivity who show differences in the scores and shapes of the PI-PB curves may be suspected of central disorders.

PB word lists are presented to the patient at a number of levels—for example, 10, 30, 70, and 90 dB above the SRT. The tests are scored and a graph may be drawn for each ear, showing the PB word scores as a function of sensation level.

If a significant difference in scores occurs (20% to 30%), it may be suspected that a central lesion is present on the side of the brain opposite the poorer score. Sometimes "rollover" of the curve occurs; that is, at some point scores begin to decrease as intensity increases (Figure 9.10). Rollover suggests a lesion on the side of the brain opposite the ear with the rollover or a lesion of the VIIIth nerve on the same side. PI-PB functions may not be helpful in detecting central lesions if a loss of hearing sensitivity is also present. The PI function may be drawn on a form, such as that shown in Figure 9.11d. A rollover ratio is derived by the following formula:

$$\text{Rollover ratio } (\%) = \frac{\text{PB Max} - \text{PB Min}}{\text{PB Max}}$$

PB Max is the highest score and PB Min the lowest score obtained at an intensity above that required for PB Max (Jerger & Jerger, 1971). Rollover ratios of .40 suggest cochlear lesions, whereas ratios of .45 or greater indicate an VIIIth nerve site. High rollover ratios are also seen in some elderly patients (Sang, 1976).

There are two factors that must be considered when determining rollover ratios. First, the procedure is not helpful if all speech discrimination scores are low. Second, for the greatest accuracy, a number of levels must be tested; establishing complete performance-intensity functions can be very time-consuming.

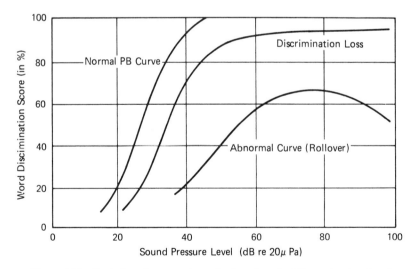

Figure 9.10 Typical performance-intensity functions for PB words, showing the normal increase in speech discrimination scores with increased intensity and the "rollover" (decreased discrimination beyond a certain level) evident in some ears contralateral to a central auditory disorder.

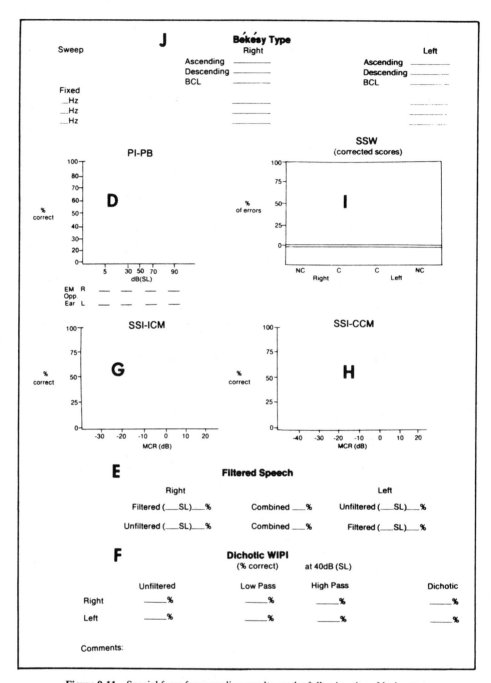

Figure 9.11 Special form for recording results on the following site-of-lesion tests: (D) PI-PB function; (E) filtered speech; (F) dichotic WIPI test for children; (G) SSI-ICM; (H) SSI-CCM; (I) staggered spondaic word test; (J) Békésy audiogram type.

The Rush Hughes Difference Score Test

Most patients with normal hearing sensitivity find speech discrimination tests using traditional PB or CNC materials relatively easy. One such test, recorded in 1948 by Rush Hughes, a professional radio announcer, used the Harvard PB–50 words but was recorded with poor quality and fidelity. Use of these materials with most patients will result in reduced discrimination scores, not because the words themselves are difficult, but because they are distorted. Goetzinger and Angell (1965) found that differences between scores on the more difficult Rush Hughes test and on easier tests of monosyllabic recognition (such as the W–22 word lists) did not normally exceed 20% to 24%, and that when differences exceeded 30%, central auditory deficiency was implied. This procedure has been suggested as a valuable test for central lesions (Goetzinger, 1972).

The *Rush Hughes Difference Score Test* is simply performed by testing speech discrimination monaurally using recorded W–22 word lists at 40 dB above the SRT and the Rush Hughes test at 50 dB above the SRT, or below the uncomfortable loudness level, whichever is lower. Because these levels may be rather high, the nontest ear must frequently be masked with a broad-band noise to avoid its participation in the test.

The difference scores of the two ears are determined by subtracting the Rush Hughes score from the W–22 score. If the scores differ by 30% or more for the same ear when hearing sensitivity is normal, a lesion in the temporal lobe contralateral to the poorer-performing ear is suspected. This procedure has not maintained high acceptance.

Filtered Speech Tests

Although standard tests for speech discrimination do not identify central lesions, distortion of the speech signal presented monaurally often results in reduced speech discrimination scores in the ear contralateral to a central lesion (Bocca & Calearo, 1963). This statement is true if the lesion does not impair the symbolization and memorization processes of the brain, which may result in much more demonstrable symptoms.

Several methods have been used to distort the speech signal for purposes of central auditory tests. Speech has been periodically interrupted, masked, compressed in time, presented at low sensation levels, and filtered. Filtering some frequencies from the speech spectrum has become the most popular of these methods.

A signal may be passed through a filter that rejects the low frequencies and passes the highs (high-pass filter), or one that rejects the high frequencies and passes the lows (low-pass filter). A signal may also be processed through a filter that rejects both high and low frequencies above and below a prescribed range so that only a band of frequencies is allowed through. This is called band-pass filtering and is usually described in terms of the range from the lowest to the highest frequencies passed.

Difficulty in discriminating filtered speech depends largely on the filter characteristics, such as whether the signal is high-pass, low-pass, or band-pass filtered; the cut-off frequency of the filter (the precise frequency above or below which the filtering takes place); and the filter rejection rate (usually expressed in decibels per octave). The steeper the rejection rate, the greater the distortion of the signal. Filtered speech tests may be performed monaurally or binaurally.

The classical work with monaural filtered speech tests was done by Bocca, Calearo, and Cassinari (1954). These researchers used low-pass filtered speech, markedly attenuating frequencies above 800 Hz. Bocca (1967) has suggested that distorted sentence materials are superior to isolated words because they put greater stress on the brain's capacity for pattern recognition.

In temporal lobe lesions, discrimination may be much the same in both ears for unfiltered speech, but it may be markedly poorer in the ear contralateral to the lesion when filtered speech is used. Jerger (1960) found this to be true using low-pass filtered PB words in cases with lesions both in the brain stem and in the temporal lobe. Similar findings for temporal lobe lesions were observed by Antonelli and Calearo (1968) and by Hodgson (1967).

Binaural Audiometry Using Filtered Speech

It has been found (Bocca, 1955) that combining a quiet undistorted signal to one ear with the same signal to the other ear, at a loud level but distorted, yields surprising results when the central auditory pathways are intact. Discrimination for soft speech is naturally poor, as is discrimination for loud distorted speech. When the two signals are presented simultaneously (soft to one ear, distorted to the other), a dramatic increase in discrimination score is observed as the two signals are fused in the brain. No such summation of scores was observed by Jerger (1960) or Calearo (1957) in patients with temporal lobe disorders.

Because no such tests are commercially available, audiologists must prepare their own material. They can do this with little difficulty by using a phonograph or tape recorder to provide the test material, which they then send through a splitter that routes the signal to two channels of a stereo tape recorder. Channel 1 of the recorder is undistorted, and channel 2 is sent through a low-pass filter. Because standardized tests are unavailable, it is difficult to specify cut-off frequency and filter rejection rate; however, Jerger's use of 500 Hz with a 17 dB/octave roll-off in the high frequencies may be satisfactory.

After the binaural tape has been prepared, it can be used to feed the inputs of a two-channel speech audiometer. Channel 1 of the tape recorder is controlled by means of channel 1 of the audiometer, and the signal is presented to one ear; channel 2 of the tape recorder is controlled by channel 2 of the audiometer, and the signal is presented to the other ear.

The test may be performed using the following steps:

1. Soft speech to only one ear. The hearing-level dial may be set to about 10 dB above the SRT.

2. Loud distorted speech to the other ear. The hearing-level dial may be set to about 45 dB above the SRT.
3. Soft speech to one ear simultaneously with loud distorted speech to the other.
4. Repetition of the three procedures just described, reversing the ears that receive the soft and loud speech.

Different word lists are used for each test, and the scores are obtained for each of the conditions.

According to Bocca (1955) and Jerger (1960), the binaural summation expected in normal-hearing subjects is lacking in patients with lesions of the auditory cortex. In such cases the binaural score may not be increased over the better monaural score.

Band-Pass Binaural Speech Audiometry

Matzker (1959) developed a test wherein different filtered portions of a speech signal are presented to each ear. Discrimination for either a low-frequency band-passed signal alone or a high-frequency band-passed signal alone yield very poor speech intelligibility. If the brain stem is normal, the two signals are fused when presented simultaneously. Matzker's low-frequency band was from 500 to 800 Hz, and his high-frequency band was from 1815 to 2500 Hz. Inability to demonstrate this binaural fusion suggests a lesion in the brain stem. Matzker's original materials were German PB words.

Similar work using high and low band-pass filtered speech was done with Japanese materials (Hayashi, Ohta, & Morimoto, 1966) using bands of 300 to 600 Hz and 1200 to 2400 Hz. Franklin (1969) used a rhyme test with passbands of 240 to 480 and 1020 to 2040 Hz. Smith and Resnick (1972) used bands of 360 to 890 Hz and 1750 to 2200 Hz. Palva and Jokinen (1975) used band widths of 420 to 720 Hz and 1800 to 2400 Hz.

The test materials are fed from a phonograph or tape recorder to the two inputs of a stereo tape recorder. One channel is sent through a low-frequency band-pass filter, and the other channel is sent through a high-frequency band-pass filter. After the recording has been made, the two channels of the recorder can then feed the two channels of a speech audiometer.

One method for this test has been described by Smith and Resnick (1969). Using one channel of a two-channel speech audiometer, the low-frequency band of PB words is presented at 30 dB SL. The high-frequency band, controlled by the hearing-level dial of the second channel, is presented 10 dB above the level set for the low band. Three test conditions exist:

1. Low band to the right ear, high band to the left ear (**dichotic**).
2. Low band to the left ear, high band to the right ear (dichotic).
3. Both bands to both ears (**diotic**).

The Smith and Resnick (1972) procedure using CNC words, which they call DBF (dichotic binaural fusion), has gained some clinical prominence. There appear to be no differences in the three scores in patients with normal hearing, cochlear lesions, or lesions of the temporal lobe. Patients with brain stem disorders show significant diotic score enhancement over one or both of the dichotic scores.

The test designed by Palva and Jokinen (1975) also utilizes three test conditions with two narrow bands of filtered words. Each band alone, of course, yields very low discrimination scores. Results are obtained (1) with both bands in the right ear; (2) with both bands in the left ear; and (3) with the high band in the right ear and the low band in the left ear. Patients with disorders of the auditory cortex show poor scores on the monaural test in the ear contralateral to the lesions, although their dichotic scores are good. Patients with brain stem lesions show poor scores in any of the three conditions, especially the one involving binaural fusion. Data on filtered speech tests can be recorded on a form like the one in Figure 9.11E.

Martin and Clark (1977) employed a comparison of diotic and dichotic presentations of the WIPI test to young children so that a picture-pointing procedure could be used as a screening test for children with auditory-processing disorders. They found that diotic presentation improved the learning-disabled children's discrimination scores by 10% and that a control group did about as well on the more difficult dichotic task as on the diotic one. This procedure appears to have merit as a screening test for children who show normal hearing on standard audiometric procedures but whose histories suggest the possibility of central deficits. For those who fail the test, referral must be made for indepth testing by professionals expert in language disorders (see Figure 9.11F).

Synthetic Sentence Identification Tests

The Synthetic Sentence Identification (SSI) test described in Chapter 4 may be used to identify lesions of the central auditory system. The sentences are made more difficult to identify by using a competing message, a recording of continuous discourse. This may be an *ipsilateral competing message (ICM)*, which is presented to the test ear along with the synthetic sentences, or it may be a *contralateral competing message (CCM)*, which is presented to the opposite ear. With the test materials (SSI) fixed at a given sensation level, the competing message may be varied in intensity so that a number of message-to-competition ratios (MCRs) are obtained (Jerger, 1973).

To perform the SSI-ICM test, a series of synthetic sentences is presented to one ear. The competing message is presented to the same earphone at a number of MCRs, beginning at +10 dB (the sentences 10 dB stronger than the competition) and increasing the intensity of the competition until the percentage of sentences identified correctly drops to 20%. The test is then repeated in the other ear.

According to Jerger (1973) normal-hearing persons will perform at the 100% level with an MCR of 0 dB, 80% with an MCR of −10 dB, 55% with an MCR of −20 dB, and 20% with an MCR of −30 dB (competing message 30 dB above the sentences). On this test, patients with lesions of the brain stem show large differences in scores between the right and left ears. With an increase in the level of the competing message, scores deteriorate more rapidly than normal when the test is performed in the ear contralateral to the lesion. For example, for a patient with a lesion of the left brain stem, SSI-ICM scores will be poorer in the right ear than in the left ear (see Figure 9.11G).

The SSI-CCM test is performed in precisely the same manner as the SSI-ICM, the only difference being that the competing message is presented to one ear and the sentences are presented to the opposite ear. The MCR is varied up to −40 dB.

Persons with normal hearing will perform very well on the SSI-CCM test, even at MCRs of −40 dB. The competition of the other ear seems to have little effect on the ability to understand the synthetic sentences. Patients with lesions of the temporal lobe perform well when the sentences are presented to the ear on the same side as the lesion while the competing message is presented to the other ear. When the sentences are presented to the ear on the unimpaired side and the competition is presented to the ear on the same side as the cortical lesion, deterioration of scores ensues. For example, in a left cortical lesion, SSI scores will be good with sentences in the left ear and competition in the right ear, but scores will be poor with sentences in the right ear and competition in the left ear. Jerger (1973) therefore believes that the use of ipsilateral and contralateral competing messages with the synthetic sentence identification test not only reveals central disorders, but actually separates out lesions of the brain stem from those in the cortex (see Figure 9.11H).

Competing Sentence Tests

Building on work begun a decade earlier, Williford (1977) has reported on the use of natural sentences in diagnosing central auditory disorders. The CST (Competing Sentence Test) is made up of natural sentences and, unlike the SSI procedure, uses an open-message set. To make the procedure useful, of course, a competing message is presented to the opposite ear.

The primary message is presented at a level 35 dB above the pure-tone average (PTA) while the competing message is presented at 50 dB above the PTA. Both sentences are of the same length and on the same subject (e.g., time, food, weather, family). Fifteen sentences are usually used. The patient is told to repeat only the primary (softer) sentence. Because many brain-injured patients have difficulty in attending to soft stimuli or those under conditions of adverse message-to-competition ratios, modifications of the original method have been developed (Bergman, Hirsch, Solzi, & Mankowitz, 1987). Examples of the CST are included in the Appendix.

Patients with lesions of the temporal lobe show the greatest difficulty when the primary sentence is presented to the ear contralateral to the lesion. Simple versions of the procedure have been used successfully to identify children with learning disabilities. Children tend to improve on this test as they get older, which is not surprising because the central auditory nervous system probably continues to mature until about nine years of age.

Rapidly Alternating Speech Perception (RASP)

A test has been designed that rapidly alternates six- or seven-word sentences between the ears (see Williford, 1977). The sentences, presented at 50 dB above the SRT, are switched back and forth every 300 milliseconds. Twenty sentences are presented. In order for the patient to understand and repeat the sentences, brain stem function must be normal, because any segment presented to one ear alone is presumably too short to allow discrimination. The procedure is called the **rapidly alternating speech perception (RASP) test.**

The Dichotic Digits Test

Musiek (1983) describes a version of the **dichotic digits test** as being useful for diagnosing both brain stem and cortical disorders, although it may not be possible to tell one lesion site from the other on the basis of this test alone. Twenty sets of two-digit pairs are presented at 50 or 60 dB above the SRT. The digit 7 is omitted because it is the only one that has two syllables. The patient hears two successive pairs of two digits and is asked to repeat all four digits. The test can also be carried out using three-digit pairs but may result in low scores in some individuals due to short-term memory difficulties. For this reason, Mueller (1987a) believes that the two-digit pair test is probably better for detection of lesions in the central auditory nervous system.

The Staggered Spondaic Word (SSW) Test

Katz (1962, 1968) developed a test of dichotic listening that has undergone more standardization on English-speaking adults than most of the other tests for central auditory disorders, and has been shown to differentiate between normal children and those with learning disabilities (Berrick, Shubow, Schultz, Freed, Fournier, & Hughes, 1984). The **staggered spondaic word (SSW) test** is a measure of dichotic listening that utilizes spondees in a suprathreshold manner. Pairs of different spondaic words are presented to each ear, with some timing overlap for both ears. The first syllable of one spondee is presented to one ear; and, while the second syllable is presented, the first syllable of the other spondee is presented to the other ear. Then the second syllable of the second spondee is presented alone. This procedure is diagrammed as shown.

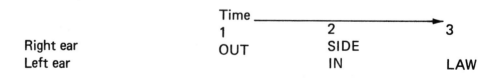

The words are recorded on two channels of a stereo tape for independent control by a two-channel speech audiometer. The items are presented so that the competing and noncompeting messages are reversed in terms of which ear is stimulated first. For example, the test may be begun as

Right (noncompeting)—Right (competing)—Left (noncompeting)

The order of the ear receiving the first spondee is alternated throughout the test, which contains forty items and takes about 20 minutes to complete.

The SSW test was designated to be performed at a level 50 dB above the SRT. If a PI-PB function has been determined, the SSW test may be delivered at the intensities in each ear at which PB Max was found. Using the PB Max intensity eliminates problems in speech discrimination posed by high-frequency peripheral hearing losses (Mueller, 1987b) or in patients with loudness tolerance problems.

During the SSW test, the patient is simply asked to repeat both spondees. Practice items are presented before the test is begun to ensure that the patient understands this unusual task. Because the SSW test is performed at relatively high sensation levels, if a hearing loss exists in one ear, no matter how mild, there is a chance that the better ear may, by contralateralization, aid in discriminating words presented to the poor ear. Naturally, the very nature of this test precludes the use of masking, but insert receivers might be useful in increasing the interaural attenuation for speech.

Scoring and interpreting the SSW test requires a special form, which is available commercially with the recording.[1] Individual errors are summed first for each ear, both for competing and noncompeting words. The total SSW score is the total number of errors obtained for both ears. Each monosyllable is given a weight of 2.5%, and the total of incorrect responses times 2.5% is subtracted from 100% to give the percentage of correct responses. In order to avoid penalizing the patient's SSW score for peripheral discrimination difficulties, the speech discrimination loss for PB words is credited to each ear by subtracting the percentage error for PB words from the percentage error on the SSW test for the same ear. Poor scores on the SSW test suggest a lesion in the higher brain centers on the side contralateral to the low-scoring ear (see Figure 9.11). Although the SSW test is very popular, one lasting complaint has been with the amount of time needed to follow the complex scoring system. At least one computer program is now available for this purpose. Mueller (1987b) has suggested that diagnosis using the SSW test may be carried out simply by computing the score for each ear on the basis of the percentage of words identified correctly.

Masking-Level Difference

The phenomenon of binaural release from masking or **masking-level difference (MLD)** has been known for some time (Hirsh, 1948). To determine the MLD, the binaural threshold is determined for a low-frequency tone pre-

---

[1]AUDITEC of St. Louis, 402 Pasadena Avenue, St. Louis, MO 63119.

sented in phase to the two ears in the presence of a binaural noise, also in phase. When the threshold is remeasured with the tones 180 degrees out of phase with the noise, a threshold improvement is found on the order of 10 to 15 dB. Abnormal MLDs in normal-hearing subjects strongly suggest a brain stem lesion (Noffsinger, Martinez, & Schaefer, 1985), but positive findings have also been observed in cases of acoustic neuroma, presbycusis, Ménière's disease, and particularly multiple sclerosis (Mueller, 1987a). MLDs have also been measured using speech signals.

Although the effects of cochlear and cortical lesions on MLD are somewhat unpredictable, there is general agreement among researchers (e.g., Olsen & Noffsinger, 1976) that the release from masking is either absent or significantly less than normal in patients with lesions in the brain stem. If the clinician has access to a device capable of shifting the phase of the pure tone without affecting the phase of the noise, simply measuring several binaural pure-tone thresholds may provide additional insight into site of lesion. The procedure is complicated by any degree of peripheral hearing loss.

Time Compressed Speech

Using special recording devices, it is possible to speed up the playback of speech stimuli without significantly creating the perception of higher vocal pitch. This **time compressed speech** has been studied using the PB words from the NU–6 lists. Central auditory lesions are best identified at 60% time compression (Kurdziel, Noffsinger, & Olsen, 1976). Kurdziel and co-workers found that in some brain lesions, time compressed speech discrimination scores were poor in the ear contralateral to the lesion, whereas in other cases scores remained normal in both ears. There has not been much information in the recent literature on the use of time compressed speech in cases of central auditory nervous system damage.

Acoustic Reflex Test

Comparison of ipsilateral and contralateral acoustic reflexes is perhaps of greater value in determining the integrity of the crossover pathways in the trapezoid body of the brain stem. If, for example, a patient has normal hearing and normal ipsilateral acoustic reflexes in both ears, it is highly probable that the cochleas, the VIIth and VIIIth cranial nerves, and the middle-ear mechanisms are intact on both sides. If, in the same individual, the contralateral reflexes are absent, the most likely explanation is that damage exists within those crossover pathways (see Figures 5.11i and j.)

Auditory Evoked Potentials

Auditory brain stem response audiometry has been useful in diagnosing central auditory disorders as long as any hearing loss in the two ears is essentially symmetrical and no more than a mild loss exists in either ear (Musiek,

1983). The presence of concomitant peripheral lesions may confound inter-pretation of ABR results if lesions are present in both the cochlea and the brain stem. Central lesions will generally slow the conduction velocity of electrical impulses sent through the nerve fibers. Musiek (1983) suggests the following general observations:

Wave I (all waves) delay Lesion in outer, middle, or inner ear
Wave I–III delay Lesion in auditory nerve or lower brain stem
Wave III–V delay Lesion in higher brain stem

In testing for lesions of the brain stem, it is useful to compare the latencies and intervals of waves I, III, and V as a function of increasing click rates. Although the ABR results may provide important diagnostic information in testing for central auditory lesions, interpretation can be difficult when it is complicated by the absence of some waves, the influence of unusual audiometric configurations, and the patient's age and body temperature.

Authorities on the subject of diagnosis of auditory brain stem lesions tend to agree with Musiek, Gollegly, Kibbe, and Verkest (1988) that the ABR is generally the most sensitive and specific test currently available for this purpose, but that the use of the complete central test battery is also extremely important (Jerger, Neely, & Jerger, 1980; Musiek & Geurking, 1982).

The P–300, or cognitive potential of the late auditory evoked response is elicited by an "oddball" paradigm, whereby the subject tries to discriminate between a frequently occurring stimulus and a rarely occurring stimulus. For example, a 1000 Hz tone burst may be presented 80% of the time, while a 2000 Hz tone burst is presented randomly 20% of the time. The subject is asked to count only the higher pitched tones. The waveform elicited by the rare (2000 Hz) stimulus shows a large positive peak with a latency of approximately 300 milliseconds. Reduction in amplitude or increase in the latencies of the P–300 have been found in elderly individuals, those suffering from dementia, and head trauma patients. This procedure is thought to hold future promise as a diagnostic procedure for other disorders of the central auditory nervous system.

SUMMARY

This chapter has dealt with the function and audiological diagnosis of lesions in the auditory nerve and central auditory nervous system. Although consid-erable mystery continues to surround the auditory system, nowhere is this mystery greater than in the higher auditory pathways. Impulses that pass from the cochlea are transmitted by means of the auditory nerve to the cochlear nuclei, which are waystations for transmission to higher centers and areas for complex frequency analysis. The cochlear nuclei also represent the highest centers at which the processing of neural stimuli represent auditory information obtained from just one ear. From the cochlear nuclei, auditory information is processed by the superior olivary complexes, the lateral lemnisci, the inferior colliculi, and the medial geniculate bodies. Impulses are finally transmitted to the cortex by the auditory radiations. Owing to the numerous decussations at higher centers, there is representation of each ear on both sides of the brain, with greater representation on the contralateral side.

Caution should always be exercised when an audiologist attempts to determine the site of a lesion affecting the auditory system. A patient may, for example, have both a cochlear and a central disorder. Most auditory tests give results that reflect primarily the first lesion reached by the stimulus (the most peripheral lesion) but can be further complicated by the more central lesion. Ruling out one anatomical area of the auditory system should not result in a diagnosis of a lesion in a specific region elsewhere.

Behavioral tests for site of lesion may be positive in patients with lesions of the auditory nerve and cochlear nuclei. However, lesions at the higher centers produce more subtle symptoms and are often insensitive to currently used tests. Special procedures have been devised for testing central disorders, but none has been demonstrated to be infallible. Much research is needed to improve techniques for detecting disorders in the central pathways and pinpointing the area of damage. There is little doubt that this is one of the most challenging areas for research in diagnostic audiology.

GLOSSARY

Acoustic neuritis Inflammatory or degenerative lesions of the auditory nerve.

Acoustic neuroma A tumor involving the nerve sheath of the auditory nerve.

Auditory nerve The VIIIth cranial nerve, which comprises the auditory and vestibular branches, passing from the inner ear to the brain stem.

Auditory radiations A bundle of nerve fibers passing from the medial geniculate body to the temporal gyri of the cerebral cortex.

Cerebellopontine angle (CPA) That area at the base of the brain at the junction of the cerebellum, medulla, and pons.

Cerebellum The lower part of the brain above the medulla and the pons. It is the seat of posture and integrated movements in the brain.

Cerebrovascular accident (CVA) A clot or hemorrhage of one of the arteries within the cerebrum. A stroke.

Commissure Nerve fibers connecting similar structures on both sides of the brain.

Computed tomography (CT) A procedure for imaging the inside of the body by representing portions of it as a series of sections. The many pictures taken are resolved by computer, and the amount of radiation to the patient is significantly less than with older procedures.

Decussation A crossing over, as of nerve fibers connecting both sides of the brain.

Dichotic Stimulation of both ears by different stimuli. This is usually accomplished under earphones from two channels of a tape recorder.

Dichotic digits test A test for central auditory disorders performed by presenting two pairs of digits simultaneously to both ears.

Diotic Stimulation of both ears with stimuli that are approximately identical, as through a stethoscope.

Dorsal cochlear nucleus The smaller of two cochlear nuclei on each side of the brain; it receives the fibers of the cochlea on the ipsilateral side.

Extra-axial Outside the brain stem.

Heschl's gyrus See *Superior temporal gyrus*.

Inferior colliculus One of the central auditory pathways, found in the posterior portion of the midbrain.

Internal auditory canal A channel from the inner ear to the brain stem allowing passage of the auditory and vestibular branches of the VIIIth nerve, the VIIth nerve, and the internal auditory artery.

Intra-axial Inside the brain stem.

Kernicterus Deposits of bile pigment in the central nervous system, especially the basal ganglia. It is associated with erythroblastosis and the Rh factor.

Lateral lemniscus That portion of the auditory pathway running from the cochlear nuclei to the inferior colliculus and medial geniculate body.

Magnetic resonance imaging (MRI) A system of visualizing the inside of the body without the use of X-rays. The body is placed in a magnetic field and is bombarded with radio waves, some of which are reemitted and resolved by computer, which allows for viewing of soft tissues and various abnormalities.

Masking level difference (MLD) The binaural threshold for a pure tone is lower when a binaural noise is 180 degrees out of phase than when the noise is in phase between the two ears.

Medial geniculate body The final subcortical auditory relay station, found in the thalamus on each side of the brain.

Medulla oblongata The lowest portion of the brain, connecting the pons with the spinal cord.

Minimal auditory deficiency syndrome Changes in the size of neurons in the central auditory nervous system caused by conductive hearing loss in early life. The result is difficulty in language learning.

Multiple sclerosis (MS) A chronic disease showing hardening or demyelinization in different parts of the nervous system.

Neoplasm Any new or aberrant growth, as a tumor.

Neurofibromatosis (NF) The presence of tumors on the skin or along peripheral nerves. Also called von Recklinghausen's disease.

Olivocochlear bundle (OCB) A grouping of nerve units in the brain stem that course to the cochlear nuclei and terminate in the cochleas. Efferent fibers from the OCB provide inhibitory connections to the auditory neurons.

Pneumoencephalography A method of visualizing the lower portions of the brain with X-rays by bubbling air up the spinal column and removing the cerebrospinal fluid.

Pons A bridge of fibers and neurons that connect the two sides of the brain at its base.

Rapidly alternating speech perception (RASP) test A test for central auditory disorders in which sentences are rapidly switched from the left ear to the right. Normal brain stem function is required for discrimination.

Reticular formation Located in the brain stem, the reticular formation communicates, with all areas of the brain and contains centers for inhibition and facilitation of afferent stimuli.

Staggered spondaic word (SSW) test A test for central auditory disorders utilizing the dichotic listening task of two spondaic words presented so that the second syllable presented to one ear is heard simultaneously with the first syllable presented to the other ear.

Superior olivary complex (SOC) One of the auditory relay stations in the mid-brain, largely comprising units from the cochlear nuclei.

Superior temporal gyrus The convolution of the temporal lobe believed to be the seat of language comprehension for the auditory system.

Temporal lobe The part of the cerebral hemispheres usually associated with perception of sound. The auditory language areas are located within the temporal lobes.

Thalamus Located in the brain base, the thalamus sends projecting fibers to and receives fibers from all parts of the cortex.

Time compressed speech A system of recording speech so that it is accelerated and therefore distorted, but the words remain discriminable.

Tonotopic Arranged anatomically according to best frequency of stimulation.

Trapezoid body Nerve fibers in the pons that connect the ventral cochlear nucleus on one side of the brain with the lateral lemniscus on the other side.

Ventral cochlear nucleus The larger of the two cochlear nuclei on each side of the brain; it receives the fibers of the cochlea on the ipsilateral side.

STUDY QUESTIONS

1. Sketch from memory the auditory pathways arising from the cochlea. Label the different waystations, and specify as far as you can the functions of each.
2. Make a list of the possible causes of hearing disorders at each of the sites just named.
3. Draw an audiogram typical of an VIIIth nerve lesion. List the results of as many site-of-lesion tests as you can remember.
4. Why are lesions of the central auditory nervous system subtle and difficult to observe on standard audiometric tests?

5. List the tests that may be performed for central auditory lesions. Discuss the shortcomings of each test listed.
6. What is evoked response audiometry? List the tests that can be done with this procedure and the areas of the auditory system involved.

REVIEW TABLE 9.1 AUDIOLOGICAL SYMPTOMS OF RETROCOCHLEAR LESIONS

VIIITH NERVE AND COCHLEAR NUCLEI	CENTRAL PATHWAYS
Negative SISI	Poor binaural fusion
No recruitment; decruitment	Low SSI-ICM scores
Marked tone decay at all frequencies	Low SSI-CCM scores
Rapid acoustic reflex decay	Increased wave III–V interval
Elevated or absent acoustic reflexes	SDS for distorted speech poor in ear
Marked increase in ABR wave V latencies	contralateral to the lesion
Békésy Type III or IV	
SDS for distorted speech poor in ear ipsilateral to lesion	

REFERENCES

ALLEN, D. V., & ROBINSON, D. O. (1984). Middle ear status and language development in preschool children. *Asha, 26,* 33–37.

ANDERSON, H., BARR, B., & WEDENBERG, E. (1969). Intra-aural reflexes in retrocochlear lesions. In C. A. Hamberger & J. Wersall (Eds.), (pp. 49–55). *Disorders of the skull base region.* New York: Wiley.

ANTONELLI, A., & CALEARO, C. Further investigations on cortical deafness. *Acta Otolaryngologica* (Stockholm), *66,* 97–100.

BERGMAN, M., HIRSCH, S., SOLZI, P., & MANKOWITZ, Z. (1987). The threshold-of-interference test: A new test of interhemispheric suppression in brain injury. *Ear and Hearing, 8,* 147–150.

BERRICK, J. M., SHUBOW, G. F., SCHULTZ, M. C., FREED, H., FOURNIER, S. R., & HUGHES, J. P. (1984). Auditory processing tests for children: Normative and clinical results on the SSW test. *Journal of Speech and Hearing Disorders, 49,* 318–325.

BLAKELY, R. W. (1959). Erythroblastosis and hearing loss: Responses of athetoids to tests of cochlear function. *Journal of Speech and Hearing Research, 2,* 5–15.

BOCCA, E. (1955). Binaural hearing: Another approach. *Laryngoscope, 65,* 1164–1175.

———. (1967). Distorted speech tests. In A. B. Graham (Ed.), *Sensorineural hearing processes and disorders* (Henry Ford Hospital International Symposium). Boston: Little Brown.

BOCCA, E., & CALEARO, C. (1963). Central hearing process. In J. Jerger (Ed.), *Modern Developments in Audiology* (pp. 337–370). New York: Academic Press.

BOCCA, E., CALEARO, C., & CASSINARI, V. (1954). A new method for testing hearing in temporal lobe tumors: Preliminary report. *Acta Otolaryngologica* (Stockholm), *44,* 219–221.

CALEARO, C. (1957). Binaural summation in lesions of the temporal lobe. *Acta Otolaryngologica* (Stockholm), *47,* 392–395.

CARHART, R. (1967). Audiologic tests: Questions and speculations. In F. McConnell & P. H. Ward (Eds.), *Deafness in childhood* (pp. 229–251). Nashville, TN: Vanderbilt University Press.

FRANKLIN, B. (1969). The effect on consonant discrimination of combining a low-frequency passband in one ear and a high-frequency passband in the other ear. *Journal of Auditory Research, 9*, 365–378.

GANG, R. P. (1976). The effects of age on the diagnostic utility of the rollover phenomenon. *Journal of Speech and Hearing Disorders, 41*, 63–69.

GOETZINGER, C. P. (1972). The Rush Hughes test in auditory diagnosis. In J. Katz (Ed.), *Handbook of clinical audiology* (pp. 325–333). Baltimore: Williams & Wilkins.

GOETZINGER, C. P., & ANGELL, S. (1965). Audiological assessment in acoustic tumors and cortical lesions. *Eye, Ear, Nose and Throat Monthly, 44*, 39–49.

GOODHILL, V. (1950). Nuclear deafness and the nerve-deaf child: The importance of the Rh factor. *Transactions of the American Academy of Ophthalmology and Otolaryngology, 54*, 671–687.

HAYASHI, R., OHTA, F., & MORIMOTO, M. (1966). Binaural fusion test: A diagnostic approach to the central auditory disorders. *International Audiology, 5*, 133–135.

HIRSH, I. (1948). The influence of interaural phase on interaural summation and inhibition. *Journal of the Acoustical Society of America, 23*, 384–386.

HODGSON, W. (1967). Audiological report of a patient with left hemispherectomy. *Journal of Speech and Hearing Disorders, 32*, 39–45.

JERGER, J. (1960). Observations on auditory behavior in lesions of the central auditory pathways. *Archives of Otolaryngology* (Chicago), *71*, 797–806.

———. (1973). Diagnostic audiometry. In J. Jerger (Ed.), *Modern developments in audiology* (2nd ed.) (pp. 75–115). New York: Academic Press.

JERGER, J., & JERGER, S. (1971). Diagnostic significance of PB word functions. *Archives of Otolaryngology, 93*, 573–580.

JERGER, J., NEELY, J., & JERGER, S. (1980). Speech, impedance and auditory brainstem response audiometry in brainstem tumors. *Archives of Otolaryngology, 106*, 218–223.

JERGER, J., OLIVER, T. A., & JENKINS, H. (1987). Suprathreshold abnormalities of the stapedius reflex in acoustic tumors. *Ear and Hearing, 8*, 131–139.

JERGER, S., & JERGER, J. (1975). Extra- and intra-axial brain stem auditory disorders. *Audiology, 14*, 93–117.

JOHNSON, E. W. (1977). Auditory test results in 500 cases of acoustic neuroma. *Archives of Otolaryngology, 103*, 152–158.

JOSEY, A. F., GLASSCOCK, M. E., & MUSIEK, F. E. (1988). Correlation of ABR and medical imaging in patients with cerebellopontine angle tumors. *The American Journal of Otology, Supplement, 9*, 12–16.

KATZ, J. (1962). The use of staggered spondaic words for assessing the integrity of the central auditory nervous system. *Journal of Auditory Research, 2*, 327–337.

———. (1968). The SSW test: An interim report. *Journal of Speech and Hearing Disorders, 33*, 132–146.

———. (1978). The effects of conductive hearing loss on auditory function. *Asha, 20*, 879–886.

KEITH, R. W. (1981). Tests of central auditory function. In R. J. Roeser & M. P. Downs (Eds.), *Auditory disorders in school children* (pp. 159–173). New York: Thieme-Stratton.

KURDZIEL, S., NOFFSINGER, D., & OLSEN, W. (1976). Performance by cortical lesion patients on 40 and 60% time compressed materials. *Journal of the American Audiology Society, 2*, 3–7.

MARTIN, F. N., & CLARK, J. G. (1977). Audiologic detection of auditory processing disorders in children. *Journal of the American Audiology Society, 3*, 140–146.

MATKIN, N. D. (1965). *Audiological patterns characterizing hearing impairment due to Rh incompatibility*. Unpublished doctoral dissertation, Northwestern University.

MATZKER, J. (1959). Two new methods for the assessment of central auditory functions in cases of brain disease. *Annals of Otology, Rhinology and Laryngology, 68,* 1185–1197.

MUELLER, H. G. (1987a). An auditory test protocol for evaluation of neural trauma. *Seminars in Hearing, 8,* 223–238.

————. (1987b). The staggered spondaic word test: Practical use. *Seminars in Hearing, 8,* 267–277.

MUSIEK, F. E. (1983). The evaluation of brainstem disorders using ABR and central auditory tests. *Monographs in Contemporary Audiology, 4,* 1–24.

MUSIEK, F. E., & GEURKING, N. A. (1982). Auditory brainstem response (ABR) and central auditory test (CAT) findings for patients with brainstem lesions: A preliminary report. *Laryngoscope, 92,* 891–900.

MUSIEK, F. E., GOLLEGLY, K. M., KIBBE, K. S., & VERKEST, S. B. (1988). Current concepts on the use of ABR and auditory psychophysical tests in the evaluation of brain stem lesions. *The American Journal of Otology, 9,* 25–35.

NOFFSINGER, D., MARTINEZ, C., & SCHAEFER, A. (1985). Puretone techniques in evaluation of central auditory function. In J. Katz (Ed.), *Handbook of clinical audiology* (3rd ed.) (pp. 337–354). Baltimore: Williams & Wilkins.

OLSEN, W. O., & NOFFSINGER, D. (1976). Masking level differences for cochlear and brainstem lesions. *Annals of Otology, Rhinology and Laryngology, 85,* 820–825.

PALVA, A., & JOKINEN, K. (1975). The role of the binaural test in filtered speech audiometry. *Acta Otolaryngologica, 79,* 310–314.

POOL, J. I., PAVA, A. A., & GREENFIELD, E. C. (1970). *Acoustic nerve tumors: Early diagnosis and treatment* (2nd ed.). Springfield, IL: Thomas.

RASMUSSEN, G. L. (1960). Efferent fibers of the cochlear nerve and cochlear nucleus. In G. I. Rasmussen & W. F. Windle (Eds.), *Neural mechanisms of the auditory and vestibular systems* (pp. 105–115). Springfield, IL: Thomas.

————. (1964). Anatomic relationships of the ascending and descending auditory systems. In W. S. Fields & B. R. Alford (Eds.), *Neurological aspects of auditory and vestibular disorders* (pp. 5–23). Springfield, IL: Thomas.

RENTSCHLER, G. J., & RUPP, R. R. (1984). Conductive hearing loss: Cause for concern. *Hearing Instruments, 35,* 12–14.

SKINNER, P. H. (1978). Electroencephalic response audiometry. In J. Katz (Ed.), *Handbook of clinical audiology* (pp. 311–327). Baltimore: Williams & Wilkins.

SMITH, B., & RESNICK, D. (1969). *An auditory test for assessing brain stem integrity: Preliminary report.* Paper presented at the annual convention of the American Speech and Hearing Association, Chicago.

————. (1972). An auditory test for assessing brain stem integrity: Preliminary report. *Laryngoscope, 82,* 414–424.

TELIAN, S. A., & KILENY, P. R. (1988). Pitfalls in neurotologic diagnosis, *Ear and Hearing, 9* (1988), 86–91.

VENTRY, I. M. (1980). Effects of conductive hearing loss: Fact or fiction. *Journal of Speech and Hearing Disorders, 45,* 143–156.

WEBSTER, D. B., & WEBSTER, M. (1977). Neonatal sound deprivation affects brain stem auditory nuclei. *Archives of Otolaryngology, 103,* 392–396.

WILLIFORD, J. A. (1977). Differential diagnosis of central auditory dysfunction. *Audiology: An Audio Journal for Continuing Education, 2.*

SUGGESTED READINGS

MAUE-DICKSON, W. (1981). The auditory nerve and central pathways, Prenatal development. In F. N. Martin (Ed.), *Medical Audiology* (pp. 371–392). Englewood Cliffs, NJ: Prentice-Hall.

MOORE, B. C. J. (1982). *An introduction to the psychology of hearing.* New York: Academic Press.

WHITFIELD, I. C. (1967). *The auditory pathway.* Baltimore: Williams & Wilkins.

Part 4:   Special Problems in Audiology

10

PSEUDOHYPACUSIS

The past four chapters have discussed anatomical areas within the auditory system and hearing losses associated with lesions in each of these areas.   The term **pseudohypacusis** describes the apparent loss of hearing sensitivity without organic disorder to explain the loss or with insufficient pathological evidence to explain the extent of the loss.

The source of patient referral, history of hearing loss, symptoms, and behavior both during and outside of hearing tests are factors to be considered before making a diagnosis of pseudohypacusis.   Patients whose hearing losses appear to be exaggerated may manifest these symptoms because they are incapable of more reliable behavior, because they are willfully fabricating or exaggerating a hearing disorder, or because they have some psychological disorder.   Observation of the patient and special tests for pseudohypacusis often lead the audiologist to the proper resolution of the problem.

CHAPTER OBJECTIVES

This chapter should alert the reader to the problem of false or exaggerated hearing loss and some of the symptoms that make its presence known.   The terms associated with this condition should be learned, as should the special tests that qualify and quantify it.

TERMINOLOGY

Not all audiologists and other specialists concerned with hearing use the term **pseudohypacusis**. Some prefer **nonorganic hearing loss**, which suggests that some or part of a claimed hearing disorder is not the direct result of an organic disorder of the hearing system. Another popular term is **functional hearing loss**. The word *functional* is often used by physicians and psychologists to describe the symptoms of a condition that is not organic. Although the term *functional* may be used to express any kind of a nonorganic disorder, the word *pseudohypacusis* has been coined to relate specifically to hearing loss. Some audiologists use the term **psychogenic** (beginning in the mind) **hearing loss** to express a nonorganic problem whose cause is psychological rather than deliberately feigned. An older term for psychogenic hearing loss is **hysterical deafness**.

One term, probably used far too often, is **malingering**. A malingerer is a deliberate falsifier of physical or psychological symptoms for some special gain. The slang military term *goldbrick* has been used to describe those persons who use the pretense of some disability to avoid undesired duty. Malingering is also frequently suspected in association with automobile and industrial accidents, when the payment of sums of money may be involved to compensate patients for damages. Many patients who are called malingerers actually have a hearing loss but exaggerate its severity to increase their gains.

Although *pseudohypacusis* and *nonorganic hearing loss* are the terms used in this book, the reader should be aware of other terminology and should know that terms such as *nonorganic hearing loss*, *functional hearing loss*, and *pseudohypacusis* are general and do not suggest cause as do the terms *malingering* and *psychogenesis*. There is no way to know for certain whether a patient with a nonorganic hearing loss (or any other kind of nonorganic disorder, for that matter) is malingering, has a psychogenic problem, or suffers from some combination of the two. Unless the patient admits to lying, or the confirmed diagnosis of psychogenicity is made by a qualified psychologist or psychiatrist, the audiologists should settle for more general terms.

PATIENTS WITH PSEUDOHYPACUSIS

Patients manifesting symptoms of pseudohypacusis may be of any age, sex, or socioeconomic background. It is probable that more adult males have been suspected of this disorder because emphasis has been placed on eliminating its possibility among men applying to the Veterans Administration for compensation for hearing loss.

Ross (1964) has described the development of nonorganic hearing loss in children under some circumstances. Very often, children with normal hearing inadvertently fail the screening tests performed in public schools. There are many reasons for failure to respond during a hearing test besides hearing loss:

Equipment may malfunction, instructions may be misunderstood, ambient room noise may produce masking at threshold, patients may have difficulty in following instructions, and so on. Children may find that as soon as school and parental attention focus on a possible hearing problem, they begin to enjoy a degree of gain in the form of favors, excuses for poor grades, and special attention. By the time some children are seen by hearing specialists, they may be committed to perpetuating the notion that they have hearing losses. Ross believes that public school referrals to otologists or audiologists should be made only after the individual responsible for the screening is fairly certain that a hearing loss is present.

There is probably a myriad of reasons why individuals might show evidence of pseudohypacusis. If a patient is, in fact, malingering or deliberately exaggerating an existing hearing loss, the motivation may be nothing more than financial gain. Other reasons may simply be to gain attention or to avoid performing some undesirable task. Because the underlying reasons for psychogenic hearing loss are more difficult to understand, this problem has been considered a form of **conversion neurosis**. Whatever the dynamics of nonorganic hearing loss, they may be deeply enmeshed in the personality of the patient, and a cursory look at them in any single book must be recognized for its superficiality.

Signs of Pseudohypacusis

There are many signs that alert the audiologist to pseudohypacusis. These include the source of referral, the patient's history, behavior during the interview, and performance on routine hearing tests. Some patients are so overt in their symptoms of nonorganicity that they are easily recognized, even by nonprofessional personnel. At times the nonorganic patient is the comic caricature of a hard-of-hearing person, appearing to have no peripheral vision when approached in the waiting room, and so on. Other patients with nonorganic problems show no such easily recognized signs.

When a patient is referred to an audiology center with the specification that there is compensation involved, nonorganicity immediately becomes of prime concern. Such referrals may be made by the Veterans Administration, insurance companies, attorneys, or physicians. To be sure, only a small number of such patients show nonorganic behavior. The incidence of nonorganic hearing loss in this group, however, is bound to be higher than in the general population.

When patients indicate a specific incident as the cause of their hearing loss, and stand to gain financially if hearing loss is proved, the audiologist's suspicion is likely to be raised. Often such patients' histories do not suggest nonorganicity, but it exists nevertheless. In many cases the manner in which information is volunteered by the patient is as revealing as the actual data. The audiologist should be alert for exaggerated hearing postures, extremely heavy and obvious reliance on lip-reading, and so on.

Performance on Routing Hearing Tests

One of the first clues to pseudohypacusis is inconsistency on hearing tests. The test-retest reliability of most patients with organic hearing loss is usually quite good, with threshold differences rarely exceeding ±5 dB. When audiologists find differences in pure-tone or speech thresholds that exceed this value, they must conclude that one or both of these measures is wrong. Sometimes, of course, the cause of such inconsistency is wandering attentiveness, and bringing the matter to the patient's attention solves the problem. In any case, the patient should be advised of the difficulty, and increased cooperation should be solicited.

One of the most common symptoms of nonorganicity is incompatibility between the pure-tone average and the SRT. In audiograms that are generally flat, the agreement should be within 5 to 10 dB. If the audiometric configuration becomes irregular, as in the sharply falling high-frequency hearing loss, the SRT may be closer to the two-frequency average or even at or better than the best of the three speech frequencies. In older patients or those suffering from abnormalities of the central auditory nervous system, the SRT is sometimes poorer than the pure-tone average. When the SRT is better than the pure-tone average, without an explanation such as audiometric configuration, nonorganicity is likely.

That the pseudohypacusic patient often shows inconsistencies between thresholds for speech and pure tones is understandable. If, for example, a person were "malingering" a hearing loss, the objective would be to respond consistently to sounds above threshold as if they were at threshold. Patients must therefore remember how loud a signal was the last time they heard it so that they can respond when the sound reaches the same level again. This is why test–retest is often so revealing. Some nonorganic patients have an uncanny ability to replicate their previous responses to speech or pure tones, but they fail in equating the loudness of the two. When spondees and pure tones are presented at the same intensities, the spondees appear louder, probably because the energy is spread over a range of frequencies.

Performance on other-than-threshold tests is sometimes helpful in detecting nonorganic hearing loss. The audiologist might wonder why a patient with a sensorineural hearing loss has excellent speech discrimination. To be consistent on this test, the nonorganic patient may merely count the number of words and remember how many were deliberately missed.

Determination of acoustic reflex thresholds was discussed in Chapter 5, and the results of this test on different kinds of auditory lesions were described in the four chapters that followed. Except in cases of cochlear damage, the acoustic reflex threshold is expected to be at least 65 dB above the behavioral threshold. When the reflex threshold is less than 10 dB above the voluntary threshold, nonorganic hearing loss is a probability (Lamb & Peterson, 1967).

Another suggestion of nonorganicity comes from the apparent lack of cross-hearing in unilateral cases. Considerable attention was paid in Chapters 3 and 4 to contralateralization of pure tones and speech. When individuals feign a loss of hearing in one ear without the knowledge of cross-hearing, they often give responses showing normal hearing in one ear and a profound (or total) loss, exceeding the normal values of interaural attenuation, for the other ear (Figure 10.1A). A lack of cross-hearing is especially noticeable for bone conduction, where any interaural attenuation is negligible. In fact, a truly profound loss of hearing in one ear would appear as a conductive hearing loss; the air-conduction thresholds would be obtained from the nontest ear with about 55 dB lost to interaural attenuation, resulting in the appearance of a fairly flat air-conduction audiogram of about 55 dB HL, with bone conduction in the normal range (Figure 10.1B). The bone-conduction signals delivered to the poor ear would be heard in the better ear at normal levels (0 to 15 dB HL) since there is virtually no interaural attenuation for bone conduction. A true, total unilateral loss is demonstrated audiometrically only with masking in the normal ear (note the masked symbols used in the audiogram shown in Figure 10.1C).

Many audiologists have noted a peculiar form of response from some nonorganic patients during SRT tests. Often these persons will repeat only

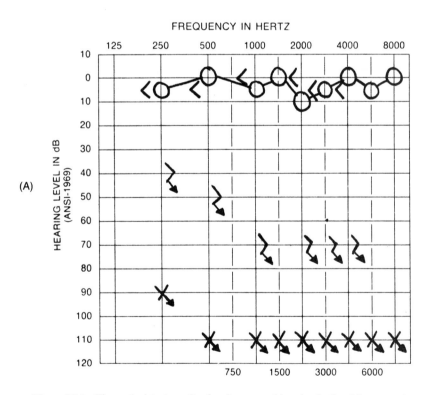

Figure 10.1 Theoretical test results showing normal hearing in the right ear and (A) a false total loss of hearing in the left ear (no evidence of cross hearing); (B) a true total loss of hearing in the left ear showing tones cross-heard in the right ear, giving the appearance of a conductive loss; and (C) a total loss of hearing in the left ear with proper masking performed in the right ear.

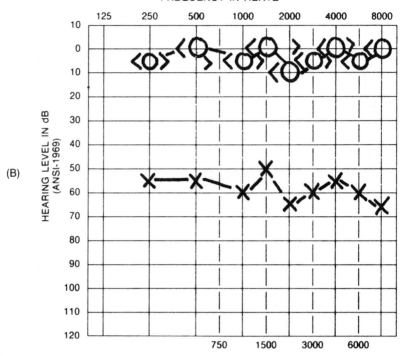

(B)

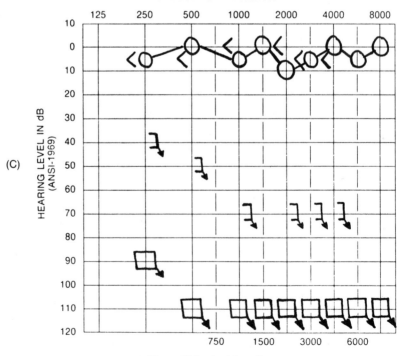

(C)

Figure 10.1 (*continued*)

half of each spondee at a number of intensities—for example, "hot" (for *hotdog*) or "ball" (for *baseball*). Why this occurs has not been explained, but it has been reported fairly often.

Suspicion of nonorganic hearing loss is by no means proof. If nonorganicity is suspected, it must be investigated further with great caution, using special diagnostic tests.

TESTS FOR PSEUDOHYPACUSIS

The primary purpose of special tests for pseudohypacusis is to provide information about the patient's hearing, even in cases in which cooperation is lacking. Behavioral tests for nonorganic hearing loss may be performed with pure tones or with speech. Some tests may be carried out with the usual diagnostic audiometer, and other tests require special equipment. Unfortunately, many of the tests are merely qualitative; that is, they produce evidence of nonorganicity but do not reveal the threshold of hearing. Other tests are quantitative and reveal information about the patient's actual thresholds.

The Stenger Test

The **Stenger test** was designed for use with unilateral hearing losses. This test is based on the Stenger principle, which states that when two tones of the same frequency are introduced simultaneously into both ears, only the louder tone will be perceived. The test works best when there is a large difference (at least 25 dB) between the admitted thresholds of the two ears. The Stenger test may be carried out on a two-channel audiometer. A single pure-tone source may be split and controlled by two separate hearing-level dials, or tones may be generated by two separate oscillators. If two oscillators are used, the tones must be locked in phase to avoid beats.

The thresholds of each ear for the desired frequencies are obtained first. Then, using one channel of the audiometer, a tone is introduced 10 dB above the threshold of the "better" ear. A response should always be obtained. A tone is then presented 10 dB below the threshold of the "poorer" ear. A response will be absent. There are two possible reasons that patients may not respond to the tone in their poorer ear. The first, obviously, is that they may not hear it. The second is that they may be unwilling (or psychologically unable) to respond to a tone that they do in fact hear. At this point, both tones are introduced simultaneously, 10 dB above the better-ear threshold reading and 10 dB below the poorer-ear threshold reading.

If patients fail to respond, it is because they hear the tone in the poorer ear, which they do not wish to admit. They will be unaware of the tone in the better ear, owing to the Stenger effect, and so will not respond at all. This is called a *positive Stenger*. If the patient responds when both ears are stimulated, this is called a *negative Stenger* and suggests the absence of nonorganicity, at least at the frequencies tested.

If a positive result is found on the Stenger test, more quantitative information may be obtained. This is done by presenting the tone at 10 dB above the threshold for the better ear and at 0 dB HL in the poorer ear. With successive introductions the level of the tone in the poorer ear is raised in 5 or 10 dB steps. The patient should always respond because the 10 dB SL tone in the better ear provides clear audibility. If responses cease, the level of the tone in the poorer ear should be noted.

The lowest intensity which produces the Stenger effect is called the **minimum contralateral interference level**. This level may be within 20 dB of the actual threshold of patients with pseudohypacusis. Although some clinicians always perform the Stenger test by finding the minimum contralateral interference level, use of the screening procedure described first in this section often saves considerable time when Stenger results are negative.

A negative result on the Stenger test is fairly conclusive evidence that there is no significant nonorganic component in the "poorer" ear. The test is useful only in unilateral cases and works best when the threshold in the better ear is normal and a large difference exists between the admitted thresholds of the two ears. A positive Stenger tells the audiologist that the threshold results obtained in the poorer ear are inaccurate, but it does not reveal the true organic thresholds, although they may be approximated.

The Speech Stenger Test

The *speech Stenger test* may be carried out with spondaic words in exactly the same fashion as with pure tones. The principle is unchanged and requires that spondees be presented by means of a two-channel speech audiometer.

The SRTs are obtained for each ear, using channel 1 for one ear and channel 2 for the other ear. Spondees are then presented 10 dB above the better-ear threshold, 10 dB below the level recorded as threshold for poorer ear, and finally at these levels simultaneously. The test is best performed using monitored live voice, so that the proper pacing can be accomplished.

Criteria for positive and negative on the speech and pure-tone Stenger tests are identical. Patients' failure to repeat words presented below the admitted threshold of the poorer ear suggests that they really do hear the words loudly enough to make them unaware that the words are presented above the threshold of the better ear at the same time.

Like the pure-tone Stenger test, the modified version often helps to identify the presence of nonorganic hearing loss but may not reveal the precise organic threshold of hearing. Positive results on this test, however, will encourage the audiologist to perform other tests to identify the true SRT. The speech Stenger test has the advantage over the pure-tone version in that there is no need for concern over the two tones beating. Determination of the minimum contralateral interference level for spondees may be made to help in estimating the SRT.

The Doerfler-Stewart Test

The **Doerfler-Stewart (D-S) test**, a confusion test that uses spondaic words and sawtooth noise, is named for the audiologist and engineer who devised it (1946). The test is performed binaurally and is contrived to confuse patients by presenting noise in their ears so that they lose their "loudness yardsticks" if their intentions are to respond consistently to the words above threshold as though they were at threshold. Menzel (1960) has recommended that the Doerfler-Stewart test be performed early in the battery of hearing tests to discourage nonorganicity in those patients whose intention it is to malinger.

The D-S test is usually performed using monitored live voice. After the first SRT is determined, patients are presented with a series of spondaic words to which they are instructed to reply. The presentation level is 5 dB above the first SRT. A noise is introduced into both ears along with the words and is increased in intensity in 5 dB steps with each word presentation. If the patient stops repeating words, the level of the noise is recorded as the *noise interference level* (NIL). The level of noise is increased and the level of the words decreased. If the limit of the audiometer is reached, the clinician begins to attenuate the noise in 5 dB steps until 0 dB HL is reached.

A second SRT is obtained and a threshold for the noise is determined (called the *noise detection threshold* or NDT). A set of norms for the differences among SRT_1, SRT_2, $SRT_1 + 5$, NIL, and NDT has been set up by Doerfler and Epstein (1956), but each audiometer should be calibrated to determine the values for NIL and NDT. When the extremes of these norms are exceeded on two or more measures, the test is considered positive and suggests that the true SRT of the patient is lower than what is volunteered.

The main problem with the D-S test is that, although it often indicates the presence of nonorganicity, it does not tell its extent, nor does it reveal the true SRT. The test is binaural and is therefore eliminated in unilateral cases. When speech discrimination scores are poor, either real or feigned, the patient may appear unable to repeat 100% of a list of spondees at any sensation level.

The Lombard Test

The **Lombard test** is based on the familiar phenomenon that people increase their vocal levels when they speak in a background of noise. If a noise is presented to the ears of speakers who do not hear the noise, they will not change the loudness of their voices. If, however, the level of a person's voice goes up as noise is added, it is obvious that the noise is audible to that person.

The subject is positioned with air-conduction receivers over both ears and is asked to read or speak aloud. A neatly typed paragraph helps to avoid some difficulties professed during performance of this kind of test. As the subject reads, a masking noise added to both ears is gradually increased in intensity. The examiner listens for increased vocal loudness. To help detect this loudness increase, the subject may be asked to read into a microphone, which is fed into the VU meter of the speech audiometer being used. The gain on the VU meter may be adjusted so that the speaker's voice peaks around −5 VU. Any increases in the loudness of the reader's voice can then be observed visually as an increase in the value of the peaks on the VU meter.

If there is an increase in the loudness of the subject's voice, noted by observing the peaks on a VU meter, it can be said that the noise was at least loud enough to cause this voice reflex. No change in loudness might suggest that the noise was not heard or was not loud enough to cause the reflex. Surely a person with a 90 dB loss of hearing should not show a positive result on the Lombard test at 75 dB, and nonorganic hearing loss is immediately suspected in such a case. Beyond this, interpretation of the Lombard test must be made only in a general way.

As was implied, the Lombard test is not a strong test for nonorganic hearing loss. All attempts at finding normal values—that is, how many decibels above threshold a noise must be to cause the reflex—have failed. Some people begin to show some changes at 25 or 30 dB above threshold, and others may speak or read with noise at 100 dB SL in both ears with no noticeable changes in the loudness of their voices.

Delayed-Speech Feedback Test

People monitor the rate and loudness of their speech through a variety of feedback mechanisms—for example, tactile, proprioceptive, and auditory feedback. Auditory feedback is probably dominant. After a phoneme is uttered, it is processed through the auditory system and the next phoneme is cued. The **side-tone** built into the ordinary telephone amplifies speakers' voices so that they hear themselves in the receivers of their own telephones along with the voices of the people with whom they speak. Some telephone side-tones are louder than others.

If a person's voice is recorded on magnetic tape, delayed 0.1 to 0.2 seconds, and played back, this **delayed auditory feedback (DAF)** causes subjects to alter their speech patterns, in some ways creating an effect similar to stuttering. Speakers may slow down, prolong some syllables, increase their loudness, or find it very difficult to speak at all. The creation of delayed feedback audiometry was inevitable as a test for nonorganic hearing loss, for surely a speaker's voice played back with a short delay can have no effect on speech production unless it is heard.

For this test, the subjects may be placed before a microphone, preferably in the patient room of a two-room audiometric suite. They wear a pair of air-conduction receivers. A prepared text that is easy to read and that can be completed in one-half to one minute is provided. The subjects are instructed to read the passage aloud and then to pause for a cue from the examiner, whereupon they read the passage aloud again, and so on. The first one or two readings should be allowed with no feedback, and the reading time should be recorded with a stopwatch. The VU meter of a speech audiometer should be adjusted so that the subject's word peaks average about −5 VU.

The delayed-speech portion of the test is begun after the preliminary steps. The test may be performed in both ears or one ear, with or without the nontest ear masked. The intensity of the signal is controlled by the hearing-level dial of a speech audiometer and is first set at 0 dB HL. After each reading, the level is raised 10 dB until a positive result is seen. A positive result is defined as any change in the reading rate (sped up or slowed down by more than 3 to 5 seconds for a short passage), an increase in vocal intensity as seen on the VU meter (the Lombard effect), or obvious hesitations or prolongations on syllables or words.

In many ways, speech DAF is interpreted like the Lombard test. When changes occur in speaking rate, it must be assumed that subjects have heard their own voices and that this has had an effect on their monitoring systems. If this effect is noted at a low hearing level, it is assumed that hearing is probably normal or near normal, at least for the low and middle frequencies. Some speech changes have been observed as low as 10 dB above the SRT.

Some persons can tolerate delayed-speech feedback at very high sensation levels with no apparent breakdowns in their speech and voice patterns. Others are apparently much more susceptible to distraction by their own slightly delayed voices. As in so many tests, positive results on speech DAF are much more meaningful than negative results. When persons have difficulty reading or speaking under the DAF condition, this must mean that they have heard the signal at the level at which it was presented. Some patients' reading abilities are so bad that the test must be abandoned.

Pure-Tone Delayed Auditory Feedback Test

The principle of delayed auditory feedback has been applied to pure tones. Ruhm and Cooper (1964) devised a technique whereby subjects tap a pattern on a silent switch with their preferred index finger. The pattern may be two taps, pause, four taps, pause, two taps, and so on. The patient's arm is placed inside a sleeve or is otherwise hidden from view. The arm is placed with the forearm down so that tapping is done primarily with the finger. In this way the subjects are deprived as much as possible of visual, tactile, and auditory feedback of their tapping performance.

Patients are seated so that they cannot see the controls on the DAF apparatus. A two-room arrangement works well for this test. Patients are instructed on how to tap on the switch and are then asked to demonstrate this ability to the examiner. Earphones are placed over the ears and the test is begun.

The DAF device is instrumented so that, if properly keyed, a brief tone (50 milliseconds) is presented to the subject's ear via an air-conduction earphone 200 milliseconds after each tap. The short delay from the tap on the key to the audibility of the tone causes subjects to modify their tapping behavior in several ways. Pure-tone DAF subjects may change their tapping rates (tap faster or slower), increase their tapping pressure on the switch, or change the rhythm or the number of their taps (e.g., from a pattern of two and four to a pattern of one and three, etc.).

A tone of desired frequency is presented by means of the audiometer through which the DAF device is keyed. The starting level should be 0 dB HL. Several tapping patterns are allowed between each increase in intensity, which is done in steps of 5 dB. The DAF threshold is the level at which any alteration of tapping performance is noted. Responses may be monitored auditorily by the examiner, or a readout may be obtained on a graphic recorder that shows the tapping performance, including in some cases, tapping pressure.

Ruhm and Cooper (1962) found that positive results on pure-tone DAF tests occur at sensation levels as low as 5 dB. The tone must be slightly above threshold for it to be audible 100% of the time. When positive results are seen, the examiner may infer that the patient's hearing threshold is no poorer than 5 dB below the DAF threshold.

Of all the tests described so far in this section, pure-tone DAF comes closest to doing what is necessary, identifying the patient's true organic threshold. Occasionally patients are seen who cannot or will not tap consistent patterns. In such cases the test cannot be performed.

Békésy Audiometry

Jerger's four types of Békésy tracings, described in Chapter 5, were illustrated for several kinds of disorder in Chapters 6 through 9. Jerger and Herer (1961) described a fifth type of tracing, wherein the pulsed-tone threshold appears to be poorer (is lower on the audiogram) than the continuous-tone threshold. Because no organic pathology is associated with such a pattern, and because this Type V tracing was first observed among patients with nonorganic hearing loss, Type Vs and nonorganicity have become associated with each other.

A number of writers have reported Type V tracings as being symptomatic of nonorganic hearing loss. When individuals are trying to respond consistently at some suprathreshold level, they must remember how loud the tone was the last time they responded. Subjects must set up their own internal standards for the loudness of a tone to be traced. For subjects with normal hearing, more intensity is required for pulsed tones than for continuous tones for the tones to appear equally loud at levels above threshold (Rintelmann & Carhart, 1964).

Hattler (1970) found that the Type V pattern was accentuated when he used a **lengthened off time (LOT)**. Instead of using the normal pulse rate of 200 milliseconds on and 200 milliseconds off, Hattler used 200 milliseconds on and 800 milliseconds off. He found that Type V patterns often appeared with this arrangement, whereas they did not with the normal 50% duty cycle. The other four Békésy patterns were unaffected by the lengthened off time.

Finding that the Type V pattern did not always appear in cases of nonorganic hearing loss, Hood, Campbell, and Hutton (1964) developed a procedure called **BADGE,** an acronym for **Békésy Ascending Descending Gap Eval-**

uation. The procedure involves the use of a fixed frequency, comparing three Békésy tracings alleged to be threshold. The first trace is obtained with a continuous tone, called a *continuous ascending* (CA) tone, that increases in intensity from 0 dB HL. The second trace is made with a *pulsed ascending* (PA) tone. The third and last trace, obtained with the tone set at 30 dB above the PA reading, is called *pulsed descending* (PD). A number of patients with nonorganic hearing loss showed sharp differences on these three one-minute tracings, which should have been identical in an organic hearing loss. Nonorganic patients who did not exhibit Type V tracings showed positive BADGE results. This comparison of ascending and descending thresholds had been described much earlier, using a conventional audiometer as a test for nonorganic hearing loss (Harris, 1958).

At this time very few clinics perform Békésy audiometry as a routine procedure (Martin & Morris, 1989). When Békésy audiometry is performed in determining site of lesion, the audiologist may be surprised by unusual or even bizarre patterns that lead to the diagnosis of pseudohypacusis. Type V tracings have also been found among patients with true organic hearing losses (Hopkinson, 1965), and so such tracings should not lead to an unqualified diagnosis of pseudohypacusis. Positive results on the LOT or BADGE test do not provide information about the patient's threshold and should be examined carefully in light of other hearing tests.

Performance of tracking behavior on an automatic audiometer requires more attention and cooperation than some patients can muster. Such tracking behavior is undoubtedly influenced by a number of interrelated factors, such as physiological and psychological readiness, fatigue, boredom, motivation, and personality. Békésy audiometry may overlook some patients with pseudohypacusis, and it may suggest that others with true organic disorders are showing some nonorganic behavior. Unless audiologists are faced with collecting evidence of nonorganic hearing loss, their primary concern is determining threshold, which is not obtainable using the Békésy audiometric procedures just described.

Swinging Story Test

Another way of confusing a patient who alleges a unilateral hearing loss is to administer the **swinging story test**. The patient is asked to listen to a story, parts of which are presented to the better ear, parts to both ears, and parts to the poorer ear. The story is read so rapidly that it is difficult for the listener to be certain what information was obtained from which ear. This test requires the use of a two-channel speech audiometer with a switch that allows for rapid switching to the left ear, right ear, or binaural position. A two-room audiometric setup is essential. Although the swinging story test is generally performed using monitored live voice, it can be prerecorded on a stereophonic tape.

Patients are advised only that they will be told a story and that they are to repeat all of the story that they can remember. The earphones are positioned

Bad Ear	Both Ears	Good Ear
1.	Lyon stalked dangerous prey	in the jungle
2. carrying his rifle confidently.	His animal instincts	and years of experience
3. enhanced by schooled intelligence	led him confidently	through the thicket.
4. Jim Lyon had been	long known as	the cleverest hunter in the jungle.
5. Except for those	on four feet.	Lyon never came home unsatisfied
6. or empty-handed.	Deer were his favorite prey	because of their succulent meats
7. and handsome pelts.		

Figure 10.2 Example of a swinging story test. (Courtesy of Ms. Mary Ann Mastroianni.)

over both ears, and the test is begun. The examiner reads (or plays through a tape recorder) one of the swinging stories, a sample of which is shown in Figure 10.2. The hearing-level dials are set so that the story will be presented 10 dB above the threshold of the better ear and 10 dB below the threshold of the poorer ear. At the completion of the test the patient is asked to repeat the story.

If the patient includes any information provided to the poorer ear only, the conclusion must be drawn that hearing in that ear is below the admitted SRT.

The swinging story test is obviously limited to unilateral cases. This test must be performed only after considerable experience if monitored live voice is to be used, because it obviously requires a great deal of dexterity and sophistication on the part of the examiner. Unfortunately, this test does not identify the true threshold in the poor ear, but it does demonstrate graphically to patients, without otherwise discussing the situation, that, if they are deliberately feigning or exaggerating a unilateral hearing loss, the examiner is aware of it. Slight modifications of the swinging story test allow it to be performed in bilateral cases by presenting the story 10 dB above and 10 dB below the SRT.

Electrophysiological Tests

Nothing could be better suited to the testing of pseudohypacusic patients than procedures that would require no voluntary responses. If the audiologist could make a determination of auditory threshold in such a manner, the very lack of required cooperation would tend to discourage patients from attempting to malinger. Some tests are available that have been designed with this objective in mind.

Acoustic Reflex Tests. An addition to the many uses already described for acoustic immittance meters is a method of estimating hearing sensitivity for patients who are unwilling or unable to cooperate. Following up on some earlier work on differential loudness summation, Jerger, Burney, Mauldin, and Crump (1974) developed what has come to be known as **Sensitivity Prediction from the Acoustic Reflex (SPAR)**.

The SPAR test is based on the fact that acoustic reflex thresholds get lower as the signal band width gets wider. Stated differently, a normal-hearing person will require greater intensity for a pure-tone than for a wide-band noise to elicit the reflex. The usual difference is about 25 dB. Patients with sensorineural hearing losses of mild to moderate degree show only a 10 to 20 dB difference, whereas patients with moderately severe losses show less than a 10 dB difference. Of course, patients with profound losses will show no acoustic reflex for either stimulus. To estimate the degree of hearing loss, the acoustic reflex thresholds (in dB SPL) at 500, 1000, and 2000 Hz are averaged and compared to the threshold for the broad-band noise.

Electrodermal Audiometry. **Electrodermal audiometry (EDA)** combines the use of Pavlovian conditioning with measurements of the psychogalvanic response. It has been known for some time that the skin serves as a conductor of electricity. By placing electrodes on the surface of the skin at two neighboring points, as at two adjacent fingertips, the electricity can be amplified and studied in terms of its electrical conductance (the Tarchinov effect) or electrical resistance (the Fere effect). For purposes of audiometry, resistance has been the more popular phenomenon studied. Skin resistance is measured in electrical ohms.

The introduction of a tone to a subject's ear may result in a drop in skin resistance, which can be read on a meter attached to a **Wheatstone bridge**. After several tonal presentations, however, the reflex disappears through adaptation. Bordley and Hardy (1949) were the first to apply psychogalvanometry to audiometry. They reasoned that by pairing a tone presented through an earphone with a small electrical shock delivered by electrodes to the fingers of the hand opposite the pickup electrodes, the patient could be conditioned to respond to the tone. Because the shock always results in a drop in resistance, tones could be followed by shocks until the subject associated the two. This conditioning, similar to the conditioning of Pavlov's dogs, results in a drop in skin resistance following a tone, even if no shock is presented. Pavlov, it will be remembered, rang a bell before presenting a piece of meat to a dog. After several such pairings, the dog was observed to salivate after hearing the bell, even without seeing or smelling the meat. In the case of EDA the electrical shock is called the *unconditioned stimulus* (UCS) because it will always evoke a response, and the tone is called the *conditioned stimulus* (CS) because it will not produce a drop in skin resistance without conditioning by pairing it with electrical shocks. The skin resistance change is called the electrodermal response (EDR). Electrodermal audiometry follows the usual learning paradigm: *stimulus* (tone), *response* (EDR), *reinforcement* (shock). Adhering to a rigid conditioning and reinforcement schedule increases the usefulness of electrodermal audiometry.

The first application of the EDR procedure to speech audiometry, or **electrodermal speech reception threshold (EDSRT)**, was made by Ruhm and Carhart (1958) and was applied to patients with nonorganic hearing loss shortly thereafter (Ruhm & Menzel, 1959). The procedure differs from the pure-tone method in that spondaic words are used as the stimuli. Using speech requires not only that the stimulus be heard by the subject, but that it be properly discriminated in order for a conditioned response to be obtained. In this way an SRT can be obtained with no cooperation on the part of the patients except that they remain awake and relatively motionless.

The days of EDA as a popular test have passed. This is partly true because the validity of the test is highly suspect in many cases. In addition, recent legislation protects individuals from being forced to receive noxious stimuli, such as electric shocks. Electrodermal audiometry has been called **objective audiometry**. It may be objective in the sense that patients do not play a voluntary role in stating when they hear a stimulus. Interpretation of responses, however, is a highly subjective matter.

Auditory Evoked Potentials (AEP). The use of AEP audiometry, described in Chapter 5, lends itself nicely to examining difficult-to-test patients, especially those with suspected pseudohypacusis. It is probable that auditory brain stem response (ABR) audiometry is increasing in popularity for such purposes (e.g., Beagley, 1973).

Naturally, the value of AEPs is determined largely by the expertise of the examiner. A procedure like ABR may have a deterring effect on pseudohypacusic behavior because patients should recognize early in the examination that determination of hearing ability may be made without their active cooperation. Of course, it must also be remembered that the stimuli used in ABR testing (clicks or tone pips) do not allow for accurate determination of threshold for discrete frequencies.

Other Confusion Tests

Often tests are administered that are designed to confuse patients suspected of nonorganic hearing loss in hopes they will abandon their lack of cooperation. A series of tones may be introduced above and below the voluntary threshold, and the patient may be asked to count the tones and tell the number that were heard (Ross, 1964). This becomes a problem for pseudohypacusic patients because they have to remember which tones they are willing to admit to hearing. The same procedure may be used to pulse the tones rapidly from one ear to the other in a unilateral case. The tones should be above the threshold of the "better" ear and below the admitted threshold of the "poorer" ear (Nagel, 1964).

The "yes–no" method described by Frank (1976) is often useful in finding pure-tone thresholds for children. The child is instructed to say "yes" when a tone is heard and "no" when a tone is not heard. An ascending method is used. Many children falsifying test results will say "no" coincidentally with tonal presentation below their admitted thresholds. This method is easy and fast and makes life simpler for the audiologist, when it works. Naturally, the more sophisticated patients are, the less likely they are to be tripped up by such an obvious subterfuge.

Nonorganic hearing loss may be identified by use of a standardized test for lip-reading ability (Utley, 1946), often with excellent results. The patient may be seated facing the examiner through the observation window separating the patient room from the control room. Lights in the patient room should be dimmed to eliminate glare. The patient wears the earphones of a speech audiometer and is given one form of the test with the hearing-level dial set well below admitted threshold but above the level estimated as threshold by the audiologist. A different form of the test is given in identical fashion but with the microphone switched off. Patients often do considerably better on the test when they hear, possibly because they are eager to prove they are good lip-readers.

MANAGEMENT OF THE PATIENT WITH PSEUDOHYPACUSIS

Creating an open confrontation with a pseudohypacusic patient rarely results in improved test validity. After all, cooperation is hardly forthcoming in the presence of hostility. Clinicians may advise the patient that test inconsistencies exist, but they should try to shift the "blame" for this to their own shoulders, using such explanations as, "Perhaps I did not make it clear to you that you are to raise your hand even if the tone is very soft. You have been waiting until the tone is relatively loud. I am sorry that I did not make this clearer before, but let us try again." This provides patients with an honorable way out, which they often take.

As may be seen from the preceding section of this chapter, a number of tests for pseudohypacusis are at the disposal of the audiologist. In most cases it is not difficult to uncover nonorganicity. Many tricks have been used. For example, audiologists may cover their mouths when speaking to a patient who professes to rely on lip reading. Patients may be given instructions through a speech audiometer below their admitted SRTs such as, "Remove the earphones, the test is over." Any movement of the hands toward the receivers tells the audiologist that the patient has heard the instruction and reacted before realizing that it was below the admitted threshold.

The greatest problem in dealing with pseudohypacusic patients concerns the determination of the true threshold and how to manage the cases. If all patients with pseudohypacusis were liars, whose dishonesty was motivated by greed or laziness, perhaps the job would be easier. It is possible, however, that many patients with nonorganic problems may be deeply troubled. As stated earlier some hearing losses may be entirely feigned, others merely exaggerated, and still others produced on an unconscious level.

One of the temptations that all professional persons must avoid in working with handicapped patients is that of making value judgments. Although we may be curious about the psychodynamics of a given situation, we cannot play psychiatrist with a patient suspected of having a psychogenic hearing loss. We also cannot play prosecutor, no matter how convinced we are that a patient is malingering. Malingering can be proved without question only if the patient admits to it.

If it is suspected that a nonorganic hearing loss is present, it may be an unwise practice to draw the audiogram. Too many persons are prone to glancing at the red and blue lines with no study of the actual results and what they mean. When nonorganicity is suspected, it may be better to write "pseudohypacusis" across the audiogram to force anyone reading it to look more carefully at the report that should accompany the results of any hearing evaluation. In writing reports, audiologists should avoid the word *malingering*, but they should not hesitate to say *pseudohypacusis* or *nonorganic hearing loss* if they believe this to be the case. Referrals to psychiatrists or psychologists are sometimes indicated, but they should be made very carefully. Exactly how a patient should be advised of test results is an individual matter and must be dictated by the experience of the audiologist.

SUMMARY

Many patients seen in audiology clinics manifest symptoms of nonorganic hearing loss. They may be malingering, exaggerating hearing losses, or have psychogenic disorders. There may also be other reasons for test results to be inaccurate. The responsibility of the audiologist is to determine the true organic thresholds of hearing, even if this must be done with less than the full cooperation of the patient.

A number of tests are available that can be performed when pseudohypacusis is suspected. Some of these tests merely confuse patients and provide evidence of nonorganicity; they might also convince the patients that they must be more cooperative. Other tests actually help determine auditory thresholds.

There is evidence (Martin & Monro, 1975; Martin & Shipp, 1982; Monro & Martin, 1977) that knowledge about the principles underlying some audiometric measures may assist the patient in "beating" a test or symptom. Some procedures are more resistant to practice or sophistication than are others. Audiologists must consider these factors in working with pseudohypacusic patients.

The audiologist has an obligation to serve the patient, even when the patient is uncooperative. The problems of writing reports and counseling are much greater with patients with nonorganic hearing loss than with those showing no evidence of this condition.

GLOSSARY

Békésy Ascending Descending Gap Evaluation (BADGE)   A test for nonorganic hearing loss using the Békésy audiometer.   The subject who exaggerates pure-tone thresholds is confused by the fact that tracings are begun above and below threshold, pulsed, and continuous.

Conversion neurosis   A Freudian concept by which emotional disorders become transferred into physical manifestations (e.g., hearing loss, blindness, etc.)

Delayed auditory feedback (DAF)   The delay in time between a subject's creation of a sound (e.g., speech) and his or her hearing of that sound.

Doerfler-Stewart (D-S) test   A test for nonorganic hearing loss using spondaic words and sawtooth noise.

Electrodermal audiometry (EDA)   A procedure for testing the hearing of some patients using an auditory signal as a conditioned stimulus and an electric shock as an unconditioned stimulus.

Electrodermal speech reception threshold (EDSRT)   The speech reception threshold obtained by using a single spondaic word as the conditioned stimulus, using the EDA paradigm.

Functional hearing loss   See *Nonorganic hearing loss.*

Hysterical deafness   An older term for *Psychogenic hearing loss.*

Lengthened off time (LOT)   A procedure for nonorganic hearing loss using the Békésy audiometer.   By increasing the off time of the automatically pulsed tone, Type V Békésy patterns become exaggerated.

Lombard test   A test for nonorganic hearing loss based on the vocal reflex (i.e., a speaker will increase the loudness of speech when a loud noise interferes with normal auditory monitoring.)

Malingering   The conscious, willful, and deliberate act of feigning or exaggerating a disability (such as hearing loss) for personal gain or exemption.

Minimum contralateral interference level   On the Stenger test, the lowest intensity of a signal presented to the poor ear that causes that patient to stop responding to the signal which is above threshold in the better ear.

Nonorganic hearing loss   The exaggerated elevation of auditory thresholds.

Objective audiometry   Procedures for testing the hearing function that do not require behavioral responses from the subject when the signal is heard.

Pseudohypacusis   See *Nonorganic hearing loss.*

Psychogalvanic response   The change in the electrical skin resistance or potential of the skin in response to an unconditioned stimulus (e.g., electrical shock) or a conditioned stimulus (e.g., a pure tone).

Psychogenic hearing loss   A nonorganic hearing loss produced at the unconscious level, as by an anxiety state.

Sensitivity Prediction from the Acoustic Reflex (SPAR)   Prediction of approximate degree of hearing impairment based on the level of pure tones versus a broad-band noise required to elicit the acoustic reflex.

Side-tone The feedback system, as in a telephone, whereby a speaker hears and monitors his or her own speech as it is uttered.

Stenger test A test for unilateral nonorganic hearing loss based on the Stenger principle.

Swinging story test A test for unilateral nonorganic hearing loss. Portions of a story are presented to the ''better'' ear, ''poorer'' ear, and both ears. If the patient repeats information presented below the admitted threshold of the poorer ear, this is prima facie evidence that the hearing loss in that ear is exaggerated.

Wheatstone bridge A device for measuring the electrical resistance of a circuit (as the skin in electrodermal audiometry). It consists of a conductor that joins two branches of a circuit.

STUDY QUESTIONS

1. What are the first symptoms of pseudohypacusis you might notice? How do they manifest during the nontest situation and the test situation?
2. Make a list of pure-tone tests for nonorganic hearing loss. Separate them into groups according to ease of performance, necessity for special equipment, identification of threshold, and so on.
3. Repeat question 2 for speech tests.
4. Consider the concepts of malingering, exaggeration, and psychogenicity as they relate to hearing loss.
5. What are the advantages and disadvantages of ABR audiometry in the diagnosis of pseudohypacusis?

SUGGESTED READING

MARTIN, F. N. (1986). The pseudohypacusic. In J. Katz (Ed.), *Handbook of Clinical Audiology* (3rd ed.) (pp. 742–765). Baltimore: Williams & Wilkins.

REVIEW TABLE 10.1 SUMMARY OF TESTS FOR PSEUDOHYPACUSIS

NAME OF TEST	TYPE OF SIGNAL		SPECIAL EQUIPMENT REQUIRED	TYPE OF LOSS		ESTIMATES THRESHOLD
	PURE TONE	SPEECH		UNILATERAL	BILATERAL	
Auditory brain stem response audiometry	X		X	X	X	X
Békésy audiometry	X			X	X	
Confusion tests	X	X		X	X	
Delayed pure-tone feedback	X	X	X	X	X	X
Delayed-speech feedback		X	X	X	X	
Doerfler-Stewart test		X			X	
Electrodermal audiometry	X	X	X	X	X	X
Lombard test		X			X	
SPAR test	X		X	X		
Stenger test	X	X		X		X
Swinging story test		X		X		

REFERENCES

BEAGLEY, H. A. (1973). The role of electrophysiological tests in the diagnosis of hearing loss. *Audiology 12*, 470–480.

BORDLEY, J. E., & HARDY, W. G. (1949). A study in objective audiometry with use of the psychogalvanic response. *Annals of Otology, 58*, 751–760.

DOERFLER, L. G., & EPSTEIN, A. (1956). The Doerfler-Stewart test for functional hearing loss. *Monograph of the Veteran's Administration*. Washington, DC: U.S. Government Printing Office.

DOERFLER, L. G., & STEWART, K. (1946). Malingering and psychogenic deafness. *Journal of Speech Disorders, 11*, 181–186.

FRANK, T. (1976). Yes–no test for nonorganic hearing loss. *Archives of Otolaryngology, 102*, 162–165.

HARRIS, D. A. (1958). A rapid and simple technique for the detection of nonorganic hearing loss. *Archives of Otolaryngology* (Chicago), *68*, 758–760.

HATTLER, K. W. (1970). Lengthened-off time: A self-recording screening device for nonorganicity. *Journal of Speech and Hearing Disorders, 35*, 113–122.

HOOD, W. H., CAMPBELL, R. A., & HUTTON, C. L. (1964). An evaluation of the Békésy ascending descending gap. *Journal of Speech and Hearing Research, 7*, 123–132.

HOPKINSON, N. T. (1965). Type V Békésy audiograms: Specification and clinical utility. *Journal of Speech and Hearing Disorders, 30*, 243–251.

JERGER, J., BURNEY, P., MAULDIN, L., & CRUMP, B. (1974). Predicting hearing loss from the acoustic reflex. *Journal of Speech and Hearing Disorders, 39*, 11–22.

JERGER, J., & HERER, G. (1961). An unexpected dividend in Békésy audiometry. *Journal of Speech and Hearing Disorders, 26*, 390–391.

LAMB, L. E., & J. L. PETERSON, (1967). Middle ear reflex measurements in pseudohypacusis. *Journal of Speech and Hearing Disorders, 32*, 46–51.

MARTIN, F. N., & MONRO, D. A. (1975). The effects of sophistication on Type V Békésy patterns in simulated hearing loss. *Journal of Speech and Hearing Disorders, 40*, 508–513.

MARTIN, F. N., & MORRIS, L. (1989). Current audiological practices in the United States. *The Hearing Journal, 42*, 25–42.

MARTIN, F. N., & SHIPP, D. B. (1982). The effects of sophistication on three threshold tests for subjects with simulated hearing loss. *Ear and Hearing, 3*, 34–36.

MENZEL, O. J. (1960). Clinical efficiency in compensation audiometry. *Journal of Speech and Hearing Disorders, 25*, 19–54.

MONRO, D. A., & MARTIN, F. N. (1977). The effects of sophistication on four tests for nonorganic hearing loss. *Journal of Speech and Hearing Disorders, 42*, 528–534.

NAGEL, R. F. (1964). RRLJ: A new technique for the noncooperative patient. *Journal of Speech and Hearing Disorders, 29*, 492–493.

RINTELMANN, W. F., & CARHART, R. (1964). Loudness tracking by normal hearers via Békésy audiometer. *Journal of Speech and Hearing Research, 7*, 79–93.

ROSS, M. (1964). The variable intensity pulse count method (VIPCM) for the detection and measurement of the pure-tone threshold of children with functional hearing losses. *Journal of Speech and Hearing Disorders, 29*, 477–482.

RUHM, H. B., & CARHART, R. (1958). Objective speech audiometry: A new method based on electrodermal response. *Journal of Speech and Hearing Research, 1*, 169–178.

RUHM, H. B., & COOPER W. A., JR. (1962). Low sensation level effects of pure-tone delayed auditory feedback. *Journal of Speech and Hearing Research, 5*, 185–193.

———. (1964). Delayed feedback audiometry. *Journal of Speech and Hearing Disorders, 29*, 448–455.

RUHM, H. B., & MENZEL, O. J. (1959). Objective speech audiometry in cases of nonorganic hearing loss. *Archives of Otolaryngology* (Chicago), *69*, 212–219.

UTLEY, J. (1946). A test of lipreading ability. *Journal of Speech and Hearing Disorders, 11*, 109–116.

11

THE PEDIATRIC PATIENT

measuring response not hearing

Most of the audiometric procedures described earlier in this text can be applied with great reliability to children. In such cases the examination is often no more difficult than it is with cooperative adults. However, there are many instances when, because of the level at which a particular child functions, special diagnostic procedures must be adopted. In many cases the challenge of how to manage children and their families during the emotional times that follow diagnosis is as great as that of the diagnosis itself.

CHAPTER OBJECTIVES

This chapter presents a variety of techniques that have proved helpful in obtaining information about the auditory function of children who cannot be tested using normal audiometric procedures. Methods are described to determine the presence, type, and extent of hearing loss in children. Some insights should be gained about cases presenting special diagnostic difficulty, such as central disorders and pseudohypacusis. Some case management strategies should be developed for dealing with the families of hearing-impaired children.

AUDITORY RESPONSES

It has been stated in this book that what is measured with hearing tests is not "hearing" itself but, rather, a patient's ability and/or willingness to respond to a set of acoustic signals. Therefore, whatever determination is made about the hearing of any individual is made by inference from some set of responses. The hearing function itself is not observed directly.

The manner of patient response to some of the tests described earlier has not been considered to be of great concern. For example, it is not important whether the patient signals the awareness of a tone by a hand signal, by a vocal response, or by pressing a button. When working with small children, however, the manner and type of response to a signal may be crucial to diagnosis. It is also important to remember that most small children do not respond to acoustic signals at threshold; rather, sounds must be more clearly audible to them than to their older counterparts. It is safe, therefore, to assume that during audiometry, small children's responses must be considered to be at their **minimum response levels (MRLs)**, which, in some cases, may be well above their thresholds.

Responses from small children may vary from voluntary acknowledgment of a signal to involuntary movement of the body, or from an overt cry of surprise to a slight change in vocalization. Response to sound may be totally unobservable except for some change in the electrophysiological system of the child being tested. If a clear response to a sound is observed by a trained clinician, it may be inferred that the sound has been heard, although the sensation level of the signal may be very much in doubt. On the other hand, if no response is observed, it cannot be assumed that the sound has not been heard.

Obviously, a number of factors contribute to the responses offered by a child. Perhaps of primary concern is the physiological and psychological state of a small child prior to stimulation. Shepherd (1971) described prestimulus activity levels as a range consisting of alert attentiveness, relaxed wakefulness, drowsiness, light sleep, and deep sleep. Shepherd also described, in interesting detail, the specific auditory, behavioral, and electrophysiological response systems. Hodgson (1987, p. 186) emphasizes that audiologists should spend time observing normal children in order to understand motor development, language and speech acquisition, and auditory behaviors.

Even though audiologists may have preferences for certain kinds of responses from a child, they must be willing to settle for whatever the child provides. Audiologists must also be willing to alter in midstream the kind of procedure used if it seems that a different system might be more effective. Examiner flexibility and alertness are essential when testing children. Modification of a procedure may be the only way to evoke responses from a child. Response to a sound may appear only once, and it can easily be lost to the inexperienced or unobservant clinician.

Speech and language are imitative processes, acquired primarily through the auditory sense. A hearing defect, either congenital or acquired early in life, can interfere with the development of concepts that culminate in normal speech and language. For a variety of reasons, many children with abnormal hearing proceed into the third year of life or beyond before a hearing problem is suspected. A hearing disorder in a child is often not detected because people believe that if their own child had a hearing loss, they would somehow know it, that he or she would be obviously different from other children.

There has also been a mistaken notion that hearing-impaired babies do not babble. It is probable that the act of babbling is a kind of vegetative activity that is reinforced by the child's tactile and proprioceptive gratification from the use of the mouth and tongue. At about age 6 months, normal-hearing children begin to notice that those interesting cooing sounds have been coming from their own mouths, and they begin to exercise some control over them by varying rate, pitch, and loudness. This second stage is called **lalling**. Often, hearing-impaired children, who do not receive auditory feedback, will gradually decrease their vocalizations. After a period of lalling, on the other hand, normal-hearing children go into stages of **echolalia**, in which they repeat in a parrotlike fashion the sounds they hear. Eventually, meaning becomes attached to sounds, and the projective use of words is initiated. Usually the normal child is speaking well before the age of 2 years, whereas the child with a severe auditory defect is not.

Surely the earliest possible identification of a hearing deficit is crucial. The earlier in the life of the child that aural habilitative measures can be applied, the greater are the chances for the successful development of speech communication. The primary source of disagreement among experts is the methodology by which early identification of hearing loss may be made. Of course, the accuracy and efficiency of these procedures must also be considered.

Infant Screening

Procedures have been recommended that include the screening of newborn babies in the earliest hours of life. Wedenberg (1956) screened 150 infants between the ages of 1 and 7 days. His test consisted of hitting a cowbell with a hammer close to the child's head. Of the infants, 149 responded with an **auropalpebral reflex (APR)**, which is a contraction of the muscles surrounding the eyes. Wedenberg subsequently used an audiometer, which powered a small loudspeaker positioned near the sleeping child's head. Testing with a variety of frequencies, he observed responses from normal-hearing infants in light sleep to range from 104 to 112 dB SPL. He observed that premature children do not respond well to external stimuli and that arousal responses depend, to a large extent, on the sleep level of the child.

Downs and Sterritt (1967) used a commercially available device (Figure 11.1) to produce a 3000 Hz **warble tone** and found that they could observe responses of most infants at about 90 dB SPL. Responses consisted primarily of APRs, movement of the hands or head, and overall startle responses. These researchers tested about 10,000 infants using this procedure, with only 150 failing, 4 of whom were subsequently identified as having hearing losses.

For a time, the kind of results just reported suggested that screening the hearing of neonates before they left the hospital might be the method by which early identification and followup could be achieved. A number of drawbacks to the procedure exist, however. The training of the individual performing the test is of paramount importance. Attendance by a separate observer is

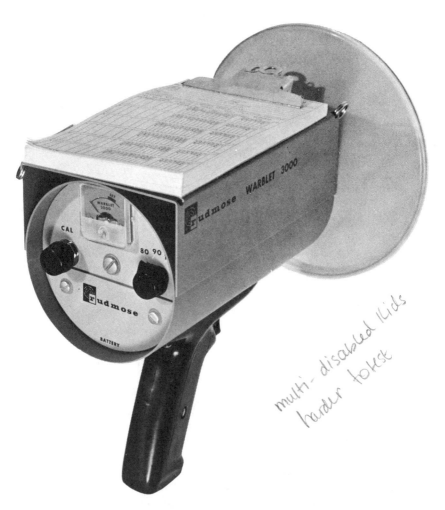

Figure 11.1 A Warblet used in neonatal screening. When the device is held 9 to 10 inches from the child's head, it emits a 3000 Hz warble tone at 80, 90, or 100 dB SPL. (Courtesy of Tracor.)

often useful, but disagreements on acceptance of responses occur. The problems of record keeping and followup are also tremendous. Because a number of children may give false negative responses, informing their parents of possible hearing loss may produce undue alarm and concern.

In 1970 a joint committee of the American Speech-Language-Hearing Association, the American Academy of Ophthalmology and Otolaryngology, and the American Academy of Pediatrics recommended against the widespread use of neonatal screening. Their guidelines, which were later revised (ASHA, 1984), suggest that, because of its many financial and other practical drawbacks, massive screening of infants is not the ideal way to proceed. They recommended that only children at risk be screened for hearing loss, and that a practical approach to this is to use the **high-risk register**. This register includes evidence of (1) family history of hearing loss; (2) viral or other nonbacterial infections during pregnancy (e.g., rubella, cytomegalovirus, herpes, syphilis, toxoplasmosis); (3) craniofacial abnormalities (e.g., cleft palate, abnormalities of the pinna or throat, etc.); (4) low birth weight (less than 1500 grams); (5) high levels of bilirubin (a bile pigment) in the fetal blood; (6) bacterial meningitis; (7) severe asphyxia, coma, seizures, or the need for continued ventilation (Gerkin, 1984a).

Since some hearing losses are hereditodegenerative, a child falling on the high-risk register because of family history may pass the screening, lulling the family into a false sense of security about the potential for later development of a hearing loss. An obvious additional difficulty in using the high-risk register lies in the fact that many hereditary hearing losses are of a recessive nature, and the genetic potential for hearing loss may exist without an obvious family history of this disorder. Evidence is beginning to emerge that suggests that the high-risk register may not be as efficient as many people believe it to be.

Recently new guidelines were published for identification of infants who are at risk for hearing loss (ASHA, 1988). ASHA's definition of "at-risk infants" coincides with the high-risk register. They recommend that evaluation of these infants be carried out, preferably while they are in the hospital after birth, but within the first 3 months of life so that habilitation can commence by age 6 months. Attempts at diagnosis should continue, along with habilitative efforts. ASHA's guidelines recommend: "(1) parent/caregiver education, (2) audiologic evaluation by ABR, and (3) a comprehensive followup and management system for those infants who fail initial ABR evaluation."

In recent years auditory brain stem response (ABR) audiometry has become increasingly popular as a neonatal testing system. Some of the disadvantages of this procedure have been discussed previously in this book—for example, the lack of frequency specificity evident when click stimuli are used. When testing infants on the high-risk register, it is important to compare responses to norms that correspond to children's gestational ages rather than to their chronological ages because immaturity of the central nervous system in a premature child can have a profound effect on results and must be taken into account. When one recalls that ABR is not a true test of hearing but, rather, a test of synchronous neural firings in response to sound, the caveat about what appear to be normal-hearing or hearing-impaired infants is instantly clear.

Although they concluded that "ABR is the most objective measure currently available with which to assess the functional integrity of the peripheral auditory system in neonates," the Committee on Hearing, Bioacoustics, and Biomechanics of the National Research Council (ASHA, 1987) also cautions that the ABR is "only a moderately effective predictor of the behavioral audiogram." This research emphasizes the need for data over a period of years to determine the percentage of false positive and false negative identifications of neonatal hearing loss based on ABR testing. Followup testing is essential when ABR results are either positive or negative for infants on the high-risk register.

A number of arguments favor postponing ABR testing of children in neonatal intensive care units until they reach the age of 3 to 6 months because of excessive costs and inaccuracies in predicting hearing loss in this population (Downs, 1982; Roberts, Davis, & Phon, 1982). Nevertheless, ABR for these infants has a number of strong advocates (Galambos, Hicks, & Wilson, 1984; Jacobson & Morehouse, 1984). It seems certain that this kind of testing will continue in many major hospitals; in fact, it will probably increase as improved technology results in better and more reliable procedures.

Gerkin (1984b) pointed out that hearing screening procedures can be justified on several bases, including cost efficiency. When compared with other disorders routinely screened for, such as phenylketonuria (PKU) or neonatal hypothyroidism, the yield is considerably higher. For example, Simmons, McFarland, and Jones (1980) found hearing loss in one out of 50 infants who graduated from an intensive-care nursery. From a purely objective and financial viewpoint, the fact that $350 million might be saved each year if early identification and habilitation of hearing impairments were in place (Downs, 1977) seems to justify neonatal hearing screening, even if the obvious humanitarian aspects are ignored.

Several devices are available for testing neonates while they are in the hospital. One, the **crib-o-gram** (see Figure 11.2) is based on the work of Simmons and Russ (1974) and Simmons (1976). A motion-sensitive transducer is placed beneath the infant's crib, and activity is monitored for 10 seconds before the presentation of the acoustic stimulus, which is a narrow-band noise centered at 3000 Hz with an intensity of 92 dB SPL. Activity is also monitored for 2.5 seconds after discontinuation of the stimulus. A series of 30 samples is obtained. If, on the basis of probability, the infant has failed the screening, a light on the instrument is illuminated and the child is referred for further testing. Although this test is easy for nonaudiologists to administer, it does take nearly an hour to perform, and problems with maintenance should be a consideration before it is adopted for routine use.

Another device, the **neonatal auditory response cradle** (Bennett, 1979), was developed in England. This procedure involves the use of a cradle with a pressure-sensitive headrest and a mattress capable of measuring startle responses to sounds in terms of movements of the head, trunk, and limbs. A belt is placed around the baby's abdomen to sense changes in respiration.

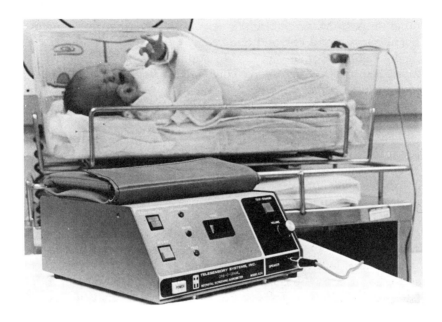

Figure 11.2 A crib-o-gram in use. (Courtesy of Telesensory Systems, Inc.)

Receivers are placed in the child's ears to deliver the sounds so that responses can be observed from the right and left ears separately, which is unlike the sound-field stimulation used with the crib-o-gram. The signal is a narrow-band noise (2600 to 4500 Hz) presented at 85 dB SPL. Between 2 and 10 trial blocks are tested (each trial block contains two sound and two no-sound elements), and monitoring takes place for at least 5 seconds before and after each sound presentation. Bennett and Lawrence (1980) found the procedure highly reliable, although a number of equipment difficulties have been reported.

TESTING CHILDREN FROM BIRTH TO ONE YEAR OF AGE

Experienced audiologists do not launch quickly into hearing tests with small children. First they spend some time casually observing each child. They should notice such factors as the children's relationships with the adults who have taken them to the clinic; their gaits, standing positions, and other indications of general motor performance; and their methods of communication. Compiling complete and detailed case histories is of paramount importance.

It has been frequently observed that, in general, the broader the frequency spectrum of a sound, the better it is at catching the attention of a small child. For this reason, many clinicians use speech or other broad-band signals in testing. One of the great dangers of accepting an obvious response to a sound with a broad acoustic spectrum lies in the fact that many children have reasonably good sensitivity in some frequency ranges and impaired sensitivity in other ranges. Many children, for example, have sharply falling high-frequency hearing losses and respond quite overtly to sounds like the clapping of hands or the calling of their names. In addition, there is a smaller but significant number of children who have congenital low-frequency sensorineural hearing losses (Ross & Matkin, 1967).

Ewing and Ewing (1944) were pioneers in the testing of young children. They used a wide variety of noisemakers, such as bells, rattles, rustling paper, and xylophones. They advocated using a spoon stirring in a cup, which produces a soft sound from a child's daily life that may evoke a response when a loud sound does not. Stress on using meaningful sounds is most closely associated with the work of the Ewings, and their influence is still evidenced in much of modern pediatric audiometry.

Hardy, Hardy, Brinker, Frazier, and Doughtery (1962) tested a large group of babies ranging in age from 4 to 8 months. The procedure they used requires two clinicians. One clinician sits before the child, who is usually seated on the mother's lap, to occupy the child's attention with a toy or puppet. The second clinician, who is behind and to the side of the mother, utters phonemes such as "S, S, S, S." Toys and other noisemakers may also be used; crinkling cellophane or onionskin paper makes the sort of soft, annoying sound that is extremely useful in techniques such as these but provides little or no information about the configuration of the hearing loss.

Often a child will turn in search of a sound. Hardy and others concluded that most children are about 8 months old before they search for a sound by turning their heads. If a child does not turn to locate a sound by the age of 8 months, it can be suspected that something is wrong, although not necessarily hearing loss. Mental retardation and some childhood symbolic disorders may manifest themselves in a similar lack of response. The general approach being described here constitutes what has been called **behavioral observation audiometry (BOA)**.

Sound-Field Audiometry

Several approaches using multiple loudspeakers in a sound-field situation have been used. Tape recordings of animal noises and baby cries have been effective in eliciting responses, even when filtered into narrow bands. Although a sound, such as a whistle, bell, drum, or some vocal utterance, may appear subjectively to represent a specific frequency range, this often turns out not to be true. What may seem to be a high-pitched sound may have equal intensity in the low- and high-frequency ranges, as verified by spectral analysis. One exception to this is the Manchester high-pitch baby rattle (Kettlety, 1987), which has been used extensively in Great Britain as a specially designed infant screening device whose intensity is primarily above 5000 Hz.

The justification for narrow-band filtering of a signal for use with a small child seems obvious. Many clinicians use the narrow-band noise generators on their clinical audiometers as stimuli to elicit responses from small children. The belief is that this provides specific frequency information if the child responds. Such an approach may be very misleading. The narrow bands on many audiometers are not very narrow at all, and they may reject frequencies on either side of the center frequency at rates as little as 12 dB per octave. This allows sufficient energy in the side bands to produce a response when a child has not heard the frequency in the center of the band. It is obvious that audiologists must understand the nature of the equipment they use and, if they elect to test with narrow bands, they should ascertain for themselves just what the band widths are.

Several kinds of responses may be observed when sounds are presented to a child from different directions in the sound field. The child may look for the sound source, cease ongoing activity, awaken from light sleep, change facial expression, or offer a vocalized response. Once again, a response to sound has considerable significance, whereas a lack of response is not necessarily meaningful. A useful setup for sound-field localization has been diagrammed by Hodgson (1987) and is shown in Figure 11.3.

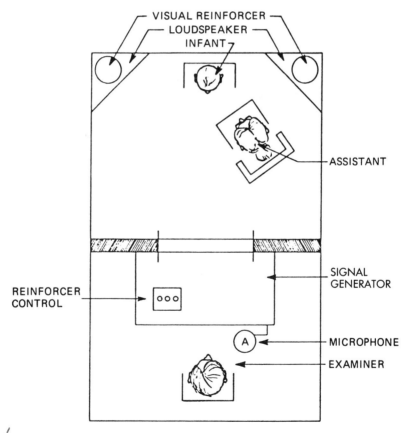

Figure 11.3 Diagram of a room useful for sound-field localization tests with small children. (Adapted from William R. Hodgson, *Hearing Disorders in Children*, ed. F.N. Martin, © 1987, p. 201. Reprinted by permission of Pro-Ed, Englewood Cliffs, New Jersey.)

Frequently, children will respond to the off-effect of a sound but not to the on-effect. Evaluation of responses to cessation of sound often goes well with the use of noisemakers, but it can be adapted to sound-field audiometry. A high-intensity pure tone or narrow noise band can be introduced for a minute or so and then abruptly interrupted. This interruption may produce a response, in terms of searching behavior, where the initial presentation of the sound will not.

It is generally the case that at age 2 months a soft voice begins to become a better stimulus than a loud voice. At 1 to 3 months, percussion instruments elicit the best responses in terms of APRs, startle responses such as the **moro reflex**, and overall activity increase or crying. At 4 months, percussion instruments are less successful than they were earlier, but the human voice gains in effectiveness. By 6 months of age much reflex activity begins to disappear.

Relying on the localization ability of normal-hearing babies more than 4 months old, Suzuki and Ogiba (1961) developed a sound-field procedure called **conditioned orientation reflex (COR)**. Children are seated between and in front of a pair of loudspeakers, each of which holds an illuminated doll within the children's peripheral vision. Pure-tone and light introductions are paired; and, after several of these paired presentations, children will begin to glance in the direction of the light source in anticipation of the light whenever a tone is presented. The introduction of the light may then be delayed until after children have glanced at the speaker; this can serve as a reinforcement for their orientation to the signal. This procedure works well with some small children and has been modified in several ways, including the "puppet in the window illuminated" (PIWI) procedure (Haug, Baccaro, & Guilford, 1967). VRA, to be discussed next, can successfully test many children as young as 6 months in developmental age.

Rewarding children's responses made to auditory stimuli with visual stimuli has led to the use of **visual reinforcement audiometry (VRA)** (Liden & Kankkonen, 1961). The reinforcer may be anything from a light to a picture, as long as it evokes the children's interests. Matkin (1973) reported that VRA works under earphones, if the children will tolerate them, as well as in the sound field, with or without hearing aids. Speech as well as tones may serve as signals.

Audiologists do not completely agree on the best acoustic stimulus for testing small children. Many but not all authorities believe that pure tones are probably not the ideal stimuli, as they are not meaningful to children. Pure tones have the obvious advantage that they supply information about children's sensitivity at specific frequencies. If, however, a child shows no interest in pure tones, other, carefully controlled acoustic stimuli may be used.

A good physical environment is essential for success in testing small children. It is usually best to have two examiners. DiCarlo, Kendall, and Goldstein (1962) describe a procedure whereby the child is tested across a small table. On the floor beside the table the clinician places a box of toys containing noisemakers, and either makes noises under the table or has an assistant stationed behind the child create the sound. The examiner must watch the child's face carefully.

A potential problem, present whenever screening responses involving high-intensity stimuli are used, is the effect of loudness recruitment on startle responses. If recruitment is present, a child could conceivably respond to a sound as if it were loud, when in fact it might be only slightly above auditory threshold. If this occurs, a child with a cochlear hearing loss with loudness recruitment may pass early screening tests because of the very nature of the disorder. The criteria for minimum response level may be very different for hearing-impaired children than for normal children.

TESTING CHILDREN 1 TO 5 YEARS OF AGE

look at child's articulation

At one year of age the hard-of-hearing child may begin to lose the potential for normal spoken language development. Lack of speech often brings the problem to the attention of the parents or other caretakers. At 18 months, the normal child usually obeys simple commands. Speech tests are useful to evaluate children at this age, as a child may give good responses to soft speech while apparently ignoring percussion instruments. It is interesting that quiet voiced speech will sometimes elicit a response when whispered speech will not. At 2 to 3 years of age, tests with voice, whispers, pitch pipes, and other special stimuli may be unnecessary on "normal" hearing-impaired children, as they can often be taught to respond to pure tones, especially warble tones.

Early reports in the literature on testing children indicated that it was not possible to get pure-tone threshold responses on children under 5 years of age. It is now quite common to test children age 3 or under. It is naturally necessary to work rapidly and smoothly to keep such a young child's attention and cooperation. A child with a "pure" hearing loss (i.e., no other significant problems) should be testable well before 3 years of age.

If a child cannot be tested using formal methods, an imitation of vocalization can be tried. The clinician can babble nonsense syllables, without the child watching, to see if the child will imitate. If imitation does take place, this indicates that hearing is good enough to perceive voice. The severely hearing-impaired child may attempt to imitate but may do so without voice. This is a most important diagnostic sign. In addition to being a strong indication of hearing loss, silent imitation indicates that the child's perceptual function is probably intact. If the child vocalizes, the voice quality can be evaluated. Although the vocal quality of the hearing-impaired individual is often different from that of the normal hearer, it must be remembered that the voice of the very young, hearing-impaired child frequently cannot be differentiated from that of the normal child.

It is possible to observe a child's reaction to examiner imitation of the child's sounds. In this case a response is made by the examiner to the child's babbling or other vocalizations. A normal child may cease vocalization and may sometimes repeat it. There are instances in which this procedure works when nothing else does, as the child may stop and listen, the interpretation being that the examiner's voice was heard. The child may also be tested by asking questions, such as, "Where is Mommy?" "Where are your hands?" The question "Do you want to go home now?" often evokes a clear response, but it should be reserved as a last resort, for if children do hear that question it may become impossible to keep them further. Often a whisper may cause 2- or 3-year-old youngsters to whisper back. If they can hear their own whisper, this may indicate good hearing for high-pitched sounds.

Speech Audiometry

Some children will not respond to pure tones and, by their almost stoical expressions, it appears that they cannot hear. A large number of these children can be conditioned to respond to speech signals. If they possess the appropriate language skills, many children will point to parts of their bodies or to articles of clothing. If this kind of response can be obtained, the clinician can recite a list of items to which the child points. The level of the signal can be raised and lowered until speech threshold is approximated.

Pictures or objects that can be named with spondaic stress can be used to test children. A child will often point to a "cowboy" or "hotdog." The clinician may first demonstrate the procedure and then reward the child's appropriate behavior with a smile, a nod, or a wink. SRTs can frequently be obtained with pictures by age 2 years. Speech discrimination tests, such as the WIPI (Ross & Lerman, 1970) described in Chapter 4, may be accomplished in the same way.

Speech audiometry has revealed hearing abnormalities or their absence in children who were unable or unwilling to take pure-tone tests. This has resulted, in many cases, in a substantial savings of time in initiating remedial procedures. Failure of children to respond during speech audiometry may, of course, occur because they do not know what the item (picture or object) is, rather than because they have not heard the word. The clinician should inquire of the adults accompanying their children to the examination whether specific words are within the children's vocabularies. It is essential to assure that it is discrimination and not receptive vocabulary that is being tested.

Pure-Tone Audiometry

Many times, in testing small children, the problem is to get them to respond. The ingenuity of the clinician can frequently solve this problem. For a child to want to participate, usually the procedure must offer some enjoyment. Some children, however, are so anxious to please that they deluge the clinician with many false positive responses on pure-tone tests, so that it is difficult to gauge when a response is valid. In such cases, slight modifications of adult-like tests may prove workable with some older children. A child may be asked to point to the earphone in which a tone is heard. The ears may be stimulated randomly, and in this way the appropriateness of the response can be determined. The same result may be achieved by using pulsed-tone procedures, asking the child to tell how many tones have been presented.

Operant Conditioning Audiometry

Many times it appears that no approach to a given child will result in reliable hearing-test results. This is particularly true of retarded children. Spradlin and Lloyd (1965) suggested that, given sufficient time and effort, no child is "untestable," and they recommended that this term be replaced by the phrase *difficult to test*.

Operant conditioning audiometry (OCA) is often practiced by using food as a reward for proper performance. A child may be seated in the test room before a table that contains a hand switch. Sounds are presented either through the sound-field speaker or through earphones. The child is encouraged to press the switch when the sound, which can be either a pure tone or a noise band, is presented. If the child's response is appropriate, a small amount of food, such as a candy pellet, some fruit juice, or a token, is released from a special feeder box. Usually, once children see that pressing the switch will result in a reward, they will continue to press it in pursuit of more. It is essential that the switch that operates the feeder be wired in series with the tone-introducer switch so that no reward is forthcoming without presentation of the sound. In this way the child gets no reinforcement for pushing the switch unless a tone is actually introduced, and, presumably, heard. Signals that are thought to be above the child's threshold must be introduced first, after which the level may be lowered until threshold is reached. A good starting point is 90 dB HL at 500 Hz, because there is a strong likelihood of hearing at this frequency and level.

Operant conditioning audiometry requires much time and patience if it is to work. Often, many trials are required before the child begins to understand the task. As in other audiometric procedures, it is essential that the signals be introduced aperiodically, for the child may learn to predict a signal and to respond to a sound that has not been heard. There are many times when operant conditioning audiometry can be successful where other procedures have failed. The term **tangible reinforcement operant conditioning audiometry (TROCA)** was coined by Lloyd, Spradlin, and Reid (1968) to describe specifics of operant conditioning to audiometry.

For a number of years clinicians have been using *instrumental conditioning* in testing young children—that is, teaching the children to perform in a certain way when a sound stimulus is heard. This requires a degree of voluntary cooperation from the children, but the clinician can select a method that will evoke appropriate responses.

A number of clever devices have been described in the literature for use in instrumental conditioning. The **peep show** (Dix & Hallpike, 1947) gives children the reward of seeing a lighted picture when they respond correctly to a tone presented through a small loudspeaker below the screen. The **pedi-**

acoumeter (Guilford & Haug, 1952) works on a similar principle, except that the child may wear earphones to increase the accuracy of the test. If the child hears a tone and responds correctly by pushing a button, one of seven puppets pops up to startle and amuse. Similar approaches have been used with animated toys, pictures, slides, and motion pictures.

A new device on the scene is the Playtone audiometer (see Figure 11.4) which is microprocessor-controlled and employs animated graphics on a color monitor. The child is shown how to respond by pressing a touch pad each time a tone is heard. The reward for a correct signal is the placement of a face in the window of a boat, train, or airplane, or the appearance of a cartoon bear putting on his clothes, one item at a time. The procedure appears to be fun for small children, who are encouraged by a color TV screen to approach the device when they might otherwise be frightened. The Playtone audiometer employs a conditioning phase, producing sounds through a small loudspeaker, and can be used in a manual or fully automated mode once the child agrees to don the earphones. A major advantage to this device is that it requires only one clinician to test a child. The final word on the Playtone audiometer

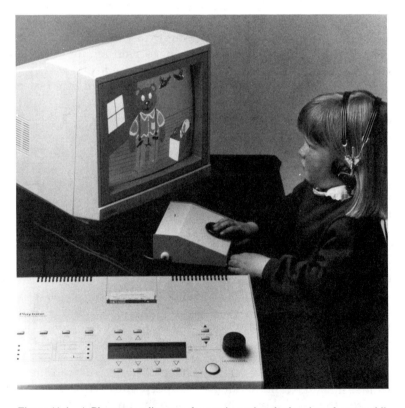

Figure 11.4 A Playtone audiometer for use in testing the hearing of young children. (Courtesy of Life-Tech, Inc.)

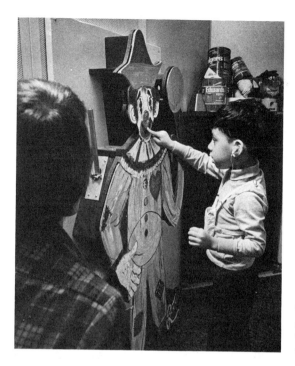

Figure 11.5 Photograph of a young hearing-impaired child being tested in the sound field for speech thresholds. The clown serves as a device for delivering a tangible reward (candy pellets) when the part of the clown named by the clinician is pressed by the child.

will be written in the research conducted on small children or other difficult-to-test populations.

Martin and Coombes (1976) applied the principles of operant audiometry to the determination of speech thresholds. A brightly colored clown was devised whose body parts (e.g., hand, mouth, nose, leg) were wired to microswitches which triggered a candy-feeder mechanism (see Figure 11.5). Children were shown how to touch a part of the clown. Reinforcement of the correct response was immediate delivery of a candy pellet to a cup, which was momentarily lighted in the clown's hand. Preprogramming of the proper switch on a special device in the control room ensured that false responses would not be rewarded. Speech thresholds were obtained on very young children in a matter of several minutes. Weaver, Wardell, and Martin (1979) found this procedure for obtaining speech thresholds useful with retarded children.

Play Audiometry

Often, using elaborate devices and procedures is unnecessary to test the hearing of young children (see Figure 11.6). Many children can simply be taught by demonstration to place a ring on a peg, a block in a box, or a bead in a bucket when a sound stimulus is introduced. The more enthusiasm the clinician shows about the procedure, the more likely the child is to join in. Children seem to enjoy the action of the game. Tones can be presented through

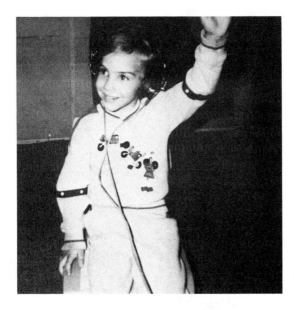

Figure 11.6 A small child taking a voluntary pure-tone hearing test.

earphones if children will tolerate them, or through the sound-field speaker if they will not. Some children will readily accept the new insert receivers because they are light and do not encumber movement.

The probable reason that some clinicians do not embrace play audiometric techniques is that they feel these techniques can easily become boring to the children and that conditioning will therefore extinguish rapidly. This is probably a case of projection of adult values since many alert children can play the "sound game" for long periods of time without boredom. When asking children to move beads or other objects from one container to another, it is a good idea to have a large supply on hand, because many children will refuse to play further once the first bucket has become empty, even if they have appeared to enjoy the game up to this point.

One problem in using play audiometry is to find suitable rewards for prompting the children to maintain interest and motivation in the test. DiCarlo, Kendall, and Goldstein (1962) felt that conditioning in audiometry depends on the following: (1) motivation, (2) contiguity (getting the stimulus and response close together in time and space), (3) generalization (across frequency and intensity), (4) discrimination (between the stimulus and any background activity), and (5) reinforcement (conveying to children that they are doing what is wanted).

It often becomes apparent to a clinician that a limited amount of time is available to test a small child and that, even though some reliable threshold results are forthcoming, the test should best be abbreviated before the child ceases to cooperate. In such cases, it may be advisable to test one frequency in each ear both by air conduction and by bone conduction. This will provide information about the relative sensitivity in each ear and about the nature of the disorder (conductive or sensorineural). If an SRT is obtained that suggests normal hearing, the frequency to be tested may be a higher one, say 3000 or 4000 Hz, to make certain that the normal SRT does not mislead in cases of high-frequency hearing loss. If only three to six thresholds are to be obtained, it is often more meaningful to get readings at one or two frequencies in each ear by both air and bone conduction than to obtain six air-conduction thresholds in one ear. Accurate threshold readings at only 500 and 2000 Hz will give some evidence of degree, configuration, and type of hearing loss.

Sometimes it is impossible, for a variety of reasons, to teach a child to take a hearing test in one session. In such cases the child should be rescheduled for further testing and observation. It is often worthwhile to employ the talents and interests of the child's parents or other adults. They can be instructed in methods of presenting sounds and evoking responses. Children may also be more amenable to training in the comfort and security of their homes than in the strange and often frightening environment of sound-treated rooms. One parent may use a noisemaker, such as a bell, in full view of the child, while the other parent responds to dropping a block in a bucket or by some other enjoyable activity. Children can be encouraged to join in the game and, after beginning to participate by following the parents' lead, can be encouraged to go first. Once they participate fully, the sound source can be gradually moved out of the line of vision so that responses can be determined to be to auditory stimulation. A few minutes a day of such activities may allow the audiologist, at the time of the next clinic appointment, to use the same procedure, preferably with the same materials, which are already familiar to the child. After professional observation of the child's responses, the audiologist can substitute other sound stimuli in an attempt to quantify the hearing loss, if any. It has also been found useful to have the parents borrow an old headband and set of earphones to accustom the child to wearing them without fear.

Small children's failure to produce observable responses to loud sounds during informal testing may or may not be due to profound hearing loss. In such cases, lack of response during formal testing, such as pure-tone audiometry, may mean either that the children have not heard the sounds or that they have not responded correctly when they have heard them. Deciding between these two possibilities is often difficult. It is sometimes advisable to teach children to respond to some other stimulus, such as to a light or to the vibrations of a hand-held bone-conduction vibrator, which delivers a strong low-frequency tone. If a child can be taught to give appropriate responses to one sensory input, the inference is that the child can be conditioned to respond and that lack of response to a sound probably means that it was not heard.

Immittance Measures

The use of acoustic immittance measurements with children has great clinical utility. Tympanometry can determine a number of middle-ear disorders in children, including abnormal middle-ear pressure, eustachian tube malfunction, effusion, thin tympanic membrane, and patency of pressure equalization tubes (deJonge, 1984). Additionally, the sensation level or absence of the acoustic reflex can give general kinds of information about a possible sensori-neural hearing loss.

The main disadvantage of immittance tests with very small children results from any movements or crying they may manifest. For a test to be accurate, the patient must be relatively motionless. Furthermore, any vocalizations— for example, crying—will be picked up by the probe microphone. An experienced team of clinicians can often work so efficiently that children are distracted and tested before they have time to object. In other cases, children can be sedated without affecting the results of the test. Immittance measurements should almost always be attempted on small children.

Electrophysiological Hearing Tests

It has been obvious for some time that objective tests for measuring hearing in young children would be highly desirable. Such tests must embody methods that require no active participation from the child, and they must result in clear-cut responses of an objective nature. An obvious approach would seem to be to monitor one or more of the child's electrophysiological mechanisms for any changes that might be induced by the introduction of a sound. Changes in pulse rate, breathing pattern, heart rhythm, skin resistance, and electrical brain activity have all been investigated.

Electrophysiological tests today primarily involve auditory evoked potentials and a great deal of satisfaction has been achieved using ABR audiometry. A primary advantage is in the fact that the procedure is effective during sleep and the child may be anesthetized with no effects on test accuracy.

For a number of years electrodermal audiometry (EDA) was very popular for testing young children (Hardy & Pauls, 1952). This popularity has waned considerably. Although some clinicians reported high correlations between electrodermal response and behavioral thresholds, others reported confusing results and poor reliability. A popular contention today is that if conventional or play audiometry will not work with a small child, the chances are that EDA will not work either (O'Neill, Oyer, & Hillis, 1961). The trauma to the child caused by the electric shocks that are used in this test as a conditioning stimulus are not justified by the presumed value of the procedure, which is rarely if ever used today (Martin & Gravel, 1989).

Differences of opinion also exist about the reliability of respiration audiometry in testing young children. Another procedure, **cardiotachometry** (Eisenberg, 1975), has been suggested. Heart rate seems to decelerate when speech stimuli are presented to a listener; no such effects are evident with nonspeech signals. Respiration audiometry and cardiotachometry have not gained the status for testing children that had been predicted.

Experts in pediatric audiology continue to disagree on the relative merits of electrophysiological hearing tests. There is little doubt, however, that continuing research will bring us closer to the goal of an efficient and reliable index of auditory function in uncooperative children. Until that goal is reached, audiologists will still have to confirm their findings with behavioral tests. The diagnosis is never complete until a voluntary hearing test is obtained.

LANGUAGE DISORDERS

Small children are frequently seen in audiology centers because they show some deficiencies in the normal development of speech and language. Because language and speech depend on interactions between the peripheral and central nervous systems, a detailed history must be taken. Special attention should be paid to such things as handedness, onset of different kinds of motor development, the age at which meaningful speech or other communication system was acquired, social development, communication of needs, and pre- and post-natal developmental factors. Pertinent data should also include prenatal diseases, the length of the pregnancy, difficulties at birth, and early distress—for example, that seen in cyanotic ("blue") babies, in babies with jaundice, and so on. Notations should be made of childhood illnesses, especially those involving high or prolonged fevers; medications taken; and developmental histories, such as ages of sitting alone, walking, and so on. Attention should be paid to any illnesses or accidents and any regressions in development associated with them. Some objective data may be obtained from tests of hearing, symbolic behavior, intelligence, and receptive and expressive language. A brief history form is illustrated in Figure 11.7.

A young child's unwillingness to cooperate may be common to all sensory modalities and could indicate a disorder or combination of disorders other than hearing loss (e.g., mental retardation or emotional maladjustment). If a child does not respond to visual stimuli, such as lights or shadows, or to touching or vibration, one might wonder whether the problem is in fact behavioral. However, if a positive response is obtained in one modality and a negative one in another, a certain patterning appears, which is more significant than a generalized response (or lack of response). When responses to sound are absent and responses to other sensory modalities are present, a strong indication of hearing loss exists.

Although long lists of possible causes have been postulated, significant language delay is usually produced by hearing loss, some congenital or early acquired symbolic disorder, mental retardation, emotional disturbance, or a psychosocial disorder such as **autism**. A common error of clinicians is to consider causes as an either–or condition and to attempt differential diagnosis to rule out all but one cause. The experienced clinician will have observed that the presence of a significant disorder in a child increases rather than decreases the probability of another disorder.

When a small child has a language disorder and hearing loss cannot be eliminated as a possible causal factor, the resources and experience of the clinician are called on for an appropriate diagnosis. The behavioral characteristics of the clinical entities mentioned here can frequently be ruled out on the

THE UNIVERSITY OF TEXAS AT AUSTIN
Division of Communication Disorders

Pediatric Case History

Date _____

Patient's Name _____ Sex _____ D.O.B. _____
         Last   First   Middle

Age _____ Home Phone _____ Address _____

School _____ Grade _____ Teacher _____

Parents' Names _____

Referred by _____

Sex and Ages of Other Children _____

Pre–Birth
    Maternal Illness, Accident, Medication _____
_____

    Rh Factor _____ Previous Miscarriages _____
    Length of Pregnancy _____

Birth
    Weight _____ Age of Mother _____ Cesarean _____
    Condition _____ Difficulty _____
    Jaundice, Anoxia, Cyanosis _____

Infancy and Childhood
    Seizures _____
    Motor Development _____
    Speech _____
_____

    Illnesses, Accidents _____
_____

    Familiar Hearing Loss _____
    Ear Infections and Surgery _____
_____

    Drugs _____
    Nephritis, Mumps, Diabetes _____
    Other Problems _____
_____

    Response to Sound _____

    Onset and Progression of Loss _____
_____

    Previous Audiograms _____
_____

    Hearing Aid: Ear _____ Type and Make _____
    Date and Place Bought _____
    Success with Aid _____
    Behavioral Problems _____
_____

    School Progress _____
    Other Comments:

_____

Clinician

Figure 11.7 Sample of a brief history form for children with hearing disorders.

basis of observation of behavior and developmental history. The problem then remains to differentiate between the hard-of-hearing and the otherwise language-disordered child. Even though the brain-injured child is said to manifest such symptoms as impatience, hyperactivity, poor judgment, **perseveration**, and **dysinhibition**, often a symbolic disorder exists without the presence of bizarre behavior.

Audiologists frequently see children who are either believed to have hearing losses or whose auditory behavior is so inconsistent as to cast doubt on the presence of normal hearing. A parent or teacher may complain that a child's responses to sound are inconsistent, that performance is better when background noises or competing messages are at a minimum, and that it is possible that the child "just doesn't pay attention." Sometimes auditory test results appear normal on such a child, and the parents are mistakenly reassured that all is fine. The audiologist must constantly be alert for auditory-processing disorders that can coexist with other learning and language disabilities. A child with such disorders should be referred to the proper specialists, such as speech-language pathologists.

So as not to over-refer cases to language pathologists, Martin and Clark (1977) developed a screening procedure using a dichotic listening task with the WIPI test as discrimination stimuli. Children with intact central auditory nervous systems seemed to do as well diotically (high- and low-frequency filtered bands to both ears) as they did dichotically (high band to one ear and low band to the other ear). Children with confirmed language-learning disorders showed significant diotic enhancement, indicating that they have difficulty in fusing the signals from the two ears. More screening tests are needed so that children with central auditory disorders, however mild, will not be overlooked but will be properly referred for complete diagnosis and therapy. Many of the tests for central auditory disorders, described in Chapter 9, can be performed accurately on children as young as age 6 years.

In the final analysis, the diagnosis of the "difficult case" must often be made subjectively by a highly qualified, experienced examiner. Despite the initial diagnosis, it must be borne in mind that until a pure-tone audiogram is accomplished on the language-impaired child, hearing loss as a possible contributory element cannot be ruled out.

PSYCHOLOGICAL DISORDERS

As stated previously, hearing loss that is congenital or acquired early in life can contribute to child language disorders. Moreover, it can have an effect on social, intellectual, and emotional development, including "egocentricity, difficulty in empathizing with others, rigidity, impulsivity, coercive dependency and a tendency to express feelings by actions rather than by symbolic communication" (Rose, 1983, p. 23). As a child continues to develop in the absence of normal hearing, the normal parent–child relationship is invariably affected, leading to further abnormality. Certainly the potential for psychological abnormality lends further justification for intervention at the earliest possible time.

IDENTIFYING HEARING LOSS IN THE SCHOOLS

The exact number of hearing-impaired school-age children is not known. Surveys that attempt to come up with figures are also confounded by such factors as geographic location and season of the year; there are more failures during cold weather (Gardner, 1988). It is probable that as many as 5% or even more of the public school population may have a hearing impairment at any given time. This does not count the students enrolled in residential and day schools for children with primarily profound hearing impairments.

Probably the most notable survey on hearing in school-age children was the Pittsburgh study (Eagles, Wishik, Doerfler, Melnick, & Levine, 1963). A large number of students in the Pittsburgh area were studied over a period of 4 years. Complete hearing testing was accomplished on carefully calibrated audiometers in adequate sound chambers, and otological examinations were obtained on all children. This study identified 1.7% of all the children tested between the ages of 5 and 10 years as having some degree of hearing impairment.

Several methods have been studied for identifying schoolchildren with hearing impairments. One is for the teacher to be alert for children with possible hearing problems. This system has not proved valid, as teachers tend to miss many of the children with hearing losses while selecting many other children with normal hearing as having hearing disorders. When identification of hearing impairments was compared between teachers and parents, the parents did slightly better but they, too, were far from accurate in their selections.

Obviously, some means of testing in the schools is necessary for identification to be accurate. Group screening procedures have the obvious advantage of testing a number of children simultaneously, decreasing the demands on personnel, space, and equipment. However, some problems do arise. The earphones used in screening procedures tend to get out of calibration easily, especially when dropped or bumped. In addition, false positive responses are a great problem in screening children because many children strive to pass for fear of nonacceptance.

The importance of equipment accuracy and the use of an acceptable workspace are mandatory. Audiometers should be calibrated annually by a factory-trained technician, with outputs checked on an artificial ear every 3 months (Patrick, 1987, p. 407). Of course, if an audiometer or its earphones are jarred or dropped, calibration should be checked before any further hearing tests are done. Listening checks should be performed at the start of every test day, with special attention to breaks in the receiver cords.

There are several methods by which the children who fail group screening tests may be followed. One way is to reschedule the child for a second group test to minimize over-referrals to specialists. Another method is to refer directly to a physician or audiologist when the child fails the first test. If a screening test is failed, the child should be given an individual threshold test, either at the time of the screening or shortly thereafter. ASHA (1984) recommends rescreening a child on the same day if possible, and otherwise within a two-week period. If a child fails a rescreening, an individual threshold test should be administered as soon as possible.

Patrick (1987, p. 402) summarizes the important questions that should be asked when planning a public school hearing screening program.

1. Can we effectively identify those children who have significant hearing loss?
2. Is it practical to screen for middle ear disorders?
3. What is the school's responsibility in implementing and maintaining these programs?

Individual Screening Tests

For the most part, school screening tests today are carried out on an individual basis. They are usually performed by fixing the intensity of the audiometer and changing frequencies. Obviously, the tests may be performed more rapidly if a restricted number of frequencies is sampled and screening is done at a level high enough to be attended to easily by small children. Some authorities have recommended screening only at 4000 Hz because this frequency is often affected by hearing loss. Other people believe that screening with immittance meters will uncover the major source of hearing disorders in the schools—otitis media. It is possible that this approach could catch middle-ear disorders in the early stages, perhaps averting any hearing loss at all. The combination of tympanometry and acoustic reflex tests is most useful for this purpose. Of course, middle-ear problems are not the *only* cause of hearing loss in schoolchildren. Cooper, Gates, Owen, and Dickson (1975) suggested a combination of pure-tone screening at 4000 Hz (to find children with high-frequency sensorineural losses) and immittance screenings (to find children with middle-ear problems).

The Pittsburgh study (Eagles, Wishik, Doerfler, Melnick, and Levine, 1963) showed several important aspects of hearing problems among school-age children. The poor correlations between positive physical findings on otological examination and hearing losses proves the obvious—that the best way to know if a hearing loss is present is through audiometry, and the best way to know if an otological abnormality is present is by otoscopic examination. Perhaps immittance measures should be considered along with otoscopy as the criteria for middle-ear disease.

In 1975 ASHA published its guidelines for identification audiometry in the schools. Proposed revisions of these guidelines that have since appeared (ASHA, 1984) state that the goals of such programs are to incorporate acoustic immittance measures with pure-tone audiometry as a means of identifying persons who are in need of audiological and medical services. Patrick (1987, p. 412) states that 80% to 90% accuracy is obtained when acoustic immittance is combined with pure-tone screenings, as compared to 60% to 70% accuracy when pure tones are used alone. New, automated, portable, easily used immittance screening devices (see Figure 11.8A and B) produce a tympanogram

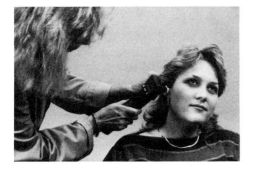

A

Figure 11.8 Portable acoustic immittance device shown in use (A) and in its holder (B) which stores, recharges the unit, and prints the tympanogram and acoustic reflexes (see Figure 11.9). (Photos courtesy of Welch-Allyn.)

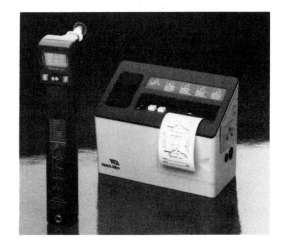

B

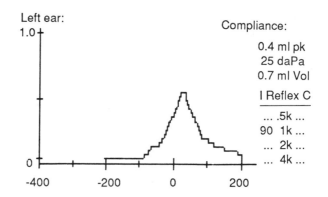

Patient name:_____

Date: 22-Aug-89   Time: 10:06

Left ear: Compliance:
1.0
                                       0.4 ml pk
                                       25 daPa
                                       0.7 ml Vol

                                       I Reflex C
                                       ─────────
                                       ... .5k ...
                                       90 1k ...
                                       ... 2k ...
0   ... 4k ...

-400   -200   0   200

American Electromedics Corp.
AE-106 Tympanometer Serial #360147
Calibration date: 30-May-89

Tester: _____
Comments:

Figure 11.9 Printout of a tympanogram and acoustic reflex screening done on a normal school-age child.

and screen for acoustic reflexes in a matter of seconds on each ear tested (see Figure 11.9). The ASHA guidelines are summarized as follows:

1. Children to be tested are from age 3 to the third grade. *read over*
2. Individual rather than group testing should be used.
3. Manual rather than automatic audiometry should be used.
4. Test frequencies should be 1000, 2000, and 4000 Hz if acoustic immittance measures are included; 500 Hz should be added in the absence of immittance measures if the ambient room noise levels allow.
5. Screening levels should be 20 dB HL.
6. Failure to respond at any frequency at the screening level in either ear constitutes a failure.
7. Children who fail the screening should be rescreened as soon as possible, but certainly within 5 weeks.
8. Referrals of children who fail the rescreening should be made to an audiologist.
9. Appropriate calibration of equipment and monitoring of background noise levels is essential.
10. Screenings may be carried out by support personnel under the supervision of a professional audiologist, who should personally perform any detailed audiometric examinations. *list – a general ?*

Testing the Reliability of Screening Tests

Any screening test carries with it the danger of misclassification. No matter how cleverly a test is designed, it is not possible to determine its shortcomings without submitting the procedure to some empirical verification. A procedure described by Newby (1948) involves the use of the **tetrachoric table** and appears to serve this purpose well (see Figure 11.10). One hundred children who have taken the screening test are selected at random and given threshold tests under the best possible test conditions. The threshold test serves as the criterion for accuracy of the group test. Cells A and D in Figure 11.10 represent agreement between individual and group tests, showing correct identification of those children with and without hearing losses. Cells B and C represent disagreement between the two tests; the larger the number in those two cells, the poorer the group test is at doing its job. Cell C seems to be the biggest offender, passing children on the group test who fail the individual test, missing their hearing losses. This suggests that criteria, such as the screening level, number of children tested at one time, and so on, are too lax. A large number in cell B shows that time and energy are being wasted by identifying normal-hearing children as having hearing losses. In such cases, test criteria may be too stringent, failing children who should have passed.

No matter how carefully a test is conceived, the number in cells B and C will probably never reach the ideal zero. If the criteria are so stringent that no child passes who should fail, the penalty is to retest a lot of normals or to

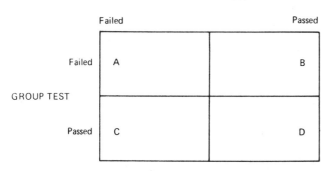

INDIVIDUAL TEST

Figure 11.10 Tetrachoric table used to test the efficiency of a group test of hearing. The children correctly identified as having hearing losses by the group test and verified by the individual test are shown in cell A. Those properly identified as having no hearing losses are shown in cell D. Those children with normal hearing incorrectly identified by the group test as having losses are shown in cell B. Cell C shows the children with hearing losses who were missed by the group test.

make many over-referrals. On the other hand, decreasing the number in cell B at the expense of missing children with hearing losses seems unthinkable.

In the real world, the person in charge of any screening program must balance factors of money, personnel, and the number of children to be tested against the efficiency of the test. There appears to be an inverse relationship between efficiency and accuracy in group screening tests if one defines efficiency in terms of the number of tests performed with the least expenditure of time and money.

PSEUDOHYPACUSIS IN CHILDREN

There are numerous reports in the literature of pseudohypacusis in children. The causes may range from misunderstanding of the test, to malingering, to psychogenic hearing loss. As a general rule it is not difficult for alert clinicians to detect nonorganicity in children and, with some clever manipulation, to determine the true organic hearing thresholds. The earlier nonorganic problems can be detected, the sooner they can be dealt with. It is important to eliminate the reliance on a false hearing loss quickly, before it becomes a crutch on which the child may lean to solve or avoid emotional, social, or academic problems.

Dixon and Newby (1959) observed a series of 40 children with pseudohypacusis. These children had normal hearing, yet they behaved on hearing tests as though they had hearing losses. The tendency seemed to be greater in girls than in boys. The children did not appear to have hearing difficulty in normal conversational situations and often showed normal speech thresholds, despite apparent hearing losses for pure tone. Dixon and Newby felt that motivation for pseudohypacusis in children may be very different from that in adults, and that psychological or psychiatric consultation may be indicated in some cases.

Although many schoolchildren try diligently to pass their hearing tests, some others manifest nonorganic symptoms. Ross (1964) has pointed out the dangers of reinforcing children's notions that they have a hearing loss. The child may consciously or unconsciously see the advantages of hearing loss and may decide that the risk is worth the secondary gains to be realized in the forms of favors and excuses. Ross advised that children should not be referred for special examinations by physicians unless the person in charge of the school tests is reasonably certain that a hearing problem exists. Most experienced audiologists can probably recall specific incidents in which a child has become committed to continued fabrication of a hearing loss, no matter how the problem got started.

Public school environments for hearing evaluations are often less than satisfactory. Often the testing is done in large rooms with poor acoustics and with considerable masking from room noise. Many children may be tested before an audiometer calibration defect is detected. Unless all the criteria for adequate testing are met, the purpose of the procedure is defeated.

MANAGEMENT OF HEARING-IMPAIRED CHILDREN

Although other conditions may be contributory to a child's delay in onset of language and normal speech, it is often determined that hearing loss itself is the primary problem. Whether a hearing loss is present at birth or develops some time afterward can have a great effect on language acquisition. When hearing losses exist before the normal development of language, they are referred to as **prelingual**. Those acquired after that time are called **postlingual**. Naturally, the later in life a postlingual hearing loss begins, the better are the chances to conserve the speech and language that the child has already learned through the hearing sense.

It is the audiologist's obligation to pursue medical reversal of a hearing loss as soon as that possibility presents itself. Determination of otologic or surgical treatment is made on the basis of medical decisions. Audiologists should make referrals immediately when otitis media or other infections are evidenced, or when there is any indication of a structural deviation that might involve the auditory system. If medical treatment of a hearing loss is impossible, or is accomplished to the extent that it leaves the child with some hearing loss, further intervention is indicated.

Counseling

Precisely how to convey to parents or caretakers the nature and extent of their children's hearing loss is not universally agreed on. Many clinicians use a system of direct information transfer; that is, they present the information, insofar as it is known, about a child's hearing loss. Often this includes descriptions of the audiogram, definitions of terms, and options for dealing with the child's needs. The intent is to educate the caretakers to the point that they can best handle the child's hearing problems. What clinicians often do not realize is that their choice of language, verbal and nonverbal, and even the amount of information provided, may have profound effects, both positive and negative, on the receiver of that information.

The reactions of parents to the realization, however gradual, that their child has a hearing impairment are not always the same. Whether externalized or internalized, it is safe to say that the effect is generally quite intense. As Moses (1979) points out, parents view their children as extensions of themselves, with hopes and dreams of perfection. When an imperfection is uncovered, these dreams are shattered. Because of its invisibility, hearing impairment often does not seem to society like a true handicap, which makes the adjustment even more difficult for the parents.

Stream and Stream (1978) reviewed the stages through which parents pass when they learn of their child's handicap. Parents initially go through a period of *denial* as a means of self-defense against very bad news. During this state it is frequently fruitless even to try to provide details of the diagnosis and recommendations for training, for parents are simply incapable of acceptance at this stage.

In what Stream and Stream (1978) called the second stage of "mourning," the parents frequently express *anger* as they relinquish their feelings of denial. "Anger may be transferred to others: loved ones, marital partner, God, physician, or audiologist; anyone and anything is vulnerable" (Stream & Stream, 1978, p. 338). Audiologists must be able to function as counselors and be able to accept this anger, even if it is directed toward them. Objectivity at this point is crucial.

When anger has subsided, it is common for parents to go through a period of *guilt*. Parents who persist in seeking explanations for the cause of the hearing loss may be looking for a way out of the awful sense that they have somehow done this to their child or are being punished for some past sin. If the guilt is projected toward the other marital partner, the foundation of the marriage may become shaky; divorce is not uncommon among parents of handicapped children. Indeed, many parents never pass beyond the guilt stage, with unfortunate consequences for the child, who may become spoiled or overprotected, or may never reach his or her full potential. Merely telling parents that they need not blame themselves is often fruitless, but the audiologist should try to avoid words or actions that promote guilt.

When parents begin to cease reeling from the impact of the bad news about their child, they seek ways to help and teach in order to maximize the child's potential. At this juncture they may be so overloaded with assignments, information, and well-meaning advice from professionals, family, and friends that they perceive themselves as inadequate to the job at hand. At this point *anxiety* increases, which must be dealt with before any form of therapy can become effective for the child.

Before parents can help their children, they must be helped themselves. They must be taught to cope with the challenge of parenting a handicapped child. They must learn to continue to give and accept love and to include the entire family in normal activities, as well as in activities prescribed for the child with the hearing loss. The audiologist, as a sensitive and empathetic listener, must learn to see beyond the words to the feelings of family members regarding a hearing-impaired child. Therapy without personal concern may be useless. Even the words used to describe the child's problems may be crucial.

For some time Luterman (1987), as well as others, has been concerned with the manner of information transfer to parents. Martin, George, O'Neal, and Daly (1987) conducted a survey in the United States and learned that parents (or other caregivers) are often not receptive to detailed information immediately after they have learned that their child has an irreversible hearing loss. Respondents to their survey indicated that initial parental reactions include sorrow, shock, denial, fear, anger, helplessness, and blame. It takes varying and sometimes prolonged amounts of time for the diagnosis of hearing loss to be accepted. Martin et al. suggest that acceptance of the diagnosis of hearing loss is easier for parents and others if they have the opportunity to observe hearing tests as they are performed on their children. Parents are often confused and disturbed by new and unusual terminology.

When presenting diagnostic information that may be painful, audiologists must temper their enthusiasm for launching habilitative efforts with patience and understanding. Reliance on feedback from parents regarding their anxiety levels during counseling may be misleading. For example, what appears to be a lax or indifferent parental attitude may be a smokescreen for fear and bewilderment.

It is also often the case that caregivers opt for a plan of action that is not what the audiologist believes to be in a particular child's best interest. Because of their background and training, many audiologists believe that the first avenue followed should employ the aural/oral approach, maximizing residual hearing with amplification and encouraging the use of communication through speech. A different decision by a parent may appear wrong to the clinician, but that opinion must be repressed.

The function of the audiologist should be to determine the times, after diagnosis, at which educational and habilitative options can best be conveyed to the parents. These alternatives should be explained carefully, objectively, and without bias, so that the caretakers themselves can make an informed decision regarding the management of their child. Opportunities for further consultation with the clinician, as well as participation in parent support groups, should be provided at the earliest possible time. Audiological counseling should be viewed as a continuing process, and parents should be made to feel that they can come to their audiologist/counselor at times when assistance is needed.

It is natural for clinicians to present diagnostic information to the adults who have accompanied a child to the hearing evaluation. When children are old enough, and have sufficient hearing to process the information, it should be given directly to them in the presence of their caretaking adults. This eliminates the resentment that many children feel when they have been excluded from discussion of matters that relate directly to them. Naturally, when children are very young or severely hearing impaired, it is the adults who should be addressed, but always with sensitivity to the child's feelings. When children are young and profoundly hearing-impaired, it is their caregivers who must decide on the means by which the children are to be educated.

Educational Options

The precise modes of communication by which profoundly hearing-impaired children should be educated continues to be debated. As mentioned earlier, many people believe that emphasis should be placed on speech, with amplification designed to take advantage of residual hearing. Strict adherents to this philosophy, often called *oralists*, believe that since all children live in a world in which communication is accomplished through speech, their adjustment is best made by teaching them to speak so that they will fit in with the majority of others.

Other experts believe that manual communication, by signs and finger-spelling, allows children with profound hearing losses to communicate more readily so that communication skills can be learned more quickly and specific subject materials can be taught. Additionally, these *manualists* often believe that satisfactory communication using speech is not attainable for many children, and that their adjustment should be made to the nonhearing world, where they will be accepted more completely.

According to Vernon and Mindel (1978), the greatest psychological danger to the profoundly hearing-impaired child is the inability of the parents, and the professional specialists with whom they deal, to understand the problems involved. Their belief is that the frequent failure of amplification, even with speechreading and auditory training, testifies to the need for the early use of manual communication. They further emphasize their philosophy that children's psychological and educational needs are not met by forcing them into artificial situations and insisting that they become something they are not — hearing persons.

Implementation of Public Law 94-142, the Education for all Handicapped Children's Law, mandated **mainstreaming** of handicapped children whenever possible. This led to more than half of the approximately 80,000 profoundly hearing-impaired children in the United States being moved away from specialized schools. Many of these specialized schools began to close as a consequence of these moves (Lane, 1987).

Lane (1987) felt that the community of the severely to profoundly hearing impaired is at odds with the very professions that were designed to help it. He states, "To achieve intellectual and emotional maturity at full participation in society most deaf children require an education conducted in their primary language, American Sign Language. . . ." Proponents of oral or combined oral and manual approaches to teaching the hearing-impaired may be just as adamant in their beliefs. Educational placement for hearing-impaired children is an issue that is passionately disputed by educators and clinicians, and is not likely to be easily resolved.

Brief descriptions follow of some of the more popular teaching methods used:

The Aural/Oral Method. Often called the multisensory or auditory-global approach, this system attempts to tap the child's residual hearing through amplification and employ auditory and speechreading (lip-reading) training. The child's output is expected to be speech.

The Acoupedic Method. This method is called *unisensory* because the emphasis is placed entirely on the use of audition and early amplification with hearing aids. The child is not allowed to develop skills at speechreading, and is actually deprived of visual cues. This system is not popular today.

Total Communication (TC). Total Communication is probably the most popular teaching system now employed for children with severe to profound hearing losses. TC is accomplished by taking the best of the aural and sign systems, placing the emphasis on both signs and speech to help the child to communicate. Proponents believe that language is learned more quickly and accurately using TC than by other methods, but critics maintain that it is unreasonable to expect some children to learn to listen, read lips, and follow signs at the same time.

Fingerspelling (Dactylology). Fingerspelling has been called "writing in the air" (Mayberry, 1978, p. 408), as it is a system by which each letter of the alphabet is represented by a precise formation of the fingers of one hand. It allows users to spell out entire words, phrases, and sentences. Although fingerspelling alone does not facilitate the development of language in a hearing-impaired child, it does preserve the rules of grammar and syntax, which are often compromised with some of the other systems. Figure 11.11 shows the manual alphabet.

American Sign Language (ASL). In American Sign Language (ASL), often called Ameslan, specific signs are created with the hands in conjunction with the face and the body, especially shifting of the shoulders. ASL also makes use of three-dimensional space. Many linguists consider it a true language, with its own syntax and morphology, and it should not be viewed as a deficient or inaccurate form of English. ASL has even been accepted by some colleges and universities as an alternative to satisfaction of the undergraduate foreign language requirement.

Signed English (SE). Signed English (Bornstein & Saulnier, 1973) is a manual system that follows the rules of English grammar. Fingerspelling augments this system when no particular sign represents a word. SE takes ASL vocabulary and places it in English word order.

Seeing Essential English (SEE 1). SEE 1 uses signs as they would appear in spoken English, with specific signs for some articles and verbs, and markers to help in identifying such aspects of English as tense and number (Paul & Quigley, 1987, p. 64). This system breaks words down into morphemes (e.g., *a-part-ment*).

Signing Exact English (SEE 2). SEE 2 (Gustafson, Pfetzing, & Sawolkow, 1987) is similar to SEE 1 but is less rigid with respect to following precise rules of English morphology, which may account for its wide use (Paul & Quigley,

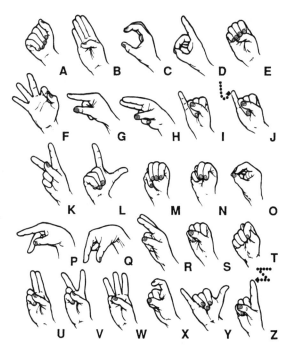

Figure 11.11 The manual alphabet.

1987, p. 65). This system breaks words down into morphemes that are individually accepted words (e.g., *cow-boy*).

Linguistics of Visual English (LOVE). This method of manual communication uses signs, as in SEE 1 and SEE 2, but employs a slightly different written system, although it follows English word order. Fingerspelling is used to show irregular tense use. LOVE is less commonly used than SEE 1 or SEE 2 (Mayberry, 1978, p. 409). *Colorado*

Pidgin Sign English (PSE). Sometimes called simultaneous communication, Pidgin Sign English is a combination of manually represented English and some grammatical features of ASL (e.g., plurality). In PSE not all words are signed; what is deleted is what is considered least informative, such as articles (Paul & Quigley, 1987, p. 66).

Cued Speech. Cued speech (Cornett, 1967) was devised to aid speech-reading and speech development and employs eight formed hand shapes in four positions, which are made close to the face of a speaker so they may supplement speechreading information. The cues assist in differentiating among sounds that appear the same on the lips (e.g., /m/, /b/, and /p/). The child must simultaneously attend to both the speechreading and the cues, for the cues by themselves are meaningless.

Know all ↑

A variety of placement options may be available for the formal education of hearing-impaired children. These include privately and publicly funded institutions, residential and day schools, and public schools. Many hearing-impaired children in the public schools are mainstreamed with nonhandicapped children. Of all children in regular classrooms requiring special educational considerations, the hearing-impaired make up the largest groups (Flexer, Wray, & Ireland, 1989). Although classroom teachers have shown an interest in knowing more about their hearing-impaired students, they admit that their present knowledge is inadequate for proper management (Martin, Bernstein, Daly, & Cody, 1988). In addition to educational management, teacher information is essential regarding classroom acoustics, individually worn amplification devices, and systems to help improve the signal-to-noise ratios for the children (see Ross, Brackett, & Maxon, 1982).

When children are mainstreamed, direct contact with the classroom teacher is the best way to see that their needs are being met. If intervention is handled diplomatically, the audiologist will find most teachers receptive and eager to learn how to help their students. Special help includes assigning preferential seating, providing a maximum of visual clues, encouraging hearing-aid use, issuing written assignments when possible, and maintaining frequent contact with the parents.

The ideal seat in the classroom is not necessarily right at the front near the teacher's desk. Each situation is different, but light, especially from windows, should be at the child's back whenever possible, so that glare and shadows are at a minimum. It should be possible for the microphone of the hearing aid to face the other students in the class. The teacher should speak distinctly to the child but should not overemphasize lip movements, which is a natural tendency when talking to any hearing-impaired person. Shouting should be avoided, and the teacher should see that the child's hearing aid is in working order. Homework and other assignments should be printed on handouts or written on the chalkboard in addition to being orally explained. Sign language interpreters, when used, should be welcomed to the classroom and their presence explained to the normal-hearing children.

Academic progress should be monitored with the parents on a more frequent basis than is done with normal-hearing students. It is axiomatic that any system of teaching hearing-impaired children in the classroom or speech and hearing clinic will be most effective if it is complemented by a strong home program.

Parental decision to follow a certain course regarding a child's training may change on the basis of the reinforcement that is received for the efforts made, and the information acquired. The responsibility of the pediatric audiologist is to remain as a source of information and support to families, to follow up the initial diagnosis with regular hearing evaluations, and to assist with hearing aids and other listening devices as needed. Insightful clinicians must develop skills that allow them to facilitate rather than to direct families in the series of decisions that are so crucial if hearing-impaired children are to reach their potentials.

The reader may have noted that a scrupulous attempt has been made throughout this book to avoid use of the word *deaf*. Ross and Calvert (1967) have pointed out that the "semantics of deafness" may have a profound effect on the ability of a family with a hearing-impaired child to cope with the problems that arise. The lay public, and to a large extent the professional community as well, has polarized people into two groups, those who hear and those who do not. When people are labeled as "deaf," it means to many that they cannot hear at all and that they will remain mute. This can inhibit the use of residual hearing and the development of spoken language. Ross and Calvert state that ignoring the quantitative nature of hearing loss may affect the child's diagnosis, interaction with the parents, educational placement and treatment, and expectations for achievement.

SUMMARY

Pediatric audiology can be time consuming and frustrating. Many times clinicians do not have the feeling, as they have with most adults, of complete closure on a case at the end of a diagnostic session. Nevertheless, the proper identification and management of hearing loss in children is one of the most solemn responsibilities of the audiologist. Truly, work with children is often carried out more as an art than a science, testing the cleverness and perseverance of clinicians and calling on all their training and experience.

Pediatric audiology includes the use of those tests and diagnostic procedures designed especially for children who cannot be tested by conventional audiometry. Approaches vary with both the chronological and mental ages of children. Some tests, designed merely to elicit some sort of startle reaction, may be carried out on children as young as several hours of age. Other tests employ play techniques or use special rewards to encourage proper performance on hearing tests. Still other procedures involve measuring changes in a child's electrophysiological state in response to sound. With some children it is possible to test by making slight alterations in the conventional audiometric techniques used with adults.

Hearing testing in children is designed to determine the nature and extent of a child's communicative problem and is virtually useless unless some habilitative path is pursued. Pediatric audiologists must muster every resource at their disposal, including interactions with caretakers and other professionals, in designing approaches that will maximize the human potential in every hearing-impaired child. To do less than this is to do a disservice to the children whose futures may be profoundly affected by such professional decisions.

GLOSSARY

Auropalpebral reflex (APR) Contraction of the ring muscles of the eyes in response to a sudden unexpected sound.

Autism A condition of withdrawal and introspection manifested by asocial behavior in infants and young children.

Behavioral observation audiometry (BOA) Observation of changes in the activity state of an infant in response to sound.

Cardiotachometry Analysis of changes in heart rate in response to sound.

Conditioned orientation reflex (COR) A technique for testing young children in the sound field by having them look in the direction of a sound source in search of a flashing light.

Crib-o-gram A motion-sensing device attached to an infant's crib. A graphic recorder indicates whether changes in the baby's motion are related to the presentation of a series of sounds.

Dysinhibition Bizarre behavior patterns often associated with brain-damaged individuals.

Echolalia A baby's meaningless imitation of others' speech sounds as a form of vocal play. A natural step in the development of speech and language.

High-risk register A set of criteria designed to help identify neonates whose probability of hearing loss is greater than normal.

Lalling The stage in speech development wherein infants coo and create vocal sounds for their own amusement.

Mainstreaming Integrating hearing-impaired (or other handicapped) children into the "least restrictive" educational setting. This often implies placement in a regular school classroom with special educational assistance where necessary.

Minimum response level (MRL) The lowest level of response offered by a child to an acoustic stimulus. Depending on a variety of circumstances, the signal responded to may be either barely audible or well above threshold.

Moro reflex A sudden embracing movement of the arms and drawing up of the legs of infants and small children in response to sudden loud sounds.

Neonatal auditory response cradle A system for assessing the hearing of newborn children by presenting narrow-band noise to their ears via ear insert devices and measuring reflexive responses in terms of head, limb, or body movements or changes in respiratory pattern.

Operant conditioning audiometry (OCA) The use of tangible reinforcement, such as edible items, to condition difficult-to-test patients for pure-tone audiometry.

Pediacoumeter A device used for pure-tone audiometry with small children. If children respond correctly to the presentation of a tone, they are rewarded by the appearance of a small puppet.

Peep show A device for sound-field pure-tone testing of small children. If children respond correctly to a tonal presentation, their reward is the appearance of a picture in a window.

Perseveration Persistent repetition of an activity.

Postlingual hearing loss Hearing loss acquired by a child after s/he has developed some language skills.

Prelingual hearing loss Hearing loss that is either congenital or acquired before language skills have been acquired.

Tangible reinforcement operant conditioning audiometry (TROCA) A form of operant audiometry using tangible reinforcers, such as food or tokens.

Tetrachoric table A table containing four cells designed to test the efficiency and accuracy of group hearing tests.

Visual reinforcement audiometry (VRA) The use of a light or picture to reinforce a child's response to a sound.

Warble tone A pure tone that is frequently modulated. The modulation is usually expressed as a percentage (e.g., a 1000 Hz tone warbled at 5% would vary from 950 to 1050 Hz).

STUDY QUESTIONS

1. What are the first five questions you would ask the parents of a small child being seen for a hearing evaluation?

2. A child under one year of age is to be seen for an evaluation. How would you prepare prior to the child's arrival in the clinic? List the procedures you would use, in the order you would use them.

3. List the pros and cons of neonatal screening.

4. What are the major steps you would take as an audiologist organizing a school hearing test program? Once begun, how would you test its efficiency?

5. Consider the major causes for the lack of speech development. List some of the typical symptoms for each cause.

6. How would you approach the counseling of parents of a hearing-impaired child?

7. List the training and educational options for a severely hearing-impaired child.

REVIEW TABLE 11.1 PROCEDURES USED IN PEDIATRIC AUDIOMETRY

PROCEDURE	AGE GROUP MOST SUITABLE	PROBABILITY OF SUCCESS
Warblet	Infants	Fair
Speech sounds	4 to 8 months	Good
COR, VRA	6 months to 2 years	Good
Imitation of vocalization	Under 1 year	Fair
Play audiometry	1 to 6 years	Good
Operant conditioning	2 to 5 years	Good
Noisemakers	Under 3 years	Fair
Immittance measures	All ages	Good
AEP	All ages	Good
Pure-tone audiometry	Over 3 years	Good

REFERENCES

AMERICAN SPEECH-LANGUAGE-HEARING ASSOCIATION. (1984). Proposed guidelines for identification audiometry. *Asha, 26,* 47–50.

_____. (1988). Guidelines for the identification of hearing impairment in at risk infants age birth to 6 months. *Asha, 30,* 61–64.

BENNETT, M. J. (1979). Trials with the auditory response cradle I: Neonatal responses to auditory stimuli. *British Journal of Audiology, 13,* 125–134.

BENNETT, M. J., & LAWRENCE, R. J. (1980). Trials with the auditory response cradle II: The neonatal respiratory response to an auditory stimulus. *British Journal of Audiology, 14,* 1–6.

BORNSTEIN, H., & SAULNIER, K. (1973). Signed English: A brief follow-up to the first evaluations. *American Annals of the Deaf, 118,* 454–463.

COMMITTEE ON HEARING, BIOACOUSTICS, AND BIOMECHANICS, COMMISSION ON BEHAVIORAL AND SOCIAL SCIENCES AND EDUCATION, NATIONAL RESEARCH COUNCIL. (1987). Brainstem audiometry of infants. *Asha, 29,* 47–55.

COOPER, J. C., GATES, G. A., OWEN, J. H., & DICKSON, H. D. (1975). An abbreviated impedance bridge technique for school screening. *Journal of Speech and Hearing Disorders, 40,* 260–269.

CORNETT, R. O. (1967). Cued speech. *American Annals of the Deaf, 112,* 3–13.

DE JONGE, R. (1984). Tympanometry and the evaluation of middle-ear disease in children. *Audiology: A Journal for Continuing Education, 9,* 75–90.

DICARLO, L. M., KENDALL, D. C., & GOLDSTEIN, R. (1962). Diagnostic procedures for auditory disorders in children. *Folio Phoniatrica, 14,* 206–264.

DIX, M. R., & HALLPIKE, C. S. (1947). The peep show: A new technique for pure tone audiometry in young children. *British Medical Journal, 2,* 719–723.

DIXON, R. F., & NEWBY, H. A. (1959). Children with nonorganic hearing problems. *Archives of Otolaryngology, 70,* 619–623.

DOWNS, D. W. (1982). ABR testing in the neonatal intensive care unit: A cautious response. *Asha, 24,* 1009–1015.

DOWNS, M. P. (1977). The expanding imperatives of early identification. In F. Bess (Ed.), *Childhood deafness: Causation, assessment and management,* (pp. 95–106). New York: Grune & Stratton.

DOWNS, M. P., & STERRITT, G. M. (1967). A guide to newborn and infant screening programs. *Archives of Otolaryngology, 85,* 15–22.

EAGLES, E., WISHIK, S., DOERFLER, L., MELNICK, W., & LEVINE, H. (1963). Hearing sensitivity and related factors in children. *Laryngoscope,* Monograph Supplement.

EISENBERG, R. B. (1975). Cardiotachometry. *Physiological Measures of the Audio-Vestibular System,* ed. L. J. Bradford. New York: Academic Press, pp. 319–348.

EWING, I., & EWING. A. (1944). The ascertainment of deafness in infancy and early childhood. *Journal of Laryngology, 59,* 309–333.

FLEXER, C., WRAY, D., & IRELAND, J. A. (1989). Preferential seating is *not* enough: Issues in classroom management of hearing-impaired students. *Language, Speech and Hearing Services in Schools, 20,* 11–21.

GALAMBOS, R., HICKS, G. E., & WILSON, M. J. (1984). The auditory brain stem response reliably predicts hearing loss in graduates of a tertiary intensive care nursery. *Ear and Hearing, 5,* 254–260.

GARDNER, H. J. (1988). Moderate vs. cold weather effects on hearing screening results among preschool children. *The Hearing Journal, 41,* 29–32.

GERKIN, K. P. (1984a). The high risk register for deafness. *Asha, 26,* 17–23.

_____. (1984b). Infant hearing screening. *Audiology: A Journal for Continuing Education, 9,* 59–73.

GUILFORD, F. R., & HAUG, C. O. (1952). Diagnosis of deafness in the very young child. *Archives of Otolaryngology, 55,* 101–106.

GUSTAFSON, G., PFETZING, D., & SAWOLKOW, E. (1980). *Signing Exact English: The 1980 edition.* Los Alamitos, California: Modern Signs Press. Found in Paul, P. V., & Quigley, S. P. (1987). Some effects of early hearing impairment on English language development. In F. N. Martin (Ed.), *Hearing Disorders in Children* (pp. 49–80). Austin, TX: Pro-Ed.

HARDY, W. G., HARDY, J. B., BRINKER, C. H., FRAZIER T. M., & DOUGHTERY, A. (1962). Auditory screening of infants. *Annals of Otology, Rhinology and Laryngology, 71,* 759–766.

HARDY, W. G., & PAULS, M. D. (1952). The test situation of PGSR audiometry. *Journal of Speech and Hearing Disorders, 17,* 13–24.

HAUG, O., BACCARO, P., & GUILFORD, F. (1967). A pure-tone audiogram on the infant: The PIWI technique. *Archives of Otolaryngology, 86,* 435–440.

HODGSON, W. R. (1978). Tests of hearing—Birth through one year. In F. N. Martin (Ed.), *Pediatric Audiology* (pp. 174–200). Englewood Cliffs, NJ: Prentice-Hall.

———. (1987). Tests of hearing—The infant. In F. N. Martin (Ed.), *Hearing Disorders in Children* (pp. 185–216). Austin, TX: Pro-Ed.

JACOBSON, J. T. & MOREHOUSE, C. R. (1984). A comparison of auditory brain stem response and behavioral screening in high risk and normal newborn infants. *Ear and Hearing, 5,* 247–253.

KETTLETY, A. (1987). The Manchester high pitch rattle. *British Journal of Audiology, 21,* 73–74.

LANE, H. (1987). Mainstreaming of deaf children—From bad to worse. *The Deaf American, 38,* 15.

LIDEN, G., & KANKKONEN, A. (1961). Visual reinforcement audiometry. *Acta Otolaryngologica* (Stockholm), *67,* 281–292.

LLOYD, L. L., SPRADLIN, J. E., & REID, M. J. (1968). An operant audiometric procedure for difficult-to-test patients. *Journal of Speech and Hearing Disorders, 33,* 236–245.

LUTERMAN, D. M. (1987). Counseling parents of hearing-impaired children. In F. N. Martin (Ed.), *Hearing Disorders in Children* (pp. 303–319). Austin, TX: Pro-Ed.

MARTIN, F. N., BERNSTEIN, M. E., DALY, J. A., & CODY, J. P. (1988). Classroom teachers' knowledge of hearing disorders and attitudes about mainstreaming hard-of-hearing children. *Language, Speech and Hearing Services in Schools, 19,* 83–95.

MARTIN, F. N., & CLARK, J. G. (1977). Audiologic detection of auditory processing disorders in children. *Journal of the American Audiology Society, 3,* 140–146.

MARTIN, F. N., & COOMBES, S. (1976). A tangibly reinforced speech reception threshold procedure for use with small children. *Journal of Speech and Hearing Disorders, 41,* 333–338.

MARTIN, F. N., GEORGE, K., O'NEAL, J., & DALY, J. (1987). Audiologists' and parents' attitudes regarding counseling of families of hearing-impaired children. *Asha, 29,* 27–33.

MARTIN, F. N., & GRAVEL, K. L. (1989). Pediatric audiological practices in the United States. *The Hearing Journal, 42,* 33–48.

MATKIN, N. D. (1973, June). *Some essential features of a pediatric audiological evaluation.* Talk presented to the Eighth Danavox Symposium, Copenhagen.

MAYBERRY, R. I. (1978). Manual communication. In H. Davis & S. R. Silverman (Eds.), *Hearing and Deafness,* 4th ed. (pp. 400–417). New York: Holt, Rinehart and Winston.

MOSES, K. (1979). Parenting a hearing-impaired child. *Volta Review, 81,* 73–80.

NEWBY, H. A. (1948). Evaluating the efficiency of group screening tests of hearing. *Journal of Speech and Hearing Disorders, 13,* 236–240.

O'NEILL, J., OYER, H., & HILLIS, J. (1961). Audiometric procedures with children. *Journal of Speech and Hearing Disorders, 26,* 61–66.

PATRICK, P. E. (1987). Identification audiometry. In F. N. Martin (Ed.), *Hearing disorders in children* (pp. 399–425). Austin, TX: Pro-Ed.

PAUL, P. V., & QUIGLEY, S. P. (1987). Some effects of early hearing impairment on English language development. In F. N. Martin (Ed.), *Hearing disorders in children* (pp. 49–80). Austin, TX: Pro-Ed.

Roberts, J. L., Davis, H., & Phon, G. L. (1982). Auditory brainstem response in preterm neonates: Maturation and follow-up. *Journal of Pediatrics, 101,* 257–263.

Rose, D. S. (1983). The fundamental role of hearing in psychological development. *Hearing Instruments, 34,* 22–26.

Ross, M. (1964). The variable intensity pulse count method (VIPCM) for the detection and measurement of the pure-tone thresholds of children with functional hearing losses. *Journal of Speech and Hearing Disorders, 29,* 477–482.

Ross, M., Brackett, D., & Maxon, A. (1982). *Hard of hearing children in regular schools.* Englewood Cliffs, NJ: Prentice-Hall.

Ross, M., & Calvert, D. R. (1967). The semantics of deafness. *Volta Review, 69,* 644–649.

Ross, M., & Lerman, J. (1970). A picture identification test for hearing impaired children. *Journal of Speech and Hearing Research, 13,* 44–53.

Ross, M., & Matkin, N. (1967). The rising audiometric configuration. *Journal of Speech and Hearing Disorders, 32,* 377–382.

Shepherd, D. C. (1971). Pediatric audiology. In D. E. Rose (Ed.), *Audiological assessment* (pp. 241–279). Englewood Cliffs, NJ: Prentice-Hall.

Simmons, F. (1976). Automated hearing screening test for newborns: The crib-o-gram. In G. Mencher (Ed.), *Proceedings of the Nova Scotia Conference on Early Identification of Hearing Loss* (pp. 171–180). Basel: S. Karger.

Simmons, F., & Russ, F. (1974). Automated newborn hearing screening: Crib-o-gram. *Archives of Otolaryngology, 100,* 1–7.

Simmons, F. B., McFarland, W. H., & Jones, F. R. (1980). Patterns of deafness in newborns. *Laryngoscope, 90,* 448–453.

Spradlin, J. E., & Lloyd, L. L. (1965). Operant conditioning audiometry with low level retardates: A preliminary report. In L. L. Lloyd & D. R. Frisina (Eds.), *The audiological assessment of the mentally retarded: Proceedings of a national conference.* (pp. 45–58). Parsons, KS: Parsons State Hospital and Training Center.

Stream, R. W., & Stream, K. S. (1978). Counseling the parents of the hearing-impaired child. In F. N. Martin (Ed.), *Pediatric audiology* (pp. 311–355). Englewood Cliffs, NJ: Prentice-Hall.

Suzuki, T., & Ogiba, Y. (1961). Conditioned orientation reflex audiometry. *Archives of Otolaryngology, 74,* 84–90.

Vernon, M., & Mindel, E. (1978). Psychological and psychiatric aspects of profound hearing loss. In D. Rose (Ed.), *Audiological assessment* (pp. 99–145). Englewood Cliffs, NJ: Prentice-Hall.

Weaver, N. J., Wardell, F. N., & Martin, F. N. (1979). Comparison of tangibly reinforced speech-reception and pure-tone thresholds of mentally retarded children. *American Journal of Mental Deficiency, 83,* 512–517.

Wedenberg, E. (1956). Auditory test in newborn infants. *Acta Otolaryngologica, 46,* 446–461.

SUGGESTED READINGS

Luterman, D. (1987). *Deafness in the family,* San Diego: College-Hill Press.

Martin, F. N. (Ed.). (1987). *Hearing disorders in children.* Austin, TX: Pro-Ed.

Northern, J. L., & Downs, M. P. (1983). *Hearing in children* (3rd ed.). Baltimore: Williams & Wilkins.

12

MANAGEMENT OF THE
HEARING-IMPAIRED PATIENT

The purpose of this book has been to introduce the reader to basic information relating to auditory disorders and their diagnoses. Clinical audiologists have responsibilities that transcend diagnosis. When a medical condition is present that causes or contributes to the patient's hearing problem, proper otological consultation must be sought. In the absence of medical treatment or after its completion, the audiologist is the logical person to take charge of the patient's total aural rehabilitation program. Also included among the audiologist's professional chores are taking proper case histories, determining appropriate referrals upon completion of the examination, writing reports, and making liaisons with related professionals.

If it is decided that a hearing aid is indicated for a patient, the audiologist should assist both in selecting the instrument and in training to ensure optimum efficiency in its use. Of tremendous importance is the counseling session that should follow each audiological assessment, for what is said to the patient or family and *how* it is said can have great psychological impact. All the preceding materials in this book have led to what must be summarized briefly in the following pages. An understanding of normal and abnormal auditory functioning, together with diagnostic procedures, is without merit unless it culminates in activities that improve the lives of hearing-impaired persons.

CHAPTER OBJECTIVES

This chapter is designed to assist the reader in various aspects of patient management, such as taking histories, writing reports, cooperating with other professionals, and promoting aural rehabilitation, including the use of amplification systems and counseling. Less emphasis is placed on precise methodologies in this chapter than in previous chapters. The intention here is to give the reader a brief overview of a number of different aspects of audiology not previously covered in detail in this book.

PATIENT HISTORIES

Dr. Dilling dors this part not James Anderson (Aud)   *case history*

Proper documentation of a patient's history is almost as important as the audiometric examination. The manner in which the history is recorded may follow one of several formats, ranging from informality to close adherence to a printed form. Some audiologists perfer to ask only questions that appear to relate to the patient's particular complaints, and to jot their remarks down informally. This approach requires much skill and experience and allows for possible omission of essential questions.

Some history forms are lengthy and contain more items than are essential for gathering data pertinent to a particular hearing problem. A short form like the one shown in Figure 12.1, has proved useful in the majority of adult cases. Although in some busy audiology centers case histories are recorded by ancillary personnel (technicians or clerks), or are mailed to the patient for completion prior to evaluation, it is best for the audiologist to ask the questions or at least to review the questionnaire with the respondent.

Any case-history form must provide space for a statement of the problem, including why the services of the audiologist were sought. It is helpful to know the patient's own attitude about the appointment. Knowing the reason for the visit to the clinic can provide powerful insight before the rest of the history has been completed or the first test has been administered. Information about the duration and degree of hearing loss should be gleaned, along with family history of ear disease or hearing impairment, noise exposure, infection, or trauma to the ear or head. History of vertigo, of past surgery related to the ear, of previous hearing tests, and so on is most important. In addition, reports of experience with hearing aids are valuable.

The manner in which questions are answered may be revealing. Often a patient hesitates in answering some questions, which may suggest that not too much credence should be given to the answers. This hesitancy sometimes reflects disagreement among family members. On the other hand, the fact that questions are answered rapidly and with apparent self-assurance does not, in itself, ensure validity. People who have repeatedly answered the same types of questions, perhaps posed by different specialists, become practiced at responding and may find themselves answering questions incorrectly with

THE UNIVERSITY OF TEXAS AT AUSTIN
Speech and Hearing Center

Adult Case History

Clinic #_____ Clinician(s) _____

Patient's Name_____ Sex_____
              Last   First   Middle

D.O.B._____ Age_____ Date_____

Address: Street_____ Phone:
                                               Home_____

          _____   Office_____
          City_____

          State_____ Zip_____

Occupation_____ Referral Source_____

I.   CHIEF COMPLAINT:_____
     _____

II. PREVIOUS HEARING EVALUATION   YES_____   NO_____
     A.   Where:_____
     B.   When:_____
     C.   Remarks:_____
          _____

III. HEARING LOSS   YES_____   NO_____
     A.   Ear: Right_____ Left_____ Both_____
     B.   Age at onset:_____
     C.   Progressive: Yes_____   No_____
     D.   Fluctuant: Yes_____   No_____
     E.   Dysacusis: Yes_____   No_____
     F.   Paracusis willisii: Yes_____   No_____
     G.   Remarks:_____
          _____

IV. FAMILY HISTORY OF HEARING LOSS   YES_____   NO_____
     A.   Who:_____
     B.   Remarks:_____
          _____

V.   EAR INFECTIONS   YES_____   NO_____
     A.   Ear: Right_____ Left_____ Both_____
     B.   Age at onset:_____
     C.   Drainage: Yes_____   No_____
     D.   Pain: Yes_____   No_____
     E.   Treatment:_____
     F.   Remarks:_____
          _____

VI. EAR SURGERY   YES_____   NO_____
     A.   Ear: Right_____ Left_____ Both_____
     B.   Date(s):_____
     C.   Type(s):_____
     D.   Remarks:_____

Figure 12.1 Sample of a short form for recording history of hearing loss and related conditions.

```
VII.  TINNITUS                              YES_____      NO_____
      A.  Ear:              Right_____    Left_____     Both_____
      B.  Description:_____
      C.  Constant:                         Yes_____      No_____
      D.  Fluctuant:                        Yes_____      No_____
      E.  Remarks:_____

VIII. VERTIGO                               YES_____      NO_____
      A.  Rotary:                           Yes_____      No_____
      B.  Lightheadedness:                  Yes_____      No_____
      C.  Nausea:                           Yes_____      No_____
      D.  Remarks:_____

IX.   HEAD INJURIES                         YES_____      NO_____
      A.  Date(s):_____
      B.  Type(s):_____
      C.  Loss of consciousness:            Yes_____      No_____
      D.  Affected hearing:                 Yes_____      No_____
      E.  Remarks:_____

X.    SYSTEMIC ILLNESSES                    Mumps_____      Measles_____
      Diabetes_____   Renal_____   Infections_____   Circulatory_____
      Other_____

XI.   MEDICATION_____
      _____
      _____

XII.  NOISE EXPOSURE                        YES_____      NO_____
      A.  Type(s):_____
      B.  Duration:_____
      C.  Remarks:_____

XIII. HEARING AID                           YES_____      NO_____
      A.  Air conduction_____      Bone conduction_____
      B.  Ear fitted:   Right_____    Left_____      Binaural_____
      C.  Type:  Body_____ Ear level_____ In-ear_____ Eyeglass_____
      D.  Make:_____
      E.  Model:_____
      F.  First worn:_____
      G.  Period worn:_____
      H.  Benefit:_____
      I.  Earmold:                          Yes_____      No_____
      J.  Remarks:_____

XIV.  AURAL REHABILITATION                  YES_____      NO_____
      A.  Remarks:_____

XV.   COMMENTS_____
      _____
      _____
      _____
```

Figure 12.1   (continued)

aplomb, simply because they have responded to the same questions many times. The clinician should try to elicit objective responses as much as possible. Statements of a diagnostic nature, such as "I have otosclerosis," or "My child has a nerve-type hearing loss," should be investigated thoroughly, because such remarks may represent the respondent's incorrect reflection of a previous diagnosis.

REFERRAL TO OTHER SPECIALISTS

Audiologists may refer their patients to other specialists for a variety of reasons. They may feel that additional help is needed for either diagnosis or treatment. The talents of such professionals as otologists, speech-language pathologists, psychologists, educators, or hearing-aid dispensers may be called upon. In any case, a proper report should be sent to provide the person who will be seeing the patient with as much pertinent information as is available. It is essentially mandatory to have the patient or guardian sign a release form authorizing the audiologist to provide such information to interested parties. The form, properly filed, may prevent possible legal difficulties.

An audiogram or other data obtained on hearing tests should not be forwarded without qualifying remarks, which should be more extensive than a mere cover letter. The audiologist should not suppose that the recipient of test results will totally understand and interpret tests correctly. At the other extreme, the audiologist should not include long, verbose reports conveying details of each and every test. Professional time is valuable and should not be occupied in reading unnecessary verbiage. In fact, it is probable that long reports are either not read at all or are only scanned for the pertinent facts.

Each report must be written specifically for the type of specialist to whom it is sent. Students should realize that reports sent about the same patient to an otologist and to a speech-language pathologist may differ greatly in the type of information included and in the manner in which statements are made. In addition, two otologists may differ in the type of information or degree of interpretation they desire. As audiologists get to know particular referral sources, they develop an awareness of how reports should be written for each one. Some may require very formal documents, whereas others will prefer informal synopses.

Briefly, the organization of a report sent to a professional person might be:

First paragraph: Identification of the patient (name, age, sex, short statement of history); the reason for referral

Second paragraph: Statement of the type and degree of hearing loss; reference to results that require special attention from the audiometric worksheets and tympanograms; interpretation of test results, where needed; implications for communication difficulties

Third paragraph: Specific recommendations, such as hearing aids, speech, language or hearing therapy, return for followup, avoidance of noise exposure, and so on

Students are often confused regarding the lengths to which they may go in written reports and letters before they cross professional boundaries and encroach upon the province of another profession. There is no formal, precise definition of these boundaries, but audiologists should exercise their expertise and voice their opinions regarding their patients. Statements of type and degree of hearing loss, interpretation of test results, and probable site of lesion are within the audiological province. Statements of cause of hearing loss begin to cross over into otology and should be made carefully. If the test battery and hearing history strongly suggest a specific condition, phrases such as "consistent with acoustic trauma" or "not unlike the findings in otosclerosis" may be used.

The clinic and/or the audiologist will, in all probability, be judged by the reports and forms they send to other professional workers. Messy audiograms and poorly written or proofread reports may cause the recipient to deduce that the audiological examination was also poorly done. Reports should be sent out as quickly as possible after patient evaluations. Audiologists represent their clinics and their profession, and good public relations may be as important to the proper management of the patient as good and accurate testing, for one reflects the other.

Liaisons with Otolaryngologists

It is obvious that the audiologist is not the person to recommend or perform surgery or medical treatment. This is the duty of the physician, preferably an otologist in the case of ear disease. On the other hand, most otologists are neither trained nor interested in the intricacies of diagnostic audiology or the nonmedical aspects of aural rehabilitation. Many cases of hearing loss are of such a routine nature that no special concern is needed for their management. In other important, difficult, or contradictory cases, however, consultation between the otologist and the audiologist is of great advantage to the patient. It is a mistake to think of the relationship between audiology and otology as one in which the audiologist merely provides audiometric services for the use of the physician in a diagnosis. In such situations, the role of the audiologist may deteriorate to that of technician. The association between medicine and audiology should be a symbiotic one, a professional relationship that leads to improved patient management.

In referring patients to a physician, audiologists should state in their reports the areas of concern and the reasons for referral. Recommendations for specific treatment should, of course, not be made. If the patient has a disorder that appears reversible (e.g., a conductive hearing loss caused by otitis media), the audiologist should reschedule the patient for testing following medical attention to ascertain the degree of hearing improvement derived. The same is true when patients with mixed hearing losses are referred. After an air–bone gap is closed, the sensorineural portion of a mixed loss may appear different from the pretreatment bone-conduction audiogram. A reevaluation of aural rehabilitation needs may be required in such cases.

Liaisons with Clinical Psychologists

Sometimes psychological tests are required because the patient's problem is at least partially complicated by an emotional disorder. The preprofessional training of most audiologists provides a sufficient vocabulary of psychological terms and association with psychological tests to permit interpretation of a psychologist's report. As in referrals to physicians, when referring a patient to a psychologist, audiologists should state their particular concerns about the patient and their reasons for referral. In addition to assistance with emotional disorders, the psychologist can provide information about the patient's performance versus potential—for example, whether a child is reaching academic potential or needs some special help. At times it is not until after consultation that it is decided whether the audiologist or the psychologist will become the central figure in the rehabilitation of the patient.

Liaisons with Speech-Language Pathologists

Although many audiologists have reasonably good academic backgrounds in speech-language pathology, most have limited clinical experience. A number of members of the American Speech-Language-Hearing Association (ASHA) hold the Certificate of Clinical Competence in both speech-language pathology and audiology, but most would not claim true competence in both areas. In any case, because of the similarities in the backgrounds and training of professionals in these two areas, an audiologist probably identifies more strongly with speech-language pathology than with other specialties.

Often an audiologist will see patients because the speech-language pathologist wishes to know if some aspect of a speech or language disorder is related to a hearing problem, as well as the extent of this relationship. In the case of young language-delayed children, the identification of a hearing disorder may play a large role in habilitation. In such cases, collaboration between specialists can result in the proper planning of remediation. Some voice or articulation disorders are directly produced by the inability to discriminate or hear in some frequency ranges.

Reports sent from audiologists to speech-language pathologists should be frank and direct. Audiologists should state their opinions regarding the type and extent of hearing impairment, and they should recommend referral to other specialists, such as otolaryngologists or psychologists, if indicated. The audiologist may state an opinion regarding the effects of hearing loss on a patient's speech, but should refrain from specific recommendations regarding therapy.

In working with some pediatric patients, an audiologist may have little more than a clinical hunch about the child's hearing. Phrases such as "hearing is adequate for speech" appear frequently in reports. In such cases, strong recommendations should be made so that followup testing is conducted at intervals until the bilateral hearing sensitivity throughout the critical frequency range can be ascertained. Honest errors made by audiologists may not be caught for some time, unless routine followup is carried out.

Liaison with Teachers of the Hearing-Impaired

Reports sent to teachers of hearing-impaired children are in many respects the same as those sent to speech-language pathologists. Events and developments of recent years have brought clinical audiologists and teachers closer together for the betterment of children with hearing disorders. This is largely due to the trend toward removing children from the self-contained environment of traditional schools for the deaf into the mainstream of education.

In order to permit hearing-impaired children to compete with their normal-hearing contemporaries, the combined efforts of the two specialties of clinical audiology and education of the "deaf" have come into closer harmony than ever before. This is largely true because of the emphasis now being placed on the use of residual hearing. As the barriers between the two groups break down, their formal educations include more overlapping course work. The harmony achieved can result in teamwork, with the children being the ultimate beneficiaries.

Teachers must learn to understand the implications of audiological management, and audiologists must learn to comprehend the difficulties in the day-to-day management of hearing-impaired children. Items of mutual concern include hearing aids, auditory training systems, and implications of classroom acoustics. Audiologists' isolation from teachers and teachers' reluctance to accept audiological intervention will disappear as the interactions between these professions continue to increase.

Liaisons with Hearing-Aid Dispensers

Some are audiologists (like Erica Lyman)

For many years hearing aids were sold through a variety of retail outlets, including drug and department stores. Those selling the instruments sometimes had little knowledge of hearing aids and how they are selected and maintained. In recent years the hearing-aid industry has made a serious effort to elevate itself professionally through in-service training programs. Consequently, many dispensers today are much more competent than their predecessors. In fact, many have degrees in audiology. Many states require that hearing-aid dispensers be licensed before they can dispense hearing aids. State licensure requires, among other things, the passage of an examination that covers such topics as audiometry, hearing-aid specifications, earmolds, and so on.

Procedures for selecting hearing aids are discussed later in this chapter. Audiologists are often asked for their professional opinions regarding specific dispensers to be used. These decisions should not be made arbitrarily. Such aspects as proximity of a dealer to the patient's home and availability of local service and repairs are important. Some dispensers enjoy better reputations in the community than do others for their willingness to follow up sales courteously with service, an important aspect of a hearing-aid purchase. Audiologists who are new in an area may check with the local Better Business Bureau or with colleagues to learn of the reputations of different dispensers.

When patients are referred directly to dispensers, they may have detailed recommendations for specific makes and models of hearing aids, or the dispensers may be asked to exercise judgment in the selection. After patients are fitted with hearing aids, they should return to the audiologist at least once for final counseling and for sound-field testing, electroacoustic measurements to ascertain that the instruments are performing properly, and scheduling of hearing-aid orientation sessions.

HEARING AIDS

When nonmedical aural rehabilitation is indicated, consideration is given to amplification in the form of hearing aids. It is true that some patients with hearing loss do not need or cannot use hearing aids. The audiologist should nevertheless examine this possibility for all hearing-impaired patients as part of the total rehabilitation program.

A hearing aid can be thought of as a miniature public address system. Sounds that strike the microphone (input transducer) are amplified and transmitted electrically to a miniature loudspeaker (output transducer) and then into the patient's external ear canal. A few hearing aids utilize a bone-conduction vibrator held to the patient's mastoid by a metal headband, much like the bone-conduction vibrator of an audiometer. Modern hearing aids accomplish their amplification with integrated circuitry, enabling the instruments to be considerably smaller than their predecessors, which required vacuum tubes or transistors to accomplish the same functions. Power for the instruments is obtained from small batteries.

Hearing aids are signal processors; that is, they alter the signal input to improve it for the wearer. Traditional hearing aids have involved analog technology, in which the changes are made by modifying a continuous electrical signal. The newer digital technology changes the continuous electrical signal, by means of an analog-to-digital converter (A/D), into a series of many separate bits (binary digits). When the signal is in digital form, advanced processing operations can be carried out. Finally, the altered bits are changed back to analog form by a digital-to-analog converter (D/A). Digital hearing aids can provide clarity of signals and improved signal-to-noise ratios, which are superior to those obtained with more traditional analog instruments.

Digital hearing-aid technology has been accepted in the market more slowly than originally anticipated because of technical problems involving instrument size and power needs. Roeser and Taylor (1988) were able to demonstrate improved speech recognition in noise with the use of digital over analog hearing aids, and their subjects preferred the sound quality of the digital instruments. Despite these findings, their subjects continued to show preference for their own aids from the perspectives of instrument size and other cosmetic considerations. Hecox and Punch (1988) have pointed out some of the many advantages of digital hearing aids and the need for clinicians to work with their patients regarding the "increased cost and cosmetic tradeoffs. . ." Levitt (1988a) warned that, despite the superiority of digital instruments, they should not be perceived by clinicians or represented to patients as a "panacea."

As part of the trend toward sophisticated signal processing abilities in modern hearing aids, noise reduction circuitry is included to improve speech recognition in the presence of background noise. There is some question as to whether this approach results in better speech discrimination than can be obtained with more traditional circuitry (Klein, 1989) and whether the increased expense is justified. Advanced versions of this circuitry will almost certainly be forthcoming.

In addition to the usual on–off switches and volume controls, many hearing aids today have internal and external adjustments to modify the amplification obtained in different frequency ranges. Some aids also contain electromagnetic coils that, when switched into the circuit, bypass the microphone so that the user can hear more clearly over the telephone. These so-called T switches have been used for improved telephone communication systems for more than forty years, and it has been mandated that all corded telephones must be compatible with hearing aids (Beck, 1989).

Characteristics of Hearing Aids

Hearing aids are usually described in terms of their electroacoustic properties, which include **saturation sound-pressure level (SSPL)**, **acoustic gain**, **frequency response**, and **distortion**. Until the **Hearing Aid Industry Conference (HAIC)** (1961, 1975), these characteristics were loosely defined, which led to a number of misconceptions. The most recent specifications for hearing aids are published by the American National Standards Institute (ANSI S3.22–1982). Measurements are made on an artificial ear using a 2 cm^3 coupler to accommodate the earmold, the external receiver of the aid, or to hold the plastic tubing that comes from the receiver. Although the 2 cm^3 coupler measurement does not represent the hearing aid's gain in a real ear, it does provide a standardized system for comparing different aids.

Saturation Sound-Pressure Level (SSPL). It is obvious that some control must be exercised by the manufacturer over the maximum sound pressure emitted from a hearing aid. If this pressure were unlimited, it could damage the wearer's hearing. The saturation sound-pressure level, previously called the maximum power **output**, is the greatest sound pressure that can be produced by an aid. The SSPL is considered one of the most important measurements; it is usually made in an acoustically treated enclosure (see Figure 12.2) using an input signal of 90 dB SPL with the aid turned to full volume (SSPL 90).

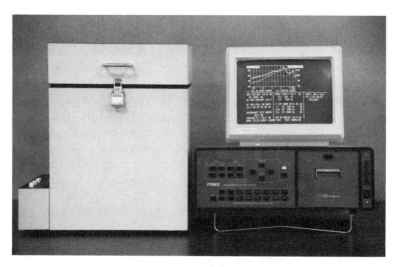

Figure 12.2 A test unit for measurement of hearing aid characteristics. (Courtesy of FONIX.)

Volume Control

Acoustic Gain. The acoustic gain of a hearing aid is the difference in decibels between an input signal and an output signal. The gain (volume) control of the aid is adjusted to its desired position, and a signal of 50 or 60 dB SPL is presented to the microphone from a special loudspeaker within the sound-treated enclosure of the hearing-aid test box. The output SPL is measured on a sound-level meter. If the output SPL is 100 dB with an input of 60 dB SPL, the acoustic gain is 40 dB. High-frequency average (HFA) full-on gain is the average gain at 1000, 1600, and 2500 Hz. Although these measurements reflect maximum gain, they do not represent a true picture of the gain of the aid on the patient because aids are rarely worn at full-volume settings. The ANSI standard is used for measuring acoustic gain below the aid's full-on position. This **reference test gain** allows for a more realistic appraisal of the way a hearing aid might perform on a patient. The two main types of gain include *functional gain*, the measured difference between aided and unaided thresholds in the sound field, and *insertion gain*, the increase in sound-pressure level delivered by the hearing aid as measured at the tympanic membrane with a probe tube microphone.

Frequency Response. The range of frequencies that any sound system can amplify and transmit is limited. In the case of hearing aids, this range is restricted primarily by the transducers (microphone and receiver) and by the earmold configuration. The frequency response of a hearing aid is determined by first measuring the reference test gain over a wide frequency range. This is best done using a sweep frequency audio oscillator on a hearing-aid test unit. In most test boxes a graph is automatically drawn that shows the response of the hearing aid over a frequency range of 125 to 10,000 Hz. Figure 12.3 shows a tracing from an in-the-ear aid that provides maximum amplification in the

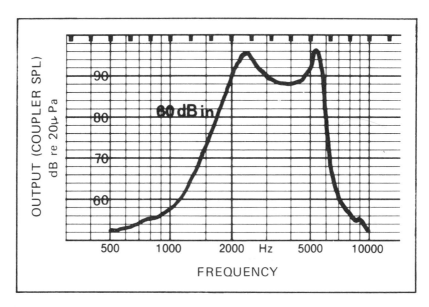

Figure 12.3 Frequency response characteristics of a typical in-the-ear hearing aid. Measurements were made with a 2 cm³ coupler and 60 dB SPL input level. (Courtesy of Starkey Laboratories, Inc.)

1500 to 6000 Hz range. Modern ear-level aids can provide wider frequency response ranges than their predecessors because of advances in technology. To determine the frequency response, a line is drawn parallel with the baseline, which is 20 dB below a level showing the average gain at 1000, 1600, and 2500 Hz. The points of intersection of this line with the response curve may be considered the frequency range of the instrument.

Distortion. When a sound leaving the hearing aid differs from the input signal, distortion has taken place. This was considered in the brief discussion on frequency response characteristics that exemplify frequency distortion. Amplitude distortion refers to the differences in the relationships of the amplitudes of the input and output signals.

When sounds of one frequency are increased in amplitude, they may cause the electronic or mechanical portions of an amplifying system to be overstressed. This **harmonic distortion** can be expressed as the percentage of distortion of the input signal. The greater the harmonic distortion of a hearing aid, the poorer the quality of the amplified sounds of speech.

Other Hearing-Aid Parameters. Modern hearing-aid test equipment allows for a number of other checks to be made on the characteristics of hearing aids. Some of these checks include: equivalent input noise level, input-output characteristics, dynamic characteristics of aids with automatic gain controls, battery drain, and the performance of telephone induction coils. Although definitions and descriptions are not presented here, the interested reader is encouraged to check the suggested reading list at the end of this chapter.

∠ Types of Hearing Aids

Hearing aids come in a variety of shapes, sizes, colors, and types. Among the hearing aids available today are traditional body-type aids, behind-the-ear aids, eyeglass aids, in-the-ear aids, and in-the-canal aids.

Body-Type Aids. Body-type hearing aids (Figure 12.4A) contain the microphone, amplifier, tone, power, and output limiting controls, and a battery case, which may be clipped to the wearer's clothing or worn in a pocket or a special case. A cord carries the electrical impulses to a receiver, which is coupled to the patient's ear through the use of a custom-fitted earmold (Figure 12.5). Body-type aids have several advantages: Sound fidelity is usually better, the controls are easy to adjust because they are relatively large, and the batteries last longer than do those for some types of aids. Battery compartments are large enough to allow easy access.

Problems with **acoustic feedback** are generally fewer with body-type aids than with the other types. Acoustic feedback is a whistling sound that is the result of a cycle when the amplified environmental sounds leave the receiver and reach the microphone. This sound is reduced by fabricating a tightly sealed earmold and by moving the receiver as far from the microphone as is practical.

Body-type aids have several disadvantages, not the least of which is the cosmetic aspect of the hearing aid. Despite attempts at public education, a stigma is often attached to hearing aids, and some people shun their use as a

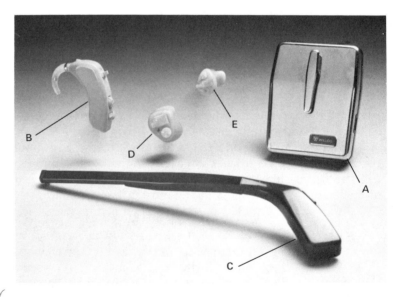

Figure 12.4 Five types of commercial hearing aids showing: (A) body-type aid; (B) behind-the-ear aid; (C) eyeglass aid; (D) in-the-ear aid; (E) in-the-canal aid. (Courtesy of Starkey Laboratories, Inc.)

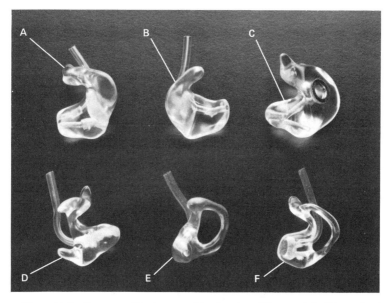

Figure 12.5 Six types of lucite earmolds, showing: (A) vented shell for reduction of low frequencies; (B) shell type for severe impairment; (C) receiver type for use with external transducer; (D) ¾ skeleton; (E) skeleton; (F) open-bore canal for enhanced high frequencies. (Courtesy of Starkey Laboratories, Inc.)

result. Not only are the cords unsightly, but they often break, causing the signal to be intermittent. In addition, when a body aid is worn under clothing, the rubbing of the microphone may cause a loud and disturbing noise. Recently, aids have been developed that can be worn on the ear and still provide the power previously found only in body-type aids; use of the latter has therefore dropped sharply.

Behind-the-Ear Aids. Hearing aids worn behind the ear (BTE) (Figure 12.4B) allow for localization of sound, especially when a separate instrument is worn on each ear (binaural). Many patients report that it is easier to focus on a sound when ear-level aids are worn.

Problems with clothing noise are eliminated with all head-worn hearing aids, as are difficulties with cords, because the receiver is built into the same case that houses the microphone and amplifier. The decreased size of the instrument makes adjustments of controls and insertion of batteries somewhat more difficult, especially for patients who are very young, elderly, or physically handicapped. As the quality of BTE aids improved and they became more powerful, their overall use increased, although, like their predecessors, they too are being overtaken in sales by the newer in-the-ear models.

Eyeglass Aids. Hearing aids may also be built into the temple bars of eyeglasses (Figure 12.4C). Patients who wear eyeglasses and hearing aids all the time used to prefer these instruments because they had less cumbersome hardware and were held more firmly than the BTE aids, which are suspended by the plastic tube that leads to the ear. The popularity of eyeglass aids has diminished considerably in recent years, due largely to the increased interest in in-the-ear aids.

In-The-Ear Aids. Instruments that are worn entirely in the concha and external auditory canal (Figure 12.4D) are very popular today. With improved technology, the gain, SSPL 90, and frequency response characteristics of these tiny devices have been vastly improved. Many people now wear in-the-ear (ITE) aids with great satisfaction; these people would not have had this option not too many years ago.

The newest type of hearing aid to have a major impact is the in-the-canal (ITC) aid (Figure 12.4E), which fits primarily in the external auditory canal with only slight protrusion into the concha. This design takes advantage of the natural acoustic properties of the pinna, which are largely ignored by the other instrument styles. Improvements in the transducers, especially the use of the **electret microphone** (also used in ITE and BTE aids), allow for broader frequency responses than were previously thought possible in a small instrument.

Many people are attracted to the canal aid because of its small size, although from the audiologist's point of view appearance is the least important criterion for selection of a hearing aid. Because the instrument is actually built into the patient's earmold, the amplified sound is closer to the tympanic membrane and thus requires less in the way of gain and output than the other models. Problems with instrument weight, wind noise, and so on are all lessened with this type of aid. Even though the canal aid is apparently a popular choice among potential hearing-aid users, its increased cost, along with considerations such as the patient's manual dexterity and canal size, limits its use in certain cases.

Any of the hearing aids just described can be worn in one ear or in both ears, barring anatomical abnormalities or restrictive hearing losses. Many audiologists have been convinced, either through the research literature, or through comments by their patients, that speech is clearer, louder, easier to understand, and less contaminated by background noises when two hearing aids are worn. In addition, localization of a sound source is usually enhanced with binaural hearing aids. In a small percentage of cases, however, speech recognition is so poor in one ear that binaural aids decrease, rather than increase efficiency.

CROS Aids. A patient with an unaidable unilateral hearing loss has a particular kind of listening difficulty, which can include soft speech from the "bad side." Little had been done in the way of amplification for such problems until Harford and Barry (1965) described a specially built instrument called **CROS**, an acronym for **contralateral routing of signals**. In this configuration the microphone of the system is mounted on the side of the impaired ear, and the signal is routed to the amplifier and receiver that are mounted on the side of the normal-hearing ear. The signal may be routed electrically through wires that are draped behind the head for BTE or ITE aids, through the front pieces of eyeglasses, or by way of FM transmitters and receivers. The signal is presented to the ear canal of the "good" ear, either through a plastic tube or through a custom earmold that contains an additional opening to allow un-amplified sounds to enter the ear canal normally. In this way patients hear from the "good" side in the usual fashion, but they also hear sounds from the "bad" side as they are amplified and led to the better ear. A volume control allows for manipulation of the sound intensity of the CROS system.

Many patients have very good results with CROS, and its popularity is such that many hearing-aid manufacturers have these instruments in their inventories. CROS has expanded beyond its original intended use for unilateral hearing loss, and it has been used both monaurally and binaurally for high-frequency losses and in other difficult cases where traditional fitting would result in chronic feedback problems. Numerous variations of the CROS system are available for these different types of hearing losses.

Cochlear Implants. An exciting addition to the variety of hearing instruments came with the development of the **cochlear implant** (House, 1982). This is the first major step in the surgical implantation of hearing aids for patients with profound sensorineural hearing losses who are unable to use conventional amplification. The internal receiver, which is implanted under the skin behind the pinna, consists of wire electrodes and a tiny coil. Active electrodes are placed in the scala tympani and ground electrodes outside the bony labyrinth or in the eustachian tube, (Figure 12.6). A small microphone, worn outside the body at the concha of the external ear, feeds electrical impulses to a speech processor, which amplifies and filters the signal. From the processor the signal goes to a transmitter, which converts it to magnetic impulses that are sent to the electrodes. An electrical signal is induced from the magnetic field in the cochlea and flows on to stimulate the auditory nerve (Figure 12.7).

Only a small number of adverse effects from implant surgery have been reported, and many of these have been corrected with revisions in the system and surgical procedures. Initially, only adults with profound hearing losses were provided with cochlear implants. A variety of tests had to be performed to ensure that the hearing losses were due to hair cell rather than nerve cell damage. The hearing losses had to have been acquired after the development of speech and language, and the patients had to be free of physical or psychological conditions that might adversely affect adjustment to the instruments. As the cochlear implant device was improved, and diagnostic tests such as ABR were expanded, candidacy for implantation grew to include children with congenital hearing losses.

Implant recipients are counseled regarding the fact that they will not be able to discriminate among many of the sounds of speech. Although frequency discrimination is far from perfect, voices may be heard at normal conversational levels; this provides sound awareness and cues such as rate and rhythm, which can assist the listener in speechreading.Many patients have reported that hearing their own voices again allows them to monitor their vocal pitch and loudness much more effectively than was possible prior to implantation.

As experience with cochlear implants increased, and as the design of the instruments improved to include multiple electrodes, the number of physicians

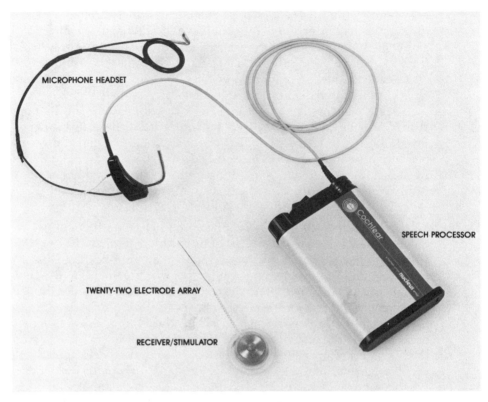

Figure 12.6 Example of a cochlear implant device showing its internal and external components. (Courtesy of Cochlear Corporation.)

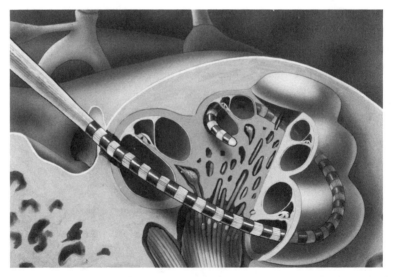

Figure 12.7 Implantation of a multi-electrode array of a cochlear implant device. (Courtesy of Cochlear Corporation.)

doing implant surgery and the number and variety of recipients has increased. The modern consensus is in agreement with Dorman, Hannley, Dankowski, Smith, and McCandless (1989), who concluded that the use of many channels provides better speech recognition than can be obtained with systems employing fewer channels.

Implantable Bone-Conduction Devices. There are many people who suffer from severe conductive hearing losses for whom surgery either has failed to improve their hearing or is not an option. Some of these people have been helped in the past by bone-conduction hearing aids, but others may prefer a relatively new option involving a magnetic device that can be surgically implanted under the skin in the mastoid area. The procedure may be performed as outpatient surgery, using either local or general anesthesia.

During surgery a screw hole is prepared following a surgical incision in the mastoid which is closed after the instrument is firmly screwed into place. After the incision has healed (about 8 weeks), the patient is fitted with the induction coil (which fits directly over the implant) and either an at-the-ear or body-worn, battery-powered processor. Initial results with this device are promising. Patients report good sound quality, elimination of acoustic feedback, and preference for this device over their previously worn hearing aids (Johnson, Meikle, Vernon, & Schleuning, 1988).

Naturally, since hearing stimulation is by means of bone conduction, patients must have significant air–bone gaps and have reasonably good bone-conduction thresholds. Yellin, Meyerhoff and Roland (1988) recommended that candidacy criteria include pure-tone averages by bone conduction no poorer than 30 dB HL, with hearing at no frequency in the testable range poorer than 40 dB HL. Time will reveal whether this procedure will become popular for conductively hearing-impaired individuals.

Vibrotactile Aids. Despite all attempts to take advantage of residual hearing through amplification, some patients simply cannot be helped by any of the devices just described. There is currently a revival of interest in instruments that amplify sound, not to augment hearing per se but to provide tactile stimulation on the surface of the skin (Downs, 1984). Levitt (1988b) stated that, in part, this renewed interest has been brought about because of (1) the recent excitement over cochlear implants, (2) the fact that vibrotactile aids are noninvasive, and (3) the fact that they pose less risk to young children than does surgery.

Tactile aids are based on the principle that vibratory patterns are generated that are directly related to the acoustic wave that strikes the microphone of the device. The tactile aid, in turn, provides cues that assist in determining the rate and rhythm of speech, thereby enhancing the patient's speechreading ability. The output transducers may be placed on the fingers, the back of the hand, or in the case of small children on the sternum (breastbone), stomach or back. Because these instruments will probably play an important role, especially in the speech and language training of some young, severely hearing-impaired children, research into the devices and their usefulness is ongoing (Downs, 1984; Roeser, Friel-Patti, & Scott, 1983).

To expect that vibrotactile aids will eventually replace hearing aids is probably a mistake, because the skin is less than an ideal receptor of vibratory information. It is advisable to explore traditional amplification thoroughly, especially with young children, before adopting vibrotactile stimulation. Modern versions of vibrotactile aids use microcomputers that assist in the perception of such cues as fundamental frequency and intonation (Young, Boothroyd, & Redmond, 1988). Although some encouraging results have been reported from experimental work with vibrotactile aids on severely hearing-impaired adults with encouraging results (Weisenberger, 1989), experimentation is needed before it is likely that these instruments will be widely adopted.

Selecting Hearing-Aid Candidates

Although many people have rules of thumb for determining whether or not a given patient should try a hearing aid, audiologists often find such rules confining and lacking in usefulness. An old common rule was to recommend a hearing aid if the average hearing loss at 500, 1000, and 2000 Hz exceeded 30 dB in the better ear. Restriction to this kind of guideline eliminates a number of critical factors, such as duration of hearing loss, speech recognition ability, audiometric contour, age, intelligence, vocation, education, financial resources, and—perhaps most important of all—motivation to use a hearing aid.

Before the modern era of middle-ear surgery, most patients wearing hearing aids had conductive hearing losses. Because patients with conductive losses usually have good speech discrimination and tolerance for loud sounds, many physicians encouraged these patients to try hearing aids. On the other hand, patients with sensorineural hearing losses were discouraged from wearing aids because of their speech discrimination difficulties. Because of the way sound must seem distorted for most patients with sensorineural losses, along with problems of loudness recruitment, such patients often appeared to be poor risks for amplification.

With advances in middle-ear surgery, the number of people wearing hearing aids who had conductive hearing losses decreased, and the number who had sensorineural losses increased, partly as a result of improvements in the instruments and partly because of the influence of rehabilitative audiology. Selecting an aid for a person with a sensorineural loss involves more than simply scrutinizing the audiogram and making a recommendation. In many cases a trial period of several weeks with a new hearing aid can be a determining factor.

SELECTING HEARING AIDS

Several methods are now in use for selecting hearing aids. Procedures include having the patient deal directly and exclusively with a hearing-aid dispenser who may not be a clinical audiologist, supplying audiometric data to the dispenser to help in selecting aids, making general recommendations for aids, making specific recommendations regarding particular instruments, and issuing hearing aids directly to the patient.

Patient Selection of a Hearing Aid

When a patient deals directly with a nonaudiologist hearing-aid dispenser, direct guidance from an audiologist is absent. Patients may select dealers arbitrarily, or they may be given lists of several dealers by an audiologist or otologist. In this way patients can shop among the dealers until they find an aid that looks and sounds acceptable and is affordable. Of course, in this way decisions are influenced to some extent by the personality and sales expertise of the dealer. Unfortunately, because some patients may suffer the confusion common to shoppers and may simply select an aid from the last dealer they see, this is not a recommended procedure.

Referrals to Hearing-Aid Dispensers

If, after audiological assessment, the audiologist feels that a hearing aid is indicated, a copy of the test results may be provided to the patient and contact made directly with a dispenser who is not an audiologist. Many audiologists feel that as long as the patient is seen by a reliable dispenser, the patient's best interests will be served. Following selection of the instrument, the audiologist should see the patient again for an aided performance check to determine the efficacy of the hearing aid selected.

Some audiologists provide their patients with general kinds of prescriptions for hearing aids. These specifications might include which ear to be aided (if only one ear is selected), the type of aid, gain, SSPL 90, frequency response, and so on. In this way the dealer selects from a stock of instruments and attempts to satisfy the needs of the patient within the confines of the recommendations.

Unless the patient returns to the audiologist after an aid has been obtained, there is no way to know whether the original recommendations have been followed by the hearing-aid dealer or whether the selected instrument is satisfactory. The audiologist and hearing-aid dealer may discuss by telephone possible modifications of the original recommendations.

Recommendations Based on Hearing-Aid Evaluations

Carhart (1946) described a procedure for hearing-aid evaluation that was used for many years and is still used by a number of audiologists in modified form. This procedure included making measurements in the sound field using a number of different tests, performed both unaided and with a variety of different hearing aids. The differences between aided and unaided scores showed the amount of improvement (or detriment) provided by the aid. Measurements included the SRT, speech discrimination scores in quiet and in the presence of background noise, most comfortable and uncomfortable loudness levels, and range of comfortable loudness, as well as subjective estimates of clarity, quality, and the like. If four to six instruments were tested, the ideal one provided the lowest SRT, the highest speech discrimination scores, a level of most comfortable loudness close to the level of normal conversation (60 to 70 dB SPL), and a broad range of comfortable loudness.

Opinions regarding the accuracy of these procedures varied. Haug, Baccaro, and Guilford (1971) found them reliable and valid. Shore, Bilger, and Hirsh (1960) drew just the opposite conclusion. In addition to doubts about the replicability of sound-field audiometry with hearing aids, other problems presented themselves. Even if a selection was felt to be proper and a specific prescription was made for an aid, there was no guarantee that the instrument purchased would have characteristics identical to the one recommended, even if manufacturer, model, receiver, and settings were the same.

A major objection to the Carhart approach to hearing-aid evaluations is that often the speech discrimination scores appear to be very similar with different instruments. One may conclude from this that the aids are performing similarly and that no significant differences exist with respect to discrimination for speech. A more likely conclusion, however, is that the instruments perform very differently from one another, but that the tests used are not sufficiently sensitive to ferret out these differences. Consequently, synthetic sentences with competition from continuous discourse, rhyme tests, connected discourse, nonsense syllables, or high-frequency emphasis PB word lists have been used instead of standard PB word lists during traditional hearing-aid evaluations. At present there is movement in the direction of hearing-aid selection based on subjective quality measurements.

One approach to hearing-aid selection is to match, as closely as possible, the acoustic characteristics of the earmold–hearing-aid configuration to the acoustic needs of the patient, thus maximizing the use of residual hearing. Through venting and special earmold designs, for example, low-frequency energy can be deemphasized for patients with hearing losses that are primarily in the higher frequencies. Midfrequency energy can be modified with acoustic dampers or filters in the tubing of the earmolds or ear hooks of the aids, and high-frequency energy can be enhanced with bell-shaped tubing and two earmold openings. Prior to the advent of this approach to acoustic modification, attempts at shaping the acoustic signals were limited to the use of electronic filters within the instruments themselves. Killion, Berlin, and Hood (1984) described a hearing-aid design that uses an open canal fitting to enhance the low frequencies for patients with "reverse ski-slope" audiograms, which are characterized by better hearing in the high frequencies than in the lows.

Knowledge of the patient's thresholds and most comfortable loudness (MCL) and uncomfortable loudness levels (UCLs) is essential to the hearing-aid selection process. If this information is not directly available from the patients themselves, the audiologist must determine their acoustic needs insofar as possible from other tests. For example, when selecting aids for small children, UCLs can be inferred from acoustic reflex thresholds when these are measurable, but this procedure is not always accurate.

Dissatisfaction with existing methods, improvements in hearing-aid design, and the ongoing desire to improve hearing health care have led to some interesting developments in recent years. Attention to preselection procedures during hearing-aid evaluations maximizes the likelihood that instruments with the greatest potential to help individual patients will be used during the selection process. Computer-based systems have been devised to simplify the various calculations required during hearing-aid evaluation procedures and to reduce potential errors when, for example, comparing gain at the tympanic membrane to gain in a hard-walled (e.g., 2 cm³) cavity, retrieving results from different instruments, or converting hearing-level to sound-pressure level values (Popelka & Engebretson, 1983). Libby (1988, p. 12) has summarized the most commonly used prescriptive hearing-aid selection procedures, and interested persons are encouraged to read this succinct but informative article.

Audiologists have come to realize that despite the important measurements made in hard-walled 2 cm³ couplers, the "real ear" behaves quite differently. Amplified sound-pressure levels in the human ear are not accurately represented by the artificial cavity. This realization has encouraged the measurement of hearing-aid characteristics within the external auditory canal of the patient using tiny probe or probe tube microphones (see Figure 12.8). Such measurements reflect not only the acoustic characteristics of the hearing aid, but also the natural individual resonance characteristics of the ear itself and the interactions among these effects (Libby, 1988). Martin (1989) made the point that probe tube information can be very valuable with respect to setting a hearing aid's SSPL 90, acoustic gain, and the like, but that measurement with speech stimuli, behavioral observation, and regular monitoring visits is essential to proper fitting when working with children. It should be stressed that real-ear measures are not a substitute for hearing tests.

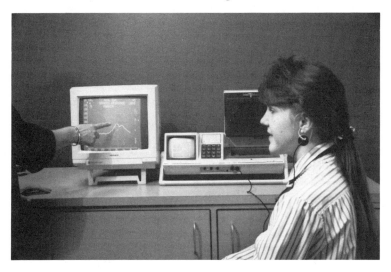

Figure 12.8 A probe tube microphone system for *in situ* measurement of hearing-aid performance. (Courtesy of Starkey Laboratories, Inc.)

Even though improved methods of collecting objective hearing-aid data continue to develop, many researchers believe that patients themselves should play more active roles in selecting their aids. With the present enthusiasm for hearing aids and the entry of many audiologists into the dispensing process, the search for improved methods of hearing-aid selection and evaluation continues.

Dispensing Hearing Aids

Hearing-aid selection procedures are carried out in most military and Veterans Administration audiology centers. Different brands and types of hearing aids are purchased on a contract basis, and several aids of each make and model are stocked. Supplies are replenished from a central depository as aids are isued. After a particular type of instrument is selected for a patient, the specific aid with which that patient was tested is issued. Issuing the aid that has been tested has many advantages.

Until the 1970s, the bylaws of ASHA did not allow its members to dispense hearing aids directly. Such sales were considered unethical because it was felt that the audiologist's objectivity might be compromised if any profit motive were injected into the selection process. The tide on this entire subject has turned. Not only are many audiologists dispensing hearing aids directly to patients, but many university training programs are preparing students for this practice.

Under proper conditions, direct dispensing of hearing aids appears to be an ideal procedure. The audiologist must be (1) aware of the characteristics and adjustments of the aids to be dispensed, (2) able to provide simple repairs, (3) capable of making and modifying earmolds, and (4) able to provide a total aural rehabilitation program suited to each individual's needs. In addition, direct dispensing provides the unique opportunity for a patient to receive an entire rehabilitation program from one highly trained professional person. Before embarking on a hearing-aid dispensing program, the audiologist must be aware of any state licensing laws pertaining to hearing-aid fitting and dispensing.

Regardless of how the hearing aid is obtained, the audiologist must be prepared to assist patients who encounter problems with their instruments. Some common problems and solutions are summarized in Table 12.1. When there appears to be no simple correction for a malfunctioning aid, factory repair may be required. The proper course can be guided by the audiologist, who must ascertain, among other things, that patients understand the terms of the new aid repair warranty.

Selecting Hearing Aids for Children

A child who is mature enough to perform behavioral hearing tests and is found to be in need of amplification may be tested by modifying certain adult selection procedures. Absence of receptive language skills, of course, precludes the use of speech audiometry in pediatric testing.

TABLE 12.1 COMMON PROBLEMS WITH HEARING AIDS AND THEIR SOLUTIONS

COMPLAINT	EXPLANATION	SOLUTION
Weak sound	Partial obstruction in earmold	Clean earmold.
	Partial obstruction in tubing	Clean tubing.
	Incorrect battery	Replace with proper battery.
	Weak battery[a]	Replace with strong battery.
Intermittent sound	Broken cord[b]	Replace cord.
	Dirty battery contacts	Roll battery around in compartment or clean contacts with emery board or fine sandpaper.
	Dirty controls	Move switches and controls through all positions to dislodge dirt. Roll volume control several times through entire range. Spray with contact cleaner.
	Weak battery[a]	Replace with strong battery.
No sound	Dead battery[a]	Replace with fresh battery.
	Battery improperly inserted	Remove and replace battery.
	Obstruction in earmold	Clean earmold.
	Obstruction in tubing	Clean or replace tubing.
	Twisted tubing	Untwist or replace tubing.
	Broken cord*	Replace cord.
	Broken receiver[c]	Replace receiver.
	Set for telephone coil	Move to microphone position.
	Improper use	Check owner's manual.
Aid works but is noisy	Acoustic feedback	Check for tight-fitting mold. Check connection between mold and receiver. Check for properly inserted mold. Check for crack in tubing or ear hook.
	Clothing noise[b]	Clear aid of clothing. Use hearing-aid harness.

[a]Use a battery tester that places a "load" on the battery.
[b]Body-type or CROS aid only.
[c]Body-type aid only.

If a child can be conditioned to take a pure-tone hearing test in the sound field, thresholds may be measured both with and without hearing aids at a number of different frequencies. The improvements in thresholds obtained in the aided condition show the functional gain provided at different frequencies. Ross and Duffy (1961) found this to be a reliable procedure, and it is still used in many clinics today. If pure tones are used in the sound field, they should be either automatically pulsed on and off, or warbled to avoid problems with standing waves (see Chapter 2). A warble tone is one that is frequency modulated—that is, modified in frequency over time. A 1000 Hz tone warbled at 5% changes systematically in frequency from 950 to 1050 Hz.

Some work is being done at this time on the use of auditory brain stem response (ABR) testing in the fitting of children's hearing aids. It should be emphasized that this work is preliminary, has a number of technical problems, and may lead to errors in fitting. The danger of incorrect hearing-aid selection for a small child is such that every precaution should be taken to ensure accuracy.

Sometimes it is felt that a small child needs amplification even though no audiometric results have been obtained. Many such children are enrolled in language stimulation programs, and they should spend some time during each therapy session being conditioned to play audiometry. The earlier the age at which amplification through a proper hearing aid, along with auditory training, can be provided, the better are the chances for development of normal language and intelligible speech and voice.

ASSISTIVE LISTENING DEVICES AND SYSTEMS (ALDS)

One of the major disadvantages of wearable hearing aids is the noise that exists between the microphone of the aid and the talker, thus creating adverse signal-to-noise ratios and decreasing speech intelligibility. The closer the talker is to the listener's hearing aids, the fewer are the effects of intervening room noise masking. In addition, the reverberative and other acoustic characteristics of any room may affect important parameters of sound waves as they travel through air. Getting talker and listener close together in space is often difficult in classrooms as well as in a variety of other listening situations.

Older auditory training units were hard-wired, meaning that the microphone and amplifier were physically connected to receivers worn by the listeners. This configuration severely restricted the person speaking to close proximity to the microphone, and limited the person listening to a fixed location at the receivers.

Telecoils in hearing aids can be used to interface in a variety of ways with assistive listening devices in classrooms, theaters, hospitals, auditoriums, retirement facilities, libraries, and personal offices and homes. Specialized systems may transmit speech from a talker's microphone, which can contain a portable transmission system that is easily worn to allow freedom of movement, to the hearing aids via one of several systems, including an induction loop system that produces an electromagnetic field worn around the neck or a frequency modulated (FM) system, which is a unit that picks up the voice of the talker from a radio frequency (RF) carrier signal. Infrared systems utilize light frequencies invisible to the human eye to carry speech signals to a receiving unit (see Ploshay & Hofman, 1984). In addition to the use of the telecoil to pick up a speech signal, there may be direct audio input from a receiving unit to the aids. Examples of several assistive listening devices may be found in Figure 12.9.

Included in the general category of assistive listening devices and systems are signaling or alerting units, which have been called "environmental adaptations" (Vaugn, Lightfoot, & Teter, 1988). These devices amplify telephones,

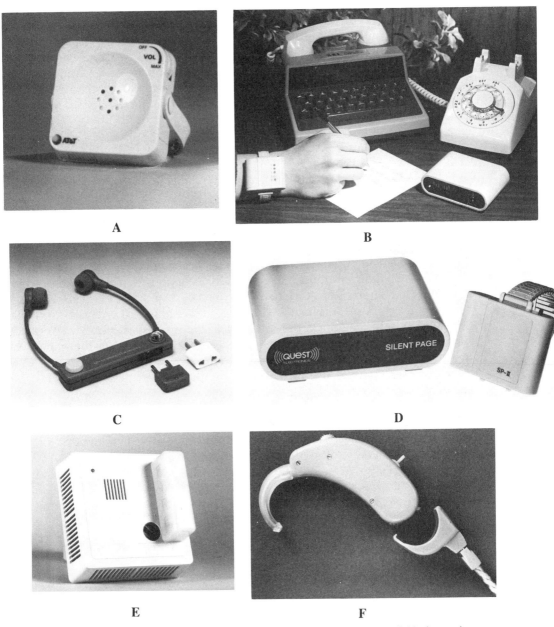

Figure 12.9 Examples of a few assistive listening devices and systems available for use by hearing-impaired individuals: (A) strap-on telephone amplifier; (B) telephone communication devices; (C) binaural headset which receives infrared carrier signal (this device can be used for interpersonal communication or in listening to television); (D) paging device with receiver designed to be worn on the wrist to alert hearing-impaired individuals to environmental sounds such as doorbells; (E) smoke detector which both sounds a loud alarm and illuminates a powerful strobe light; (F) one type of direct audio input device, bypassing the microphone of a behind-the-ear hearing aid. (Photographs courtesy of Siemens Hearing Instruments, Inc. and HARC Mercantile Limited).

flash lights, or otherwise alert individuals who cannot use hearing to be aware of emergency signals such as the sounding of smoke or fire alarms, babies crying, or such mundane but important signals as telephones, timers, doorbells, and alarm clocks. Also included are telecaptioning decoders and telecommunication devices for the deaf (TDDs). Modern technology and microcircuitry have created instruments that can markedly improve the quality of life for the hearing-impaired.

MANAGEMENT OF TINNITUS

Tinnitus has been mentioned several times in this book. Complaints of ear or head noises go back through recorded history and accompany, to some degree, almost every etiology of hearing loss. Many people experience tinnitus even though they have normal hearing, and a significant number suffer from severe and near-debilitating tinnitus. Figure 12.10 summarizes many of the causes of tinnitus, which has been variously described by such adjectives as "ringing," "crickets," "roaring," "hissing," "clanging," "swishing," and a host of others.

With the formation of the American Tinnitus Association (DeWeese & Vernon, 1975), professional consciousness has been raised on the subject of tinnitus. Professionals have learned to heed the complaints of tinnitus sufferers. Other than the use of masking sounds to cover up the tinnitus—for example, a clock radio or white sound generator at night, or a hearing aid during the day—little was available until about a decade and a half ago to help these people. Treatment has included drugs, such as vitamins and vasodilators; surgery, such as labyrinthine or vestibular nerve destruction; nerve blocks; and cognitive therapy, all with mixed success.

The principles of biofeedback have also been applied to tinnitus relief. Biofeedback allows individuals to monitor their own physiological activity by attaching recording electrodes to specific parts of the body; these permit the subject to observe and to control the activity. Some patients have learned to monitor and suppress their tinnitus through the use of biofeedback techniques.

The wearable tinnitus masking unit has enjoyed some marginal popularity. Most such devices are similar to behind-the-ear hearing aids (see Figure 12.4B) and are manufactured by some hearing-aid companies. The tinnitus masker, designed as a miniature masking unit, produces a band of noise that surrounds the frequency of the tinnitus. When no specific frequency or noise band is reported as characteristic of the individual's tinnitus, a broad-band signal may be used as the masker. With patience and gradual adjustments, a close match to a patient's tinnitus can be obtained. Special devices called tinnitus audiometers have been developed to enable audiologists to determine patients' specific masking spectral needs, along with the intensities required to mask their tinnitus. It is interesting that despite patient complaints of the extreme loudness of their tinnitus, when matched to signals of similar acoustic spectra, the sensation levels of the head noises are rarely more than 10 dB.

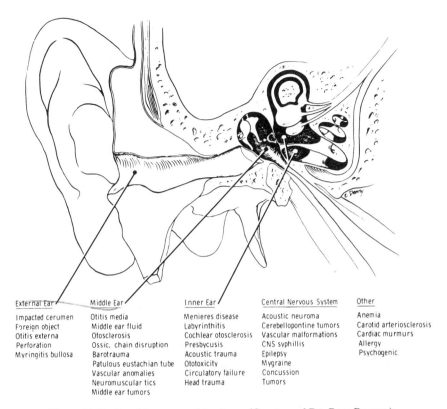

External Ear	Middle Ear	Inner Ear	Central Nervous System	Other
Impacted cerumen	Otitis media	Menieres disease	Acoustic neuroma	Anemia
Foreign object	Middle ear fluid	Labyrinthitis	Cerebellopontine tumors	Carotid arteriosclerosis
Otitis externa	Otosclerosis	Cochlear otosclerosis	Vascular malformations	Cardiac murmurs
Perforation	Ossic. chain disruption	Presbycusis	CNS syphillis	Allergy
Myringitis bullosa	Barotrauma	Acoustic trauma	Epilepsy	Psychogenic
	Patulous eustachian tube	Ototoxicity	Mygraine	
	Vascular anomalies	Circulatory failure	Concussion	
	Neuromuscular tics	Head trauma	Tumors	
	Middle ear tumors			

Figure 12.10 Possible causes of tinnitus. (Courtesy of Dr. Ross Roeser.)

Most patients have given disappointing reports on the effects of tinnitus maskers, but a few are extremely satisfied with the results. Some claim that not only is the tinnitus relieved by what they observe to be external sounds preferable to their own tinnitus, but also that the tinnitus is relieved after the masking device is removed. Although it is not completely understood, this effect may be explained by some residual inhibition in the auditory system. If a hearing loss is present, a mild gain hearing aid often serves as an effective tinnitus masker. In any event, the phenomenon of tinnitus continues to be perplexing.

COUNSELING

One of the greatest responsibilities of the audiologist is to ensure that test results and diagnostic impressions are imparted adequately to patients and their families. Accurate test results are of paramount importance, but the tests serve merely as instruments to help the clinician give advice and counsel to patients and their significant others. Many people in our society have been conditioned to accept the recommendations of professionals without understanding the underlying reasons for these recommendations.

To a large degree, the specific approach used, and the details included in counseling a patient or family, are determined by the audiologist's interests and professional experience. Certainly, the type and degree of loss should be explained, and the audiogram should be discussed in some detail. The particulars of special tests are sometimes not well understood, but if some interest is shown in these tests, the results should be explained in detail, using the clearest terms possible.

In some cases it is necessary to avoid more than perfunctory explanations of test results. Examples of such cases may be the presence of pseudohypacusis or the involvement of potentially serious medical conditions. An audiologist must not engage in discussions with patients regarding acoustic tumors and the like; this is the responsibility of the physician. On the other hand, if an audiologist suspects a potentially reversible condition for which a referral is made to an otologist, the patient is entitled to know the reason for the referral.

When discussing test results, the audiologist must create an atmosphere of calm professionalism. This is often the basis for the extent of the patient's confidence in the clinician. The amount of time spent in counseling depends, in large measure, on the motivation of the patient. After an explanation of the test results and recommendations, the audiologist should solicit questions from the patient and try to answer them in appropriate detail.

Often it is the unasked questions that the audiologist must sense and answer. Patients and their families are frequently fearful of inquiring about possible progression of hearing loss. Many older patients fear that it is only a matter of time before they will lose their hearing entirely. Although progression of hearing loss may or may not have been demonstrated by repeated hearing evaluations over time, it is possible for the audiologist to play a calming and reassuring role.

When specific recommendations are made, the importance of patient follow-through should be stressed, but excessive optimism should be avoided lest eventual disappointment be the result. It is possible to provide guidance in an encouraging yet realistic manner.

The matter of counseling the parents or caretakers of hearing-impaired children was discussed in Chapter 11. It has been known for some time that the diagnosis of hearing loss in children may be met with a number of emotional reactions, some of which may interfere with the very habilitative measures that the audiologist intends. Many people have inferred that adults with acquired hearing loss do not suffer the same shock, disappointment, anger, sadness, and range of other reactions, because they are more or less expecting the diagnosis they hear. Apparently, however, this is far from true in many cases, and hearing-impaired adults may be much more emotionally fragile than had been supposed (Martin, Krall, & O'Neal, 1989). As with parents, it is often difficult to distinguish those adults who receive what they perceive to be bad news about irreversible hearing loss in a matter-of-fact way from those for whom the same news is catastrophic.

It is almost always desirable to ask new patients to be accompanied to their hearing evaluations by a significant other person, such as a spouse. Observing the tests, as well as the responses given (particularly on speech recognition tests), allows for insights into the nature of the hearing handicap that are difficult to comprehend when explained. In all cases it is the adult patient who should be addressed directly during postevaluation counseling. Elderly people in particular resent the exclusion they suffer when they are ignored and discussed in their very presence. The use of stock hearing aids or assistive listening devices may be very useful in helping the patient through the counseling process.

Audiologists face a dilemma in that, following the pronouncement that a hearing loss is probably irreversible, their patients have difficulty in understanding and processing subsequently presented technical aspects of their hearing disorder and explanations of test results. At the same time, patients complain that they desire to learn much more at the time of diagnosis than audiologists, physicians, and hearing-aid dealers usually provide (Martin, Krall, & O'Neal, 1989). A major complaint by patients is that they feel rushed while in the clinician's office. One solution to this problem is to ask patients individually what they know about their problems and what they wish to be told. It should be emphasized that further counseling is available, and patients should be encouraged to call for more indepth discussion of their hearing problems. After people have had a chance to compose themselves, they often think of many pertinent questions or details that they want explained.

Many adults find that support groups are of great assistance in dealing with their hearing losses. One such group is Self Help for Hard of Hearing, Inc., which publishes its own consumer-oriented journal for hearing-impaired adults. What the hearing-impaired are asking for is no more than they are entitled to—a concerned and compassionate clinician who is willing to give sufficient time and express appropriate interest in what to many people is a profound and disturbing handicap.

MANAGEMENT OF THE HEARING-IMPAIRED ADULT

Adult patients requiring audiological management of their hearing problems are usually adventitiously impaired. Although some hearing losses are sudden—for example, the result of drug therapy or some illness—most are gradual, almost insidious. The management of these patients is often called *aural rehabilitation*. In recent years there has been increasing emphasis on the rehabilitative aspects of audiology.

While medical science has advanced in the treatment of diseases that cause hearing loss, similar advances have served to prolong life, with the result that for the first time in history, the population of the United States consists of more older people than younger people. Because hearing loss is the almost inevitable result of aging, the number of adults with acquired hearing loss is increasing. Audiologists must be prepared to meet this challenge.

Before an aural rehabilitation program can begin, it is essential that the patient's hearing handicap be assessed. It has been customary to make this assessment on the basis of objective audiometric data alone. The information provided earlier in this book is essential to patient management, but it does not supersede other information which may also be critical, such as the patient's own view of the handicap, individual needs and preferences, socioeconomic status, education, vocation, and a host of other important considerations.

A number of attempts to assess the degree of hearing handicap have been made. These have been based both on audiometric data and on scales computed with the assistance of the patient. A review of hearing handicap scales is provided by Giolas (1982). Although none of these methods is perfect, they assist the audiologist in compiling data about how the hearing impairment affects the individual who is the central figure in the rehabilitation process. After all, it does little good to insist that a patient needs to wear hearing aids when the patient has no such intention and therefore minimizes the effects of the hearing loss.

The goal of adult aural rehabilitation is always to make maximum use of residual hearing. Residual hearing is useful hearing, and it is not always easily discernible by looking at an audiogram, spondee threshold, or speech discrimination score. The patient's residual hearing is the difference in decibels between the auditory threshold and the uncomfortable loudness level. This is the dynamic range of hearing. The broader the dynamic range, the better candidate the patient is for a hearing aid and aural rehabilitation.

A number of decisions must be made after the handicap has been assessed. The decision on hearing aids must be made, and proper selection and orientation should be arranged. The nature of the orientation must be selected—that is, whether therapy should be done individually or in groups, who should constitute the specific group, what visual cues should be emphasized, how speech can be conserved, and so on. Rehabilitative efforts must be geared to the individual, whose curiosity and ability to comprehend should not be underestimated. The patient should be educated as fully as possible about hearing loss in general and about the specific handicap in particular. How the ear works and what has gone wrong, the effects of the loss on speech communication, implications for progression of the loss, and interactions with family and friends must all be discussed openly and honestly with the patient, with a close friend or family member present whenever possible.

Patients should be taught to maximize their communicative skills, in part by managing their environments. People should be encouraged to be in the same room with and facing others with whom they speak. Position in the room should be manipulated to take advantage of lighting, room noise should be minimized during conversation, and assistive listening devices should be used when this is appropriate.

Ideally, at least some portion of aural rehabilitation is performed in the audiology center in a group setting, but this is not always possible. In some cases the patient is homebound or in a home for the elderly and cannot visit the clinic. Arrangements should be made to meet the needs of each patient whenever possible.

Many audiologists are more comfortable in the role of diagnostician than therapist. Modern audiology demands that the clinician be facile in both of these areas. The reader is encouraged to explore the Suggested Readings list at the end of this chapter for more information about dealing with the handicap of acquired hearing loss.

AUDITORY TRAINING

A major task of the rehabilitative audiologist or therapist is to train the hard-of-hearing patient in the maximum use of residual hearing through **auditory training**. There are obvious differences in the approaches to prelingually and postlingually impaired patients. Children who have suffered hearing loss from birth or early childhood cannot call upon the memory of speech sounds and so must begin training in special ways. The term *auditory retraining* is more appropriate to the adult or older child who must be reeducated in listening for specific sounds.

Auditory Training with Children

Hearing-impaired children vary considerably in the enthusiasm with which they accept amplification. A great deal of the acceptance depends on the

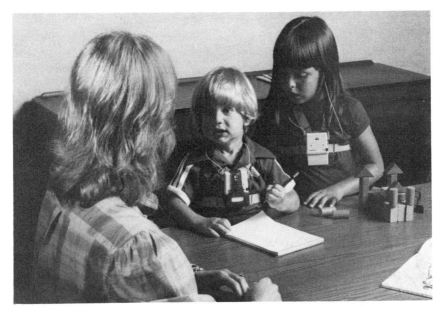

Figure 12.11 Two hearing-impaired children wearing FM auditory training units. (Courtesy of Phonic Ear.)

approach made by the family and therapist. The sudden presentation of loud and distorted sounds can be frightening to children. They may be confused and annoyed by the earmold, receiver, or cord. For the small child there is no way for explanations to precede the wearing of the aid. It goes without saying that the more readily the aid is accepted, the sooner training can begin (see Figure 12.11). Auditory training programs may be quite comprehensive, and specific goals and objectives should be established for auditory training based on individual needs.

Working with school-age children is often easier than working with younger children. The main problem, again, is the children's acceptance of their hearing aids or the receivers of auditory training units. The approach can make a great and lasting difference in the children's attitudes toward amplification. The therapist and family should show enthusiasm for the project, but it is important that children not learn to use their aids as instruments of punishment against their elders. Children have been known to pull hearing aids from their ears and throw them to the floor when they become angry with their parents.

Auditory Retraining with Adults

There is considerable disagreement among experts on the best approach to training hearing-impaired adults. Beginning training with an auditory trainer affords higher quality of sound and better discrimination. Some audiologists, however, believe that the patient should learn early to discriminate among sounds using the limited properties of a wearable instrument.

The vast majority of persons attending organized classes for auditory training do so with the objective of improved hearing-aid use. Many patients with sensorineural hearing losses cannot make the adjustment to aids or refuse to attempt to do so.

For both children and adults, auditory training may be given in groups or individually. Naturally, individual therapy allows for greater personal attention, but work in the group has a psychotherapeutic value that cannot be underestimated. Many adults, particularly older people become depressed over their hearing losses. They feel persecuted and alone. Although they may realize on an intellectual level that their problems are not unique, emotionally they feel quite isolated. The mere experience of being with persons of their own age and with similar problems may lift their spirits and aid in their rehabilitation.

Professional attitudes on the value of auditory training vary. Although there is little evidence to prove that periods of professional training increase speech discrimination scores, either with or without hearing aids, most audiologists are in favor of such programs. The educational and emotional values of therapy can only be approximated. Auditory training with hearing aids provides a period of orientation that is essential to the effective use of residual hearing when it is predicated on individually developed programs.

SPEECHREADING

It is the mistaken concept among many laypersons, and among some professionals as well, that if hearing becomes impaired, it can be replaced by **lip-reading**, a means by which the words of a speaker may be recognized by watching the lips. In recent years the term **speechreading** has been used to replace *lip-reading*, because it is recognized that the visual perception of speech requires much more than attending to lip movements alone. Recognition of facial expressions, gestures, body movements, and so on contributes to the perception of speech.

It has generally been agreed for some time that much of the speech signal may be visually perceived. Many speech sounds are produced so that they may be recognized on the lips alone, at least in terms of their general manner and place of production. Some sounds, such as /p/, /m/, and /b/, are produced in such fashion as to make them difficult to differentiate on the basis of visual cues alone. Other sounds, such as /g/, /k/, and /h/, cannot be perceived visually.

Although much has been done to investigate the value of speechreading, and a number of methods are available to teach this skill to hearing-impaired persons, it is still a considerably misunderstood concept. It is a gross error to believe that speechreading alone can replace hearing in the complete understanding of spoken discourse. It is also an error to believe that more than about 50% of the sounds of speech may be perceived through speechreading alone.

In order for speechreading to be of maximum value to the patient, it should be taught in conjunction with auditory training, so that the combined effects of vision and residual hearing may be gained. When the two senses are used simultaneously, they interact synergistically; that is, the combined effect on discrimination for speech is greater for watching and listening together than for either watching alone or listening alone.

Speechreading Training with Children

Speechreading for small, hearing-impaired children should begin early in life. The children should be encouraged to watch the faces of their parents and others. Speech to these children should be slow, simple, and carefully articulated without exaggeration. The error committed by many parents is to mouth speech without voice, in the belief that the exaggerations will help the children speechread and that voice is unnecessary since the children are "deaf." Using voice allows the production of the speech sounds to be more natural and, it is hoped, provides some auditory cues if the children's residual hearing has been tapped by using amplification.

Speechreading Training with Adults

Many people believe that speechreading is an art that requires an innate talent possessed more by some persons than by others. It is probably true that some people are more visually oriented than others. Some people do better on speechreading tests without training than do other people who have had a number of speechreading lessons.

The methods of teaching speechreading to adults vary considerably in their philosophy and implementation. Some include an analytic approach to the movements of the speaker's lips, whereas others are more synthetic in their approach. Research is under way on computer-assisted training in speechreading, using the latest in video disk technology. Suffice it to say in this brief discussion that speechreading should be made as natural to the patient as possible, utilizing residual hearing through a hearing aid if this is indicated.

SUMMARY

Diagnosis of the type and degree of a patient's hearing loss is an essential beginning to aural rehabilitation. For proper management, the audiologist must become sophisticated in the intricacies of history taking. Audiologists also must maintain good relationships with other professional workers who may be involved in the rehabilitation of the patient. Proper relationships are strongly influenced by the exchanges among professionals, such as letters and reports.

Audiologists should be responsible for the total program of aural rehabilitation of the hearing-impaired patient. They must make the determinations of the need for special measures, such as tinnitus therapy, speechreading, auditory training, and the acquisition of hearing aids. If a hearing aid is indicated, the audiologist should figure prominently in the selection procedure.

The importance of a proper professional relationship between the audiologist and the patient (or family) cannot be overstated. Advising and counseling sessions greatly affect the overall management of the hearing-impaired.

GLOSSARY

Acoustic feedback The whistling sound that is created when the signal leaving the receiver of a hearing aid leaks back into the microphone and is reamplified.

Acoustic gain The difference in decibels between the intensity of the input signal and the intensity of the output signal in a hearing aid.

Auditory training The training of the hearing-impaired patient in the optimum use of residual hearing.

Cochlear implant A coil and series of electrodes surgically placed in the mastoid and inner ear. It is designed to provide sound to an adult with a profound hearing loss by means of a processor and external coil.

CROS (contralateral routing of signals) A hearing aid originally developed for patients with unilateral hearing losses. The microphone is mounted on the side of the poorer ear, and the signal is routed to the better ear and presented by means of an "open" earmold.

Distortion In a hearing aid, the result of the output signal's being an inexact copy of the input signal. Distortion is usually caused by the microphone, speaker, and/or amplifier.

Electret microphone A device for converting the mechanical energy of sound into an electrical signal by the use of capacitors, rather than magnets or crystals. The many advantages of this kind of microphone include its small size and excellent frequency response.

Frequency response The frequency range of amplification (as in a hearing aid) expressed in Hertz, from the lowest to the highest frequency amplified.

Harmonic distortion The distortion created when harmonic frequencies are generated in an amplification system. Usually expressed in percentage of distortion.

Hearing Aid Industry Conference (HAIC) An organization, consisting of hearing-aid manufacturers, that provides standardization of measurement and reporting on hearing-aid performance data.

Lip-reading See *Speechreading*.

Output The maximum power emitted from a hearing aid, regardless of input level.

Reference test gain The acoustic gain of a hearing aid as measured in a hearing-aid test box. The gain control of the aid is set to amplify an input signal of 60 dB SPL to a level 17 dB below the SSPL 90 value. The average values at 1000, 1600, and 2500 Hz determine the reference test gain.

Saturation sound-pressure level (SSPL) The newer term for maximum power output of a hearing aid. The highest sound-pressure level to leave the receiver of a hearing aid, regardless of the input level.

Speechreading The use of visual (primarily facial) cues to determine the words of a speaker.

Vibrotactile hearing aids Devices that deliver amplified vibratory energy to the surface of the skin by means of special transducers. They are designed for patients whose hearing losses are so severe that assistance in speechreading cannot be obtained from traditional hearing aids.

STUDY QUESTIONS

1. In what ways do the approaches to aural rehabilitation differ for children and adults?
2. List and describe the electroacoustic characteristics of hearing aids.
3. What are the advantages and disadvantages of different types of hearing aids?
4. What measurements are made in a hearing-aid evaluation?
5. List the data you would include in a report sent to different specialists with a common interest in your patient. In what ways are the reports similar and dissimilar?
6. List the first five questions you would ask when recording a patient's history.
7. Design a case history form that might be suitable for
   a. the adult patient;
   b. the pediatric patient.

8. How may tinnitus be treated?

9. How might acceptance of an acquired hearing loss be improved?

REFERENCES

AMERICAN NATIONAL STANDARD FOR SPECIFI-
CATION OF HEARING AID CHARACTERISTICS.
(1982). ASA STD7–1976 (ANSI S3.22–1982).
New York: American National Standards Institute.

BECK, L. B. (1989, January–February). The
"T" switch: Some tips for effective use. *Shhh*,
pp. 12–15.

CARHART, R. (1946). Tests for selection of
hearing aids. *Laryngoscope, 56*, 780–794.

DEWEESE, D., & VERNON, J. (1975). The
American Tinnitus Association. *Hearing Instruments, 18*, 19–25.

DORMAN, M. F., HANNLEY, M. T., DANKOWSKI,
K., SMITH, L., & McCANDLESS, G. (1989).
Word recognition by 50 patients fitted with
the Symbion multichannel cochlear implant.
Ear and Hearing, 10, 44–49.

DOWNS, D. (1984). Tactile aids: New help for
the profoundly deaf. *The Hearing Journal, 37*,
20–24.

GIOLAS, T. G. (1982). *Hearing-Handicapped
Adults.* Englewood Cliffs, NJ: Prentice-Hall.

HARFORD, E., & BARRY, L. (1965). A rehabilitative approach to the problem of unilateral hearing impairment: The contralateral
routing of signals (CROS). *Journal of Speech
and Hearing Disorders, 30*, 121–138.

HAUG, O., BACARO, P., & GUILFORD, F. R.
(1971). Differences in hearing aid performance. *Archives of Otolaryngology, 93*, 183–185.

HEARING AID INDUSTRY CONFERENCE (HAIC).
(1961). *Standard Method of Expressing Hearing-
Aid Performance.* New York: Author.

———. (1975). *Standards for Hearing Aids.*
New York: Author.

HECOX, K. E., & PUNCH, J. L. (1988). The
impact of digital technology on the selection
and fitting of hearing aids. *American Journal
of Otology, 9*, 77–85.

HOUSE, W. F. (1982). Surgical considerations
in cochlear implants. *Annals of Otology, Rhinology, and Laryngology, 91*, 15–20.

JOHNSON, R., MEIKLE, M., VERNON, J., &
SCHLEUNING, A. (1988). An implantable
bone conduction hearing device. *American
Journal of Otology, 9*, 93–100.

KILLION, M. C., BERLIN, C. I., & HOOD, L.
(1984). A low frequency emphasis open canal
hearing aid. *Hearing Instruments, 35*, 30–66.

KLEIN, A. J. (1989). Assessing speech recognition in noise for listeners with a signal
processor hearing aid. *Ear and Hearing, 10*,
50–57.

LEVITT, H. (1988a). Digital hearing instruments: A brief overview. *Hearing Instruments, 39*, 8–12.

———. (1988b). Recurrent issues underlying
the development of tactile sensory aids. *Ear
and Hearing, 9*, 301–305.

LIBBY, E. R. (1988). Hearing aid selection
strategies and probe tube microphone measures. *Hearing Instruments, 39*, 10–15.

MARTIN, D. (1989). Probe microphones, prescriptions and children. *Hearing Instruments,
40*, 28–29.

MARTIN, F. N., KRALL, L., & O'NEAL, J. (1989).
The Diagnosis of Acquired Hearing Loss: Patient Reactions. *Asha, 31*, 47–50.

PLOSHAY, K. L., & HOFMAN, C. L. (1984). Infrared listening systems—A buzzword in the
making. *Hearing Instruments, 35*, 6–47.

POPELKA, G. R., & ENGEBRETSON, A. M. (1983).
A computer-based system for hearing aid assessment. *Hearing Instruments, 7*, 6–44.

ROESER, R. J., FRIEL-PATTI, S., & SCOTT, B. L.
(1983). Development and evaluation of a
tactile aid for the reception of speech. *Audiology: A Journal for Continuing Education, 8*,
79–94.

Roeser, R. J., & Taylor, K. (1988). Audiometric and field testing with a digital hearing aid. *Hearing Instruments, 39*, 14–22.

Ross, M., & Duffy, J. K. (1961). *Clinical uses of pure-tone soundfield audiometry.* Paper presented at the annual convention of the American Speech and Hearing Association, Chicago.

Shore, I., Bilger, R. C., & Hirsh, I. J. (1960). Hearing aid evaluation: Reliability of repeated measurements. *Journal of Speech and Hearing Disorders, 25*, 152–170.

Vaugn, G. R., Lightfoot, R. K., & Teter, D. L. (1988). Assistive listening devices and systems (ALDLS) enhance the lifestyles of hearing impaired persons. *American Journal of Otology, 9*, 101–106.

Weisenberger, J. M. (1989). Evaluation of the Siemens Minifonator vibrotactile aids. *Journal of Speech and Hearing Research, 32*, 24–32.

Yellin, W., Meyerhoff, W. L., & Roland, P. S. (1988). A new development for conductive hearing loss. *Tejas, 14*, 44–45.

Young, E. J., Boothroyd, A., & Redmond, C. (1988). A wearable multichannel tactile display of voice fundamental frequency. *Ear and Hearing, 9*, 342–350.

SUGGESTED READINGS

Libby, E. R. (1988). Hearing aid selection strategies and probe tube microphone measures. *Hearing Instruments, 39*, 10–15.

Skinner, M. W. (1988). *Hearing aid evaluation.* Englewood Cliffs, NJ: Prentice-Hall.

Appendix **I**

INSTRUCTIONS
FOR TAKING
THE HEARING EXAMINATION

As a part of your examination you will receive several different hearing tests. The results of these tests will help us determine the type and degree of hearing impairment you have so that we may best advise you regarding your hearing difficulties.

The tests are divided into three parts: (1) hearing for speech, (2) hearing for tones, and (3) measurements of eardrum function. Here are a few simple instructions to make these tests go more quickly and easily for you and to ensure the accuracy of the test results.

You will be seated in a sound-treated room. A pair of earphones will be placed over your ears or a button will be held to your forehead or behind your ear by a metal or plastic strap. This equipment will fit snugly but should not be uncomfortable.

For your first speech test you will hear some two-syllable words like *sunset* or *airplane*. Please repeat each word you hear, even if you have to guess. Some of these words will be too faint to hear, but try to repeat as many as you can. Do not be concerned over missing some of the words since it is expected that this will happen. Please do not watch the examiner's face because this may interfere with the accuracy of the test. From this examination we can determine your **speech reception threshold**, which tells us how loud speech must be before you can barely understand it. You will find an alphabetical list of the words which will be used below. Please familiarize yourself with this list.

For the next tests you will be asked to listen closely and respond to some very soft tones in one ear. The test will be repeated in your other ear. As soon as you barely hear each tone please signal the clinician. You may be asked to press a button, raise your hand, or give a verbal response. There will be a series of such tones of different pitches, first in one ear and then in the other. Each time you are aware of a tone, even faintly, please signal. On the basis of this test we can determine your hearing levels for **air conduction** and **bone conduction**, so that we can draw your pure-tone **audiogram**. The audiogram gives us information about how well your ear hears sounds across a wide range of pitches.

You will than be given a list of 50 one-syllable words, which you will be able to hear at a comfortable loudness level. Each word will be preceded by the phrase "Say the word . . ." You are asked merely to say the last word of the phrase. For example, if the examiner says "Say the word *boy*," you simply repeat "*boy*." If you are not certain of the word, please try to guess and repeat the word that it most sounds like. This test may be repeated at a louder level. This will give us your **speech discrimination** or word understanding score for each ear.

It may be necessary to introduce a continuous wind-like noise into one ear while your other ear is being tested. This noise, while loud, is harmless, and will help to ensure that the ear not being tested does not take part in the test. Simply try to ignore the noise and concentrate on the test signal.

Another routine test will measure the movement of your eardrum. Your ear will first be examined with a special light called an otoscope. Then a tightly fitting plastic piece will be inserted into one ear. An earphone will be placed over your other ear. You will note the following sensations: a humming sound, a sensation of slight pressure, and a series of loud tones. There is no danger to your ears or to your hearing from this procedure. Although this test takes only a few minutes, it provides us with a great deal of information about your eardrum, your middle ear, and the nerves that go from the ear to the brain and back. This procedure is called **acoustic immitance** and requires only that you sit quietly. No response on your part is necessary.

The examining audiologist will be glad to answer any questions you might have regarding these instructions or the test results. These instructions will be explained in greater detail during the testing session.

Please feel free to ask questions at any time.

The words used to test your **speech reception threshold** will be taken from the following list. You do not need to memorize these words, but please look over the list.

airplane	armchair
birthday	doormat
eardrum	farewell
iceberg	mousetrap
mushroom	northwest
playground	railroad
sidewalk	stairway
sunset	

WORD LISTS FOR USE IN SPEECH AUDIOMETRY

SPONDAIC WORDS

CID Auditory Test W–1[1]

LIST A

1. greyhound	10. duckpond	19. baseball	28. oatmeal
2. schoolboy	11. sidewalk	20. stairway	29. toothbrush
3. inkwell	12. hotdog	21. cowboy	30. farewell
4. whitewash	13. padlock	22. iceberg	31. grandson
5. pancake	14. mushroom	23. northwest	32. drawbridge
6. mousetrap	15. hardware	24. railroad	33. doormat
7. eardrum	16. workshop	25. playground	34. hothouse
8. headlight	17. horseshoe	26. airplane	35. daybreak
9. birthday	18. armchair	27. woodwork	36. sunset

[1]The lists from Tests W–1 and W–22 are reproduced by permission of Technisonic Studios and the Central Institute for the Deaf. (Twelve-inch LP recordings of the CID word lists are available from Technisonic Studios, Inc., 1201 Brentwood Boulevard, St. Louis, Missouri 63117.)

PB WORD LISTS

CID Auditory Test W–22

LIST 1A

1. an	14. low	26. you (ewe)	39. none
2. yard	15. owl	27. as	(nun)
3. carve	16. it	28. wet	40. jam
4. us	17. she	29. chew	41. poor
5. day	18. high	30. see (sea)	42. him
6. toe	19. there	31. deaf	43. skin
7. felt	(their)	32. them	44. east
8. stove	20. earn (urn)	33. give	45. thing
9. hunt	21. twins	34. true	46. dad
10. ran	22. could	35. isle (aisle)	47. up
11. knees	23. what	36. or (oar)	48. bells
12. not (knot)	24. bathe	37. law	49. wire
13. mew	25. ace	38. me	50. ache

LIST 2A

1. yore (your)	13. move	25. air (heir)	38. new (knew)
2. bin (been)	14. new	26. and	39. live (verb)
3. way	15. jaw	27. young	40. off
(weigh)	16. one	28. cars	41. ill
4. chest	(won)	29. tree	42. rooms
5. then	17. hit	30. dumb	43. ham
6. ease	18. send	31. that	44. star
7. smart	19. else	32. die (dye)	45. eat
8. gave	20. tare (tear)	33. show	46. thin
9. pew	21. does	34. hurt	47. flat
10. ice	22. too (two, to)	35. own	48. well
11. odd	23. cap	36. key	49. by (buy)
12. knee	24. with	37. oak	50. ail (ale)

LIST 3A

1. bill	11. out	21. done	30. do
2. add (ad)	12. lie (lye)	(dun)	31. hand
3. west	13. three	22. use (yews)	32. end
4. cute	14. oil	23. camp	33. shove
5. start	15. king	24. wool	34. have
6. ears	16. pie	25. are	35. owes
7. tan	17. he	26. aim	36. jar
8. nest	18. smooth	27. when	37. no (know)
9. say	19. farm	28. book	38. may
10. is	20. this	29. tie	39. knit

40. on	**43.** glove	**46.** though	**49.** ate
41. if	**44.** ten	**47.** chair	(eight)
42. raw	**45.** dull	**48.** we	**50.** year

LIST 4A

1. all (awl)	**14.** leave	**27.** art	**40.** jump
2. wood (would)	**15.** of	**28.** will	**41.** pale (pail)
3. at	**16.** hang	**29.** dust	**42.** go
4. where	**17.** save	**30.** toy	**43.** stiff
5. chin	**18.** ear	**31.** aid	**44.** can
6. they	**19.** tea (tee)	**32.** than	**45.** through
7. dolls	**20.** cook	**33.** eyes (ayes)	(thru)
8. so (sew)	**21.** tin	**34.** shoe	**46.** clothes
9. nuts	**22.** bread (bred)	**35.** his	**47.** who
10. ought (aught)	**23.** why	**36.** our (hour)	**48.** bee
11. in (inn)	**24.** arm	**37.** men	(be)
12. net	**25.** yet	**38.** near	**49.** yes
13. my	**26.** darn	**39.** few	**50.** am

KINDERGARTEN PB WORD LISTS

Haskins Lists[2]

LIST 1

1. please	**14.** rag	**27.** bath	**40.** neck
2. great	**15.** put	**28.** slip	**41.** beef
3. sled	**16.** fed	**29.** ride	**42.** few
4. pants	**17.** fold	**30.** end	**43.** use
5. rat	**18.** hunt	**31.** pink	**44.** did
6. bad	**19.** no	**32.** thank	**45.** hit
7. pinch	**20.** box	**33.** take	**46.** pond
8. such	**21.** are	**34.** cart	**47.** hot
9. bus	**22.** teach	**35.** scab	**48.** own
10. need	**23.** slice	**36.** lay	**49.** bead
11. ways	**24.** is	**37.** class	**50.** shop
12. five	**25.** tree	**38.** me	
13. mouth	**26.** smile	**39.** dish	

LIST 2

1. laugh	**4.** plow	**7.** gray	**10.** fat
2. falls	**5.** page	**8.** park	**11.** ax
3. paste	**6.** weed	**9.** wait	**12.** cage

[2]Reproduced by permission of Ms. Harriet L. Haskins.

13. knife	23. bless	33. freeze	43. fresh
14. turn	24. suit	34. race	44. tray
15. grab	25. splash	35. bud	45. cat
16. rose	26. path	36. darn	46. on
17. lip	27. feed	37. fair	47. camp
18. bee	28. next	38. sack	48. find
19. bet	29. wreck	39. got	49. yes
20. his	30. waste	40. as	50. loud
21. sing	31. crab	41. grew	
22. all	32. peg	42. knee	

LIST 3

1. tire	14. else	27. thick	40. frog
2. seed	15. nest	28. if	41. bush
3. purse	16. jay	29. them	42. clown
4. quick	17. raw	30. sheep	43. cab
5. room	18. true	31. air	44. hurt
6. bug	19. had	32. set	45. pass
7. that	20. cost	33. dad	46. grade
8. sell	21. vase	34. ship	47. blind
9. low	22. press	35. case	48. drop
10. rich	23. fit	36. you	49. leave
11. those	24. bounce	37. may	50. nuts
12. ache	25. wide	38. choose	
13. black	26. most	39. white	

CNC WORD LISTS

NU Auditory Test No. 6 (Alphabetized)[3]

LIST I

1. bean	11. gap	21. knock	31. pool
2. boat	12. goose	22. laud	32. puff
3. burn	13. hash	23. limp	33. rag
4. chalk	14. home	24. lot	34. raid
5. choice	15. hurl	25. love	35. raise
6. death	16. jail	26. met	36. reach
7. dime	17. jar	27. mode	37. sell
8. door	18. keen	28. moon	38. shout
9. fall	19. king	29. nag	39. size
10. fat	20. kite	30. page	40. sub

[3]Reproduced by permission of Dr. Tom W. Tillman.

41. sure
42. take
43. third

44. tip
45. tough
46. vine

47. week
48. which

49. whip
50. yes

LIST II

1. bite
2. book
3. bought
4. calm
5. chair
6. chief
7. dab
8. dead
9. deep
10. fail
11. far
12. gaze
13. gin

14. goal
15. hate
16. haze
17. hush
18. juice
19. keep
20. keg
21. learn
22. live
23. loaf
24. lore
25. match
26. merge

27. mill
28. nice
29. numb
30. pad
31. pick
32. pike
33. rain
34. read
35. room
36. rot
37. said
38. shack
39. shawl

40. soap
41. south
42. thought
43. ton
44. tool
45. turn
46. voice
47. wag
48. white
49. witch
50. young

LIST III

1. bar
2. base
3. beg
4. cab
5. cause
6. chat
7. cheek
8. cool
9. date
10. ditch
11. dodge
12. five
13. germ

14. good
15. gun
16. half
17. hire
18. hit
19. jug
20. late
21. lid
22. life
23. luck
24. mess
25. mop
26. mouse

27. name
28. note
29. pain
30. pearl
31. phone
32. pole
33. rat
34. ring
35. road
36. rush
37. search
38. seize
39. shall

40. sheep
41. soup
42. talk
43. team
44. tell
45. thin
46. void
47. walk
48. when
49. wire
50. youth

LIST IV

1. back
2. bath
3. bone
4. came
5. chain
6. check
7. dip
8. dog
9. doll

10. fit
11. food
12. gas
13. get
14. hall
15. have
16. hole
17. join
18. judge

19. kick
20. kill
21. lean
22. lease
23. long
24. lose
25. make
26. mob
27. mood

28. near
29. neat
30. pass
31. peg
32. perch
33. red
34. ripe
35. rose
36. rough

37. sail	41. such	45. tire	48. wheat
38. shirt	42. tape	46. vote	49. wife
39. should	43. thumb	47. wash	50. yearn
40. sour	44. time		

CALIFORNIA CONSONANT TEST ITEMS[4]

LIST 1

Samples

1. bag
2. nice
3. seen
4. dale
5. leash
6. tail

Test Items

1. gage	21. shin	41. kick	61. tan	81. match
2. pail	22. much	42. tin	62. chore	82. pass
3. cup	23. reap	43. bus	63. sis	83. faith
4. mush	24. back	44. date	64. cuss	84. rig
5. face	25. same	45. lass	65. rat	85. chief
6. kill	26. tore	46. hitch	66. till	86. shore
7. leap	27. rage	47. sick	67. pick	87. cop
8. seep	28. pill	48. leaf	68. page	88. map
9. fake	29. chop	49. cheat	69. core	89. dive
10. babe	30. muss	50. ridge	70. lease	90. peep
11. pays	31. dale	51. thin	71. than	91. hip
12. kick	32. peach	52. hiss	72. sheep	92. kin
13. laugh	33. rap	53. pave	73. can	93. catch
14. cheap	34. have	54. hit	74. batch	94. hack
15. gaze	35. tick	55. sick	75. fail	95. dies
16. beep	36. share	56. beach	76. budge	96. sin
17. mass	37. beak	57. hat	77. tail	97. rove
18. patch	38. beat	58. chin	78. robe	98. jail
19. gave	39. cheap	59. sail	79. lash	99. leash
20. thick	40. cuff	60. sun	80. pin	100. raise

[4]Reproduced by permission of Dr. Elmer Owens.

HIGH-FREQUENCY CONSONANT DISCRIMINATION WORD LIST[5]

LIST 1

1. kits	10. hicks	18. fixed
2. sip	11. skits	19. kiss
3. tipped	12. kit	20. skit
4. sis	13. pit	21. spit
5. tip	14. hick	22. hits
6. kick	15. picks	23. ticked
7. skips	16. hit	24. fit
8. ticks	17. six	25. sipped
9. hiss		

LIST 2

1. kicked	10. skipped	18. thick
2. hips	11. hip	19. hissed
3. fits	12. sips	20. spits
4. fix	13. sit	21. sick
5. stick	14. stiff	22. kicks
6. its	15. fist	23. sits
7. tick	16. skip	24. picked
8. tips	17. pits	25. kissed
9. pick		

CHILDREN'S PICTURE-IDENTIFICATION TEST

WIPI Test[6]

1. school	broom	moon	spoon
2. ball	bowl	bell	bow
3. smoke	coat	coke	goat
4. floor	door	corn	horn
5. fox	socks	box	blocks
6. hat	flag	bag	black
7. pan	fan	can	man
8. bread	red	thread	bed
9. neck	desk	nest	dress
10. stair	bear	chair	pear

[5]Harvey J. Gardner, "Application of a High Frequency Consonant Discrimination Word List in Hearing-Aid Application," *Journal of Speech and Hearing Disorders*, 36, August 1971, 354–355. Reprinted by permission.

[6]Reproduced by permission of Dr. Mark Ross and Stanwix House, Inc.

11. eye	pie	fly	tie
12. knee	tea	key	bee
13. street	meat	feet	teeth
14. wing	string	spring	ring
15. mouse	clown	crown	mouth
16. shirt	church	dirt	skirt
17. gun	thumb	sun	gum
18. bus	rug	cup	bug
19. train	cake	snake	plane
20. arm	barn	car	star
21. chick	stick	dish	fish
22. crib	ship	bib	lip
23. wheel	seal	queen	green
24. straw	dog	saw	frog
25. pail	nail	jail	tail

SYNTHETIC SENTENCES[7]

1. Small boat with a picture has become
2. Built the government with the force almost
3. Go change your car color is red
4. Forward march said the boy had a
5. March around without a care in your
6. That neighbor who said business is better
7. Battle cry and be better than ever
8. Down by the time is real enough
9. Agree with him only to find out
10. Women view men with green paper should

COMPETING-SENTENCE TEST[8]

_____ 1. a. I think we'll have rain today.
　　　　b. There was frost on the ground.

_____ 2. a. This watch keeps good time.
　　　　b. I was late to work today.

_____ 3. a. I'm expecting a phone call.
　　　　b. Please answer the doorbell.

_____ 4. a. The bus leaves in five minutes.
　　　　b. It is four blocks to the library.

[7]Reproduced by permission of Dr. James Jerger.
[8]Reproduced by permission of Dr. Jack A. Williford.

_____ 5. a. My mother is a good cook.
b. Your brother is a tall boy.

_____ 6. a. Please pass the salt and pepper.
b. The roast beef is very good.

_____ 7. a. There is a car behind us.
b. This road is very slippery.

_____ 8. a. Leave the keys in the car.
b. Fill the tank with gas.

_____ 9. a. It's always hot on the Fourth of July.
b. Christmas will be here very soon.

_____ 10. a. We had to repair the car.
b. You should really take a taxi.

_____ 11. a. The ice-cream sundae is very good.
b. We have chocolate and strawberry today.

_____ 12. a. Fasten your seat belt.
b. Get ready for take-off.

_____ 13. a. I think you need a band-aid.
b. You should see a doctor.

_____ 14. a. This is the latest style.
b. That fits you perfectly.

_____ 15. a. I will be back after lunch.
b. You may take this Saturday off.

_____ 16. a. I have seen this movie before.
b. This movie is not like the book.

_____ 17. a. Air-mail will get there faster.
b. Please answer on a postcard.

_____ 18. a. I think we have met before.
b. You probably don't remember me.

_____ 19. a. This train is going west.
b. All the cars are air-conditioned.

_____ 20. a. The children are playing baseball.
b. Football is an exciting game.

_____ 21. a. Let's sit down on this bench.
b. Get me a chair so I can rest.

_____ 22. a. The office will be closed tomorrow.
b. You should come to work on Monday.

_____ 23. a. I read that in the newspaper.
b. The man on the radio said it.

_____ 24. a. I wonder what time it is.
b. I think it is time to leave.

_____ 25. a. The traffic is getting worse.
b. I hate the rush hour traffic.

COMMON AUDIOLOGICAL PREFIXES, SUFFIXES, AND ABBREVIATIONS

PREFIXES

a(n)- without, absense

ante- before

anti- against

audio- related to hearing

centi- one-hundredth

de- remove

deci- one-tenth

dermo- skin

dys- disordered, abnormal

ecto- on, outside

encephalo- brain, head

endo- in, inside

ento- within, inner

hema- blood

hyper- excessive

hypo- deficient

inter- between

intra- within

kilo- one thousand times

macro- large

meso- middle, intermediate

micro- small

milli- one one-thousandth

myo- relating to muscles

neuro- relating to nerves

os- bone

oto- relating to the ear

peri- around, about

retro- located behind

sub- under

vaso- blood vessel

SUFFIXES

-cide kill

-cise cut

-ectomy excision, removal

-genesis development of

-itis inflammation of

-oma tumor of

-oscopy look into

-osis condition of

-otomy cut into

-plasty surgical formation of

-sclerosis hardening of

-tomy incision

ABBREVIATIONS

ABLB Alternate binaural loudness balance (test)

ABR Auditory brain stem response

AC Air conduction

AMLB Alternate monaural loudness balance (test)

ANSI American National Standards Institute

APR Auropalpebral reflex

ART Acoustic reflex threshold

ASHA American Speech-Language-Hearing Association

BADGE Békésy ascending-descending gap evaluation

BC Bone conduction

BCL Békésy comfortable loudness

BER Brainstem evoked response

BOA Behavioral observation audiometry

CCM Contralateral competing message

CGS Centimeter-gram-second

cm Centimeter

cm/sec Centimeters per second

CNC Consonant-nucleus-consonant (words)

COR Conditioned orientation reflex

CPA Cerebello-pontine angle

cps cycles per second

CR Conditioned response

CS Conditioned stimulus

CVA Cerebral vascular accident

d Dyne

DAF Delayed auditory feedback

D-S Doerfler-Stewart (test)

e Erg

EAC External auditory canal

ECochG Electrocochleography

EDA Electrodermal audiometry

EDR Electrodermal response

EEG Electroencephalogram

EM Effective masking

ENG Electronystagmography

ERA Evoked response audiometry

f Frequency

FFR Frequency following response

GSR Galvanic skin response

HAIC Hearing Aid Industry Conference

HL Hearing level

Hx History

ICM Ipsilateral competing message

J Joule

k Kilo

λ (Lambda) Length

LER Late evoked response

LOT Lengthened off-time (test)

m Meter

M Mass

μ (Micro) One-millionth

MAF Minimum audible field

MAP Minimum audible pressure

MCL Most comfortable loudness

MCR Message-to-competition (ratio)

ME Middle ear

mks Meter-kilogram-second

MLD Masking-level difference

MLV Monitored live voice

mmho Millimho

m/sec Meters per second

msec Millisecond

mV Millivolt

Mx Medicine

N Newton

NDT Noise-detection threshold

NIL Noise-interference level

NIOSH National Institute for Occupational Safety and Health

OCA Operant conditioning audiometry

OE Outer ear

OM Otitis media

Ω(Omega) Ohm

OSHA Occupational Safety and Health Administration

Pa Pascal

PBK Kindergarten PB (words)

PB Phonetically balanced (word lists)

PD Pulsed descending

P.E. Pressure equalization (tube)

PI-PB Performance intensity (function) for PB words

PTA Pure-tone average

PVT Physical volume test

R Resistance

RCL Range of comfortable loudness

Rx Prescription

S Stiffness

SAI Social adequacy index

SAL Sensorineural acuity level

SBLB Simultaneous binaural loudness balance (test)

SDT Speech-detection threshold

SI Système International

SISI Short increment sensitivity index

SL Sensation level

S/N Signal-to-noise (ratio)

SOM Secretory otitis media

SPAR Sensitivity prediction from the acoustic reflex

SPL Sound-pressure level

SRT Speech reception threshold

SSI Synthetic-sentence identification

SSPL Saturation sound-pressure level

SSW Staggered spondaic word (test)

ST Spondee threshold

STAT Suprathreshold adaptation test

TRA Tinnitus research audiometer

TROCA Tangible reinforcement operant conditioning audiometry

UCL Uncomfortable loudness

UCR Unconditioned response

UCS Unconditioned stimulus

ULCL Upper limits of comfortable loudness

VRA Visual reinforcement audiometry

VU Volume unit

WDS Word discrimination score

WIPI Word intelligibility by picture identification (test)

Z Impedance

AUTHOR INDEX

Page numbers in *italics* refer to complete reference

A

Alexander, G. C., 137, 141, *151*
Alford, B., 299, *320*
Allen, D. V., 344, *359*
Alleyne, B. C., 304, *321*
American Academy of Ophthalmology and
    Otolaryngology (AAOO), 78, 79, *112*
American National Standard for Specification of
    Hearing Aid Characteristics, *460*
American National Standards Institute (ANSI), 44,
    46, 47, 49, 50, *62*, 64, 77, 78, *112*, 167, 177,
    212, 433
American Speech and Hearing Association
    (ASHA), 80, *112*, *151*, *212*
American Speech-Language-Hearing Association
    (ASHA), 75, 76, 79, *112*, 117, 120–21, 125,
    151, 177, 389, 406, 407, 409, *421*
American Standards Association (ASA), 33, *62*
Anderson, E. E., 252, *280*
Anderson, H., 94, *113*, 194, *212*, 298, *320*, 332, *359*
Angell, S., 347, *360*
Antablin, J. K., 136, *154*
Antonelli, A., 348, *359*
Atkinson, C. J., 116, *153*

B

Baccaro, P., 394, 422, 444, *460*
Bailey, H. A. T., 127, *153*, *280*
Bamford, J., 136, *151*
Baran, J. A., *213*, 292, *321*
Barany, E. A., 83, *112*
Barr, B., 194, *212*, 252, *280*, 298, *320*, 332, *359*
Barry, L., 438, *460*
Barry, S. J., 128, *151*
Bartels, D., 167, *213*
Beagley, H. A., 378, *384*
Beasley, W. C., 33, *62*
Beattie, R. C., 120, 129, 135, *151*, *152*
Beauchaine, K., 285, *321*
Beck, L. B., 433, *460*
Békésy, G. V., 65, *112*, 291, 294, *320*
Bell, D. W., 136, *153*
Bench, J., 136, *151*
Benigno Sierra-Irizarry, M. A., 201, *212*
Bennett, M. J., 390, 391, *421*
Benson, R. W., 118, 133, *152*
Berger, K. W., *151*
Bergman, M., 306, *321*, 351, *359*
Berlin, C. I., 444, *460*

Bernstein, M. E., 417, *422*
Berrick, J. M., 352, *359*
Berry, G. A., 127, *153*
Berry, R. C., 141, *151*
Bess, F. H., 135, *154*
Bierman, C. W., 242, *280*
Bilger, R. C., 137, *151*, 444, *461*
Bilger, R. D., 34, *62*
Blakely, R. W., 342, *359*
Blegvad, B., 175, *212*
Blosser, D., 90, *113*, 129, *153*
Blythe, M., 125, *153*
Bocca, E., 347, 348, 349, *359*
Boothroyd, A., 442, *461*
Bordley, J. E., 377, *384*
Bornstein, H., 415, *421*
Borton, T., 298, *320*
Brackett, D., 417, *423*
Bragg, V., 107, *112*
Brey, R. H., 197, *212*
Brinker, C. H., 392, *422*
Brookhouser, P. E., 285, *321*
Brunt, M. A., 177, *212*
Burke, L. E., 119, *151*
Burney, P., 377, *384*
Burns, P., 100, *113*
Butler, E. C., 100, *113*

C

Calearo, C., 347, 348, *359*
Calvert, D. R., 417–18, *423*
Campbell, R. A., 374, *384*
Carhart, R., 76, *112*, 123, 134, 135, 141, *151*, *154*, *155*, 168–69, 171, *212*, 263, 264, *280*, 341, 342, *360*, 374, 378, *384*, 443, *460*
Carteretta, E. C., 147, *153*
Cassinari, V., 348, *359*
Chaiklin, J. B., 90, *112*, 119, 120, *151*
Clark, J. G., 350, *360*, 405, *422*
Clark, J. L., 67, *112*
Cody, J. P., 417, *422*
Coles, R. R. A., 90, *113*, 159, *213*
Collins, F., 107, *112*
Committee on Hearing, Bioacoustics, and Biomechanics, Commission on Behavioral and Social Sciences and Education, National Research Council, 390, *421*
Conn, M., 119, *151*
Coombes, S., 399, *422*
Cooper, J. C., 407, *421*
Cooper, W. A., Jr., 373, '374, *384*
Cornett, R. O., 416, *421*
Cox, J. R., Jr., 34, *62*
Cox, R. M., 137, 141, *151*
Craig, C. H., 134, *152*
Crump, B., 377, *384*
Cyr, D. G., 285, *321*

D

Daly, J. A., 413, 417, *422*
Dancer, J., 119, *151*
Danford, R., Jr., 107, *113*
Danhauer, J. L., 129, 135, *151*, *152*
Dankowski, K., 441, *460*
David, E. E., 51, *62*
Davis, H., 118, 133, 134, 142, *151*, *152*, 160, *212*, 390, *423*
Davis, L. A., 120, *154*
De Jonge, R. R., 252, *280*, 401, *421*
Devald, J., 304, *321*
DeWeese, D., 450, *460*
DiCarlo, L. M., 394, 400, *421*
Dickson, H. D., 407, *421*
DiGiovanni, D., 127, *153*
Dirks, D. D., 120, 147, *153*, *155*, 175, *212*
Dix, M. R., 397, *421*
Dixon, R. F., 410, *421*
Doerfler, L. G., 371, *384*, 406, 407, *421*
Domico, W. D., 177, *212*
Dorman, M. F., 441, *460*
Doughtery, A., 392, *422*
Dowdy, L. K., 121–22, *153*
Downs, D. W., 390, *421*, 441, *460*
Downs, M. P., 78, *113*, 388, 390, *421*
Doyle, K. J., 135, *151*
Duffy, J. K., 134, *151*, 447, *461*
Dufresne, R. M., 304, *321*
Dugmundsen, G. I., 92, *113*

E

Eagles, E., 406, 407, *421*
Edgerton, B. J., 129, 135, *151*, *152*
Egan, J. P., 122, 132–33, *152*
Eisenberg, R. B., 402, *421*
Eldert, E., 118, 133, *152*
Eldert, M. A., 134, *152*
Elliot, L. L., 136, 137, 141, *152*, *153*
El-Mofty, A., 306, *321*
Elpern, B. S., 84, *113*, 135, *152*
Engebretson, A. M., 445, *460*
Engelberg, M., 142, *152*
Epstein, A., 371, *384*
Everberg, G., 301–2, *321*
Ewertson, H. W., 304, *321*
Ewing, A., 392, *421*
Ewing, I., 392, *421*

F

Fairbanks, G., 136, *152*
Ferraro, J. A., 196, *212*
Fifer, R. C., 201, *212*
Fitzgerald, P. G., *213*
Fletcher, H., 50, *62*, 123, *152*

Flexer, C., 417, *421*
Forbis, N. K., 121, *153*, 177, *213*
Forrester, P. W., 120, *151*
Fournier, S. R., 352, *359*
Fowler, E. P., 160, *212*
Frank, T., 119, 134, *152*, 378, *384*
Franklin, B., 349, *360*
Frazier, T. M., 392, *422*
Freed, H., 352, *359*
French, M. R., 132, *152*
Frick, L. R., 293, *321*
Friel-Patti, S., 441, *460*
Furukawa, C. T., 242, *280*

G

Gaddis, S., 128, *151*
Gaeth, J. H., 313, *321*
Galambos, R., 390, *421*
Gang, R. P., 345, *360*
Gardner, H. J., 134–35, *152*, 406, *421*, 471
Gardner, M. B., 107, *113*
Gasaway, D. C., 107, *113*
Gates, G. A., 407, *421*
George, K., 413, *422*
Gerkin, K. P., 389, 390, *421*
Geurking, N. A., 355, *361*
Giebink, G. S., 242, *280*
Gilkerson, M. R., 298, *321*
Gilmore, C., 137, 141, *151*
Giolas, D., 454, *460*
Gladstone, V. S., 255, *280*
Glasscock, M. E., 168, *214*, 340, *360*
Goetzinger, C. P., 129, 142, 143, *152*, 347, *360*
Goldstein, R., 394, 400, *421*
Gollegly, K. M., 201, 204, *213*, 355, *361*
Goodhill, V., 342, *360*
Goodman, A. C., 160, *212*
Goodman, J., 141, *151*
Graham, S. S., *280*
Gravel, K. L., 402, *422*
Green, D. S., 169, 171, 172, *212*
Greenfield, E. C., 331, *361*
Greetis, E. S., 141, *151*
Grimes, A. M., 182, *213*
Grogan, F., 107, *113*
Grubb, P., 135, *152*
Guilford, F. R., 394, 398, *421*, *422*, 444, *460*
Gurdjian, E. S., 313, *321*
Gustafson, G., 415, *422*

H

Hahlbrock, K. H., 129, *152*
Hallpike, C. S., 397, *421*
Hammed, H., 306, *321*
Hannley, M. T., 441, *460*
Hardy, J. B., 392, *422*
Hardy, J. G., 298, *321*

Hardy, W. G., 377, *384*, 392, 402, *422*
Harford, E. R., 163, 165, *212*, *213*, 438, *460*
Harris, D. A., 375, *384*
Harris, J. D., 219, *232*
Haskins, H., 133, *152*
Hattler, K. W., 374, *384*
Haug, C. O., 398, *421*
Haug, O., 394, *422*, 444, *460*
Hawkins, J. E., 118, *152*, 304, *321*
Hayashi, R., 349, *360*
Hearing Aid Industry Conference (HAIC), 433, *460*
Hecker, M. H. L., 136, *152*
Hecox, K. E., 433, *460*
Helmholtz, H. L. F. von, 291
Herbert, F., 175, *212*
Herer, G., 174, *212*, 374, *384*
Hicks, G. E., 390, *421*
Hillis, J., 402, *422*
Hirsch, S., 351, *359*
Hirsh, I., 118, 133, 137, *152*, *154*, 353, *360*, 444, *461*
Hodgson, W. R., 348, *360*, 386, 393, *422*
Hofman, C. L., 448, *460*
Hood, J. D., 97, *113*, 160–61, *212*
Hood, L., 444, *460*
Hood, W. H., 374, *384*
Hopkinson, N. T., 375, *384*
Hosford-Dunn, H., 135, *152*, 299, *321*
House, A. S., 136, *152*
House, W. F., 439, *460*
Hudgins, C. V., 118, *152*
Huff, S. J., 120, *152*
Hughes, J. P., 352, *359*
Huntington, D. A., 133, *154*
Hutton, C. L., 374, *384*

I

Igarashi, M., 304, *321*
International Organization for Standardization, *62*
Ireland, J. A., 417, *421*

J

Jacobson, J. T., 390, *422*
Jauhiainen, T., 175, *213*
Jenkins, H., 189, *212*, 332, *360*
Jerger, J. F., 76, *112*, 116, 119, 137, 140, 141, *151*, *152*, *154*, 157, 163, 165, 170, 172, 174, 175–76, 185, 189, 207, *212*, *213*, 264, *280*, 332, 343, 344, 345, 348–51, 355, *360*, 374, 377, *384*
Jerger, S., 116, 140, *152*, 157, 170, 175–76, 207, *212*, *213*, 343, 344, 345, 355, *360*
Johnson, C., 141, *151*
Johnson, E. W., *14*, 330, *360*
Johnson, K., 116, 140, *152*
Johnson, L. G., 304, *321*
Johnson, R., 441, *460*

Johnson, S. J., 299, *321*
Jokinen, K., 349, 350, *361*
Jones, F. R., 390, *423*
Josey, A. F., 168, *214*, 340, *360*

K

Kalikow, D. M., 137, 141, *153*
Kamm, C., 147, *153*
Kankkonen, A., 394, *422*
Karja, J., 175, *213*
Karlin, J. E., 118, *152*
Karmody, C., 299, *321*
Katz, D. R., 136, *152*, *153*
Katz, J., 343, 352, *360*
Keith, R. W., 344, *360*
Kemink, J. L., 201, *213*
Kemp, D. T., 292–93, *321*
Kendall, D. C., 394, 400, *421*
Kettlety, A., 392, *422*
Kibbe, K. S., 201, *213*, 355, *361*
Kibbe-Michal, K., 204, *213*
Kileny, P. R., 201, *213*, 340, *361*
Killion, M. C., 92, *113*, 444, *460*
Klein, A. J., 433, *460*
Klockhoff, I., 309, *321*
Klodd, D. A., 135, *152*
Koch, L. J., 167, *213*
Koenige, M. J., 120, *154*
Konkle, D. F., 117, 127, 132, *153*
Kopra, L. L., 129, *153*
Koval, A., 136, *151*
Kraemer, M. J., 242, *280*
Krall, L., 452, 453, *460*
Kreul, E. J., 136, *153*
Kryter, K. D., 136, *152*, *153*
Kurdziel, S., 354, *360*

L

Lamb, L. E., 366, *384*
Lane, G. I., 93, *113*
Lane, H., 414, *422*
Lang, J. S., 136, *153*
Larson, V. D., 135, *154*
Lawrence, J., 299, *321*
Lawrence, M., 309, *321*
Lawrence, R. J., 391, *421*
Lehiste, I., 134, *153*
Lempert, J., 264, *280*
Lerman, J., 136, *154*, 396, *423*
Levine, H., 406, 407, *421*
Levitt, H., *153*, 433, 441, *460*
Lezak, R., 141, *153*
Libby, E. R., 445, *460*
Liden, G., 94, *113*, 394, *422*
Lightfoot, R. K., 448, *461*
Lilly, D. J., 184, *214*

Lloyd, L. L., 397, *422*, *423*
Luterman, D. M., 413, *422*
Lynn, G., 135, *153*

M

McCandless, G., 441, *460*
McCracken, G. H., 298, *321*
McFadden, D., 304, *321*
McFarland, W. H., 390, *423*
McLemore, D. C., 129, *153*
McPhillips, M. A., 119, *152*
Mahaffey, R. B., 143, *155*
Malachowski, N., 299, *321*
Mankowitz, Z., 351, *359*
Margolis, R. H., 123, *155*, 184, *214*
Martin, D., 445, *460*
Martin, F. N., 83, 89, 90, 94, 98, 99, 100, *113*, 120,
   121–22, 125, 127, 129, 135, 138, 140, *153*,
   177, 207, *213*, 325, 350, *360*, 375, 380, *384*,
   399, 402, 405, 413, 417, *422*, *423*, 452, 453,
   460
Martin, N. D., *360*
Martinez, C., 354, *361*
Matkin, N. D., 342, *360*, 392, 394, *422*, *423*
Matthies, M. L., 293, *321*
Matzker, J., 349, *361*
Mauldin, L., 175, *212*, 377, *384*
Maxon, A., 417, *423*
Mayberry, R. I., 415, *422*
Meikle, M., 441, *460*
Melnick, W., 406, 407, *421*
Menzel, O. J., 371, 378, *384*
Merrill, H. B., 116, 129, *153*
Meyer, C. R., 107, *113*
Meyerhoff, W. L., 242, 262, 273–74, *280*, 441, *461*
Miller, K. E., 135, *154*
Mindel, E., 414, *423*
Moller, A. R., 198, *213*
Moller, C. G., 285, *321*
Monro, D. A., 380, *384*
Montgomery, P., 135, *152*
Morehouse, C. R., 390, *422*
Morgan, D. E., 120, 147, *153*, *155*
Morimoto, M., 349, *360*
Morris, L. J., 120, 121, 125, 129, 135, 140, *153*, 207,
   213, 375, *384*
Moses, K., 412, *422*
Mueller, H. G., 352, 353, 354, *361*
Munson, W. A., 50, *62*
Musiek, F. E., 201, 204, *213*, 292, *321*, 340, 352,
   354–55, *360*, *361*
Myers, D. K., 120, *154*
Myers, E. N., 304, *321*

N

Nagel, R. F., 378, *384*
Naunton, R. F., 84, *113*

Neely, J., 355, *360*
Nerbonne, C. P., 141, *151*
Nerbonne, M. A., 119, 120, *151*, *152*
Newby, H. A., 409, 410, *421*, *422*
Nielsen, D. W., *62*, 157, *214*
Nilsson, G., 94, *113*
Niparko, J. K., 201, *213*
Nixon, J. C., 136, *153*
Nober, E. H., 89, *113*
Noffsinger, D., 169, 171, 172, *213*, 354, *360*, *361*
Norris, J. D., 175, *212*
Northern, J. L., 182, *213*
Nuetzel, J. M., 137, *151*

O

Occupational Safety and Health Administration (OSHA), 306, *321*
Ogiba, Y., 394, *423*
Ohta, F., 349, *360*
Oliver, T. A., 189, *212*, 332, *360*
Olsen, W. O., 120, *154*, 169, 171, 172, *213*, 354, *360*, *361*
O'Neal, J., 413, *422*, 452, 453, *460*
O'Neill, J. 402, *422*
Owen, J. H., 407, *421*
Owens, E., 136, *153*, 170, *213*
Oyer, H., 402, *422*

P

Palfavi, L., 304, *321*
Palva, A., 175, *213*, 349, 350, *361*
Palva, T., 175, *213*
Pappas, J. J., 127, *153*
Parker, C., 141, *155*
Paryani, S., 299, *321*
Pascoe, D. R., 135, *153*
Patrick, P. E., 406, 407, *422*
Paul, P. V., 415–16, *422*
Pauls, M. D., 402, *422*
Pava, A. A., 331, *361*
Peterson, G. E., 134, *153*
Peterson, J. L., 366, *384*
Pfetzing, D., 415, *422*
Phon, G. L., 390, *423*
Pick, G. F., 294, *321*
Picton, T. W., *213*
Pierce, J. R., 51, *62*
Pierson, W. E., 242, *280*
Plattsmier, H. S., 304, *321*
Plester, D., 306, *321*
Ploshay, K. L., 448, *460*
Pool, J. I., 331, *361*
Popelka, G. R., 182, 184, *213*, 445, *460*
Porter, L. S., 123, *151*
Preslar, M. J., 51, *62*
Priede, V. M., 90, *113*, 159, *213*
Proctor, B., 313, *321*

Proud, G. O., 129, 142, *152*
Punch, J. L., 433, *460*
Pusakulich, K. M., 137, 141, *151*

Q

Quigley, S. P., 415–16, *422*

R

Rabinowitz, W. M., 137, *151*
Raffin, M. J. M., 135, 142, *154*
Rasmussen, G. L., 328, *361*
Reddell, R. C., 136, *154*
Redmond, C., 442, *461*
Reesal, M. R., 304, *321*
Reger, S. N., 65, *113*, 163, *213*
Reid, M. J., 397, *422*
Rentschler, G. J., 343, *361*
Resnick, D., 135, *154*, 349–50, *361*
Reynolds, E., 118, 133, *152*
Richardson, M. A., 242, *280*
Rintelmann, W. F., 117, 132, 133, 136, *153*, *154*, 374, *384*
Roberts, J. L., 390, *423*
Robinson, D., 120, *154*
Robinson, D. O., 197, *212*, 344, *359*
Rock, E. H., 255, *280*
Roeser, R. J., 67, *112*, 207, *213*, 432–33, 441, *460*, *461*
Roland, P. S., 441, *461*
Rose, D. E., 135, *154*, 175, *213*
Rose, D. S., 405, *423*
Rosen, S., 268, *280*, 306, *321*
Rosenberg, P. E., 169, 171, *214*
Ross, M., 133, 136, *154*, 364, 378, *384*, 392, 396, 410–11, 417–18, *423*, 447, *461*
Ruby, B. K., 120, *151*
Ruhm, H. B., 373, 374, 378, *384*
Runge, C. A., 135, *152*
Rupp, R. R., 167, *213*, 343, *361*
Russ, F., 390, *423*
Ruth, R. R., 196, *212*
Rzeczkowski, C., 137, *151*

S

Sanders, J. W., 168, *214*
Sanderson-Leepa, M. E., 133, 136, *154*
Sataloff, J., 78, *113*
Sataloff, R. T., 78, *113*
Saulnier, K., 415, *421*
Sawolkow, E., 415, *422*
Schaefer, A., 354, *361*
Schiff, M., 255, *280*
Schleuning, A., 441, *460*
Schreurs, K. K., 135, *154*

Schubert, E. D., 136, *153*
Schuknecht, H. F., 304, 313, *321*
Schultz, M. C., 352, *359*
Schwartz, D. M., 135, 136, *154*
Scott, B. L., 441, *460*
Sever, J. L., 298, *321*
Shanks, J. E., 184, *214*
Shapiro, G. G., 242, *280*
Shea, J. J., 268, *280*
Shedd, J., 165, *213*
Shepard, N. T., 201, *213*
Shepherd, D. C., 386, *423*
Shipp, D. B., 380, *384*
Shore, I., 444, *461*
Shubow, G. F., 352, *359*
Sides, D. G., 83, 94, *113*, 177, *213*
Silverman, S. R., 118, 133, 137, *152, 154*
Simmons, F. B., 390, *423*
Sivian, L. J., 50, *62*
Sjoblom, J., 175, *213*
Skinner, P. H., 344, *361*
Smith, B., 349–50, *361*
Smith, L., 441, *460*
Solzi, P., 351, *359*
Speaks, C., 137, 141, *152, 154*
Spearman, C., 121, *154*
Spradlin, J. E., 397, 422, *423*
Srinivasson, K. P., 129, *154*
Stach, B. A., 107, *113*, 143–44, *154*
Stark, E., 298, *320*
Stauffer, M. L., 120, 121, *153*
Steinberg, J. C., 132, *152*
Sterritt, G. M., 388, *421*
Stevens, K. N., 137, 141, *153*
Stevens, S. S., 118, *152*
Stewart, J. L., 51, *62*
Stewart, J. M., 78, *113*
Stewart, K., 371, *384*
Stream, K. S., 412, *423*
Stream, R. W., 412, *423*
Studebaker, G. A., 82, 89, 94, *113*
Summers, R., 51, *62*
Surjan, L., 304, *321*
Surr, R., 136, *154*
Sutherland, H. C., Jr., 107, *113*
Suzuki, T., 394, *423*

T

Talbott, R. E., 225, *232*
Taylor, K., 432–33, *461*
Telian, S. A., 340, *361*
Teter, D. L., 448, *461*
Thomas, W. G., 51, *62*
Thornton, A. R., 135, 142, *154*
Tillman, T. W., 119, 120, 134, 141, *151, 154*
Tobias, J. V., 135, *154*
Trammell, J. L., 137, *152*
Turner, R. G., 157, *214*

U

Utley, J., 379, *384*

V

Valente, M., 252, *280*
Van Bergeijk, W. A., 51, *62*
Vassallo, L. A., 78, *113*
Vaugn, G. R., 448, *461*
Ventry, I. M., 119, 120, *151*, 344, *361*
Verkest, S. B., 201, 204, *213*, 355, *361*
Vernon, J., 441, 450, *460*
Vernon, M., 414, *423*

W

Wall, L. G., 120, *154*
Wardell, F. N., 399, *423*
Weaver, N. J., 399, *423*
Weber, S., 136, *154*
Webster, D. B., 343, *361*
Webster, J. E., 313, *321*
Webster, M., 343, *361*
Wedenberg, E., 194, 212, 298, *320*, 332, *359*, 387, *423*
Wegel, R. L., 93, *113*
Weisenberger, J. M., 442, *461*
Weiss, N. S., 242, *280*
Wever, G., 292, *321*
White, S. D., 50, *62*
Wilber, L. A., 50, *62*, 92, *113*, 134, *154*
Wiley, T. L., 184, *214*
Williams, C. E., 136, *152*
Williams, P. S., 255, *280*
Williford, J. A., 351, 352, *361*
Wilson, M. J., 390, *421*
Wilson, R. H., 120, 123, 136, *154, 155*, 184, *214*
Wischik, S., 406, 407, *421*
Wittich, W. W., 89, *113*, 143, *155*
Wolfe, D. L., 129, *153*
Wood, T. J., 143, *155*
Worthington, D. W., 206, 207, *214*
Wray, D., 417, *421*
Wright, H. N., 175, *214*

Y

Yeager, A. S., 299, *321*
Yellin, W., 441, *461*
Ylikoski, J., 175, *213*
Yost, W. A., *62*
Young, E. J., 442, *461*
Young, I. M., 175, *212*
Young, L. L., 141, *155*

SUBJECT INDEX

Page numbers in *italics* refer to glossary definition

A

Abbreviations, common, 476–78
Acceleration, 23, 60, 282
Acoupedic method, 415
Acoustic, common units of measurement, 60
Acoustic feedback, 436, *458*
Acoustic gain, 433, 434, *458*
Acoustic immittance, 177–95, 207, *208*, 464
   children, 401–2
Acoustic impedance, 177, *207*
Acoustic neuritis, 341, *356*
Acoustic neuroma, 331, 338, 340, *356*
Acoustic reflex, 179, 186–94, *207*, 354, 377
Acoustic reflex arc, 187
Acoustic reflex threshold (ART), 187, *207*, 210, 211,
   275, 316
Acoustic trauma notch, 304, 305, *316*
Acquired immune deficiency syndrome (AIDS),
   242, 299, *316*
Action potential (AP), 290, *316*
Active electrode, 197, 198, *207*
Acute, 243, *275*
Aditus ad antrum, 235, *275*
Afferent, 290, *316*
Air–bone gap, 85–88, *109*

Air conduction (AC), 1, 3, *10*, 14, *109*, 464
   masking methods, 94–98
Air-conduction audiometer, 40–41, 64
Air-conduction audiometry, 73–79
Alternate binaural loudness balance (ABLB) test,
   160–62, 205, 206, *207*, 210, 211
Alternate monaural loudness balance (AMLB) test,
   163–64, 205, *207–8*, 210, 211
American Academy of Ophthalmology and
   Otolaryngology (AAOO), 389
American Academy of Pediatrics, 389
American Medical Association:
   percentage of hearing loss, 78–79
American National Standards Institute (ANSI), 34
American Sign Language (ASL), 415
American Speech-Language-Hearing Association
   (ASHA), 389, 430
American Standards Association (ASA), 33, 34
American Tinnitus Association (ATA), 450
Amplitude, 23, 26, 27, *55*
Ampulla, 282, *316*
Anechoic chamber, 53, *55*
Angular acceleration, 282
Annulus, 219, *230*
Anotia, 221, *230*
Anoxia, 299–300, *316*

485

Antihelix, 216
Antitragus, 216
Anxiety, parental, 412
Aperiodic wave, 35, *55*
Area, 60
Arteriosclerosis, 342
Articulation-gain function, 133–34
Artificial ear, 47, *55*
Artificial mastoid, 49–50, *55*
Ascending auditory pathways, 324–28
Assistive listening devices and systems (ALDS), 448–50
Athetosis, 296–98, *316*
Atresia, 221–22, *230*
Attenuation, 3, *10*
Audiogram, 76, *109*, 464
  interpretation, 85–91
Audiometer, 39–44, *109*
  air-conduction, 40–41, 64
  automatic, 65–66
  bone-conduction, 41, 42, 64
  calibration, 47–51
  playtone, 398–99
  pure-tone, 39–41, 64–66
  sound field, 44
  speech, 42–44, 114, 115, *148*
Audiometric Bing test, 101
Audiometric response simulator, 107–8, *109*
Audiometric Weber test, 102–5, *109*
Audiometry, 63
  air-conduction, 73–79
  automatic, 105–6
  behavioral observation, 392, *419*
  binaural, 348–50
  bone-conduction, 79–85
  brief tone, 175, *208*
  computerized, 107, *109*, 143–47
  electrodermal, 377–78, *381*, 383, 402
  immittance, 194–95
  objective, 378, *381*
  operant conditioning, 397–99, *419*
    tangible reinforcement (TROCA), 397, *420*
  play, 399–401
  pure-tone. *see* Pure-tone audiometry
  school, 406–10
  sound field, 392–95
  speech. *see* Speech audiometry
Auditory, 1, 2, *10*
Auditory brainstem response (ABR), 195, 198–201, 202, 206, 207, *208*, 210, 211, 316, 354–55, 383, 439, 448
  children, 389–90
Auditory cortex, 2, 328
Auditory event-related potentials, 195, 204, *208*
Auditory evoked potentials (AEP), 195–205, *208*, 354–55, 378
  children, 402
Auditory middle latency response (AMLR), 195, 201–2, 204, *208*
Auditory nerve, 2, *10*, 324–26, *356*
  development, 329

disorders, 330–41
  tumors, 331–40
Auditory placode, 294, *316*
Auditory radiations, 327–28, *356*
Auditory tract, 1
Auditory training, 455–56, *458*
  children, 455–56
Aural/oral method, 414–15
Aural rehabilitation, 424–61
  for adults, 453–55
  assistive learning devices and systems (ALDS), 448–50
  auditory training, 455–56, *458*
  counseling, 411–13, 451–53
  hearing aids, 275, 432–48
  patient histories, 425–28
  referral to other specialists, 428–32
  speechreading, 457–58, *459*
  tinnitus, 450–51
Auricle (pinna), 216–17, *230*
  disorders, 221, 231
Auropalpebral reflex (APR), 327, 387, *418*
Autism, 403, *418*
Automatic audiometry. *see* Békésy audiometry
Autophony, 258, *275*
Average velocity, 23
Axon, 289, *316*

B

Babbling, 387
Band-pass binaural speech audiometry, 349–50
Barotrauma, 242, 303
Basilar membrane, 286–87, 288, *316*
Beats, 26, *55*
Behavioral observation audiometry (BOA), 392, *419*
Békésy Ascending-Descending Gap Evaluation (BADGE), 374–75, *381*
Békésy audiometry, 105, 106, *109*, 172–77, 194, 206, 207, *208*, 210, 229–30, *275*, 316, 374–75, 383
  cross hearing and masking, 174–75
  and tone decay, 176
  variations, 175–76
Békésy comfortable loudness (BCL) test, 176, *208*
Békésy types, 172–74
Bel, 29, *55*
Bell's palsy, 250, *275*
Binaural, 115, *147*, 437
Binaural audiometry, 348–50
Bing test, 9, *11, 13*
  audiometric, 101
Biofeedback, 450
Boilermaker's disease, 304–6
Bone-conduction audiometer, 41, 42, 64
Bone-conduction audiometry, 79–85
Bone conduction (BC), 1, 2, 3, *11*, 14, *109*, 464
  distortional, 81, *110*
  inertial, 82, *110*

masking methods, 98–102
osseotympanic, 82, *110*
Bone-conduction speech discrimination testing, 142–43
Bone-conduction speech recognition threshold, 128–29
Brainstem evoked response (BER). *see* Auditory brainstem response (ABR)
Brief tone audiometry (BTA), 175, *208*
Brownian motion, 16, *56*

C

Calibration, 47–51, 67, 92–93, *109*
of speech-masking noises, 126–27
California consonant test, 136, *147*, *470*
Caloric test, 283, *316*
Cancellation, 26, *56*
Cardiotachometry, 402, *419*
Carhart notch, 263, *275–76*
Carhart tone decay test, 168–69
Carotid artery, 234, *276*
Carrier phrase, 118–19, *147*
Cell body, 289, *316*
Centimeter gram second (CGS) system, 16
Central auditory disorders, tests, 344–55
Central auditory nervous system, 324–56
development, 329
Central masking, 93–94, *109*, 127, 139
Cerebellopontine angle (CPA), 325, 340, *356*
Cerebellum, 325, *356*
Cerebral palsy, 296–98, *316–17*
Cerebrovascular accident (CVA), 342, *356*
Cerumen, 217, 225–27, 230
Children. *see* Pediatric patient
Cholesteatoma, 248–50, *276*
Chorda tympani nerve, 240, *276*
Chronic, 243, *276*
Cilia, 234–35, *276*
Clinical decision analysis (CDA), 157, *208*
Cochlea, 2, *11*, 285–314, *317*
development, 294
disorders, 295–314
duct, 286, *317*
efferent system, 290–91
emissions, 292–93
fluids, 290
frequency analysis, 293–94
functions, 287
physiology, 288
Cochlear implants, 439–41, *458*
Cochlear microphonic (CM), 290, *317*
Cochlear nucleus, 326
disorders, 341–43
Cold running speech, 118–19, *147–48*
Commissure, 326, *356*
Competing sentence test (CST), 351, 472–73
Complex noise, 91–92, *109*, 126
Complex sounds, 35–36

Complex wave, 36, *56*
Compliance, 177, *208*
static, 179, 181–84, *209*, 210, 211
Component, 35, *56*
Compression, 16, *56*
Computed tomography (C-T), 338, 340, *356*
Computerized audiometry, 107, *109*, 143–47
Computerized vestibulography, 283–85
Concha, 216
Conditioned orientation reflex (COR), 394, *419*
Conditioned stimulus (CS), 377
Conductive hearing loss, 3, 4, *11*, 12
Conductive mechanism, 3
Condyle, 217–18
Connected speech. *see* Cold running speech
Connected Speech Test (CST), 137–38, *148*
Consonant-nucleus-consonant (CNC) words, 134, *148*, 349–50, 468–70
Contralateral acoustic reflex test, 190–93
Contralateral competing message (CCM), 350
Contralateralization. *see* Cross hearing
Contralateral response pathway, 187, 188, 189
Contralateral routing of signals (CROS), 438–39, *458–59*
Conversion neurosis, 365, *381*
Corti
arch of, 287, *317*
organ of, 286, 288, *317*
Cosine wave, 19, *56*
Counseling, 451–53
parents, 411–13, 452
Crib-o-gram, 390, *419*
Crista, 282
Critical band, 92, *109–10*
Cross hearing, 89–91, *110*
Békésy audiometry, 174–75
lack of, 366–67
most comfortable loudness, 129–30
SISI, 166–67
speech discrimination, 138–39
in speech recognition threshold tests, 125
tone decay tests, 170
uncomfortable loudness, 130
Crura, 236, *276*
Crus, 236, *276*
Cued Speech, 416
Cyanosis, 391
Cycle, 19, 21, *56*
Cycle per second. *see* Hertz (Hz)
Cytomegalic inclusion disease (CID), 299
Cytomegalovirus (CMV), 299, *317*

D

Dactylology, 415
Damage risk criteria, 306–7, *317*
Damping, 21, *56*
Deafness, semantics of, 418
Deceleration, 23

Decibel (dB), 29–35, 53, *56*
  hearing level, 33–34, *56*
  intensity level, 31, *57*, 61
  logarithms, 29–31, *57*
  sensation level, 35, *58*, 61
  sound-pressure level, 32–33, 55, *58*, 61
Decruitment, 160, 205, *208*
Decussations, 326, *356*
Delayed auditory feedback (DAF), 372–74, *381*
  pure-tone, 373–74, 383
  speech, 372–73, 383
Dendrite, 289, *317*
Denial, parental, 412
Density, 16, *56*
Descending auditory pathways, 328–29
Dichotic, 349–50, *357*
Dichotic digits test, 352, *357*
Difference limen for intensity (DLI), 164, *208*
Difference tone, 26, *56*
Differential intensity discrimination, 164–68
Digital hearing-aid technology, 432–33
Diminished Schwabach, 7
Diotic, 349–50, *357*
Diplacusis binauralis, 295, *317*
Diplacusis monauralis, 295, *317*
Discrimination, differential intensity, 164–68
Discrimination testing, speech, 131–43
Displacement, 288
Distortion, 433, 435, *459*
Distortional bone conduction, 81, *110*
Doerfler-Stewart (D-S) test, 371, *381*, 383
Dorsal cochlear nucleus, 326, *357*
Down's syndrome, 221, *230*
Ductus reuniens, 286, *317*
Duration, 61
Dynamic range (DR) for speech. *see* Range of
  comfortable loudness (RCL)
Dyne (d), 27, *56*
Dysacusis, 295, *317*
Dysinhibition, 405, *419*

E

Ear, anatomy and physiology, 2
Ear, inner, 2, *11*, 281–322
  anatomy, 2
  auditory mechanism, 285–94
  development, 294–95
  disorders, 295–314
    perinatal causes, 299–300
    postnatal causes, 300–314
    prenatal causes, 296–99
  hearing loss, 12, 295–314
  vestibular mechanism, 282–85
Ear, middle, 2, *11*, 233–80
  anatomy, 2, 234–40
  cleft, 234, *277*
  development, 241
  disorders, 241–75
  fracture, 274

  hearing loss, 12
  negative pressure, 254–57, *279*
  serous effusion, 258–61, *277, 279*
  tumors, 275
Ear, outer, 2, *11*, 215–32
  anatomy, 216–20
  development, 220
  disorders, 221–29
  hearing loss, 12, 220–21
Eardrum membrane. *see* Tympanic membrane
Earphone attenuation devices, 66–67
Echolalia, 387, *419*
Ectoderm, 220, *230*
Educational options, 414–18
Effective masking (EM), 77, 93, *110*, 112
Efferent, 290–91, *317*, 328–32
Efficiency, test, 157
Elasticity, 16, *56*
Electret microphone, 438, *459*
Electrocochleography (ECochG), 195, 197, *208*
Electrodermal audiometry (EDA), 377–78, *381*, 383
  children, 402
Electrodermal speech reception threshold (EDSRT),
  378, *381*
Electroencephalic (EEG), 195
Electroencephalograph (EEG), 195–97
Electronic voltmeter, 93, *110*
Electronystagmograph (ENG), 283, 284, 285, *317*
Electrophysiological tests, 376–78
  children, 402–3
Encephalography, positive-contrast, 340
Endolymph, 282, 290, *317*
Endolymphatic hydrops, 309
Entoderm, 220, *230*
Environmental adaptations, 448–50
Environmental sound, 51
Epitympanic recess, 234, *276*
Equivalent volume, 181, 182, *208*
Erg (e), 28, *56*
Eustachian tube, 234, 235, 254–55, *276*
  blocked, 259–60
  patulous, 258
Evoked otoacoustic emission, 293, *317*
Exponent, 29, *56*
External auditory canal, 216, 217–18, *230*
  disorders, 221–27, 231
  tumors, 225
  wax, 225–27
External otitis, 222–25, *230*
Extra-axial, 343, *357*
Extrinsic redundancy, 330

F

Facial nerve, 239–40, *276*
Fallopian canal, 239–40, *276*
False negative response, 71, *110*, 116
False negative Rinne, 8
False positive response, 71, *110*, 116
Far field, 50

Fascia, 271, *276*
Fenestration, 264–68, *276*
Fere effect, 377
Filtered speech tests, 347–49
Fingerspelling, 415
Fistula, 271, *276*
Footplate, 236, *276*
Force, 26–27, *56*, 60
Forced vibration, 20, 21, *56*
Foreign bodies in external ear canal, 222
Formant, 36, *56*
Fourier analysis, 36, *56*
Free field, 53, *56*
Free vibration, 20–21, *56*
Frequency, 19, 21–22, 53, 54, *56*, 61
  effects of length, 21–22
  effects of mass, 22
  effects of stiffness, 22
  fundamental, 35, *56*
  resonant, 22–23, *58*
Frequency analysis in cochlea, 293–94
Frequency response, 433, 434–35, *459*
Frequency theories of hearing, 291–92, *317*
Functional hearing loss. *see* Pseudohypacusis
Fundamental frequency, 35, *56*
Fungus infections, 222

G

German measles, 298–99
Glue ear, 262
Glycerol test, 309, *317*
Goldbrick, 364
Green tone decay test, 169
Ground electrode, 198, *208*
Guilt, parental, 412

H

Hair cells, 288, 292
Harmonic distortion, 435, *459*
Harmonics, 36, *56*
Head trauma, 313–14
Hearing, theories of, 291–94
  frequency, 291–92, *317*
  place, 291, *318*
  resonance, 291, *318*
  resonance-volley, 292, *318*
  traveling wave, 291, *319*
  volley, 292, *320*
Hearing Aid Industry Conference (HAIC), 433, *459*
Hearing aids, 275, 432–48
  candidates, 442
  characteristics, 433–35
  common problems with, 447
  dealers, 431–32, 443
  dispensing, 446
  evaluations, 443–46

  selection, 442–48
    children, 446–48
  types, 436–42
Hearing examination, instructions for taking, 463–64
Hearing level (HL), 33–34, *56*
Hearing loss, 3, *11*
  conductive, 3, 4, *11*, 12
  hereditodegenerative, 296, *317*
  mixed, 4–5, *11*, 300, 301, *318*
  noise-induced, 303–7
  postlingual, 411, *419*
  prelingual, 411, *419*
  psychogenic, 364, *381*
  sensorineural, 3, 4, *11*, 12, 295–314, *319*
Hearing tests, early, 5. *see also* Test
Helicotrema, 285–86, *317*
Helix, 216
Hemotympanum, *276*
Hereditodegenerative hearing loss, 296, *317*
Hertz (Hz), 21, 22, 55, *57*
Heschl's gyrus. *see* Superior temporal gyrus
High-frequency emphasis word lists, 134–35
High risk register, 389, *419*
Human immunodeficiency virus (HIV), 299, *317–18*
Hypacusis, 295, *318*
Hyperrecruitment, 159, *208*
Hysterical deafness, 364, *381*

I

Immittance, 177–95, 207, *208*, 464
  children, 401–2
Immittance audiometry, 194–95
Impedance, 36–39, *57*, 61, 177
  acoustic, 177, *207*
Implantable bone-conduction devices, 441
Implants, cochlear, 439–41, *458*
Incus, 236, 237, *276*
Inertial bone conduction, 82, *110*
Infant hearing screening, 387–91
Inferior colliculus, 326, 327, *357*
Initial masking, 95, *110*, 112, 127, 150
Inner ear. *see* Ear, inner
Insert earphones, 67–68, 92, 197
Instantaneous velocity, 23
Intensity, 26–29, 53, 54, *57*, 60, 61
Intensity level (IL), 31, *57*, 61
Interaural attenuation (IA), 90, *110*
Interference, 25–26
Internal auditory canal, 324–25, *357*
International Organization for Standardization (ISO), 34
International system of units, 16
Intra-aural muscle reflex, 187, *209*. *see also* Acoustic reflex
Intra-axial, 343, *357*
Intrinsic redundancy, 330
Inverse square law, 28, *57*

Ipsilateral competing message (ICM), 350
Ipsilateral response pathway, 187, 188, 189

J

Joule (J), 28, *57*
Jugular bulb, 234, *276*

K

Kernicterus, 342, *357*
Kinetic energy, 19–20, *57*

L

Labyrinth, 281, *318*
Labyrinthitis, 302, *318*
Laddergram, 158, *209*
Lalling, 387, *419*
Language disorders, 403–5
Late evoked response (LER), 195, 202–4, 205, *209*
Lateralization, 9, *11*
Lateral lemniscus, 326, 327, *357*
Lateral line, 233
Length, 60
Lengthened off time (LOT) test, 374, 375, *381*
Le systeme international d'unites (SI), 16
Linear acceleration, 282
Linguistics of Visual English (LOVE), 416
Lipreading. *see* Speechreading
Lobule, 216
Localization, 53, 54, *57*
Logarithm, 29–31, *57*
Lombard test, 371–72, *381*, 383
Lombard voice reflex, 263, *276*
Longitudinal wave, 17, *57*
Loudness, 53, 54, *57*, 61
Loudness discomfort level. *see* Uncomfortable
  loudness level (UCL)
Loudness level, 53, 54, *57*, 61
Loudness recruitment. *see* Recruitment
Lues. *see* Syphilis

M

Macula, 282
Magnetic resonance imaging (MRI), 338, *357*
Mainstreaming, 414, 417, *419*
Malingering, 364, 365, 366, *381*
Malleus, 219, 236, 237, *276*
Management of hearing-impaired patient. *see* Aural
  rehabilitation
Manubrium, 236, *276*
Masking, 44, 53–54, *57*, 64–65, 91–102, *110*
  air conduction, 94–98
  Békésy audiometry, 174–75

bone conduction, 98–102
central, 93–94, *109*, 127, 139
effective, 77, 93, *110*, 112
initial, 95, *110*, 112, 127, 150
maximum, 95–96, 97, 99, *110*, 139
minimum, 94–95, 97, 99
most comfortable loudness, 129–30
overmasking, 94, 96, 97, 100, *110–11*, 112, 150
plateau, 97–98, 99, *111*, 128
SISI, 166–67
speech discrimination, 138–39
speech recognition threshold, 126–28
tone decay, 170
uncomfortable loudness, 130
undermasking, 97, 99, 100, *111*
Masking level difference (MLD), 353–54, *357*
Mass, 22, 27, 60
Mass reactance, 39
Mastoid, 235
Mastoidectomy, 251–52, *276*
Mastoiditis, 243, *276*
Mastoid process, 7, 11, 235, *276*
Maternal rubella syndrome, 298–99
Maximum masking, 95–96, 97, 99, *110*, 139
Measles, 300–301
Meatus, 216, *230*
Medial geniculate body, 327–28, *357*
Median plane localization, 163, *209*
Medical imaging, 338–40
Medulla oblongata, 325, *357*
Mel, 52, 55, *57*
Ménière's disease, 308–12, *318*
Meningitis, *318*
Meniscus, 258, *277*
Mesenchyme, 220, *230*
Mesoderm, 220, *230*
Meter kilogram second (mks) system, 16
Microbar, 32, *57*
Microtia, 221, *230*
Middle ear. *see* Ear, middle
Minimal auditory deficiency syndrome, 343–44, *357*
Minimum audible field (MAF), 50
Minimum audible pressure (MAP), 50
Minimum contralateral interference level, 370, *381*
Minimum masking, 94–95, 97, 99
Minimum response level (MRL), 386, *419*
Mixed hearing loss, 4–5, *11*, 300, 301, *318*
Modified rhyme test, 136
Modiolus, 286, *318*
Monaural, 115, *148*
Monitored live voice (MLV), 115, *148*
Moro reflex, 394, *419*
Most comfortable loudness (MCL), 129–30, *148*,
  150
Mucous membrane, 219, *230*, 234, *277*
Multiple sclerosis, 341, *357*
Mumps, 300–302
Myofacial pain dysfunction (MPD) syndrome, 218
Myringitis, 225, *230*
Myringoplasty, 229, *230*
Myringotomy, 251, *277*

N

Narrow-band noise, 92, *110*
Nasopharynx, 234, *277*
Natural sentence tests, 351
Necrosis, 243, *277*
Negative Rinne, 8
Neonatal auditory response cradle, 390–91, *419*
Neoplasm, 331, *357*
Neurofibromatosis (NF), 331, *357*
Neuron, auditory, 289, *318*
Newton (N), 27, *57*
Noise
  acceptable levels, 44, 46
  complex, 91–92, *109*, 126
  narrow-band, 92, *110*
  pink, 92, *111*
  sawtooth, 126, *148*
  used in masking for speech, 126–27
  white, 92, *111*, 126
Noise detection threshold (NDT), 371
Noise-induced hearing loss, 303–7
Noise inference level (NIL), 371
Nonorganic hearing loss, *381. see also*
  Pseudohypacusis
Nonsense-syllable lists, 135
Normal Schwabach, 7
Northwestern University Children's Perception of
  Speech (NU-CHIPS) test, 136–37
Nuclear deafness, 342
Nuclear magnetic resonance (NMR) imaging, 338
Nystagmus, 271, 283, *318*

O

Objective audiometry, 378, *381*
Occlusion effect (OE), 9, *11*, 83–84, 100–101, *110*
Occupational Safety and Health Administration
  (OSHA), 306
Octave, 52, *57*
Ohm, 39, *57*
Olivocochlear bundle (OCB), 329, *357*
Olsen-Noffsinger tone decay test, 169–70
Operant conditioning audiometry (OCA), 397–99,
  419
Oralists, 414
Organ of Corti, 286, 288, *317*
Oscillation, 19, *57*
Osseocartilaginous junction, 217, *230*
Osseotympanic bone conduction, 82, *110*
Ossicles, 236–39, *277*
Otalgia, 218, *230*
Otitis externa. see External otitis
Otitis media, 241–48, 250–52, *277*
  antibiotic treatment, 250–51
  dormant, 251
  mucous, 261–62
  suppurative, 241–48, 279
  surgical treatment, 251–53

Otocyst, 204, *318*
Otolaryngologist, 429–30
Otoplasty, 221, *230*
Otorrhea, 250, *277*
Otosclerosis, 262–74, *277*, 279, 303
Otoscope, 219, *230*
Otospongiosis. *see* Otosclerosis
Ototoxic, 302–3, *318*
Outer ear. *see* Ear, outer
Output, 433, *459*
Oval window, 236, *277*
Overmasking, 94, 96, 97, 100, *110–11*, 112, 150
Overrecruitment. *see* Hyperrecruitment
Overtone, 35, *57*

P

P300, 202–4
Paracusis willisii, 262–63, *277*
Parents, counseling of, 411–13, 452
Pars flaccida, 219, *231*
Pars tensa, 219, *231*
Partial recruitment, 158–59, *209*
Pascal (Pa), 28, *57*
Patient histories, 425–28
PB max, 134, *148*, 345
PB min, 345
Pediacoumeter, 397–98, *419*
Pediatric patient, 385–423
  auditory evoked potentials, 402
  auditory responses, 386
  auditory training, 455–56
  from birth to one year of age, 391–95
  electrophysiological tests, 402–3
  hearing aid selection, 446–48
  identifying hearing loss in school, 406–10
  immittance, 401–2
  infant hearing screening, 387–91
  language disorders, 403–5
  management of hearing-impaired children,
    411–18
  from one to five years of age, 395–403
  pseudohypacusis in, 410–11
  psychological disorders, 405
  speech audiometry, 396
  speechreading, 457
Peep show, 397, *419*
Performance-intensity function for PB words
  (PI-PB), 133–34, *148*, 206, 207, 344–46
Perilymph, 282, 290, *318*
Period, 21, *57*
Periodic wave, 35, *57*
Permanent threshold shift (PTS), 303, *318*
Perseveration, 405, *419*
Pharyngeal arches, 220, *231*
Phase, 24–26, 53, 54, *57*
Phon, 44, 53, 55, *57*
Phonemic regression, 313, *318*
Phonetically balanced (PB) words, 132–34, *148*,
  466–68

Physical volume test (PVT), 261, *277*
Picture identification task (PIT), *148*, 471–72
Pidgin Sign English (PSE), 416
Pink noise, 92, *111*
Pinna. *see* Auricle (pinna)
Pitch, 51–52, *58*, 61
Place theory of hearing, 291, *318*
Plateau, 97–98, 99, *111*, 128
Play audiometry, 399–401
Playtone audiometer, 398–99
Pneumoencephalography, 338–40, *358*
Pneumonia, 300
Politzerization, 255, *277*
Pons, 325, *358*
Positive-contrast encephalography, 340
Positive Rinne, 8
Postlingual hearing loss, 411, *419*
Potential energy, 19–20, *58*
Power, 28, *58*, 60
Predictive value, 157
Prefixes, 475–76
Prelingual hearing loss, 411, *419*
Prematurity, 300
Presbycusis, 313, *318*
Pressure, *58*, 60
Pressure-equalizing (P.E.) tubes, 260–61, *277*
Prolonged Schwabach, 7
Promontory, 236, *277*
Protensity, 61
Pseudohypacusis, 363–84
   children, 410–11
   management, 379–80
   performance on routine hearing tests, 366–69
   signs, 365
   terminology, 364
   tests, 369–79
Psychoacoustics, 51–54
Psychogalvanic response, 377, *381*
Psychogalvanometer, 377
Psychogenic hearing loss, 364, *381*
Psychological disorders, 405
Psychological perceptions of sound, factors
      contributing to, 61
Psychologist, clinical, 430
Psychophysical tuning curve (PTC), 294, *318*
Public Law 94–142, 414
Pure tone, 19, *58*
Pure-tone audiogram, 122–23
Pure-tone audiometer, 39–41, 64–66
Pure-tone audiometry, 63–113, 396–97
   air conduction, 73–79
   audiogram interpretation, 85–91
   audiometric response simulators, 107–8, *109*
   Audiometric Weber test, 102–5, *109*
   automatic, 105–6
   bone conduction, 79–85
   clinician's role, 71–73
   computerized, 107
   masking, 91–102
   patient's role, 70–71

Pure-tone average (PTA), 76–78, *111*
Purulent, 242, *277*

Q

Quality, 36, *58*, 61
Quinine, 303

R

Range of comfortable loudness (RCL), 131, *148*, 150
Rapidly alternating speech perception (RASP) test,
   352, *358*
Rarefaction, 16, *58*
Ratio, 29–31, *58*
Reactance, 38–39, *58*, 179, *209*
   mass, 39
   stiffness, 39
Recruitment, 158–64, 205, *209*, 211, 316
   SISI and, 167
Reference electrode, 198, *209*
Reference test gain, 434, *459*
Referrals, 428–32
Reflex decay, 189–94, *209*
Rehabilitation. *see* Aural rehabilitation
Reissner's membrane, 286, *318*
Reliability, 157
Resistance, 36, 38, *58*
Resonance, 22–23, 38, *58*
Resonance theory of hearing, 291, *318*
Resonance-volley theory of hearing, 292, *318*
Resonant frequency, 22–23, *58*
Reticular formation, 326, *358*
Reverberation, 53, *58*
Rh factor, 296, *318–19*, 342
Rhyme test, 136
Rinne test, 7–9, *11*, 13, 63
Rollover ratio, 345
Rosenberg tone decay test, 169
Round window, 236, *277*
Rubella, 298–99
Rubeola, 300–301
Rush Hughes Difference Score Test, 347

S

Saccule, 282, *319*
Saturation sound-pressure level (SSPL), 433, *459*
Sawtooth noise, 126, *148*
Scala media, 286, *319*
Scala tympani, 285, 286, *319*
Scala vestibuli, 285, 286, *319*
School hearing screening program, 406–10
Schwabach test, 7, *11*, 13, 63
Schwartze sign, 262, *277*
Screening tests, school, 406–10

Seeing Essential English (SEE 1), 415
Self Help for Hard of Hearing, Inc., 453
Semicircular canals, 282, *319*
Sensation level (SL), 35, *58*, 61
Sensitivity prediction from the acoustic reflex (SPAR) test, 377, *381*, 383
Sensitivity test, 157
Sensorineural hearing loss, 3, 4, *11*, 12, 295–314, *319*
Sensorineural mechanism, 3
Serous effusion, 258–61, *277*, 279
Short increment sensitivity index (SISI), 165–68, 206, *209*, 210, 211, *230*, 275, 314
   cross hearing and masking, 166–67
   modifications, 167–68
   and recruitment, 167
   scoring and interpretation, 167
Shrapnell's membrane, 219, *231*
Side tone, 372, *382*
Signal-to-noise (S/N) ratio, 141, *148*
Signed English (SE), 415
Signing Exact English (SEE 2), 415–16
Simultaneous binaural loudness balance (SBLB) test, 163, *209*
Sine wave, 17–19, 20, *58*
Sinusoid, 19, *58*
Site of lesion, 156–214, *209*
   acoustic immittance, 177–95, 207, *208*
   auditory evoked potentials, 195–205, *208*
   Békésy audiometry, 172–77, 194, 206, 207, *208*, 210
   differential intensity discrimination, 164–68
   loudness recruitment, 158–64, 205, *209*, 211
   tone decay, 168–72, 176, 206, *210*, 211
Social adequacy index (SAI), 142, *148*
Sone, 53, 55, *58*
Sonic boom, 23
Sound
   complex, 35–36
   defined, 16
   environmental, 51
   psychological perceptions of, factors contributing to, 61
Sound field audiometer, 44
Sound field audiometry, 392–95
Sound-isolated chambers, 68–69
Sound-level meter, 32, 44, *58*
   weighting networks, 44, 45
Sound measurement, 15–62
Sound-pressure level (SPL), 32–33, 55, *58*, 61
   saturation, 433, *459*
Sound velocity, 23
Spectrum, 36, 54, *58*, 61
Speech audiometer, 42–44, 114, 115, *148*
Speech audiometry, 114–55
   bone-conduction SRT, 128–29
   children, 396
   clinician's role, 117
   computerized, 143–47
   masking for SRT, 126–28

most comfortable loudness level, 129–30, *148*, 150
   patient's role, 116–17
   speech discrimination testing, 131–43, 464
   speech threshold testing, 117–29
   test environment, 115
   uncomfortable loudness level, 130–31, *149*, 150
Speech awareness threshold (SAT), 117
Speech detection threshold (SDT), 117–18, *148–49*, 150
Speech discrimination loss, 133
Speech discrimination score (SDS), 132, 133, *149*, 150, 194, 229, 275
Speech discrimination testing, 131–43, 464
   bone-conduction, 142–43
Speech-language pathologist, 430–31
Speech noise, 126
Speech perception in noise (SPIN) test, 137, *149*
Speechreading, 457–58, *459*
   adults, 457–58
   children, 457
Speech reception threshold, 463, 464. *see also* Speech recognition threshold (SRT)
Speech recognition score (SRS), 132
Speech recognition threshold (SRT), 117, 118–29, *149*, 150, 366
   bone conduction, 128–29
Speech threshold testing, 117–29
Spiral ligament, 286, *319*
Spondaic words (spondee), 118, 119–22, *149*, 465
   staggered spondaic word test, 352–53, *358*
Spondee threshold, 121, 122
Spontaneous otoacoustic emission, 293, *319*
Staggered spondaic word (SSW) test, 352–53, *358*
Stapedectomy, 268–74, *277*
Stapedius muscle, 186, *209*, 240, *278*
Stapedotomies, 271
Stapes, 236, 237, *278*
Stapes mobilization, 268, *278*
Static compliance, 179, 181–84, *209*, 210, 211
Stenger principle, 10, *11*
Stenger test, 369–70, *382*, 383
   speech, 370
Stenosis, 222, *231*
Stereocilia, 288, *319*
Stiffness, 22, *58*
Stiffness reactance, 39
Stria vascularis, 286, *319*
Subluxation, 252, *278*
Suffixes, 476
Superior olivary complex (SOC), 326, 327, *358*
Superior temporal gyrus, 328, *358*
Support groups, 453
Suppurative, 243, *278*
Suppurative otitis media, 241–48, 279
Suprathreshold adaptation test (STAT), 170, 207, *209*
Surgical complications, 308
"Swimmer's ear," 222
Swinging story test, 375–76, *382*, 383

Synapse, 289, *319*
Syndrome, 296, *319*
Synthetic sentence identification (SSI), 137, *149,*
  350–51, 472
Syphilis, 285, 342

T

Tactile responses, 89, *111*
Tangible reinforcement operant conditioning
  audiometry (TROCA), 397, *420*
Tarchinov effect, 377
Teachers of the hearing impaired, 431
Tectorial membrane, 288, *319*
Temporal integration, 175, *209*
Temporal lobe, 328, *358*
Temporary threshold shift (TTS), 303, *319*
Temporomandibular joint (TMJ) syndrome, 218,
  231
Tensor tympani muscle, 186, *209–10,* 240, *278*
Test
  audiometric Bing, 101
  audiometric Weber, 102–5, *109*
  Bing, 9, *11,* 13
  pseudohypacusis, 369–79
  Rinne, 7–9,*11,* 13, 63
  Schwabach, 7, *11,* 13, 63
  tuning fork, 1, 5–10, 13
  Weber, 9–10, *11,* 13
  see also Tone decay tests
Test environment, 66–69
Tetrachoric table, 409–10, *420*
Thalamus, 327, *358*
Thalidomide, 298
Theories of hearing. *see* Hearing, theories of
Threshold, 35, 39, *58,* 70, *111*
  speech awareness, 117
  speech detection, 117–18, *148–49,* 150
  speech recognition, 117, 118–29, *149,* 150, 366
  spondee, 121, 122
Threshold of discomfort (TD). *see* Uncomfortable
  loudness level (UCL)
Time compressed speech, 354, *358*
Tinnitus, 262, *278,* 450–51
  causes, 451
  management, 450–51
  maskers, 450–51
Tolerance level. *see* Uncomfortable loudness level
  (UCL)
Tone decay, 168–72, 176, 206, *210,* 211, 229, 275
Tone decay tests, 168–70
  Carhart, 168–69
  cross-hearing and masking, 170
  Green, 169
  Olsen-Noffsinger, 169–70
  Rosenberg, 169
  STAT, 170, 207, *209*
Tonotopic, 326, *358*
Total communication (TC), 415

Toynbee maneuver, 255, *278*
Tragus, 216
Transduce, 281, *319*
Transverse wave, 17, 18, *58*
Trapezoid body, 326, *358*
Traveling wave theory, 291, *319*
Treacher-Collins syndrome, 223
Trigeminal nerve, 240, *278*
Tumors
  auditory nerve, 331–40
  external auditory canal, 225
  middle ear, 275
Tuning forks, 1, 5–10, *11*
Tuning fork tests, 1, 5–10, 13
Tympanic membrane, 218–20, 229, *231,* 238–39
  perforation, 227–29, 231, 279
  thickening, 229, 231
Tympanogram, 184, 185, 194, *210*
Tympanometry, 179, 184–86, *210,* 211
Tympanoplasty, 252, *278*
Tympanosclerosis, 229, 262, *278*

U

Umbo, 219, *231*
Uncomfortable loudness level (UCL), 130–31, *149,*
  150
Unconditioned stimulus (UCS), 377
Undermasking, 97, 99, 100, *111*
Upper limits of comfortable loudness (ULCL), 141
Utricle, 282, *319*

V

Validity, 157
Valsalva, 255, *278*
Vascular accidents, 342
Vasospasm, 308, *320*
Velocity, 23, *58,* 60, 288
Ventral cochlear nucleus, 326, *358*
Vertigo, 282, *320*
Vestibule, 282–85, *320*
  abnormality, 283–85
Vestibulography, 283–85
Veterans Administration, 364, 365
Vibrations, 19–21, *58*
  forced, 20, 21, *56*
  free, 20–21, *56*
Vibrotactile hearing aids, 441–42, *459*
Viral infections, 298–302
  postnatal, 300–302
  prenatal, 298–99
Visual reinforcement audiometry (VRA), 394, *420*
Volley theory of hearing, 292, *320*
Volume unit (VU) meter, 118
Von Recklinghausen's Disease. *see*
  Neurofibromatosis (NF)

W

Warble tone, 388, *420*
Watt, 31, *59*
Wave, 16–19, *59*
   aperiodic, 35, *55*
   complex, 36, *56*
   cosine, 19, *56*
   longitudinal, 17, *57*
   periodic, 35, *57*
   sine, 17–19, 20, *58*
   transverse, 17, 18, *58*
Wavelength, 22–24, *59*
Wax (cerumen), 217, 225–27, *230*

Weber test, 9–10, *11*, 13
   audiometric, 102–5, *109*
Wheatstone bridge, 377, *382*
White noise, 92, *111*, 126
Word discrimination testing. *see* Speech
   discrimination testing
Word intelligibility by picture identification (WIPI)
   test, 136, *149*, 350, 471–72
Work, 28, *59*, 60

Y

Yes-no test, 378–79